S0-BOL-586

INTRODUCTION TO COUNSELING

Voices from the Field

SEVENTH EDITION

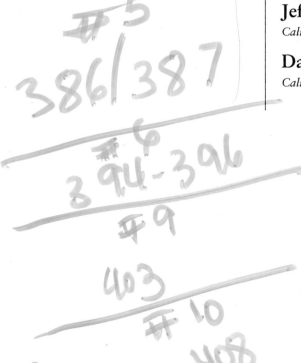

Jeffrey A. Kottler
California State University, Fullerton

David S. Shepard
California State University, Fullerton

BROOKS/COLE
CENGAGE Learning™

Australia • Brazil • Japan • Korea • Mexico • Singapore • Spain • United Kingdom • United States

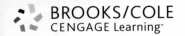
BROOKS/COLE
CENGAGE Learning™

Introduction to Counseling: Voices from the Field, Seventh Edition
Jeffrey A. Kottler and David S. Shepard

Publisher/Executive Editor: Linda Schreiber-Ganster

Acquisitions Editor: Seth Dobrin

Editorial Assistant: Rachel McDonald

Technology Project Manager: Dennis Fitzgerald

Production Manager: Matt Ballantyne

Manufacturing Buyer: Linda Hsu

Manufacturing Manager: Marcia Locke

Marketing Manager: Trent Whatcott

Marketing Assistant: Darlene Macanan

Marketing Communications Manager: Tami Strang

Art Director: Caryl Gorska

Permission Acquisition Manager – Image: Leitha Etheridge-Sims

Rights Acquisition Account Manager – Text: Roberta Broyer

Content Project Management: Pre-PressPMG

Production Service: Pre-PressPMG

Cover Designer: Lisa Buckley

Cover Image: Thomas Northcut, Jupiterimages, Siri Stafford

Compositor: Pre-PressPMG

© 2011, 2008, 2004 Brooks/Cole, Cengage Learning

ALL RIGHTS RESERVED. No part of this work covered by the copyright herein may be reproduced, transmitted, stored or used in any form or by any means graphic, electronic, or mechanical, including but not limited to photocopying, recording, scanning, digitizing, taping, Web distribution, information networks, or information storage and retrieval systems, except as permitted under Section 107 or 108 of the 1976 United States Copyright Act, without the prior written permission of the publisher.

For product information and technology assistance, contact us at **Cengage Learning Customer & Sales Support, 1-800-354-9706**

For permission to use material from this text or product, submit all requests online at **cengage.com/permissions**
Further permissions questions can be emailed to **permissionrequest@cengage.com**.

Library of Congress Control Number: 2009944106

ISBN-13: 978-0-8400-3323-9

ISBN-10: 0-8400-3323-0

Brooks/Cole
20 Davis Drive
Belmont, CA 94002
USA

Cengage Learning is a leading provider of customized learning solutions with office locations around the globe, including Singapore, the United Kingdom, Australia, Mexico, Brazil, and Japan. Locate your local office at: **international.cengage.com/region**

Cengage Learning products are represented in Canada by Nelson Education, Ltd.

For your course and learning solutions, visit **academic.cengage.com**

Purchase any of our products at your local college store or at our preferred online store **www.CengageBrain.com**

Printed in the United States of America
1 2 3 4 5 6 7 14 13 12 11 10

Brief Contents

Contents

CHAPTER 12 **Addictions Counseling and Psychopharmacology** 344

PREFACE

This text was originally created out of a very personal need to create a student-centered introduction to our field. We felt frustrated at times because the personalized warmth and sensitivity that are the basis of our profession have not been reflected in academic experiences. Too often, education emphasizes theoretical knowledge and scholarly inquiry to the exclusion of student involvement. It has been our intention that this book would not only meet the stringent demands of scholarship but also provide a lively and dynamic overview of the counseling profession that fully engages the student in the process.

This text speaks directly to you, the student; it challenges you to explore your personal motives for choosing counseling as your area of interest, and helps you to personally integrate much of the research and theoretical concepts. More than ever before, the voices of beginning and experienced counselors are used to reflect the realities of practice, make the ideas come alive, and help you personalize the content in such a way that it becomes immediately applicable to your life. In fact, there is no other profession that not only allows you to personalize concepts to your own life, but encourages you to do so; almost everything you read about in this text has implications and applications to what you do on a daily basis. You will find innumerable ways to improve immediately not only your counseling skills but also your personal relationships.

WHAT YOU CAN DO

One of the distinguishing features of this text, which makes it unique in the field, is its student-oriented focus on the *realities* of counseling practice. In addition to presenting the major historical, theoretical, and research foundations in a highly readable style, we try to engage you in a dialogue about the counseling profession, its underlying concepts, and your personal goals for the future.

It is so often the relationships we develop with people that become the foundation for a meaningful effort to change. This is as true in relationships between authors and readers as it is between a counselor and clients, or between an instructor and students. More than ever before, we strive to connect with readers in such a way that they are likely to explore the process of counseling as well as its content.

In order to make the complex conceptual ideas of counseling come alive, the book contains over 150 "Voices from the Field." In these excerpts from interviews, beginning and experienced practitioners speak openly and honestly about the challenges they face and the ways they have resolved difficulties. They present practical advice based on their experiences. When these voices are added to those of the authors, readers are exposed to the realities of counseling practice in such a way that they can make informed choices about where and how to practice new skills and knowledge. You would be well advised to use this material as a springboard for your own interviews with practitioners.

One of the assignments we routinely give when we teach this class is to ask students to interview a minimum of 6 to 10 counselors in the field, representing at least three different specialty areas. We can think of few other learning experiences that are more revealing than talking to people who are doing what you someday hope to do yourself. Ask them for advice. Find out what they love and hate about their work. It is not unusual that you will even make contacts that may someday turn into an internship placement or even a job offer.

The end of each chapter contains a series of experiential and reflective exercises that will further help you to personalize material. These introspective activities can be a used as a structured journal in which you can apply to your own life the concepts discussed in class and in the text. In addition, these activities may be helpful as questions to be explored in cooperative learning groups in class. Whether you use the exercises or not, you will find it helpful to use a journal throughout the semester to keep track of important ideas, make sense of complex ideas, and personalize material in a way that is useful to you.

WHAT TO EXPECT

Introduction to Counseling: Voices from the Field is designed for initial courses in human service programs that have titles such as "Principles of Counseling," "Professional Orientation," "Counseling Theory and Practice," "Introduction to Helping," and "Human Resource Development." The book emphasizes the development of a professional identity, ethical standards for practice, basic process skills, the counseling relationship, personal theory building, and understanding of meaningful research. We are also especially concerned with presenting a contemporary "cutting-edge" focus on the practical realities of counseling. Too often students complain that their courses and texts did not prepare them for the daily grit and grind of what it means to be a counselor.

Particular attention is devoted to the major specialties and diverse settings in which counseling takes place, such as schools and clinics and medical, industrial, mental health, community agency, and private-practice settings. We quite deliberately made the size of the book realistic for a semester's work and planned the number and length of chapters to be manageable for the student struggling to digest a new world of terminology and concepts.

The book is organized into four broad focus areas: professional identity factors, theoretical and research foundations, counseling applications, and issues in professional practice. Whereas the first two sections (Chapters 1 through 8) help you to learn the foundations of counseling, the latter two sections (Chapters 9 through 15) apply these concepts to the various specialties within the field. You are thus encouraged to master the field's basic theory and research, become familiar with the generic counseling skills, and begin thinking about the realities of developing a flexible specialty, making yourself marketable, finding suitable employment, and staying passionately committed to the profession.

WHAT'S NEW

One of the most exciting and disorienting aspects of counseling is how rapidly the field changes. This evolution in theory and research parallels the changes that practitioners experience so often. As professional counselors, we sometimes wish we could send "recall notices" to all the clients we've seen in the past, notifying them that however we may once have helped them, the method is now obsolete and they should return for new, improved methods that no longer resemble the ways we once operated.

Consistent with the mood of our times, we continue to emphasize a philosophy of counselor education and training that Jeffrey and his friend and coauthor, Bob Brown (now deceased), first proposed a number of years ago—one that is integrative and pragmatic and that seeks to combine the best of existing approaches. As in previous editions, the text includes detailed discussions on today's major issues: multicultural sensitivity, historical roots of our profession, current counseling interventions, licensure and credentialing, constructivist thinking, family violence, sexism and age discrimination, computer applications, managed care and brief therapies, legal and ethical conflicts, and gender issues, to name a few.

For this edition, we have added a number of new and exciting features:

- We have included a DVD with 14 video chapters, each corresponding to a topic in the text. The DVD has been designed so that you can view individual chapters to enhance your understanding of the reading; or you can watch the entire video as a stand-alone documentary about the field of counseling. We created this DVD to reflect both the content and the spirit of the text in its honest and spirited reflection of the realities of our profession. You will see beginning and experienced clinicians talk about what it means to be a counselor—their joys and passions, their struggles and frustrations, how they have been influenced by counseling's evolutionary figures, and how they work with clients now. In addition, the DVD contains role-playing exercises illustrating basic counseling techniques, theory-based interventions, assessment and diagnosis, and ethical decision-making. Ultimately, this DVD is both a teaching tool and a medium for bringing the counseling profession to life.
- The chapter on insight-oriented theories has been significantly expanded to include narrative and postmodern counseling, reflecting the increasing impact

narrative theory is having on our field as both a unitary theory and as a source of interventions that can be integrated into a variety of approaches.

- The chapter on integrating theory and counseling skills has a new section indicating which approaches are receiving research support for treating specific mental health disorders. We have provided this information in keeping with the movement in our profession towards evidence-based practice and the need for even beginning counselors to familiarize themselves with those theories and models demonstrated to be effective by empirical research.

- The chapter on action-oriented approaches has been expanded to include a new section on mindfulness-based counseling models. The use of "mindfulness" as a treatment intervention for a variety of emotional difficulties has emerged as one of the significant trends in our profession.

- The chapter on career counseling now includes a section we have called "Career Counseling in Hard Times." At some point in a counselor's professional journey, he or she will be called upon to help people get through times of job loss and economic insecurity. Counselors can play an invaluable role during these periods, and this new section introduces the reader to how counselors can fill this role.

- The entire book has been completely updated with over 150 new references and expanded lists of suggested readings that include fiction, nonfiction, and films, in addition to counseling and social science literature.

ACKNOWLEDGMENTS

We want to thank the "Voices from the Field" who agreed to be interviewed for this book and who were willing to be so honest and open about their experiences in the trenches. More than anything else in this text, it is your stories that give life and realism to the theory, research, and concepts presented.

We are grateful for the assistance of Steve Bornstein, Jennifer Cunningham, Parastoo Erdogan, Meghan McNeil, Michelle Parize, and Jane Thomas, who helped with the research for this edition.

We appreciate the helpful suggestions of those who reviewed the manuscript: Chaunda Scott (University of Detroit), Mercy Sally Hage (Columbia University), Cyrus Ellis (Governors State University), Lisa Hawley (Oakland University), Mike Chaney (Oakland University), Jesse DeEsch (Rider University), and Trevor Milliron (Lee University).

We are also grateful to the following faculty members who provided input and feedback: Dana Comstock (St. Mary's University), Leila Vaughn (Troy University), Frank Browning (Troy University), Conni Sharp (Pittsburg State University), Jean Jirovec (Lakeland College), Casey Tobin (Troy University), Sandra Lopez-Baez (University of Virginia), Mary Kesler (Winona State University), Karen Estrella (Lesley University), Bill Schiller (Northeastern State University), Shane Haberstroh (University of Texas at San Antonio), Shawn Spurgeon (Western Kentucky University), Kan Chandras (Fort Valley State University), Bill McManus (North Greenville University), Joy Whitman (DePaul University), Yolanda Turner (Eastern University), Debra Wilson (Troy University), David Kleist (Idaho State University), Heather Lyons (Loyola College in Maryland), Donald Nims (Western Kentucky University), Nancy Nolan (Vanderbilt University), and Adam Zagelbaum (Sonoma State University).

ABOUT THE AUTHORS

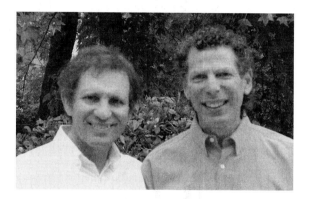

Jeffrey A. Kottler has authored over 80 books in the field for counselors, therapists, teachers, and the public, including *On Being a Therapist, Making Changes Last, Counseling Skills for Teachers, Bad Therapy: Master Therapists Share Their Worst Failures, The Client Who Changed Me: Stories of Therapist Personal Transformation, Changing People's Lives While Transforming Your Own: Paths to Social Justice and Global Human Rights,* and *The Assassin and the Therapist: An Exploration of Truth in Psychotherapy and in Life.*

Jeffrey has worked as a teacher, counselor, and therapist in a preschool, middle school, mental health center, crisis center, university, community college, and private practice. He has served as a Fulbright Scholar and Senior Lecturer in Peru and Iceland, teaching counseling theory and practice. He has also served as a visiting professor in New Zealand, Australia, Hong Kong, and Nepal. He is currently Professor of Counseling at California State University, Fullerton and head of the Madhav Ghimire Foundation which provides educational scholarships to at-risk girls in Nepal.

David S. Shepard has been practicing as a counselor in the Los Angeles area for almost two decades, working with the full range of issues clients bring to counselors, including adjustment problems, relationship issues, struggles with substance abuse, depression, anxiety, and personality disorders. Prior to his counseling career, David worked as a screenwriter in the film and television industry, where he specialized in children's animation. He is currently Associate Professor of Counseling at California State University, Fullerton, where he does research on men's issues in counseling, as well as on the uses of film for teaching counseling.

THE PROFESSIONAL COUNSELOR

WHAT COUNSELING IS AND HOW IT WORKS

CHAPTER I

KEY CONCEPTS

- Personal motives for altruism
- Making a difference in others' lives
- Countertransference
- Informed consent
- Tolerating anxiety
- Personal growth and professional development
- Neutral posture
- Subjugating personal needs
- Tolerating ambiguity and uncertainty
- Process definition of counseling
- Movement toward synthesis and integration
- Significance of self

WHY BE A COUNSELOR?

See Companion DVD
Advice for Starting

It is both interesting and useful to begin the systematic study of the counseling profession by exploring your own motives for entering the profession. The decision to become a counselor is just as complex and multifaceted as any of the issues your clients might bring to you. You will expect—even demand—that your clients be completely honest with themselves, that they confront their self-deceptions, ambivalence, and motives behind actions. It is only fair that you attempt to be honest with yourself as well.

Students enter the counseling field, as they do any other profession, for a variety of reasons. Some people genuinely wish to save the world; others, more modestly, wish to save themselves. Many deliberately choose this field because there are so many opportunities to apply classroom and book studies to their own lives. Others quite unabashedly admit that it was a toss-up for them between going to see a counselor for their own problems and becoming one.

The personal motives behind career decisions are indeed important to examine as we begin this introduction to counseling. Such an understanding will permit a more thoughtful and clear-headed approach to the material presented. A typical class often includes students who see themselves as missionaries. They choose to study counseling because they have a strong desire to help others: to make a difference in the lives of those who are suffering. They frequently have a kind of empathy that comes from personal experience. They suffered and were saved; now the roles can be reversed. They wish to make the world a bit more civilized. Perhaps this reason belongs, even slightly, to any of us who select this path; it certainly plays a huge role in people's decisions to become a helping professional. You might be enrolled in this program for a variety of reasons, all related to making a difference in the world (Kottler, 2003; 2009):

1. You have some natural talent or interest toward helping others. Maybe you have served that role throughout your life.
2. You enjoy touching others' lives, knowing that you have influenced or impacted someone.
3. You derive tremendous satisfaction from the kind of close, intimate relationships that take place in helping encounters.

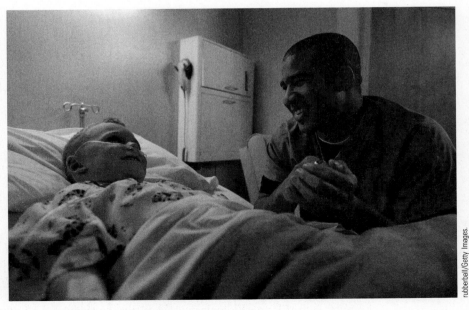

People choose to be counselors for a variety of reasons, foremost of which is that they wish to make a difference in the world, to help those who are most in need. It is through helping others learn and grow that we are often permitted to do so ourselves.

VOICE FROM THE FIELD

I always knew that I wanted to help people, though thought originally about a medical career. It wasn't until I faced the realities of what was involved in getting into and graduating from medical school that I began considering alternatives. You see, ever since I was a kid my worth was measured by what I could do for others. You might consider this part of my family culture. It is just understood that each of us will do something that involves helping others.

I would not be altogether truthful if I didn't mention that being a counselor means a heck of a lot more to me than helping people. That is important and all but so are some other reasons that I don't ordinarily admit. For instance, I have this thing about being in control. I have often felt that way in most of my relationships, so I am excited about learning ways to build trust with people. This will help me in my work but I know it will also help me with my friends and my boyfriend. I quite like the idea that after I graduate I will be much better at getting people to like and respect me.

I am also somewhat of a busybody, meaning I like to know what other people are up to. When I find out that somebody else is having problems or doing strange things, in a perverse way it makes me feel better, that maybe I'm not so strange myself. I think it is really exciting that we get to hear about people's most intimate secrets.

4. Your own problems seem diminished in comparison to those of your clients.
5. You are able to gain broadened perspectives on the meaning of life as a result of your searching conversations with others.
6. You are able to give something back to your community, to use your own learning experiences to benefit others.
7. You pass on a legacy to others as part of your commitment and dedication to service.
8. You help yourself by helping others.

Yet there are many other reasons people choose counseling as a profession. The selection could be pragmatic: Grades or test scores may prevent a move into what is perceived as a more highly competitive medical or legal education. Or the time commitments required by some disciplines may seem excessive or overwhelming. Counseling seems a reasonable compromise; the program can be completed in a few years and then the credentials will permit practice in many attractive settings.

It is also true that some people have very self-centered motivations for entering the helping professions. The counselor is able to satisfy unfulfilled nurturing needs by rescuing people with problems—and able to participate in intimate relationships as well—while always maintaining control (Herron & Rouslin, 1984; Kottler, 2010; Robertiello, 1978). Some people are attracted to counseling because they enjoy the power they can wield in influencing other people's lives (Hoyt, 2005). Counselors and other therapeutic practitioners have, in many ways, become power brokers in our society. They have become the oracles, the witch doctors, the gurus, the wizards, the mentors. In almost every culture of the world, there are professionals designated as counselors or shamans whose main job is to promote healing by harnessing forces of the natural, spiritual, physical, and psychological domains. They listen with compassion and speak with authority. They have the answers and, although they may not reveal them directly, if clients behave and do what they are supposed to, they will be gently prodded to discover truth for themselves.

I had a lot of grief at a young age. Since then I've felt drawn to those who are hurting, especially those who are dying. I know this sounds morbid, but I really do like working at the hospice with cancer patients and their families. I'm so impressed with the ones who die with dignity and good humor.

Early on, I thought my motivations were purely altruistic. Hah! I know better now. I'm more realistic and honest about what drives me and also what pushes my buttons. The truth is that this work makes me feel needed. This is especially true with my dying patients. If this work ever stops meeting my needs, I'll stop doing it.

Students also select counseling for many of the same practical reasons that lead to any other career. They need the degree for a pay raise or promotion. During tough economic times they can't find suitable employment. They are after prestige and status. The courses are offered at convenient times. Tests are infrequent or the program doesn't appear too demanding. And, indeed, counseling does not at first glance seem as rigorous as training in engineering, nuclear physics, or neurosurgery.

But don't be fooled. A counseling program is about the most challenging emotional experience a student can undertake. Although some counseling programs may not create intense academic pressure, all emphasize skill mastery and performance competencies. Counseling programs are not only interested in your ability to succeed at academic tasks but also your ability to translate book and classroom learning into action. The bottom line for success in a counseling program is what you can do and what you can deliver.

Another large part of the work you do will involve addressing your own personal reactions to your work, often called *countertransference* reactions. This refers to the phenomenon, originally described by Sigmund Freud (1912), in which clinicians lose their objectivity and clarity because of their own personal issues, which interfere with their work. Their perceptions of their clients become distorted and their interpretations polluted by their own personal stuff. While countertransference is often not addressed nearly as much in training as it should be, it is absolutely critical that you have a handle on your own biases, unresolved issues, and strong emotional reactions that may interfere with your ability to think clearly and respond helpfully to clients (Bemak & Epp, 2001; Hackney & Cormier, 2009; Maroda, 2004; Wishne, 2005).

It is also important to understand that the personal reactions you have to your clients can become a therapeutic benefit, as well as a delightful side effect of being a member of the counseling profession. In one study of how famous therapists were changed by their clients (Kottler & Carlson, 2005a), a number of leaders in the field described a multitude of new ways in which they were challenged to grow—not just professionally but also personally. In many ways, their clients became their best teachers.

Just consider, for example, some of the opinions or values you hold as most sacred. How do you feel about the death penalty, or abortion, or gun control, or gay rights, or even your deepest religious (or nonreligious) convictions? Now imagine

VOICE FROM THE FIELD

I don't have kids, and I don't think I ever will. But there are hundreds, probably thousands of children, whom I have worked with during the past years. I'd like to think some of them will remember me for a very long time. Maybe until the day they die.

I know that there are several mentors and teachers who influenced me in ways that I'll never forget. They live inside me. Their words still echo in my mind. At times I even smile when I catch myself saying something just the way that they would.

It gives me chills to think that others might someday feel so grateful for my efforts to help them. Maybe long after I'm not around anymore I will still live inside the children I worked with.

---

that someone walks in your office door and presents a point of view that is the direct opposite of what you believe. Will you be able to respond to this person with compassion and caring, free from personal biases that may cloud your judgments?

The constant and often difficult inward journey necessary for growth and counseling skill development are well worth the effort. This profession offers the student more advantages on both a personal and a professional level than almost any other field. Where else can all life experiences—books, films, travels, relationships, fantasies, jobs, losses, disasters, and triumphs—help the professional to be more effective? Everything and everyone teaches a counselor to understand the human world better, to have more compassion, to be a better communicator, to comprehend more completely the intricate complexities of behavior. Every experience allows you to teach from what you know.

In one study conducted with first-year counseling students (Melton, Nofzinger-Collins, Wynne, & Susman, 2005), participants were asked to record their innermost thoughts and feelings during simulated sessions with a client. Consistently, the students reported struggles with controlling their anger and frustration when clients didn't cooperate or meet their expectations, and reported having to manage their disappointment over missed opportunities for deeper exploration. They described fears over feeling incompetent, and elation over feeling that they were helpful in some way. These are typical reactions that you will learn to deal with over time, assuming that you remain reflective and self-critical in constructive ways.

What other profession teaches skills and competencies applicable to work that can also be so easily applied to your personal world? Counseling trains people to be more passionate consumers of life. Intensive training in observing nonverbal behavior, analyzing motives, handling confrontations, and reflecting feelings helps counselors to be more attractive human beings, helps them be experts at efficiently developing trusting, productive relationships. If counselors can do that in their offices, they can certainly do it with their friends, colleagues, children, siblings, partners, spouses, and parents.

Counseling inspires the student to be a knowledgeable generalist, a Renaissance scholar, a devourer of "truth" in any palatable form. We are not restricted to our texts for learning. We read literature, history, anthropology, sociology, biology, biochemistry, education, psychology, and philosophy, and they are all beneficial—even necessary—if we are truly to understand this abstract thing called the human mind.

Counseling permits practitioners to make a difference in people's lives and to see the results in their own lifetimes. One of the ways in which we attempt to confront our own mortality is by preserving our spirit long after physical death. Certainly the principal reward for a dedicated teacher, counselor, or therapist is the knowledge that a generation of clients will remember and use the help that was offered, even after we are gone. Our profession allows us to productively face our own fears of death by leaving behind those who, because of our efforts, feel less pain.

Counselors become more wise and self-aware with every client they see. Each presented concern forces us to consider introspectively our own degree of stability. Every discussed problem reminds us of those issues that we still have not fully resolved. A client complains of periodic urges to break out of the mold and run away, while the counselor silently considers his or her own rebellious impulses. A boring relationship, fear of failure, career stagnation, sexual frustrations, loneliness, parental dependence—all subjects that are commonly presented—force the counselor to resolve them, once and for all, in his or her own life. The profession thus continually encourages its practitioners to upgrade their personal effectiveness.

Counseling enables us to appreciate how we are all interconnected. A client shares a painful experience or difficult conflict in her life, and we think to ourselves, "It's so amazing that this person's story so relates to my own life." And then we realize that it is no coincidence, but rather a reminder that despite the fact that we and our clients may have important differences in our life experiences and backgrounds, we are all struggling together to make meaning of our lives and reach our fullest potential. David Orlinsky, a well-known therapist and author, wrote, "I would even say that doing psychotherapy provides an opportunity to worship, to celebrate our fundamental and energizing interdependence. There are moments in therapy when this energy and human beauty meet ... and where, when they meet, a healing influence resonates in all directions, into the therapist as well as the patient, and to others closely involved in the patient's life" (Orlinsky, 2005, pp. 1005–1006).

At this very moment you may want to examine your personal motives for studying counseling. (*Note*: This is one of several reflective questions that you may wish to address in your journal.) Better yet, talk to other students about what motivates them as well—not just the socially acceptable and politically correct reasons, but also the deeper, more personal drives. Although you may never fully understand all the factors, needs, interests, values, and unconscious processes that are influencing your decision, the quest is nevertheless valuable. It is likely that only years after graduation—and perhaps after your own experiences as a client—will you have a focused picture of your honest motives. This process of self-inquiry, once begun, is self-perpetuating because of the growth it fosters. And the beginning is *now*.

TO BE A COUNSELOR

Choosing counseling as a career sets into motion a chain of events and leads to a series of direct and indirect consequences, the impact of which is often initially unclear. The choice to be a counselor, for example, not only dramatically affects the

VOICE FROM THE FIELD

I was filled with so much anxiety almost every moment of my beginning years as a counselor. First, I wondered constantly if I had whatever it took to be good at this job. I compared myself to others and usually found myself wanting in some way. I wasn't smart enough. I couldn't express myself as well as others. I didn't have nearly the same life experiences, or academic background, as those who seemed so far ahead of me.

And then when I started seeing clients, I felt so anxious that I wouldn't be able to help them. I didn't know if I'd say or do the right thing. I had this vision that even though I was pretending to know what I was doing, the client would see right through me and know I was clueless.

Even after all these years I still feel anxious every time a new client walks in. I wonder if I can help him or her. I worry about whether I know enough, or whether someone else might do a better job. So you see, the anxiety lessens a bit but it never goes away.

See Companion DVD
To Be a Counselor

education, training, and molding of the student who made the decision but also affects that individual's family and friends. Imagine, for example, that you simply studied the impact of birth order on personality development. How can you *not* look at your life and your relationships with family members differently after that? Or consider the very real possibility that, in any given week in your professional life, you will listen to clients struggle with fears of dying, infidelity, loneliness, dependency, boredom, suicidal thoughts, and a hundred other issues that have haunted you throughout your life.

We have always thought that if we were to present you with a fully disclosing "informed consent" (an ethical concept you will learn about later that refers to disclosure of risks so you can make knowledgeable decisions about your participation), we would have to tell you that deciding to be a counselor has huge implications for your life in a number of ways. For one thing, *all* your relationships will change. You will develop new expectations and standards for intimacy. You will learn skills that enable you to develop closer levels of intimacy with others, and you will want to use that newfound ability to enrich your family and work relationships. In a sense, you will be ruined—forever dissatisfied with superficial encounters. After all, how can you settle for rather inane interactions when you talk to people daily about their most intimate secrets, their most powerful insights, and their most meaningful feelings? The truth is that your love relationships may very well change forever and many of your friendships may be outgrown. You are not only choosing a new profession but a new way of being, a new way of relating to yourself, to others, and to the world.

Choosing to be a counselor means opening yourself up to intense self-scrutiny and personal growth. It means examining your strengths and limitations as a human being, exploring your vulnerabilities, and identifying those aspects of your functioning that you need to improve. All these changes emerge as the consequence of simply selecting studies in counseling. A number of other implications flow from choosing to be a counselor.

VOICE FROM THE FIELD

One risk of being a counselor that I never considered is how my skills would change all my relationships. In my program, I've learned how to be pretty good at listening to people, reflecting back what they would say to me, or sometimes just being silent. At first, my spouse would get kinda pissed off at me when I did it with her. "Will you just stop being a counselor and be my husband again?" she'd say. For a while I actually worried that this counseling thing would break us apart. But after a while, she started catching on to what I was doing, and she started listening better, too. Not that we don't still fight like any couple does, but we seem to get past it faster, and feel a whole lot closer.

DEALING WITH ANXIETY

We are not referring yet to the anxiety of your clients but rather your own internal pressure and apprehensions about this work. Anxiety is not only an expected condition of life for a counseling student but a normal one. You will feel anxious about so many aspects of your training:

- Are you smart enough, or capable enough, to make it in this field?
- Is this the right job for you? Are you wasting your time?
- Will you ever know enough to be able to help someone?
- Will others find out how inadequate you really feel inside?
- Will your personal issues interfere with your ability to help people?
- Will you hurt someone because of some lapse or mistake?
- Will you be forced to look at things that you would rather avoid?

The answers to these questions cannot be addressed in a single sitting. You will likely continue to struggle with them throughout your whole career.

MAKING A COMMITMENT

To be a counselor means making a commitment to a profession and a lifestyle. For every spectacular success there are also disappointments and failures. Counselors must learn not only to temper their exhilaration after witnessing phenomenal change but also to cope with the frustrations of resistant clients, rigid institutional policies, limited budgets, overworked administrators, irate parents, and confusing laws. Although there are few greater victories than the feeling of knowing that a person has been helped as a direct result of our efforts, often clients do not accommodate our wishes or cooperate with our interventions. They may stubbornly insist on staying miserable in spite of our best attempts at helping them to find another way.

At times a counselor will do everything perfectly: patiently build a trusting relationship with a client and gently lead her through the successive counseling stages—exploring, reflecting, analyzing, interpreting, and confronting—and then, finally, the time comes for action. Let's say the client agrees that a divorce is imminent. The marriage has become destructive, her husband abusive. She realizes she cannot grow further while handcuffed. She has worked through her guilt over deserting him, her fear of disapproval by mutual friends, and her fear of making it on her own without a man to lean on. She is ready—or so she says. But time is up

VOICE FROM THE FIELD

The other day I was helping someone sort out the reasons why she was so isolated and lonely in her life. I was giving her feedback on what she does to create barriers in her relationships and keep others at a distance. I was specifically highlighting what behaviors she favors that are most annoying and I was telling her all this stuff in the most gentle way that I could.

This happens more often than I'd like to admit but the woman was hardly listening to me. What I was saying was too threatening for her to hear. Or maybe she wasn't ready to hear it yet. I don't know.

But the really weird thing is that I realized I was talking to myself as much as I was talking to her. I happen to have a similar problem of keeping myself isolated. I use my work to do that. I blame my schedule. But damn, I realized at that moment that my frustration towards my client for not listening was really directed towards myself: I wasn't listening either!

---

for this week's session. She will do her homework and be prepared by next week to make the commitment to beginning her new life as a single woman.

Eagerly, the counselor awaits the report next week. He tries hard not to pat himself on the back because he does feel proud. He has done good work. The next week arrives. The counselor waits in his office ... and waits. The client doesn't show. She doesn't return!

The counselor calls her, only to receive the cold announcement, without any explanation, that she will no longer be coming back for sessions. That's it. Before the counselor can sort out the mess, there is a knock on the door. His next client is waiting impatiently for the session.

STRIVING FOR EXCELLENCE

To be a counselor means taking responsibility for your own growth and striving for excellence in your personal behavior.

Every client presents a novel challenge. Five people who are depressed will act differently as a result of the symptoms they may call depression. One person is lethargic and drained, whereas another appears agitated and emotionally overwrought. One client has lost 14 pounds and reports being able to sleep only fitfully; another has gained considerable weight and seems to sleep all the time. One person talks constantly about suicidal fantasies, whereas another is incensed that you would even bring up self-destructive behavior. Yet among these diverse experiences, depression is the central theme.

Even though depression is but one of a dozen major problems that frequently present themselves to a counselor, there are endless variations on those themes. To be optimally helpful to each client, you will have to understand the issues thoroughly and have had some experience in handling them. Although much of this expertise will come from class lectures and readings, your own personal experiences will prove invaluable.

Whereas a male counselor cannot directly relate to the struggle of a female client considering an abortion and can never have worked through it himself, it is likely that this counselor has accumulated rich personal experiences in resolving similar value conflicts. And although a female counselor can never know the shame

VOICE FROM THE FIELD

On my first day of my internship, I was anxiously describing a new case to my supervisor, when he interrupted me and said, "Okay, why do you think this client was sent to you?" I looked at him, puzzled—I frankly didn't know what he was talking about. He went on: "You got this client because there was something for you to learn about yourself. It's no coincidence this client is sitting in the room with you." Now, you have to understand, I'm pretty much a very rational guy, and I knew my supervisor was, too. I sputtered, "I don't get it … I was assigned this client by the agency. It was totally random."

He was an older man, kind of grandfatherly, and he smiled at me. "Look, you don't have to believe in cosmic coincidences if you don't want to. I'm asking you to do something different. Reflect on what you can learn from this client; your work with her is not just about what you can do for her—she has much to teach you as well. Look for where her story mirrors your own issues, see how she deals with them, reflect on the lessons she may be teaching you about life. She's not some 'case.' She's a gift to help you grow." Those words changed how I view every client I've worked with since. They aren't a sum of symptoms, an example of some psychological disorder. They have all been gifts, and in so doing, have helped me see myself more clearly, helped me become a better counselor.

that her impotent male client feels, she does know the awful dread of being unable to perform adequately.

The consensus among many counselors is that each client provides them an opportunity after the session to look inward, personalize the material, and ask the question: *To what extent is this a problem for me?* When a client complains of stagnation in life, of too many predictable routines and boring people, how can the counselor not examine this pattern in his or her own life? Fears of growing old, of failure, of rejection, of loving, of hating—all hit a familiar chord. And the degree to which the counselor has successfully struggled with any of these themes will determine, to some extent, his or her capacity for understanding the client's fears and resolving them.

A client complains of a bad temper and uncontrolled explosive outbursts. But the counselor knows, not just theoretically but personally, the value of a bad temper—how it provides an instant excuse for abusing others: "Sorry. I couldn't help it. I have a bad temper." Beyond such insight, the counselor also knows personally just how to control his or her own anger.

In one study of master therapists who were nominated by their peers as being at the top of their profession, they were found to have a number of characteristics that went beyond mere professional competence (Jennings & Skovholt, 1999). Of course they had excellent relationship skills, but they were also very committed to working on their own emotional health. They were voracious learners, driven to excel in as many facets of life as they could. In another study that interviewed prominent counseling theorists about their best work, most of them were extraordinarily reflective about their lives and their helping efforts. They saw their clients as their best supervisors, helping them to achieve greater excellence by continually adapting, changing, and evolving (Kottler & Carlson, 2005b). Finally, extraordinary practitioners spend more time reflecting on their work and thinking about their sessions constructively than do other colleagues (Miller, Hubble, & Duncan, 2007).

Counselors, then, are constantly striving for more mastery in their lives, applying the technology of psychological helping to themselves. At any moment in time the counselor ought to be able to articulate three or four specific personal areas in need of upgrading—and be actively involved in the process.

ADOPTING A NEUTRAL POSTURE

To be a counselor implies a dedication to helping other people without having a vested interest in the particular directions that they may choose.

Based on his or her particular religious beliefs, cultural upbringing, lifestyle preferences, and value system, every counselor has a notion about what is generally good for people, whether it be brown rice, lots of exercise, plenty of fresh air, a God-fearing home, or good loving. Clients, therefore, present the counselor with the dilemma of which way to influence them: in a way that is consistent with the counselor's own beliefs or in quite another direction—one that the client may genuinely prefer.

In the social world, people are quite liberal in dispensing their opinions on a variety of issues; in the counseling session, such casually stated advice can be harmful, especially if it contributes to clients feeling like they need someone to tell them what to do because they aren't smart enough to figure things out for themselves. Counselors are interested in creating neither disciples nor dependents. They will understand that, by answering the client's persistent question, "What should I do?" they fall into one of two traps. Either they offer poor advice, which then teaches the client to resent the professional forever and not to take responsibility for the negative outcome, or worse—they offer sound advice, giving the client the clear message that the thing to do with a difficult question is just to run back to the counselor for help.

Yet a counselor often has strong personal opinions on whether clients should join the army or go back to school, get a divorce or endure the marriage, tell off nosy parents or buy them a present, turn themselves in to the authorities or learn to be more discreet, punt or go for a touchdown. Counselors are hardly all-knowing experts, creative problem solvers, or detached, objective professionals; we bring our own biases, our own unique histories, our own personal stories to the relationship. As such, the counseling relationship is a moral and political enterprise rather than a strictly neutral one, in spite of our best interests to rein in our biases (Bacaigalupe, 2002).

It is first necessary for the counselor to be aware of his or her own values and then, as far as is humanly possible, to block their effects on a client's decisions. Neutrality is the catchword of a therapeutic relationship. Although counselors may feel strongly about choices that clients make, their role is only to help clients examine the potential consequences, positive and negative, and then accept the clients' right to choose. This caution does not mean that counselors attempt to hide their true feelings from clients, using the mask of professional distance and neutrality. Rather, counselors work toward conquering the need for an investment in client decisions beyond a professional responsibility.

VOICE FROM THE FIELD

Hey, I know that I'm supposed to be paying attention to what clients are saying during sessions. I learned a long time ago how important listening skills are and how critical it is that clients feel heard and understood. Maybe even once upon a time, I did focus almost all the time.

But here's a secret: In my experience, no matter how much I concentrate and how hard I try, I don't think I'm really giving full attention more than half the time. Furthermore, I think this is better than what most counselors do.

Of course, my clients don't know how much my mind wanders and how often my attention drifts. There is just so much to think about, and so much to do, and so many buttons that are pushed in any session, that it's almost impossible to stay on track all the time. I think what makes a really exceptional counselor, though, is someone who works harder and harder to control personal stuff and give clients as much as we can.

SUBJUGATING PERSONAL NEEDS

To be a counselor involves controlling your own needs, desires, and preferences in favor of the best interests of the client.

One reason counseling is such difficult work is that the professional makes a deliberate decision to suspend all distractions—both internal and external—while in session. Whether the phone rings in another room or a siren blares through the streets, counselors do their best to block out all stimuli that are extraneous to the task at hand.

Even more difficult to banish are internal distractions. To be most helpful to the client, to focus all of your energy therapeutically, you must immerse yourself totally in the helping role. Attention to a grumbling stomach or an ingrown toenail will reduce your concentration. To daydream or indulge in fantasy while pretending to listen is obviously counterproductive. And to permit yourself the luxury of liking or disliking clients during a session can only further reduce effectiveness. The counselor therefore becomes quite adept in the meditation-type skills of gently pushing aside distracting thoughts, indulgent feelings, and any other internal behavior that reduces concentration, without sacrificing the genuineness of being human. In this sense doing counseling is very much an exercise in mindfulness in which you totally immerse yourself in the present moment (Kabat-Zinn, 2005; Segal, Williams, & Teasdale, 2001; Turner, 2008).

A rationale for the necessity to receive some compensation in exchange for delivering a therapeutic service is that it does require such extraordinary effort to stifle your natural urges. It is for this reason that counseling is an activity that is far from "natural." It is highly unnatural to push aside your urges of attraction, indulgence, and selfishness.

COPING WITH DISCOMFORT

To be a counselor requires that you learn to become comfortable in the presence of others' discomfort.

One goal of counseling is often to make people squirm. Until clients become dissatisfied with themselves, disgusted by their self-sabotaging behaviors, they will

VOICE FROM THE FIELD

I was leading a group and the members were all playing the game, "Is it safe here?" Each person was testing things, trying to decide if it was safe enough to risk sharing themselves in an authentic way. We'd been going on like this for some time. One person was saying, "I'll do it if you will," and another was responding with, "Well, if you go first then I'll follow," and a third was saying, "Maybe I'll go later, but only if you guys go first."

I had this choice to let this go on, or really push them to a deeper level. I've got to tell you: it would have been a heck of a lot easier to just let things stay on the surface. I knew that if I challenged them I'd get some flack. And sure enough, it took a lot of work to confront their caution. But that's my job, that's why I get paid to do this stuff. I know that if they stay comfy and chatty not much useful is going to happen.

rarely change. Counselors often help to intensify this discomfort as a means of encouraging continued flight toward mental health. Confrontation is intended to force the client to face discrepancies, incongruence, and inconsistency. And the counselor must get used to despair. The one place in the world where people feel safe to cry and honestly express their pain is in the counselor's office. Often the feelings of desperation are even exaggerated because the therapeutic environment is so nurturing and accepting. Clients will complain and show rage and hurt. They will cry and scream and stamp their feet. And counselors take the full force of this emotional energy.

Counselors need to become proficient at facing outbursts calmly. Often they must reinterpret psychological discomfort as a sign that things are going according to plan rather than as a signal to retreat. Only when clients are uncomfortable may we be certain they are seriously working on themselves. They do not come for a good time.

DEALING WITH LOSS AND GRIEF

To be a counselor requires that you not only sit with other people's grief, but help them access intense levels of emotional pain. Indeed, it can be argued that facilitating the expression of grief and the process of mourning is an essential component of what we do with many of our clients, regardless of their presenting issue. Mourning means coming to terms with loss, and life is saturated with losses, small and large, some necessary, some unexpected and tragic. For example, there are small losses inherent to every decision a person makes. When clients complain about feeling "stuck" (a quite common complaint in our field) regarding an important choice, their distress can be traced to a fear of facing the loss of "the road not taken." The teenager struggling with whether to try drugs in order to feel accepted by peers is afraid of losing a sense of belonging. The college student undecided whether to major in business or premed must deal with the reality that choice may mean loss of one career path. Committing to a relationship partner is terrifying for so many clients because it entails loss of the possibility that there might be other attractive mates. The decision to start a family entails a huge loss of personal freedom.

Then there are the truly significant losses: the crushing blow to self-esteem and sense of security when a client is laid off from a seemingly safe job; the grief that accompanies the breakup with a partner; the loss of physical capacity as a person deals with age or illness; and the ultimate loss—the death of a loved one.

As counselors, our role is sometimes a fairly simple one. What clients need most during these difficult times is to not experience their mourning alone; human connection in times of distress can be a significant buffer against incapacitating grief, ensuring that the pain does not cross the line into clinical depression or unmanageable anxiety. Counselors provide the connection simply by being fully present and providing the safety our clients need to experience whatever reactions are present.

If this sounds like gloomy and depressing work, this is hardly the case. Helping people mourn a loss is one of the most gratifying parts of the job. As witnesses to grief, we stay connected to the poignancy of life, reminded time and time again of the old wisdom that you cannot experience life's joys unless you are willing to feel its pain. However, this work does mean that listening to clients stirs up memories of our own losses, or warns us of potential losses to come. We can only sit with our client's pain if we are unafraid to face our own. This is not only true with respect to the losses, disappointments, and grief that we have already experienced in our lives but, eventually, the losses associated with our clients when they are ready to leave.

DEALING WITH AMBIGUITY

To be a counselor requires that you function well with abstract ideas and ambiguous circumstances.

Counselors inhabit a professional world characterized by uncertainty and ambiguity. Clients are often not fully aware of their real problems. They report discomfort, vague and abstract, but circle relentlessly when the counselor attempts to help them focus. Very often clients want counseling because they are experiencing a true dilemma wherein no answer or response is truly satisfactory. Consider, for example, the man who has met a woman he deeply loves and with whom he wishes to spend his life. But she has a child, and he—after some traumatic past experiences—has realized that he is not comfortable in the parenting role. He wants to be with her yet is unable to share her role as a parent. The dilemma is real, and no alternative is completely satisfying. He comes for counseling, and your job is to help him resolve this thorny issue.

Counselors must develop empathy for clients who seem unfocused, who vacillate daily, and who seem unhappy but don't know why. In a sense, counselors (and other social scientists) must abandon their search for cause and effect and come to terms with ambiguity and uncertainty, which reflect the reality of the individual. Counselors must relinquish the quest for answers and instead relish the challenge of helping clients with their abstractions and the uncertainty inherent in being human. To be a counselor means dedicating yourself to the resolution of conflicts that are often irreconcilable, solving problems that have no right answers, and mediating disputes among parties who may enjoy fighting.

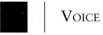 VOICE FROM THE FIELD

One of the biggest mistakes I ever made was when a client came back beaming, obviously helped by our sessions together. He went on at some length about the ways his life was now different. I sat there preening, just feeling so good about my skills and ability.

As I listened to him make his report, I reviewed in mind all the things I thought might have helped him. The previous week, for instance, I tried a new kind of interpretation in which I reframed his problem differently. Pretty cool, I thought at the time. And sure enough, I was confident this was what made the difference.

Almost as an afterthought, as he was about out the door, I asked him, "By the way, what did I do that you found so helpful?" Imagine my surprise, and disappointment, when he recited some obscure thing that I never remembered saying in the first place. How humbling to realize that I often don't know what I do that matters most.

DEFINITIONS OF COUNSELING

Counseling is indeed an ambiguous enterprise. It is done by persons who can't agree on the best treatment approach and often can't figure out what was most helpful to their clients. We debate among ourselves whether counseling should deal with feelings, thoughts, or behaviors; whether it should be primarily supportive or confrontational; whether it should focus on the past, present, or the future; whether it should involve a brief or long-term relationship; whether the counselor should take a role that is active and directive or one that is far more cautious and indirect. Further, the consumers of counseling services often can't exactly articulate what their concerns are, what counseling can and can't do for them, or what they want when it's over.

Practitioners also sometimes struggle with trying to articulate what counseling is and how and why it works. The truth is that in spite of our best intentions and solid grounding in theory, research, and technique, we don't always know what makes the greatest difference with our clients. Even our clients are not altogether certain what helped them the most, or even if the positive changes resulted from something completely unrelated to the sessions.

As a beginner, it is very important for you to realize that proper training and education will prepare you to do a number of things that research has indicated are consistently useful with some clients, presenting some complaints, in some situations. Nevertheless, you must also be prepared to live with a certain amount of ambiguity and uncertainty, not only about what is going on with your clients but also what is going on within the counseling process. In time, good counselors do have a way of sorting things out. Such positive outcomes begin with the way you set the stage for treatment.

At several points in your professional life—if not on the comprehensive examinations you may have to pass, then certainly with every astute client—you will be asked to define what it is that you do. This definition ought to be as specific as possible, describing in detail what it is that you do, why you do it, and how it works.

This definition, like counseling itself, should be a process—one designed to stimulate thinking so that ideas can ferment, evolve, and grow into a personal conception. Textbook definitions, although elegant, incisive, and comprehensive, almost always lack one essential ingredient: personalized meaning. As a beginner in this complex field—one who is already somewhat confused about what counseling is—the last thing in the world you need is another academic-sounding description of something that you don't really understand but that nevertheless sounds good to others (who may not understand it either). The definition of counseling that follows is presented in a way that most people in the field can live with, regardless of differences in their personalities, work settings, and preferred approaches. Further, this definition is offered in such a way that, after you have studied it a bit, you can actually describe to someone else what counseling is and give a fairly intelligible explanation of why and how it works. (We would even suggest you try this to boost your confidence.)

Counseling is:

- A profession with a history and set of standards that are distinct from other related disciplines such as social work, psychology, and psychiatry.
- An activity that is designed to work primarily with those who are experiencing developmental or adjustment problems (but also to work with those who struggle with forms of mental illness).
- A relationship, whether in a group, family, or individual format, that is constructed in a way to promote trust, safety, support, and lasting change.
- Multidimensional, dealing with human feelings, thoughts, and behaviors, as well as with the past, present, and future.
- A process that has a series of sequential steps:

  1. Helping people to articulate why they are seeking help
  2. Formulating goals and expectations for treatment
  3. Teaching clients how to get the most from the counseling experience
  4. Developing a high degree of trust and favorable expectations for change
  5. Diagnosing those concerns and dysfunctional areas in need of upgrading
  6. Exploring the client's world, including past and present functioning
  7. Understanding the cultural context (gender, ethnicity, race, religion, socioeconomic class, sexual orientation, etc.) of the client's experience
  8. Examining the underlying family and systemic factors that are both contributing to the problems and providing potential resources
  9. Discussing underlying issues and concerns, as well as their meanings
  10. Supporting and accepting the client as a person while selectively reinforcing those behaviors that are most fully functioning
  11. Confronting inconsistencies in the client's thoughts, language, and behavior
  12. Challenging assumptions that are inappropriate, self-destructive, counterproductive, or irrational
  13. Uncovering hidden and unconscious motives behind actions
  14. Encouraging clients to accept greater responsibility for their choices and actions
  15. Developing more options, as well as narrowing alternatives to those that are most suitable

VOICE FROM THE FIELD

I'm an elementary school counselor and it's often challenging to explain to younger kids what counseling is all about and how it all works. I usually say something like this when someone new comes in:

"I have a way cool job! I'm a person who gets to talk to kids like you! When you come here you get to talk about whatever is on your mind, whether it's happy stuff or sad stuff. When you come to visit me we can play and talk about what's going on with you. This isn't like going to the doctor. When you come here, I won't stick you with anything or make you do anything you don't want to do. And what we talk about in here is just between you and me, unless someone is hurting you or something like that."

16. Providing honest, constructive feedback
17. Structuring opportunities for practicing new ways of acting and being
18. Facilitating greater independence in the client so that counseling ends in the most efficient period of time

This description of counseling may seem to be unusually detailed, but remember—one goal was to construct a definition that almost everyone could agree with. Once you become more familiar with the major theoretical approaches in the field, you will recognize many of them reflected in the description above. And yes, this definition *is* long—and certainly too cumbersome to memorize and spit back exactly as you read it. But remember that the objective is for you to be able to describe this wonderful and complex process in your own unique way. The following example illustrates how a counselor would actually use this definition in his or her work.

CLIENT: My mom thinks I should come to see you, but I don't really know what you can do. (*This confusion is not unusual in a first interview.*)

COUNSELOR: What is it that your mother thinks I can do to help you? (*Rule number one in counseling is: When you don't know what else to do, put the ball back in the client's court to buy time until you can think of something else to say.*)

CLIENT: I don't know. She mentioned that maybe you could hear my problem and then fix it for me. (*Again, it is pretty typical that clients believe we have magic wands.*)

COUNSELOR: Without knowing exactly what problem you are referring to, maybe it would be helpful for you if I could explain a bit about what I do. The people that I see want to learn about themselves, about why they do the things they do; they want to understand better why they keep repeating the same mistakes over and over. (*The client looks perplexed. I'd better bring this more down to earth.*)

People come to see me because they feel safe here. They can talk about anything they want and know that I will listen carefully and I won't ever criticize them. I will keep whatever we talk about private, unless they seem inclined to hurt themselves or someone else. Most people also appreciate the fact that I am completely honest. (*Aha. This seems to be hitting home.*)

But just as important as being a good and safe listener, my job is to help you identify changes you want and need to make in your life and then help you get there. Ultimately, this experience will be useful to the extent that it helps you reach your desired goals.

Although this definition-in-action is hardly as specific and clear an explanation of counseling as a client (or you) might like, this still illustrates the value of being able to describe the process in a personal way. It also raises other questions; notably, how and why counseling works in the first place.

WHY DOES COUNSELING WORK?

Although at this juncture the jury has not yet returned to deliver its ultimate verdict, we do know that counseling probably works as the result of a combination of factors that many theorists find significant. You will learn in later chapters about how person-centered theorists believe that the nurturing relationship between counselor and client plays the biggest role in facilitating change; the behaviorists have evidence to indicate that reinforcement, modeling, and structured practice make the greatest difference; the psychoanalytic practitioners prefer to emphasize unconscious desires; the constructivists emphasize different perceptions of reality; the relational/feminist theorists examine issues of power and oppression in client experience; and the cognitive clinicians claim that counseling works by teaching people to think more rationally. And so on. By now it must have occurred to you that in this first chapter (or in a beginning course), it is not likely that you are going to get a completely acceptable answer to the question, "Why does counseling work?" Have patience.

On a more optimistic note, for the last half-century, researchers studying the effectiveness of counseling have repeatedly come to the conclusion that it does indeed work (Eaves & Erford, 2010). Somewhat less definitive, however, is the identification of which factors in counseling have the most positive impact. One predictor of success may be largely determined by variables related to clients, such as their motivation, severity of symptoms, and personal attitudes (Bohart, 2006; Duncan, Miller, & Sparks, 2004). That isn't to say that what we do and how we act as counselors aren't important, but merely that our best efforts should be directed toward matching our approach to the specific circumstances of each client.

In counselor training, as well, there is a strong movement across the nation toward standardization of curricula through accreditation and the development of generic training models. Professional organizations such as the American Counseling Association (ACA), American Association for Marriage and Family Therapy (AAMFT), National Association of Social Workers (NASW), and the American Psychological Association (APA) have been instrumental in developing relatively universal principles and content that should be included in the preparation of any clinician. These organizations have been so proactive and effective in their efforts, that licensure laws have been passed in almost every state and province making it possible for counselors and therapists to practice independently (or under supervision) and receive third-party reimbursement for their services.

In the case of theory development as well, efforts are directed toward finding common factors that operate in all helping systems as well as toward combining the advantages of several therapeutic approaches into a unified model (Capuzzi & Gross, 2007; Corey, 2009; Evans & Gilbert, 2005; Goldfried, 1982; Kleinke, 1994; Kottler, 1991; Lazarus, 1995; Prochaska & Norcross, 2007). Efforts have been directed toward finding common variables associated with constructive

VOICE FROM THE FIELD

I do different things on different days. On some days I'm a farmer—I till soil within people so that their own seeds of wisdom can grow. Some days, I'm a one-man rescue operation, carefully moving someone back from the brink of self-destruction. Some days, I'm a one-man band, playing accompaniment for someone who walks to the beat of a different drum. At times I'm a mirror, trying to reflect what I understand. I'm at my best when I'm a sponge—being present, listening, and soaking up the essence of another person and the hurt inside. I am frequently privileged to be a traveler—a visitor to exotic lands in the client's worlds. But on most days, I'm a struggler, trying to find my way, and trying to help others do the same.

therapeutic change (Kaslow & Lebow, 2004; Greenberg, Constantino, & Bruce, 2006; Kraemer, 2006; Maione & Chenail, 1999; Tryon, 2002). These can be sorted according to factors related to the client (expectations, personality, symptoms, honesty), factors related to the counselor (experience, training, skills, personality, confidence), administrative factors (waiting list, length of treatment, setting), and those factors related to the quality of the relationship that is established.

Eclecticism, pragmatism, and integrationism have become the watchwords of the profession. Many years ago, several writers (French, 1933; Kubie, 1934; Rosenzweig, 1936; Dollard & Miller, 1950; Thorne, 1950; Truax & Carkhuff, 1967; Frank, 1973; Strupp, 1973; and Wachtel, 1977) began to look at the common elements of various helping approaches in an effort to find the essence of what makes counseling and therapy most helpful. You must understand that prior to these years, and even up to the present, there were furious debates—even outright wars—among various theoretical camps, each convinced that it had cornered the market on what is "truth." You may even sense disagreements within your own department wherein each instructor may present a different version of what constitutes "good" counseling. Such conflicting opinions offer rich opportunities for you to sort out for yourself what you believe is most significant in helping others, based of course on supporting research, clinical experience, and reflective thought.

SIGNIFICANCE OF THE SELF

What counseling is and how it works are important concepts that can be defined and illustrated. But any explanation of counseling, however precise, exists only in a static sense. Life can be given to a definition, vitality breathed into a process, only in the context of a person—the *self* of the counselor.

You only have to consider the power of the self with respect to your own learning processes. Think about the times in your life you were most impacted by a class. Certainly the content was interesting and the subject appealing, but just as important, it was the *person* of the teacher that made the material come alive. It was the essential self of this mentor or instructor that captivated your interest and motivated you to learn. It was the connection you felt to this person that led you to work hard, to study and practice, to become devoted to the subject. The same is no less true in counseling: It is primarily through the self as an instrument that we are able to understand and influence others (Combs & Gonzalez, 1994).

According to this perspective, the most effective counselors are able to perceive primarily from an internal rather than an external frame of reference. They tend to perceive others as being capable, as internally motivated, and they do this in positive but realistic terms. They identify themselves strongly with others and feel an affinity with the human race. Additionally, they perceive their mission as altruistic rather than self-indulgent, as freeing rather than controlling, and as self-revealing rather than self-concealing.

Each of these characteristics aids in organizing personal reality and serves as a foundation from which the counselor's self mediates the counseling process. In a classic study, Fiedler (1950) illustrated the importance of the self in the counseling process by comparing the quality of the therapeutic relationships in psychoanalytic, nondirective, and Adlerian therapies. He found that the style and personal relationships of the experts in each of the three approaches were more similar than different. He also found that the nonexperts were more different from one another in relationship style than were the experts and, further, that the nonexperts tended to be less similar than the experts in their own orientation. He therefore concluded that theoretical orientation was not the distinguishing variable separating expert from nonexpert therapists; rather, the difference was more related to personal style independent of conceptual affiliation. A common thread unified the expert therapists, particularly with regard to relationship variables. In those instances in which there is a difficulty creating an alliance in counseling, it is due more often to the counselor's personality than to the client's motivation.

Effective counselors, regardless of their setting, gender, culture, and preferred approach, demonstrate certain human qualities that make them attractive and influential to others. Those counselors who are expert at using the self as an instrument—and who are powerful models with the capacity for influencing others—tend to cross theoretical boundaries. In spite of how they label themselves—as behaviorists, psychodynamic clinicians, humanists, constructivists, feminists, Adlerians, Gestaltists, or cognitive practitioners—the most dynamic practitioners are intensely aware of the potential influence their selves can wield: as modelers of personal expertness, as reinforcers of appropriate behavior, and as nurturers of warmth and support.

Thus the self is the most significant dimension in counseling; what counseling is and how it works depend to a large extent on the personal characteristics of the counselor. Quite a number of writers (Corey & Corey, 2009; Gladding, 2008; Hazler & Kottler, 2005; Skovholt & Jennings, 2004) have compiled lists of those qualities they feel are necessary for the counselor's self to be in proper operating condition. A composite of these personality characteristics includes self-confidence, high energy level, sense of humor, neutrality, flexibility, emotional stability, experience in risk taking, analytic thinking, creativity, enthusiasm, honesty, and compassion.

In reviewing these personal attributes, you cannot help but evaluate the extent to which you possess them and reflect on how much personal growth lies ahead. Yet in counselor training, the development of self as a more effective person parallels the evolution of therapeutic skills. The self becomes refined and nurtured as a sensitive and operative component of the counseling process. As the self evolves, the counselor becomes more aware of personal assets and limitations, biases, and areas in need of upgrading. Actually, this opportunity to examine your own personal functioning is the greatest benefit of joining the counseling profession. On a daily basis, you not only have the opportunity to make a difference in other people's lives, but you can also continue to work on improving the quality of your own existence.

SUMMARY

In this chapter you have explored the decision to enter the field of counseling from a personal perspective. Honesty and self-awareness are themes that you will encounter again in this book and throughout your daily practice as a counselor; in this field, there is simply no place to hide. Your personal awareness and understanding of the motives and payoffs for choosing counseling as a career objective will affect the energy, vitality, and commitment you bring to this introductory course and, ultimately, to the field.

In this relatively young profession there are many opportunities for creative individuals to make an impact. But this flexibility of roles also results in confusion among the public as to exactly what counseling is, how and why it works, and how it differs from other mental health disciplines. It is therefore necessary for the beginning counselor to define the counseling process and profession assertively, to both carve out a useful identity and provide a realistic and explicit portrait for clients who wish to know what services can and will be delivered.

SELF-GUIDED EXPLORATIONS

1. The choice to be a counselor, or even to take a course on the subject, sets in motion a number of consequences that may affect your relationships, financial situation, sleep and lifestyle habits, family life, and self-image. Mention several ways that you are already aware of in which aspects of your life are changing as a result of your decision to study counseling.

2. Even from your limited experiences thus far in learning about the profession of counseling, you already have the barest glimmering of how and why counseling works. It may be quite interesting for you, some years in the future, to look back on your definition of counseling, as articulated in the beginning of your training. What would you say to a friend who asks you: "You're studying to be a counselor? I've always wondered how that works. What *is* counseling, anyway?"

3. List some of your fears and apprehensions about training to be a counselor. Describe some of your self-doubts. Talk to classmates you trust about your anxiety and share common themes in your experiences.

4. a. If you are completely honest with yourself, what are the real reasons you are considering counseling as a career? Apart from helping others, what aspects of your motivation have to do with helping yourself in some ways? Within a group, or on your own, brainstorm as many personal motives as you can think of to explain why you are interested in this work.

   b. Take all your reasons and organize them into three main categories that make sense to you. Give each grouping a name.

   c. What do you conclude based on this analysis of motives?

5. Read any counseling textbook, and one word you are unlikely to see is *love*. Perhaps the reason is that the word has associations with passion and sexuality, feelings that have no place in a counseling relationship (and when

acted upon by counselors, cause great harm to their clients). But in understanding what makes counseling effective, it is worth reflecting on the meaning of love, in a higher, purer sense of the word. Imagine an intimate relationship in which you are putting your own needs aside, focusing completely on the needs of the person with you, listening attentively to this person's every word without judgment or giving advice, and devoting yourself with all the energy you can muster to this person's growth. Can the case be made that this is really a form of love? Perhaps the most important reason counseling works is that we give to our clients something that everyone yearns for and rarely receives, even from those who truly care about them.

Reflect on this idea in a journal, or in conversations with classmates or in small groups. Do you think that the feelings that take place within the context of counseling—the relationship between client and counselor—constitute a kind of love? Why or why not?

6. A composite of some personal qualities associated with effective counselors is listed below. For each of these characteristics that you believe is crucial to successful professional functioning, rate where you see yourself now versus where you would like to be.

Personal Quality	Where I Am Now	Where I Want to Be
Self-confidence	1 2 3 4 5 6 7	1 2 3 4 5 6 7
High energy	1 2 3 4 5 6 7	1 2 3 4 5 6 7
Sense of humor	1 2 3 4 5 6 7	1 2 3 4 5 6 7
Flexibility	1 2 3 4 5 6 7	1 2 3 4 5 6 7
Risk taking	1 2 3 4 5 6 7	1 2 3 4 5 6 7
Emotional stability	1 2 3 4 5 6 7	1 2 3 4 5 6 7
Honesty	1 2 3 4 5 6 7	1 2 3 4 5 6 7
Compassion	1 2 3 4 5 6 7	1 2 3 4 5 6 7
Dependability	1 2 3 4 5 6 7	1 2 3 4 5 6 7

How are you going to move from where you are now to where you would like to be?

FOR HOMEWORK

Interview several counselors in the field who work in different settings and specialty areas. Ask them about: (1) what they like most and least about their work, (2) how their training best and least prepared them for the realities of what they do, (3) what they face as their greatest frustrations and challenges, and (4) what advice they would offer you as a beginner to the field.

SUGGESTED READINGS

Conyne, R. K., & Bemak, F. (Eds.). (2005). *Journeys to professional excellence: Lessons from leading counselor educators and practitioners.* Alexandria, VA: American Counseling Association.

Corey, M. S., & Corey, G. (2007). *Becoming a helper* (5th ed.). Belmont, CA: Wadsworth.

Gladding, S. T. (2009). *Becoming a counselor: The light, the bright, and the serious* (2nd ed.). Alexandria, VA: American Counseling Association.

Kottler, J. A. (2010). *On being a therapist* (3rd ed.). San Francisco: Jossey-Bass.

Kottler, J. A., & Carlson, J. (2006). *The client who changed me: Stories of therapist personal transformation.* New York: Brunner/Routledge.

Pipher, Mary (2005). *Letters to a young therapist.* New York: Basic Books.

Ram Dass, & Gorman, P. (1985). *How can I help? Stories and reflections on service.* New York: Knopf.

Yalom, I. (2003). *Gift of therapy: An open letter to a new generation of therapists and their patients.* New York: HarperCollins.

FOUNDATIONS OF COUNSELING

CHAPTER 2

KEY CONCEPTS

Professional identity

Allied mental health professions

Developmental orientation

Medical model

Freud's "talking cure"

Integrative movement

Accreditation standards

Scientist-practitioner model

Evidence-based practice

Counselor as researcher

Quantitative paradigm

Qualitative paradigm

BASICS OF HISTORY AND RESEARCH

In most disciplines, history and research are often relegated to those requirements that everyone thinks are necessary but very few students relish studying. Who cares, after all, about what some obscure philosopher or educator said a hundred years ago? You just want to help people. Of what value is some research study with a bunch of charts and numbers, when all you want to do is figure out how to help some poor kid stop trying to kill himself?

Yet the past is the basis for the present and future, and research is the foundation for everything we know. One of the first tasks that occur in every counseling endeavor, regardless of the practitioner's theoretical preferences, is taking a thorough client history and collecting systematic research on the nature of the presenting problem. We explore childhood experiences, medical history, and family lineage. We track aspects of the client's social, emotional, physical, religious, educational, and vocational background in order to develop a complete portrait of functioning.

After this personal history is initiated, next begins a research process to familiarize yourself with the literature related to your client's concerns, cultural background, and particular life circumstances. In order to formulate some sort of treatment plan, you also review the research related to the issues presented in your own work setting. Whether you're aware of it or not, you've also been doing your own research, systematically keeping track of what has worked in the past, under which circumstances, with which clients. All of this review of the past helps you to gain some sort of grasp on what is happening in the present.

And if personal history is important to understanding and helping the client, then knowledge of the profession's history is necessary if you are to function as a literate professional—if you are to understand how counseling fits within the context of other helping professions.

THE IDENTITY OF COUNSELING

As you may already be aware, there are tremendous disagreements regarding professional identity and who has the superior education and training to provide the best possible help. Psychiatrists, social workers, psychiatric nurses, psychologists, marriage and family therapists, counselors, pastoral care workers, and human service specialists all claim that their particular approach to psychological concerns is the best way to relieve emotional distress. Depending on the school attended or the state in which the clinician practices, various titles are used to describe the work of helping others. Yet among these divergences there is a central core, an essence of effective practice, regardless of how it is labeled.

The "Voice from the Field" on page 27 is not far wrong in expressing her confusion over the identity of counseling as distinct from other disciplines. While there is considerable overlap between the various mental health groups—and certainly commonality in their history and research base—there are also some distinct differences.

Among the various groups in Table 2.1, matters are made more complex by the different degrees that are offered. In some parts of North America, depending on the state or province and rural or urban setting, a clinician may need a doctoral degree to practice; in others a master's degree, bachelor's degree, or even associate's degree is sufficient. Which type of program you are enrolled in and which type of degree you are seeking will depend not only on the state or province you reside in, but also your career aspirations.

There are estimated to be well over a half-million mental health care providers (counselors, family therapists, social workers, and psychologists) in the United States (Robiner, 2006). When pastoral workers and clergy who practice counseling are also included in the professional group, that figure doubles in size. Some states are dominated by marriage and family therapists (California), others by social

VOICE FROM THE FIELD

I've been so confused about what the differences are between one kind of counselor or another. In one place you're called an LPC [Licensed Professional Counselor], then you cross the state line and the license they have is an MFT [Marriage and Family Therapist]. I've got one friend who has the same degree I have but because she lives in another part of the country, she's called an LLP [Limited Licensed Psychologist]. I mean, give me a break!

Then, to make matters worse, each of the different specialties have different exams you have to pass, different theoretical preferences, and even a different scope of practice. They're supposed to specialize in different areas, but really they all fight for the same clients. And I don't think anyone could watch a counselor or therapist in action and be able to figure out what kind they were. It sure makes it difficult for someone to figure out what the best kind of training is to help people.

workers (Alabama, Illinois, Iowa, New York, Wisconsin, and Nevada), others by psychologists (Tennessee), and still others by counselors (Ohio, Texas, and Florida). Although in theory, each of these professions has a unique and distinct heritage and style of training, in practice they may do very similar things, depending on how licensure defines the scope of practice.

Depending on which type of program you are currently enrolled in, it would be helpful for you to understand some of the unique facets of your own professional identity even if we all share common theoretical frameworks, ethical concepts, and

TABLE 2.1 | ALLIED MENTAL HEALTH PROFESSIONAL GROUPS

Professional Group	Specialization
Counselors	Therapeutic interventions with relatively normal functioning clients who are experiencing adjustment reactions, developmental issues, and problems of daily living including career, education, family, personal, and esteem issues.
Psychologists	Diagnosis, treatment, and clinical management of persons with psychopathological symptoms and other severe mental disturbances.
Psychiatrists	Medical management of patients with clinically significant psychological problems; use of medication, hospitalization, and therapy to restore normal functioning.
Social Workers	Social casework and therapy to mediate relationships with social structures like schools, agencies, and health care facilities.
Family Therapists	Systemic approach to diagnosing and treating problems in a family context. Extensive use of more active/directive interventions to realign family structures.
Pastoral Care	An approach to helping that is embedded in religious, spiritual, or ministerial work, combining theology with community service.

standards of practice. The two of us have been licensed as psychologists, family therapists, and counselors, with different titles in different states; nevertheless, we have always appreciated and preferred thinking of the work we do as "counseling."

Many people use the term counseling interchangeably with "therapy," and in many ways the two words do refer to essentially the same sort of professional helping activity. Yet using the term counseling has allowed us to emphasize the particular nature of our work that specializes in:

1. Preventing rather than only fixing problems
2. Using a developmental rather than psychopathological model of diagnosis
3. Focusing on adjustment issues and developmental concerns rather than more severe psychopathology
4. Doing relatively short-term rather than long-term work
5. Practicing in the community rather than in medical settings

These sorts of generalizations are misleading and, to some extent, inaccurate. Psychiatrists and psychologists are often known to prefer working with relatively normal people who present adjustment disorders; such individuals are more verbal, articulate, and grateful, and they pay their bills on time. Likewise, although the focus of training in most counseling, human service, and family therapy programs is on doing relatively brief interventions with moderate- to high-functioning people,

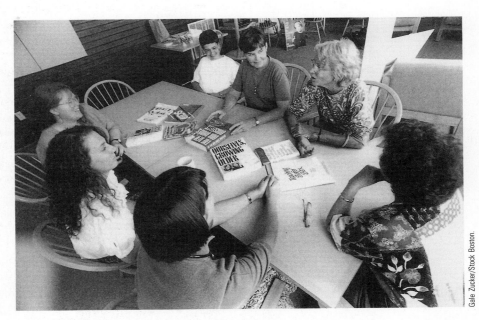

Gale Zucker/Stock Boston.

A staff meeting in action in which a diverse group of mental health professionals collaborates in case planning and treatment. In ideal settings, counselors, psychologists, social workers, psychiatric nurses, and psychiatrists work together, pooling their talents and expertise for the benefit of client welfare.

VOICE FROM THE FIELD

I ended up doing an internship at the Salvation Army. Here I was seeing people who are dual diagnosed—they are both mentally ill and addicted to one or more substances. The thing is, practically all the people I worked with in role-plays, and then in my practicum, were supposedly relatively high-functioning clients with adjustment reactions. I saw a lot of mild depression, career indecision, that sort of thing. At first, I was really angry at my program—I thought they hadn't prepared me for the "real world." You know, there were psychology and social worker

interns all at my agency, and I thought, "They must have gotten better training than me—maybe I picked the wrong specialty." But pretty soon, I caught on that the psychology and social work interns all were feeling the same way. It was actually kind of a relief to know we were all pretty much equally overwhelmed. Whatever they teach you in grad school, by the time you get through all the hours and hours licensing boards require, it really doesn't matter what kind of school you went to—you come out knowing the same thing.

many graduates end up working with severely disturbed, dual-diagnosed populations. To complicate matters further, some specialties, such as "counseling psychology," combine features of both disciplines, placing more emphasis on cultural diversity, career development, and community involvement than traditional clinical psychology does.

We don't wish to confuse you about some of the similarities and differences between counseling and therapy, or between any of the mental health professions, but just want to alert you that such distinctions exist. For the purposes of this textbook, we will use the term counseling, and speak about the profession of counseling, but you will find that many of the concepts apply equally well to other disciplines.

Counselor education will provide a solid grounding in developmentally based theory and interventions, as well as training in skills related to building effective therapeutic relationships, whether in individual, group, or family settings. This training makes you ideally qualified to work with a wide range of people: those who are struggling to cope with difficult life stressors and transitions, as well as those suffering from a variety of true emotional disorders. There was a time when counselors focused specifically on "adjustment reactions"—anxiety and depression related to specific events and developmental passages. Psychologists focused on psychopathology, with specialized training in assessment and diagnosis, whereas social workers primarily provided administrative and supportive services for the poor, aged, severely mentally ill, and the homebound. However, in our current mental health climate, these distinctions have become muddled; regardless of their professional identity, counselors, psychologists, family therapists, and social workers may find themselves working side by side, seeing the same kinds of clients, in community mental health settings as well as in private practice.

Nevertheless, counseling may be the only helping discipline that has both a preventive/developmental orientation and a remedial model that makes use of diagnosis and treatment. This focus means that we are trained to prevent problems as much as we can by intervening within an early developmental context, as well as to assess and treat problems that have already arisen. Perhaps the allied professional groups can best be thought of as forming a mental health treatment team that responds to various clients who experience problems within their areas of specialization. The team concept recognizes the responsibility of professionals to provide relevant services within their respective areas of competence and, further, demands effective communication and cooperation among professionals.

HISTORY OF COUNSELING

A unique aspect of counseling as a profession is that its foundation is grounded in so many other disciplines; it is a hybrid of knowledge from philosophy, education, psychology, psychiatry, sociology, and family studies. Even today, programs that train counselors are found in academic units as diverse as colleges of education or health sciences, departments of psychology or family studies, schools of human services, and religious institutions.

Counseling and its related disciplines of psychiatry, psychology, social work, and guidance have experienced an uneven progression of development. In the days of our Paleolithic ancestors, the first mental health professionals were fond of drilling holes in a client's head to permit demons to escape. Through the days of ancient Mesopotamia and Persia, the classical Greek and Roman eras, and into modern times, early counselors were primarily philosophers, physicians, or priests.

The primitive days of the 19th century spawned the first real counselors, the experts who attempted to heal by talking (even if they did so in ways we now find a bit bizarre). It is incredible to think that 100 years ago, counseling as we know it did not exist. And it has been only in the past 50 years that counseling has emerged as a distinct field apart from its related mental health disciplines.

The "talking cure" is a concept that we take for granted today, yet a century ago it was a revolutionary idea that was not only unaccepted but held in disrepute, smacking of witchcraft and the occult. The cathartic method of talking out problems was pioneered by Sigmund Freud at the turn of the century as a method for treating persons with psychological problems. Although the concept had existed for many years, it took Freud to build credibility for the technique. Today most people agree that talking over problems is helpful, sharing feelings and concerns is useful, and professional helpers are reasonable alternatives for those faced with problems or difficult situations. Interpersonal communication and verbal interaction form the heart of counseling, albeit in a substantially different format from what Freud envisioned. Counselors, clients, and the person in the street all believe that constructive change can occur when a counselor and a client work together toward identified, realistic goals.

THE ANCIENT PHILOSOPHERS

The first counselors were leaders of the community who attempted to provide inspiration for others through their teachings. They were religious leaders such as Moses (1200 B.C.), Mohammed (A.D. 600), and Buddha (500 B.C.). They were also philosophers such as Lao-tzu (600 B.C.), Confucius (500 B.C.), Socrates (450 B.C.), Plato (400 B.C.), and Aristotle (350 B.C.).

Many of these philosophers and religious leaders functioned as "counselors" in that they worked with a group of disciples, trying to impart wisdom to stimulate emotional, spiritual, and intellectual growth. Although their approaches to helping are considerably different from those of most contemporary counselors, we have inherited a few of their basic tenets:

- There is no single right answer to any question worth asking.
- There are many possible interpretations of the same experience.
- Any philosophy is worthless if it is not personalized and made relevant to everyday life.

These same principles, spoken in the forums of Rome, Athens, and Mesopotamia, are very much a part of what today's counselors work with on a daily basis—helping clients to find their own path to inner peace.

THE FIRST PSYCHIATRISTS

Besides those who sought to "heal" others' suffering through educational and spiritual paths, other pragmatic practitioners tried to combine philosophy with what they observed about human behavior. Foremost among these medical philosophers was Hippocrates (400 B.C.), who introduced many ideas that we now take for granted, including the concepts of *homeostasis* (the natural balance of the body) and *prognosis* (the prediction of outcomes).

Hippocrates emphasized the importance of obtaining a complete life history before undertaking any treatment (which unfortunately was usually bloodletting) and devised the first comprehensive classification of mental disorders. He is also credited with developing—over 2,000 years ago—the first counseling interventions, relying on many techniques that are still in use today: systematic diagnostic interviews, detailed history taking, trust building in a therapeutic relationship, and even dream interpretation and acknowledgment of repressed feelings.

There really were not many improvements on Hippocrates's theories until the last century or two. (Remember, the favored "treatment" in the Middle Ages for those suffering from emotional problems was being burned at the stake.) But when Sigmund Freud and his colleague Joseph Breuer evolved their "talking cure" of healing through catharsis, the professions of counseling and psychotherapy were truly born. Freud was not only a talented physician, writer, teacher, thinker, and astute observer of the human condition, but he was also remarkably persuasive as an influencer of others. He recruited into his camp a flock of followers from all over the world to spread the word about his newfound cure for emotional suffering. Many of their names may be familiar to you: Carl Jung, Alfred Adler, Wilhelm Reich, and even his own daughter, Anna Freud.

The 19th century produced a number of great philosophers who had a significant impact on the development of Freud and his students. Such thinkers as Søren Kierkegaard, G. W. F. Hegel, and Friedrich Nietzsche were just as influential in this new profession as were Freud's own colleagues in medicine. In addition, a number of brilliant mentors had instructed Freud in the intricacies of the brain as well as introduced him to the technique of hypnosis as a means of accessing the mind's inner secrets. Add to that training Freud's own penchant for philosophy, literature,

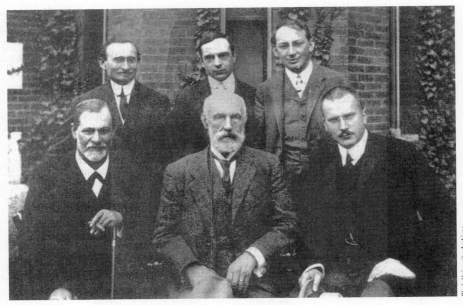

Clark University Archives.

In September 1909, Sigmund Freud was invited to the United States to give a series of lectures on his new method of psychoanalysis. This was the first systematically structured counseling approach, one that emphasized uncovering unconscious motives and allowing clients to express their innermost thoughts and feelings. Freud is pictured here (bottom left) sitting next to influential American psychologist G. Stanley Hall and colleague Carl Jung. In the top row (from left to right) are three of Freud's disciples: A. A. Brill, Ernest Jones, and Sandor Ferenczi.

and archaeology, and he was ideally suited to pull all this knowledge together into the first comprehensive model for understanding and changing human behavior.

Over the course of a prolific life in which he churned out volume after volume of meticulously documented theories on the human condition, Freud accomplished several remarkable feats, including:

- Plotting the anatomy of the human nervous system
- Developing the first form of local anesthesia for eye surgery
- Adapting the technique of hypnosis for studying the inner world
- Formulating models of personality development and psychopathology
- Emphasizing unconscious motives behind human behavior
- Suggesting that dreams have meanings that can be uncovered and interpreted
- Studying the underlying structure of society
- Developing the first formal methodology of counseling

Although it is popular nowadays to ridicule many of Freud's ideas and call him obsolete, sexist, controlling, sexually obsessed, neurotic, and a host of other names, it must be remembered that he was the primary mentor of the first generation of counselors. Many of the most famous names in the field, names representing quite diverse approaches—Albert Ellis, Murray Bowen, Fritz Perls, Alfred Adler, Carl

Rogers, Eric Berne—were all at one time practicing Freudian analysts. It would be difficult, therefore, to underestimate Freud's importance in the development of counseling, even if contemporary practitioners no longer employ his methods the way they were originally intended. (But then, how many techniques in *any* profession remain intact after a hundred years?)

INFLUENCES FROM PSYCHOLOGY

About the same time that Freud was laying the foundation for psychiatric counseling, another discipline was making its own contribution: the burgeoning field of psychology. As was the case with the first psychiatrists and counselors, all the first psychologists were philosophers. Beginning with René Descartes (1596–1650), who was among the first to study the mind as distinct from the body and soul, and continuing through the British empirical philosophers such as John Locke (1632–1704), George Berkeley (1685–1753), David Hume (1711–1776), and John Stuart Mill (1806–1873), the discipline of philosophy gave rise to the new science of psychology.

Every undergraduate psychology major memorizes the fact that the discipline was born when Wilhelm Wundt (1832–1920) founded the first experimental laboratory in 1879. However, it was really the American philosopher William James (1842–1910) who was the first to be awarded the title "Professor of Psychology." For our purposes, James's ideas are more relevant to the development of counseling as a separate discipline. He was intensely interested in the concepts of free will, consciousness, and adaptive functioning and believed humans to be creatures of emotion and action as well as thought and reason. He was also instrumental in developing the philosophy of "pragmatism," which is very much alive today in the spirit of flexibility and integration that permeates the development of new helping models. According to James (1907), the pursuit of knowledge is best directed toward finding useful tools that can be both applied to practical situations and scientifically validated. You will find that almost 100 years after his treatise on the subject, James's idea of pragmatism is still a guiding force in what we do.

Of course, many other names are associated with the development of psychology, such as G. Stanley Hall, who received the first doctorate in psychology and became the bridge between this new science and the field of education. Certainly the behaviorists, led by John Watson and B. F. Skinner, also made significant contributions to the understanding and management of human behavior through their experimental studies of reinforcement. A number of other experimental psychologists, such as Max Wertheimer and Wolfgang Kohler, approached things from quite a different perspective. From their studies of how apes solve problems, they concluded that learning does not necessarily follow an orderly progression; sometimes sudden insights play a part, and all at once a person conceptualizes the whole as greater than the sum of its elemental parts.

THE GUIDANCE ERA

In the early part of the 20th century, a completely different movement was taking place. It was a time of significant social reform, and there was an emerging

| VOICE FROM THE FIELD

Okay. Enough is enough! This is just about all the history I can take. What's with all these names and dates? Am I supposed to be able to remember all this stuff? Is this going to be on the test?

I mean, give us a break! I'm trying to sort all this stuff out, figure out who is really important and which of these dead, white guys you just stuck in to impress us. I'm all for history and all, but I've got my limit. This is just overwhelming.

I guess the big picture isn't the specifics but just that counseling comes from a lot of different places. I can see that what we do is like what philosophers do. Doctors, too. It's interesting that all these names you're throwing at us are familiar, but I've never thought of them as being part of this profession.

recognition that social forces and individual development could be assisted, directed, and—more important—guided. This awareness was especially evident in the field of education and the specialty of career guidance.

The industrial age was then flourishing; technical training and skilled workers were becoming necessary, and new programs in vocational guidance attempted to respond to these needs. Although there were a number of pioneers who took the initiative in this field, Frank Parsons is often credited as the founder of the vocational guidance movement. In his book *Choosing a Vocation* (Parsons, 1909), he described a three-part model for career counseling: (1) an analysis of one's own personal interests, abilities, and aptitudes; (2) an exploration of available occupations; and (3) the application of a systematic reasoning process to find a good match between the two. This procedure, Parsons believed, would place individuals in work settings most appropriate to their skills and education.

Parsons and several colleagues applied their new technology of testing and interviewing to help Boston's unemployed youth identify interests and abilities and find suitable work. Thus the vocational guidance field became respectable, enabling counselors to specialize in a particular aspect of human conflict. It carved a niche for guidance personnel in educational settings; however, it also prevented the integration of the structured teaching model of vocational guidance into the mainstream of counseling. For the next 60 years counselors were seen primarily as school specialists who helped children make educational and occupational decisions.

In addition to the school guidance movement, several other influences during this time contributed to the development of counseling as a profession. These included:

1. The development of standardized testing during World War I as a means to measure aptitudes, abilities, and even personality traits
2. The birth of the Veterans Administration after World War II, which resulted in the recruiting of professionals to help aid the adjustment of soldiers
3. The National Defense Education Act, the passage of which channeled more youth into the sciences after the Soviet Union launched Sputnik and thereby demonstrated that they were ahead in the space race

4. The evolution of vocational rehabilitation (working with those who are disabled) as a specialty
5. The creation of the first counseling services on college campuses
6. The establishment of a comprehensive mental health system
7. The launching of the American Personnel and Guidance Association as the first professional organization for counselors
8. Federal legislation such as the Americans with Disabilities Act, Vocational Education Act, and Work Incentives Improvement Act that mandated assistance to those with disabilities
9. The influence of accreditation by the Council for the Accreditation of Counseling and Related Educational Programs (CACREP), the American Association for Marital and Family Therapy (AAMFT), the Council on Rehabilitation Education (CORE), and the American Psychological Association (APA)
10. The spread of licensure laws across states and provinces, which granted greater legitimacy to counselors and family therapists
11. Increased cultural diversity in population through immigration, which required expertise in fostering greater harmony and adjustment
12. The managed care movement, which recognized the cost-effectiveness of using nonmedical practitioners to treat mental health problems

THE COUNSELING ERA

Not all of the contributors to the mental health movement were philosophers, psychiatrists, psychologists, or educators. One of the most influential figures in the early part of the 20th century was an abused mental patient. In *A Mind That Found Itself*, Clifford Beers (1945) described his harrowing experiences at the hands of an insensitive system that treated him as a lunatic rather than as a human being. In this classic work (which eventually led to the establishment of the National Association for Mental Health), Beers proposed that what the emotionally disturbed person needs most of all is a compassionate friend. It was the field of therapeutic counseling that finally responded to his plea.

The prevailing "medical model" espoused by psychiatrists and some psychologists had reigned supreme. This framework emphasized the diagnosis of psychopathology. Patients who sought therapeutic services were viewed as afflicted with a form of mental illness that could be treated by a number of medical options—electroconvulsive shock treatment, psychosurgery (frontal lobotomies), psychopharmacology, and, as a last resort, medical psychotherapy, which usually took the form of long-term psychoanalysis with sessions three to four times a week for a half-dozen years or more. To this day, the medical model is still at the core of many diagnostic systems, such as those used in a variety of clinical settings.

At the midpoint of the 20th century, a lone voice was heard above the throng of psychiatrists and psychologists. Carl Rogers (1902–1987) began to argue persuasively that the traditional doctor/patient pattern of interaction proposed by the medical model was not appropriate for working with the vast majority of human beings. According to Rogers, people with emotional problems are not "sick" or "mentally ill"; most people simply need a safe environment in which to work out their difficulties. He maintained that the most effective vehicle for accomplishing this task was within the context of a therapeutic relationship.

In spite of the initially cool reception given to the ideas of client-centered theory, Carl Rogers emerged as a significant force in the field of counseling and changed previous thinking about the nature of the healing alliance—not only with regard to therapeutic relationships, but also with regard to education and even the political realm. In retrospect, it seems difficult to imagine counseling today without the impact of Rogers and his ideas about the importance of relationship variables.

Person-centered counseling became the theoretical focus of many counselor education programs during the 1950s and early 1960s. On the whole, Rogers was enthusiastically embraced and legions of counselors were trained in nondirective, person-centered techniques. But in spite of the general acceptance of person-centered counseling, some concerns were emerging that questioned the nature of this approach and criticized its relevance for many client populations. Additionally, the operational difficulties involved in defining the tasks of the counselor and the difficulties inherent in the process of gathering empirical evidence to support the person-centered approach caused further questioning and exploring.

The 1960s and early 1970s saw much change and refocusing in the counseling field. The wide acceptance of the Rogerian approach came under increased scrutiny. Carkhuff and Berenson (1977) and Krumboltz (1966) wrote books that were

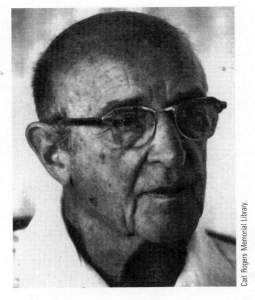

Carl Rogers Memorial Library.

Carl Rogers had a huge impact on the development of counseling as a profession, not only through his empirical research on therapeutic relationships, but also through his advocacy on behalf of empathy, education, and world peace. Rogers has the distinction not only of being a world-class scholar, teacher, documentarian, and counselor, but also of being nominated for a Nobel Peace Prize.

quite influential in challenging the field to move toward a more behavioral slant, whereas Albert Ellis (1962), Aaron Beck (1967), and other cognitive therapists emphasized the role of thinking in the counseling process. Other theorists with other ideas joined the defection. Gestalt therapy, transactional analysis (TA), values clarification strategies, reality therapy, and other concepts and approaches all clamored for attention and vied for influence.

From this rich field of inquiry and challenge there seemed to emerge a focus that gained wide credibility in counselor education. Robert Carkhuff and several collaborators (Carkhuff & Berenson, 1977; Truax & Carkhuff, 1967) imposed a systematic and generalist approach to the task of helping. Carkhuff suggested that counselors must be skilled, reliable, and capable of delivering effective levels of core counseling skills. He defined the skills and developed methods of assessing effectiveness. The work of Carkhuff is now widely accepted, with much counselor training emphasizing the development of generic skills that provide a base for effective helping relationships. In a class on techniques of counseling you are likely to follow one of several systematic skills models (Cormier & Hackney, 2008; De Jong & Berg, 2008; Egan, 2007; Murphy & Dillon, 2007; Young, 2009) that were patterned after Carkhuff's identified "core conditions." Today, counseling is built on the work of Carkhuff, who has developed a base for the skill-development process; Rogers, who emphasized the importance of the relationship dimension in counseling; and Freud, who gave credibility to the idea of treatment through talking.

In a sense, this represents the generic foundation for training in therapeutic counseling. To achieve maturity as a professional, it is necessary to integrate the various counseling approaches within the generic model used in most training. It is a mistake to assume that minimal generic skills will prepare a person to function as a counselor. Therefore, in your training you will first learn the basic skills of reflecting, confronting, summarizing, attending, and goal setting and will then expand on this base using the diverse sources of theory and technique available to counselors.

Table 2.2 summarizes the contributions of many individuals to the field of counseling. These are included not to overwhelm you with a bunch of names you will quickly forget but to impress you with the long and distinguished list of notable figures who have contributed to contemporary practice. We also wish to stress how truly interdisciplinary the profession of counseling really is, that it encompasses the work of medicine, philosophy, education, and the social sciences, as well as the more recent contributions from the various mental health specialties.

THE ERA OF COUNSELING

At one time, 80% of all students enrolled in counseling programs were following a school-based employment track. Now that trend has shifted, and the majority of new counselors are targeting themselves for employment in various agencies as community counselors, clinical counselors, mental health counselors, couples counselors, or family counselors. Clearly, the focus of counseling is now less educational and more therapeutic. This fact is reflected in the progressive name changes of the American Counseling Association (ACA), which a few years ago was called the

TABLE 2.2 | HISTORICAL FIGURES IN COUNSELING PLUS CONTRIBUTORS FROM PHILOSOPHY, EDUCATION, MEDICINE, LITERATURE, AND SOCIAL SCIENCE

400 B.C.	Hippocrates	Classified types of mental illness and personality disorders
450 B.C.	Socrates	Encouraged self-awareness as purest form of knowledge
400 B.C.	Plato	Postulated human behavior in terms of internal states
350 B.C.	Aristotle	Designed first rational psychology to manage emotions
400	St. Augustine	Prescribed introspection to master emotions
1500	Niccolo Machiavelli	Brought attention to group dynamics and social interaction
1550	Johann Weyer	Documented case histories of depression
1600	William Shakespeare	Created a literature of psychologically complex characters
1625	René Descartes	Attempted to resolve dualism of mind and body
1675	John Locke	Theorized that all knowledge originates from experience
1675	Baruch Spinoza	Developed an integrative personality theory
1800	Johannes Muller	Plotted the physiology of the nervous system
1800	Philippe Pinel	Described various forms of neurosis and psychosis
1800	Anton Mesmer	Used hypnotic suggestion to cure psychological symptoms
1850	Charles Darwin	Set forth an evolutionary theory of individual differences
1850	Jean Charcot	Scientifically studied hypnosis to give it respectability
1850	Søren Kierkegaard	Developed existential philosophy of creating meaning
1880	G. Stanley Hall	Began first child guidance clinic
1890	James Cattell	Coined the term *mental tests*
1890	Jesse Davis	Became first school counselor
1900	Emil Kraepelin	Systematized the classification of mental disorders
1900	William James	Postulated comprehensive theory of emotions
1900	Ivan Pavlov	Described behavioral theory of conditioned reflexes
1900	Sigmund Freud	Devised first systematic form of therapeutic counseling
1905	Alfred Binet	Invented first intelligence test
1910	Frank Parsons	Established field of vocational guidance
1910	Clifford Beers	Published autobiography of experiences as a mental patient
1920	Carl Jung	Proposed theory of collective unconscious
1920	Alfred Adler	Authored theory of individual psychology
1920	J. L. Moreno	Invented psychodrama
1920	John Watson	Developed notions of prediction and control of behavior
1930	Robert Hoppock	Studied levels of job satisfaction
1940	B. F. Skinner	Formulated theory of operant conditioning
1940	E. G. Williamson	Published standard text on school counseling
1945	Gregory Bateson	Emphasized family influences in mental problems

(Continued)

TABLE 2.2	HISTORICAL FIGURES IN COUNSELING PLUS CONTRIBUTORS FROM PHILOSOPHY, EDUCATION, MEDICINE, LITERATURE, AND SOCIAL SCIENCE (CONTINUED)

1945	Kurt Lewin	Used training-group format for personal development
1950	Viktor Frankl	Emphasized search for meaning in human experience
1950	Milton Erickson	Focused on linguistic aspects of therapeutic encounter
1950	Carl Rogers	Emphasized importance of relationship in counseling
1955	Rollo May	Developed framework for existential therapy
1955	Abraham Maslow	Researched what makes people most healthy
1955	Donald Super	Introduced theory of vocational decision making
1955	Rudoph Dreikurs	Developed Adlerian theory into popular treatment
1960	Joseph Wolpe	Devised systematic theory of behavior therapy
1960	Jay Haley	Began strategic family therapy
1960	Albert Ellis	Developed cognitive-based therapy
1960	Jean Piaget	Studied children's unique moral and cognitive patterns
1960	Frederick Thorne	Created integrative theory of helping
1965	William Glasser	Developed reality therapy
1965	Fritz Perls	Popularized Gestalt therapy
1965	Robert Carkhuff	Organized and researched the skills of helping
1965	John Krumboltz	Published theory of behavioral counseling
1965	Murray Bowen	Brought attention to family-of-origin issues
1965	Virginia Satir	Described communication theory in family therapy
1970	Jerome Frank	Authored seminal work on persuasion in healing
1970	Salvador Minuchin	Developed structural basis for family therapy
1970	Aaron Beck	Developed cognitive therapy for depression
1975	Allen Bergin	Edited first comprehensive handbook on therapy
1975	Heinz Kohut	Contributor to development of self-psychology
1975	Helen Kaplan	Published classic work on sex counseling
1980	Paul Pedersen	Championed cause of diversity issues
1980	John Norcross	Represented new movement toward integration of theories
1980	Irvin Yalom	Synthesized current theory on existential counseling
1980	Carol Gilligan	Pioneered research on gender differences in development
1980	Arnold Lazarus	Developed multimodal therapy
1985	Rachel Hare-Mustin	Represented feminist approaches to counseling
1985	Paul Watzlawick	Shifted emphasis from objectivism to social constructivism
1985	Steve de Shazer	Promoted brief forms of intervention
1985	Allen Ivey	Devised developmental/multicultural model for practice
1985	Norman Gysbers	Created developmental guidance program for schools

(Continued)

TABLE 2.2 | HISTORICAL FIGURES IN COUNSELING PLUS CONTRIBUTORS FROM PHILOSOPHY, EDUCATION, MEDICINE, LITERATURE, AND SOCIAL SCIENCE (CONTINUED)

1990	Michael White	Developed narrative approaches to counseling
1990	Francine Shapiro	Developed method for treating traumatic stress
1990	John Gottman	Developed research base for doing marital counseling
1990	Monica McGoldrick	Plotted role of family life cycle in counseling
1990	Derald Sue	Spearheaded multicultural counseling competencies
1990	Jeffrey Zeig	Organized conferences to promote synthesis of approaches
1995	Daniel Goleman	Introduced construct of emotional intelligence
1995	Jean Baker Miller	Helped develop relational counseling
1995	Johnson & Greenberg	Developed emotionally focused therapy
1995	William Miller	Introduced motivational interviewing for addictions
2000	Daniel Siegel	Developed field of interpersonal neurobiology
2000	Martin Seligman	Pioneered field of positive psychology
2000	Jon Kabat-Zinn	Developed mindfulness therapy
2000	Clara Hill	Developed consensual qualitative research methodology
2005	Bradford Keeney	Studied indigenous healing practices around the world to find universal concepts
2005	Nancy McWilliams	Representative of new generation of pragmatic, integrative, relational psychodynamic practitioners
2005	Robert Neimeyer	Applied constructivist approach to grief issues, reframing loss as a "new" relationship

American Association for Counseling and Development (AACD), and a few years before that was known as the American Personnel and Guidance Association (APGA). It is evident in the rapid growth of organizations like the American Mental Health Counselors Association (AMHCA) and the International Association of Marriage and Family Counselors (IAMFC). And this trend toward a more clinical focus can be seen in the emergence of licensing and credentialing for professional counselors in virtually every state.

In today's climate of "managed care," in which health insurance agencies and large employers are attempting to control costs associated with mental health treatment, counselors are playing a bigger role in many regions because of our emphasis on brief treatment and our cost effectiveness in comparison with other professionals. In spite of these changes, there are still considerable doubts about whether such a managed-care movement will ultimately be good for either our profession or the consumers of our services. Regardless of our preferences, the counseling profession has now become strongly influenced (and controlled) by the values associated with managing costs. We are now asked not only to help people but to do so in the most efficient and cost-effective way possible, as well as to document these outcomes. While this does compromise a certain degree of independence and freedom in how we practice, there have also been several positive effects that have led to increased accountability and the development of more efficient methods.

This cadre of new counselors is still using the core skills of practice that have been identified for some time—but is also drawing heavily from other fields while researching, developing, and expanding the intervention base. The emphasis is on approaches that are developmentally oriented and that use relatively short-term strategies designed to reduce symptoms, eliminate self-defeating behaviors, and increase self-esteem, self-efficacy, and self-management skills. Counselors focus on developing a solid relationship with clients, identifying core issues, understanding clients from a developmental perspective, and employing interventions best suited to the particular client and clinical situation.

The latest movement within the helping professions has been a drive toward identifying those helping models that are proven by empirical research to be effective. As a result, counselor training programs are becoming more standardized across North America as researchers demonstrate with increasing accuracy which theoretical approaches appear to work with specific emotional disorders. Another movement that is growing in its influence is the application of counseling to diverse populations, with special emphasis on increasing our responsiveness to underserved groups such as oppressed minorities, the aged, and the disabled.

Licensing and Regulation in Counseling

The best evidence of how far we have developed in our history is found in the progress made in the credentialing of counselors across the country. There was a time, just a few decades ago, when there were no standards for the preparation of counselors, no licensure laws, no certifications for specialties in any area. As a result, counselors did not enjoy the professional autonomy and respect granted to our colleagues in social work, psychology, and psychiatry.

Efforts to standardize counselor training and to regulate the practice of clinicians began in 1973, when the Association for Counselor Education and Supervision (ACES) developed a knowledge base to provide the foundation for future licensing efforts (Brooks & Gerstein, 1990). Before we could decide who should be allowed to practice counseling, we needed to establish minimum standards of training and education. Soon after this report was created, a number of states in succession, beginning with Virginia, passed licensing laws. Since that time, the field has enacted a number of different licensure, certification, and regulatory bodies, many of which are in direct competition with one another and present a confusing array of options for practitioners. As we remarked earlier, depending on the jurisdiction in which you live, you could very well become licensed as a counselor, family therapist, social worker, or psychologist.

The licensure initiative must be understood in the context of two other attempts to legitimize counseling as a profession that evolved simultaneously. In 1981, the American Counseling Association established an independent agency to accredit training programs in the field. This Council for the Accreditation of Counseling and Related Educational Programs (CACREP) developed minimum requirements for graduate programs at the master's and doctoral levels, including specialties in mental health, school counseling, student personnel, community/agency counseling, and marriage and family counseling. Other professional organizations such as the American Psychological Association (APA) and American Association for Marriage and Family Therapy (AAMFT) have developed similar standards in which certain core content and curricular experiences are required.

More and more counselor preparation programs are structuring their curricula around content areas and clinical experiences that may seem familiar to you in your own program. Although the core requirements can be met in different ways, generally the following content areas are either represented as separate courses or infused into several classes throughout the program:

1. Professional orientation, introducing you to the identity of your profession and specialty
2. Human growth and development, concentrating on the background you will need to understand how people learn and grow
3. Social and cultural foundations, providing much of the theoretical background necessary for functioning effectively with diverse populations
4. Therapeutic relationships, covering the process and skills involved in developing alliances that are likely to lead to constructive learning and change
5. Group work, preparing you to understand the dynamics, stages, and processes of counseling in groups
6. Career development, focusing on the theory and practice of vocational decision making
7. Assessment, including methods of gathering information, formulating diagnoses and treatment plans, and administering and interpreting tests
8. Research and evaluation, helping you to make sense of the professional literature, to read studies critically, and to construct legitimate evaluation methods in your work
9. Family systems theory and practice, preparing you to work with couples and families
10. Ethics, teaching you how to make decisions grounded in ethical principles and in the ethics codes of your professional associations and state regulatory agencies
11. Clinical specialty areas in addictions, psychopharmacology, child and adolescent counseling, sex abuse, and other areas

In addition to this general preparation, there are also various specialty areas such as couples and family therapy, mental health counseling, school counseling, rehabilitation counseling, student personnel, and addictions counseling. Finally, depending on program accreditation and jurisdictional licensure requirements, you are expected to have certain supervised clinical experiences, including documented hours in practice and internships.

As a result of this standardization of training, counselors are earning greater respect and recognition from colleagues in other fields, and from clients who prefer to work with practitioners employing a developmental rather than a medical model. Our legitimacy is even attested to by our eligibility for third-party reimbursement from clients' insurance companies. Although being able to participate in managed care, employee assistance, and preferred provider programs was seen at one time as a major victory, now many practitioners are beginning to wonder

VOICE FROM THE FIELD

It really amazes me how much things have changed in the past several years. Becoming licensed as a counselor is a big deal in my state. I can do so many things now that just weren't possible in earlier years.

Yeah, it means a lot to be eligible for third-party reimbursement, so I can compete in the marketplace with other professionals, but more than that, licensure means that I'm taken so much more seriously.

I just wish the laws were standardized from one place to another; it makes things kind of difficult when you want to relocate. That's why accreditation is becoming more and more important.

whether we are increasingly losing control over our case management decisions because of third-party intrusions.

It is probably a very good idea, even this early in your program, to begin researching the licensing requirements in your own area as well as the certification options that will be available to you on graduation. For example, neighboring states may have quite different licenses available to practitioners at the master's level. Those you will see most frequently include (1) Licensed Professional Counselor (LPC), (2) Marital and Family Therapist (MFT), and (3) Limited Licensed Psychologist (LLP). Almost every region has a unique professional climate, and each specialty you consider—whether in schools, agencies, rehabilitation settings, religious organizations, private practices, universities, or industry—will have different requirements in course content, internships, and supervision.

RESEARCH FOUNDATIONS OF COUNSELING

The foundations of the counseling profession are certainly built on a history of ideas. Yet the origins of this knowledge, and almost everything we know and understand about how counseling works, have been constructed primarily from a systematic investigation process known as research.

Research and the practice of counseling have typically been seen as two discrete functions within the same profession. Practitioners and scientists are generally viewed as approaching a common problem from different directions. The practitioner actually works with clients and learns from the clients. The practitioner bases decisions about treatment on his or her experience and knowledge about what has been effective in previous clinical work. The scientist often has little or no involvement with direct service but studies human behavior in controlled experimental situations. In actuality, one of the most dominant models of effective practice in the field is one in which both research and clinical work are linked closely together.

COUNSELORS AS SCIENTIST-PRACTITIONERS

The scientist-practitioner model suggests that counselors engage in research while delivering direct services to clients (Erford, 2008; Maddux & Riso, 2007; Stoltenberg & Pace, 2007). Many practicing counselors see value in this concept because they are often faced with questions about the counseling process that can only be

VOICE FROM THE FIELD

I'm completing my internship hours for licensure, so I still see myself as a student at this point. Researching new ideas, client problems, psychotropic drugs, or a new technique is perfectly natural for someone like me in a learner's role. What's changed for me, though, since I left school, is that this is no longer an academic activity; research has become for me a practical extension of what I do as a good counselor.

I don't want this to sound like I keep my nose to some researcher's grindstone all the time. I'm not just a counselor. I'm a busy mom and wife, a committee chair, and a dozen other things. I have a life! But I do adopt a mindset and an active learning approach to my work. I'm pretty good at what I do but the only way that I can get better is to keep asking questions, digging for answers, learning new things, and trying out new things. That's what research is all about.

answered by research. This helps them to determine which interventions work with individual clients or particular client populations. Eldridge (1982) and Strupp (1989) have noted that the roles of the counselor and researcher can fit together effectively, making it possible for the practitioner to become literate in both areas.

Counseling is a process of helping clients change ineffective and maladaptive behaviors. For this to work well, as a counselor, you must be able to assess the impact of any intervention; otherwise you will have no way to know if what you are doing is helpful or harmful. Imagine, for example, that a client with whom you have been working for some time has not been responding to your best intentions. You have tried your favorite method, in this case a low-key relationship-oriented approach, but to no avail. At what point do you abandon your strategy and try something else? If you are to move on to a different treatment plan, which path is most likely to prove successful, at least based on the prior experience of others who have worked in this area?

In order to function effectively, you will want to know precisely the effects of any given theory, attitude, or action so that you may reliably duplicate the intervention in the future. This is called evidence-based practice and is grounded in the idea that solid, empirical research, as well as clinical experience, should inform professional decision making and interventions (Goodheart, Kazdin, & Sternberg, 2006). Knowing which counseling skills are most likely to produce desirable results is critical, especially if you want to make a positive difference in people's lives on a consistent basis.

RESEARCH FOR THE COUNSELOR

Three aspects of research are important for counseling students to learn. First is the terminology and language of the research field, which makes communication possible with other professionals. Many terms such as *hypothesis*, *variance*, and *extraneous variable* are used in everyday discussions.

Second is knowledge of the classic studies of the field and their implications for clinical work (see Table 2.3). Counselors who are knowledgeable about the research that supports the process of counseling are able to engage in relevant conversations

TABLE 2.3 | A SAMPLING OF CLASSIC RESEARCH IN COUNSELING

Date	Author(s)	Title	Contribution
1920	Watson & Rayner	Conditioned Emotional Reactions	Demonstrated that emotional reactions to stimuli can be conditioned or learned
1938	Skinner	The Behavior of Organisms	Demonstrated the principles of instrumental conditioning
1950	Dollard & Miller	Personality and Psychotherapy	Applied learning theory to the therapy process
1950	Fiedler	A Comparison of Therapeutic Relationships	Suggested that personal variables other than the therapists' theoretical orientation determine counseling effectiveness
1952	Eysenck	Effects of Psychotherapy	Suggested that persons receiving therapy did not improve more than persons not receiving therapy
1956	Bateson et al.	Toward a Theory of Schizophrenia	Brought attention to the influence of families on psychological conditions
1963	Truax	Effective Ingredients in Psychotherapy	Suggested that therapist-offered conditions would result in either improvement or deterioration
1966	Holland	The Psychology of Vocational Choice	Presented the hexagonal model to describe the relationship between personality and occupational interests
1968	Strong	Counseling: An Interpersonal Influence Process	Suggested that counselors promote personal change through social forces
1969	Bandura	Principles of Behavior Modification	Clarified the effects and empirical basis of behavior modification
1969	Carkhuff	Helping and Human Relations	Summarized research on core conditions of counseling
1971	Ivey	Microcounseling	Presented a training system for interviewers based on "giving skills" and feedback
1977	Smith & Glass	Meta-Analysis of Psychotherapy Outcome Studies	Used meta-analysis techniques to describe the effectiveness of psychotherapy
1985	Gelso & Carter	The Relationship in Counseling and Psychotherapy	Definitively reviewed literature related to components and processes of the relationship in counseling
1989	Heppner & Claiborn	Social Influence Research	Reviewed and critiqued studies dealing with power in counseling
1992	McNamee & Gergen	Therapy as Social Construction	Compiled major contributions to constructivist approach to counseling
1994	Dawes	House of Cards	Challenged clinical assumptions and treatment methods currently in use

(Continued)

TABLE 2.3 | A SAMPLING OF CLASSIC RESEARCH IN COUNSELING (CONTINUED)

Date	Author(s)	Title	Contribution
1995	Rennie	Clients' Deference in Psychotherapy	Representative of using "grounded theory" in qualitative research for studying client experience
1997	Hill et al.	A Guide to Conducting Consensual Qualitative Research	Provided methodological standards for gathering qualitative data
1998	Gottman et al.	Predicting Marital Happiness and Stability	Studied the interactional patterns of newlyweds to predict likelihood of divorce
2000	Wampold et al.	Meta-Analysis of Component Studies in Counseling and Psychotherapy	Examined common factors operating in most theoretical systems
2003	Miller, et al.	Outcome and Session Ratings Scales	Emphasized continuous client consultations about satisfaction with counseling outcomes

with other professionals and are able to understand how the counseling profession developed and grew over time. Furthermore, as consumers of research, counselors must be capable of critical analysis of the various methodologies, statistical procedures, arguments, and conclusions of their professional literature (Roth & Fonagy, 2006). This analysis will not only provide you with useful knowledge but will also train you to think analytically, intentionally, and systematically about problems.

The third reason for learning about research is that you will gain the ability to conduct systematic studies on topics that have professional meaning to you as a student and as a professional counselor. By understanding that research can be quite focused and can be done using a small population, practitioners who want to determine effectiveness in their work environment can proceed to engage in systematic study. Once research is understood and demystified, many practitioners recognize ways to use applied and descriptive research to help in their daily work (Berrios & Lucca, 2006; Galluzzo, Hilldrup, Hays, & Erford, 2008; Heppner, Kivlighan, & Wampold, 2006).

You will be expected, before becoming a professional counselor, to have a good working knowledge of basic research skills in addition to your counseling skills. At the very minimum, you must be able to pose good research questions, use clear definitions of terms, understand sources of confusion and ambiguity and how they may be controlled, be aware of problems associated with observation and measurement, understand the value of documentation in the literature, and, above all, be knowledgeable about the process of research and be motivated to learn more about it throughout your professional life.

TWO DIFFERENT APPROACHES TO RESEARCH

You will be expected to have sufficient familiarity with the two main research paradigms in counseling: quantitative and qualitative methods. Both approaches rest on different philosophical assumptions about how we "know" about people's emotional and cognitive experiences, the motivations underlying their behavior, and how these phenomena are affected by counseling interventions.

QUANTITATIVE RESEARCH: MEASURING EXPERIENCES

You probably already have some knowledge of quantitative research, especially if you have ever taken a class in statistics. The paradigm involves using the same scientific methods applied in the natural sciences: The researcher begins with a theory of how something works, develops a hypothesis that can be tested, conducts a controlled experiment, uses statistical procedures to evaluate whether the hypothesis was supported or rejected, interprets the results in light of both the hypothesis and the broader theory that generated it, and examines the findings' implications for conducting effective counseling. Central to this paradigm is the notion that understanding human phenomena requires that researchers find a way to "quantify" people's experiences. This is often accomplished through the use of questionnaires or scales on which subjects might rate their experience.

Proponents of quantitative research argue that the use of statistics and mathematical formulae for testing hypotheses is the best way we have of obtaining reasonable certainty that a certain counseling treatment is effective, or that one treatment is more effective than another.

Given that the vast majority of counseling and psychology research in the last 100 years has been quantitative, you can see why understanding its methodology is critical—regardless of whether you are contemplating carrying out your own research, or reflecting on a study you are reading (Ponterotto, 2005). Furthermore, the movement in the field of counseling toward a "best practices" approach, often defined as using interventions validated by quantitative studies, means that ethical counseling requires continual evaluation of the most current quantitative studies testing the efficacy of treatment approaches.

QUALITATIVE RESEARCH: EXPLORING EXPERIENCES

Qualitative research rests on a very different paradigm, one that explores the "lived experiences" of people. The emphasis is on elucidating the richness and complexity of inner life. Indeed, one assumption of the qualitative research method is that we can never know exactly what people experience; at best, we know the meanings they give to what goes on inside their minds, according to the words they use to define and explain them. Thus, the data collected by qualitative researchers are not numbers but rather what people say about their lives. Interviews or observations are often conducted in which participants are invited to share their experiences. After the interviews are recorded, the researcher "codes" the transcripts in order to identify meaningful themes that capture the essence of the communications.

Perhaps you can recognize the advantages and limitations of each paradigm. Quantitative methods in counseling attempt to study large groups of people and then generalize to a given client, while qualitative methods study a relatively small number of people in depth and then try to theorize what might be evident for others. For example, this was the tradition first introduced by Sigmund Freud,

Voice from the Field

I was trained in quantitative research like most of my colleagues. I studied factor analysis, analysis of covariance, and really enjoyed the purity and beauty of attempting to identify variables that most contribute to change efforts. Over time, I noticed remarkable similarity between what I do as a counseling practitioner and what is involved in the qualitative method; that is, basically talking to people about what they do and what meaning they ascribe to these experiences. I still enjoy quantitative research, but since I've been doing qualitative research, I've noticed the ways it has improved my counseling. There are some major differences between doing counseling and research interviews, of course, but both involve investigating what people think, feel, and do, as well as what sense they make of these experiences. Likewise, when doing the coding and analysis of the interviews, I find that I am using a lot of my counseling training to find underlying themes—not only within a single conversation but across all the interviews I've conducted.

Jean Piaget, Milton Erickson, Alfred Adler, and other theoreticians who developed their ideas based on the sample of their own clients.

As you might expect, proponents of the two paradigms often debate one another over which approach is a more legitimate way to understand human behavior; perhaps a more reasonable approach would be to value the strengths of both models, while also appreciating their limitations (Creswell, 2007).

Despite the overwhelming preponderance of quantitative research in counseling and psychology journals, the qualitative paradigm has taken a definite foothold in the counseling research arena. You will encounter an increasing number of qualitative studies in the journals you read as part of your ethical mandate to stay current with research in the field. In some of the major counseling journals, up to one-sixth of the articles are qualitative, and that number is likely to increase (Berrios & Lucca, 2006).

What's particularly interesting to us as counselors is the way in which both of these very different methods of data analysis overlap with how counselors work with and think about their clients. The qualitative model is a virtual guide to how we interact with clients, while the quantitative approach speaks to how we conceptualize clients' problems. In that sense, both models serve as frameworks for conducting counseling.

Polkinghorne (2005), for example, describes the following steps for conducting an interview for a qualitative study, some of which will have obvious parallels to counseling:

1. Establish a trusting, open relationship with the participant.
2. Focus on the meaning of what the participant says, rather than the accuracy of his or her memory.
3. Move past the participant's surface responses by making it safe for the person to disclose deeper feelings and more precise descriptions of his or her experience.
4. Stay present with the participant, using listening skills to facilitate the participant's involvement.
5. Pay attention to facial gestures, posture and bodily movements, clothing, and other nonverbal information.

After the researcher has conducted several interviews, the next task is to examine the transcripts carefully, noting common themes as well as discrepancies, and to reflect on the meanings and implications of the participant's words. At the same time, the qualitative researcher (just like a good counselor) must remain aware of her or his own issues and biases, and how they influence interpretations of the meanings extracted from the participant's descriptions (Minichiello & Kottler, 2009).

COUNSELING AND RESEARCH PROCESS

We have already mentioned how a quantitative researcher takes a systematic approach to both testing the efficacy of counseling treatments and understanding human emotions, cognitions, behaviors, and their interrelationships. Note how the steps taken by a researcher using this paradigm equate with the way in which many counselors follow a systematic process of conceptualization and intervention.

Researcher	Counselor
1. Become aware that a problem exists	Develop awareness of client's presenting
2. Gather and review relevant research studies	Gather relevant data on problem and background
3. Formulate a research question	Formulate a diagnosis
4. Generate hypothesis	Generate a treatment plan
5. Test hypothesis	Initiate interventions
6. Analyze results	Observe results
7. Interpret results	Make adjustments as needed

You can readily see the parallels that guide both researchers and counselors in their investigative efforts. You may not imagine yourself as an active researcher in your career, and perhaps you will not choose to carry out publishable studies, but make no mistake: You will continually conduct research, in a number of ways, as part of your job. You will frequently undertake literature reviews every time a client presents an issue or problem about which you are unfamiliar. You will constantly test hypotheses, attempt to measure the results of your interventions, and improve your professional effectiveness in light of what you have learned previously. Even if you choose not to submit your results for publication in a professional journal, you will "publish" your new knowledge as you present lectures and supervise other counselors later in your career.

BECOMING AN INFORMED CONSUMER OF RESEARCH

Even if you never conduct systematic research studies as part of your work, you will still become a consumer of research as it informs your counseling. You will be required to understand research publications in order to engage in the best and most current practices of the profession. Studying and understanding research methodology and analyses will assist you in reading and synthesizing the volumes

VOICE FROM THE FIELD

I work as a school counselor, but I am the only one on my staff who actually enjoys doing counseling as opposed to all the other crap we have to do—scheduling, discipline problems, and the like. I don't have that many people to talk to about the kids I see. There's nobody I can really go to for supervision. So I live for the in-service workshops the district schedules every month or so when I can meet with other colleagues. I also subscribe to as many journals as I can afford and devour the articles—at least the ones I can understand. I'm kind of weak in the statistics stuff, and I'm not really all that up-to-date on the research methods, but I still get a lot out of reviewing what is new in the field. I've gotten a lot of good ideas from reading stuff in the journals.

of manuscripts published every year. You will be able to determine whether certain interventions, although statistically significant in a research article, are actually meaningful and likely to work with your specific client populations (Jones & Kottler, 2005; Ogles, Lunnen, & Bonesteel, 2001).

Consider yourself fairly warned: Counseling is sometimes a very lonely profession. Much of the time is spent alone in your office, insulated from the rest of the world. You are cut off from all distractions, separated from those you care most about, and immersed totally in the world of other people in great pain who demand your total attention. Furthermore, counseling work can become stale and predictable after a period of time. After seeing a hundred kids who won't go to class, or a hundred men who won't express feelings to their partners, or a hundred women who feel trapped in their lives, many of the issues may seem the same. One of the ways that counselors are able to remain energized in their work is by creating a larger audience for their experimental efforts. It is one thing to help a single person, or even a dozen people with a similar problem, but if you can publicize your systematic work in such a way that others may have access to your data, you will not feel so isolated; you will be part of a larger community of scholars and practitioners who pool their efforts to make sense of what is going on in their offices.

Every time you read about a new technique or model, you will use your knowledge of results to evaluate the probability of success in your work situation. Being knowledgeable about research will assist you in reading critically and evaluating the quality of the published results. You will be able to determine whether the outcomes are descriptive, important, significant, and, most importantly, useful to you.

As a member of professional associations, you will receive many journals and other literature. You will hear presentations and attend workshops where new ideas will be presented. You will participate in discussions on the Internet. With a basic knowledge of research, you will be able to ask penetrating questions and determine whether the ideas are based on sound scientific principles. Just as importantly, research training will prepare you to *plan* what you intend to do with your clients, *discover* what others have done under similar circumstances, *measure* the impact of your interventions, and *publicize* what occurred so that others can learn from your mistakes and successes.

SUMMARY

Counseling is an interdisciplinary profession that has evolved from fields such as education, philosophy, medicine, and social sciences. Although all helping professionals share similarities in what they do—such as their emphasis on the therapeutic relationship, their interest in fostering client growth, and their use of interpersonal skills and research methodology—there are also several important distinctions. The counseling profession is unique in that we (1) work toward prevention rather than the remediation of problems, (2) follow a developmental rather than a psychopathological model of assessment and treatment, (3) attempt to intervene within relatively short time periods rather than establish lengthier treatments, and (4) specialize in helping people through normal life transitions and adjustments rather than only during times of major dysfunction.

Although the power and rights that we have earned through legislative acts are still not where most of us would like them to be, counselors now enjoy an unprecedented degree of professional autonomy and respect.

SELF-GUIDED EXPLORATIONS

1. Who are the characters and personages from history—in the arts, literature, science, religion, politics, social science, and education—who have been most inspirational to you? How have they influenced your development?
2. You find yourself in a social situation in which a number of other helping professionals (a psychiatrist, psychologist, and social worker) begin to demean what counselors can do versus what these other professionals are trained to do. Set them straight by explaining how your profession makes a unique and significant contribution.
3. Describe a piece of research that you find especially meaningful and relevant to your life. What is it about this study that you most appreciate?
4. If you were going to do an original research study that is driven by a strong personal motive of yours or that is related to an ongoing issue in your life, what would you choose to look at? How would you carry out the study?
5. Conduct a small qualitative study: Ask three classmates to describe to you the reasons they chose to become counselors. Write down carefully (or record and transcribe) what they say. What common themes emerged in their narratives? How did their stories compare with your own reasons for pursuing this career?

FOR HOMEWORK

Go to the library and look through the professional journals in the field. To start out, you might consider the general ones such as: *Journal of Counseling and Development, Journal of Counseling Psychology, Counseling Psychologist, Psychotherapy, Canadian Journal of Counseling,* and *Psychotherapy Networker*. Next, consider those journals most relevant to the work setting or specialty areas you are considering, whether those areas concern school, mental health, military, rehabilitation, or other settings. Review those journals too that focus on specialty areas such as multicultural counseling, group work, assessment and testing, brief counseling, substance abuse, and family counseling, to mention just a few. Because there are hundreds of such publications, you might consult with your instructor for recommendations.

Based on your brief survey, what are your initial impressions of the status research plays in counseling practice?

SUGGESTED READINGS

Beers, C. (1945). *A mind that found itself*. New York: Doubleday.

Creswell, J. W. (2007). *Qualitative inquiry and research design* (2nd ed.). Thousand Oaks, CA: Sage.

Goodheart, C. D., Kazdin, A. E., & Sternberg, R. J. (2006). *Evidence-based psychotherapy: Where practice and research meet*. Washington, DC: American Psychological Association.

Heppner, P. P. (Ed.). (1991). *Pioneers in counseling and development: Personal and professional perspectives*. Alexandria, VA: American Counseling Association.

Heppner, P. P., Kivlighan, D. M., & Wampold, B. E. (2008). *Research design in counseling* (3rd ed.). Belmont, CA: Brooks/Cole.

Hock, R. R. (2008). *Forty studies that changed psychology: Explorations into the history of psychological research* (6th ed.). Upper Saddle River, NJ: Prentice Hall.

Hubble, M. A., Duncan, B. L., & Miller, S. D. (Eds.). (1999). *The heart and soul of change: What works in therapy*. Washington, DC: American Psychological Association.

Jones, W. P., & Kottler, J. A. (2005). *Understanding research: Becoming a competent and critical consumer*. Upper Saddle River, NJ: Prentice Hall.

Luborsky, L., & Luborsky, E. (2006). *Research and psychotherapy: The vital link*. Northvale, NJ: Jason Aronson, Inc.

Minichiello, V., & Kottler, J. A. (2009). *Qualitative journeys: Student and mentor experiences with research*. Thousand Oaks, CA: Sage.

McLeod, J. (2003). *Doing counselling research* (2nd ed.). Thousand Oaks, CA: Sage.

Pope, M. (2005). *Professional counseling 101: Building a strong professional identity*. Alexandria, VA: American Counseling Association.

Roth, A., & Fonagy, P. (2006). *What works for whom? A critical review of psychotherapy research* (2nd ed.). New York: Guilford.

Settings for Counselors

CHAPTER 3

KEY CONCEPTS

Professional identity

Generic skills

Mediation

Developmental orientation

Remedial orientation

Managed care

E-therapy

Flexible specialty

Future orientation

STUDENT: Where can I work after I get my counseling degree?

PROFESSOR: Nowhere and everywhere.

STUDENT: Huh?

PROFESSOR: You're feeling confused and frustrated because the question is more complex than you thought.

STUDENT: Actually, I'm angry because you're evading my question with that active listening stuff.

PROFESSOR: What would you like to do with your degree?

STUDENT: See what I mean? There you go again.

PROFESSOR: Okay. The reason I answered your question the way I did is that I wanted to be honest with you.

STUDENT: Yes. I appreciate that. But I'm putting all this time and work into my studies. I have a right to know what my degree will qualify me to do.

PROFESSOR: Yes, you have a right to know. You may not see that many job openings in the paper under the heading "Counselor." People often confuse the title with others like a "therapist," "psychologist," and "psychiatrist."

STUDENT: This I already know. I looked in the Yellow Pages under "Counselor" and found astrologers, dieticians, palm readers, personal coaches, finance companies, and employment agencies—not to mention the usual assortment of mystics and guidance people.

PROFESSOR: That's true. However, there are also a number of fairly specific slots for counselors to fit in and a virtually unlimited market for creative professionals to develop needed services. Although your degree may not necessarily qualify you to do one particular job, there are a hundred different ways that you could put your training to work.

STUDENT: But outside of school counselors and ministers and perhaps a crisis center, college dormitory, or probation department, I've never heard of any other places where counselors can work. I mean, we're not exactly like psychiatrists—everyone knows what they do and where they are supposed to work.

PROFESSOR: That's just it. Counselors aren't as limited to working in specific settings, such as hospitals or clinics, or with specific populations, such as the personality disordered or psychotic. Counselors work with people in so many different places, from playgrounds to corporate boardrooms.

STUDENT: I know I'm supposed to get better at dealing with ambiguity and abstractions, but couldn't you be a little more specific?

PROFESSOR: Sure. But the possibilities that I name are limited by my own meager imagination. Counselors create jobs for themselves in industry, for example. It's not that difficult to convince corporate executives that profit can be increased if morale is improved among workers. We've had graduates hired to reduce absenteeism, drug abuse, and interpersonal conflicts in companies. Sometimes they also get jobs in public relations or personnel offices. In fact, what training could possibly be better for people in management at any level? Counseling teaches you to be sensitive to others' feelings, to respect their rights, and to selectively reinforce productive behavior. You learn to confront people nondefensively, to stimulate creativity, and to encourage growth at all levels. You tell me where counselors could work.

STUDENT: But I always thought of counselors as psychotherapists with another name. When I saw my own therapist, I knew that's what I wanted to do. Are you telling me I can't?

PROFESSOR: Not at all. You can do the kind of therapy you're talking about. Licensed professional counselors and marriage and family therapists are all doing therapy. You'll have to do an internship when you graduate, and then pass a licensing exam, and then you're all set. But don't limit your thinking to just that one way of using your training. There are lots of ways counselors are helpers besides doing traditional "therapy."

STUDENT: I just thought about all the creative roles counselors could play in a hospital, for instance. Patients don't exactly feel good about being there. Maybe a counselor-at-large could help prepare people psychologically for their operations.

PROFESSOR: Exactly. Graduates have been hired to do just that. Counselors also work as part of teams in other settings. They work with medical personnel in mental health clinics, with teachers, with attorneys, and with administrators. They work everywhere and anywhere that they can persuade people their services are helpful.

STUDENT: Now I'm really confused. How can I possibly decide which direction I should go in?

VOICE FROM THE FIELD

I found that becoming a counselor was like becoming a part of a new culture. When I pass someone in the corridor of the agency where I work, we exchange smiles that seem to say, "Yes, we both know we belong to a separate species." We are people who struggle all day with questions like, "Is what I do really helpful?" "How can I be sure?" "Maybe that client would be just better off with some medication, and they're wasting their time with me." But there's also something else. We all know that we share this same privilege, hour by hour—hearing people's deepest secrets, being with them in their painful feelings of shame or loss. Even the act of simply listening all day long is an experience you have to do to really appreciate. My friends often ask me, "How can you sit there and listen to people complain without getting bored?" I always give them some kind of answer, how I was taught about focusing on process, not content, or how I'm just trying to be present. But I suspect the real answer is that for us counselors, it's just in our bones.

One of the major changes in the field over the last decades has been the increasing opportunities for counselors to work in a variety of health-related arenas. As the population ages, as technology and cultural changes occur more rapidly, and as people face greater stress in their lives, the need for counselors is growing in mental health, medical, educational, business, and governmental settings. Whereas once upon a time counselors only worked in schools, then moved into agency and institutional positions previously reserved for psychologists and social workers, now counselors have carved out additional territory of their own that makes it possible to offer help in diverse places.

In addition to the traditional settings in which counselors have worked (schools and community agencies), new specialties are emerging in private practice, consultation, personal coaching, the criminal justice system, and technologically based interventions. As never before, practitioners are finding jobs in rehabilitation, substance abuse, the mental health system, student personnel, industry, and a hundred other areas. Even more innovative, counselors are finding more and more ways to use the telephone, webcams, and the Internet to operate in more efficient and convenient ways (Lester, 2008; Reese, Conoley, & Brossart, 2006; Shaw & Shaw, 2006). There really are almost limitless possibilities for employment depending on the imagination, resources, and motivation of the counselor.

WHAT COUNSELORS HAVE IN COMMON

The needs and requirements of a particular environment determine, at least in part, the adaptations and behavior of organisms in that setting. As Charles Darwin discovered in his travels, a staggering variety of species have successfully adapted to their environments—20,000 different butterflies, 40 kinds of parrots, and 300 species of hummingbirds. There is also potentially an endless variety of counselors, each species having successfully adapted to the demands of the work environment. Every client population, geographical area, cultural heritage, institutional policy, physical facility, and psychological climate subtly shapes a new species of counselor. It is even difficult, on the basis of the everyday practice of professionals, to recognize that they are nevertheless members of the same evolutionary family. Even so, there are probably more similarities than differences among counselors in

VOICE FROM THE FIELD

To people who ask what I do, I tell them many things. I've moved around a lot because of my husband's job transfers so I hold several different licenses. In one state I'm an MFT [Marriage and Family Therapist], in another I'm an LPC [Licensed Professional Counselor], and in still another I'm an LLP [Limited Licensed Psychologist]. I've gone through training in play therapy, hypnosis, conflict mediation, EMDR [Eye Movement Desensitization Reprocessing], and about a dozen other specialties. I get lots of different journals and go to many different conferences, depending on where they happen to be located in any given year. So when people ask me what I do it seems simpler just to say I'm a counselor. It's easier to "sell" what I do that way to prospective clients.

various settings. Before we explore the roles of counselors in the places where they work, it will be helpful to review what they all share in common.

A UNIQUE IDENTITY

All counselors, irrespective of their work settings, identify themselves as part of a shared profession that is distinguished from other helping disciplines. As we mentioned in the previous chapter, counseling is *not* the same as social work, psychology, guidance, psychiatry, or education—even though those other professionals often practice counseling in some form. Each field, however similar in its methods and goals, arises out of quite different settings. Psychiatry is a specialty of medicine. Social work came from the streets, psychology from the university, and counseling from the schools. In spite of their recent trends toward convergence, each helping profession is indelibly marked by its birthplace.

Exploring and articulating your own professional identity is absolutely critical, not only to ground yourself in a discipline with its own set of standards, culture, rituals, research, and theoretical base, but also to be able to explain who you are, and what you do, to your clients and to the public. The roles you take on—as a scholar, teacher, consultant, mediator, diagnostician, interventionist, systems analyst, and so on, all contribute to your professional identity. Likewise, the setting in which you work, the organizations to which you belong, the conferences you choose to attend, and the licenses and certifications you hold also shape your dominant self-image as a professional.

MANY DIFFERENT ROLES

As would already be evident, counselors have varied roles, depending on the setting in which they practice. Some jobs demand more diagnostic and assessment skills while others require specializations in group work, or family counseling, or consultation. Generally, the most common counselor roles may be grouped into several categories.

1. *Individual assessment* comprises observation, information seeking, and interpretation of a person's behavior in areas that include performance, achievement, aptitude, personality, and interests. The results of assessment are

VOICE FROM THE FIELD

I'm working with a woman today whose 71-year-old mother is dying of uterine cancer and her 78-year-old father is binge drinking to cope with his grief. This woman is recently divorced, separated from her children, and away from her home and her friends while she tends to her parents. As if that isn't enough, she just learned that she too has cancer. She is depressed and overwhelmed.

In a situation like this, my role as a counselor is somewhat fluid. I have to pull out all the stops. I am a social worker, a psychologist, a mother, a trainer, a friend, a janitor, a nurse, a spiritual advisor, a shoulder, an ear, and a counselor. This may not be typical, but "typical" around here tends to be redefined frequently. You just have to be fluid to go with the flow.

valuable for screening, placement, diagnosis, evaluation, and planning of treatment approaches.

2. *Individual counseling* consists of those one-to-one interactions with clients in which the therapeutic process is applied to resolving personal concerns, career and educational decisions, problems of human adjustment. In many areas of the country, counselors are also expected to work with more severe emotional disorders (e.g., depression and anxiety). More and more, counselors are called on to initiate brief interventions that very quickly and efficiently change attitudes and behavior.

3. *Family counseling* focuses on the interaction patterns that lead to dysfunctional behavior. By thinking in terms of the family system to which a client belongs, the counselor is able to intervene by understanding and changing communication patterns and coalitions of power.

4. *Couples counseling* helps partners articulate their vulnerable feelings to each other, with the goals of enhancing their intimacy, resolving conflicts, or clarifying the decision of one or both partners to end the relationship. Counselors help such couples to have productive conversations on topics that usually lead to fights at home. Interventions include blocking hurtful exchanges, translating partners' harshly worded statements into softer language, and facilitating the expression of underlying emotions.

5. *Group work* structures may be used to accomplish more efficiently the goals of individual counseling. Participants have the added advantages of interaction. Counselors also work in guidance groups in which they serve a more active role, designing educational exploration experiences, providing information, and stimulating personal awareness and growth.

6. *Consultation* activities involve initiating changes on an organizational level, often by working on program development. Counselors consult with the human and organizational components of systems to help the individual parts make a more unified whole. Counselors, as human relations specialists, will intervene to fix or prevent the problems that arise from interpersonal conflict.

7. *Coaching* focuses on helping individual clients tap into existing skills or develop new skills in order to achieve specific objectives. *Executive coaches*, using both their counseling abilities and knowledge of corporate organizations, help business executives communicate more effectively to their colleagues, improve team performance, increase their own productivity, and achieve greater

VOICE FROM THE FIELD

One of the things I love best about my job is that I get to do so many different things in any given day. Today I spent a few hours in the morning leading a group, then working on a grant that I'm writing with two other colleagues. We're trying to generate some more funds that will free us up to continue doing outreach rather than just being stuck in our offices all day.

I've had jobs before where I was seeing client after client—six, seven, eight a day. Burnout city, if you ask me. As far as I'm concerned, the more variety of things I can do, the more stimulation I feel in my work. But I was so unprepared for this stuff. In my counseling program, I mostly learned how to do one-on-one counseling with reasonably cooperative people who were motivated to get help. What I wouldn't give for such a client now! The truth is that I don't do that much individual counseling anymore—almost all groups and family work. But I got a good foundation to learn the rest on my own.

professional-personal development (Sperry, 2008). *Personal (a.k.a. life) coaches* work with individuals to help them identify their strengths and passions and to facilitate actualizing their personal goals (Dean, 2001; Senior, 2007).

8. *Mediation* is used to help couples, business partners, or others involved in a disagreement settle their differences in an expedient and respectful way. Although this activity is often initiated at the recommendation of the court during divorce, child custody, or civil disputes, mediation can be employed as a form of structured conflict resolution and problem solving in a variety of situations (Milne, Folberg, & Salem, 2004). Other forms of mediation focus primarily on helping people to understand one another and make compromises that are mutually acceptable (Bush & Folger, 2004; Winslade & Monk, 2008; Young & Basham, 2010).

9. *Administration* plays a part in many counselors' work; it involves directing the activities of a school, agency, or organization. Public relations, quality control, fundraising, the conducting of meetings, paperwork processing, and decision making are major components of this kind of work.

10. *Supervision* gives experienced practitioners a significant role in helping those who are less capable. The counselor may conduct in-service workshops and provide individual or group supervision sessions that may be either emotionally or behaviorally focused. Responsibility for staff training and development may also include attention to improving staff morale.

11. *Computer technology* is now a crucial aspect of the counselor's daily life that includes using chat rooms, distance therapy, online self-help groups, Web-based programming, and Internet communications (Evans, 2009; Lieber, Archer, Munson, & York, 2006; Tate & Zabinski, 2004). Practitioners are expected to be sufficiently computer literate to take care of word processing functions (writing reports, handling correspondence) and other routine matters. For example, school counselors use computers to handle all record keeping and scheduling, and mental health counselors use software packages that help with diagnosis and case management. Counselors must be fluent enough with the Internet that they can access needed information and communicate with colleagues.

12. *Research* is an important part of measuring professional effectiveness. Counselors are frequently required to justify their existence and to demonstrate to funding agencies, regulatory commissions, citizens' advisory groups, and boards of trustees that they are earning their salaries. Research is also crucial in communicating the results of experimentation to other professionals so that the field can continue to grow.

A Set of Generic Skills

Regardless of their work settings, theoretical orientation, training program, and client population, most counselors use basically the same intervention skills. A later chapter will review in detail these universal helping skills that are employed by human service professionals in a variety of settings and contexts.

Counseling skills are divided into several broad categories:

1. *Diagnostic skills* involve questioning and assessment strategies to figure out what is going on with a client; for example, identifying a possible emotional disorder. Example: *When you say you are depressed, what exactly do you mean by that? Please say more about when you started feeling that way, how long the condition has lasted, and what it is like for you.*

2. *Exploration skills* are used to understand the client's world and collect needed information that will be helpful in later efforts. Example: *Describe what a typical day is like for you.*

3. *Relationship skills* work to build a supportive alliance with clients that is conducive to openness, trust, and respect. Example: *After I asked you how you felt about what happened I notice that you started withdrawing—you visibly pulled back, crossed your arms, and started to scowl. It seemed like a way to put distance between us and that is exactly what you said your girlfriend complains about when she is with you.*

4. *Conceptualization skills* help to promote self-awareness and deep-level investigations into the nature of a client's presentation of concerns and their larger meaning. These investigations are often based in a particular theoretical framework that helps to both explain the sources of the client's distress and be a guide for the formulation of a treatment plan. Example: *Depression like this can often signal an underlying sense of helplessness. Men who express anger the way you do, and who attempt to self-medicate themselves with alcohol, may be trying to mask feelings that have been difficult to express.*

5. *Action skills* help to translate identified problem areas and new understanding into sequential steps toward desired goals. Example: *You said that you are ready to break out of your isolation and sense of loneliness. What, specifically, do you intend to do in the next week to make a small step of progress in this area?*

6. *Group process skills* are employed in family, organizational, and consultation settings to resolve conflicts and work toward team objectives. Example: *Just a minute ago you said you don't trust anyone in your life. Yet I've noticed that there have been several times in this group that you've put yourself on the line with others. Who in here would be an exception to your general rule?*

7. *Evaluation skills* are used to measure the effects of intervention efforts and, if necessary, make adjustments. Example: *When you talk about feeling better*

about things, maybe you could say more about what you have noticed is unusual for you. An example would really help to demonstrate what you are doing differently.

You could observe any mental health or human service professional—whether working in a school, agency, company, hospital, or private practice; whether licensed as a counselor, psychologist, social worker, or psychiatrist—and regardless of theoretical orientation or training, you would still notice the use of these generic skills. They are the basis for developing any therapeutic relationship, as well as promoting change efforts.

A SET OF COMMON GOALS

Goals that are common to all counselors and that serve to clarify professional identity include helping clients to:

1. Work constructively toward life/career planning
2. Anticipate, plan, and react constructively to developmental issues and transitions
3. Integrate thinking, feeling, and behavior into a congruent expression of self
4. Respond productively to stress and reduce its negative impact on their lives
5. Develop effective interpersonal skills so that relationships with peers, family, and colleagues can have constructive potential
6. Assess strengths and identify weaknesses so that they may develop more personal awareness
7. Become aware of the holistic nature of life and integrate effective principles of living into psychological, physical, and social aspects of their lives
8. Develop more choices in their lives, with accompanying skills to make constructive decisions
9. Become independent of the counseling in the shortest time possible

This last point is particularly important in that the object of all counseling efforts is to teach clients to take care of themselves in the future. It is one thing to help people to resolve their presenting problems, but quite another to help them to generalize what they've learned so that they can apply new skills to future challenges they will face.

BOTH DEVELOPMENTAL AND REMEDIAL ORIENTATION

Counselors are interested in and trained for helping individuals to anticipate issues and concerns, develop adaptive life skills, respond constructively to issues and problems, and work toward psychological growth and increased personal mastery. Counselors choose and prize their role because of its orientation toward life/skill development, and its emphasis on improved problem-solving abilities and decision-making skills—as opposed to an orientation that focuses exclusively on diagnosis, evaluation, and remediation.

Although counselors can and do use their knowledge of personality theory, psychopathology, and emotional dysfunctions to work therapeutically, they often

VOICE FROM THE FIELD

I have the same goals with almost all the kids I see. Of course, each of them comes in for a different reason and purpose. Sometimes they're having problems keeping up with class, or fighting with their parents, or maybe they're just depressed. Regardless, though, of why they come in, they all need one thing—a place where they can vent their feelings, complain about their parents or siblings, say anything they want, without fear of being criticized or reported on. Kids think we're going to be authority figures just like every other adult in their lives. You should see the light on their faces when they realize all I'm going to do is listen and understand! It's like, "Wow, there really is a grown-up who I can tell absolutely anything to?"

focus on prevention of problems before they become severe. Counselors tend to distinguish themselves as well-trained experts working with those who don't necessarily have severe symptoms. As we mentioned previously, many counselors operate within the mental health system doing remedial work. The principal advantage of counseling practitioners, in contrast to social workers, psychologists, and psychiatrists, is their training in helping people who aren't stigmatized as dysfunctional. For example, counselors are the only mental health professionals who usually learn about career counseling, one of the areas in "normal" life that many people struggle with.

The role of the counselor is not to instruct but to stimulate the natural growth and potential inherent in human beings (American Counseling Association, 2005; Ivey, Ivey, Myers, & Sweeney, 2004). As people develop, they have the capability to initiate, expand, and maintain psychological growth. In fact, many consider this capacity to be an essential feature of adult development (Broderick & Blewitt, 2006; Goodman, Schlossberg, & Anderson, 2006; Newman & Newman, 2009; Sheehy, 1995). The crystallization of a client's irreconcilable conflict and the client's resulting discomfort are tools often used by counselors. The client can resolve that anxiety by moving to a more mature developmental stage, which will allow for an integration of the conflict and subsequent reduction in personal discomfort.

Counselors rely heavily on the work of developmental theorists as they attempt to stimulate clients to initiate developmentally relevant growth. Developmental work focuses on client issues and may include psychosexual development (Freud, 1924), cognitive development (Piaget, 1926), conceptual development (Vygotsky, 1934/1986, 1978/2006), language development (Chomsky, 1968/2006), psychosocial development (Erikson, 1950), career development (Super, 1957), moral development (Kohlberg, 1969), religious development (Fowler, 1981), relational development (Jordan, 1997), empathy development (Siegel & Hartzell, 2003), ego development (Loevinger, 1976), cultural identity development (Sue & Sue, 2008), sexual identity development (Horowitz & Newcomb, 2001), or gender development (Comstock, 2005; Shepard, 2005), among many possibilities.

This core of knowledge implicit in these developmental theories may be described as follows:

1. Human development proceeds in a series of progressive stages leading to increasingly complex behaviors.

VOICE FROM THE FIELD

"I want to quit my job, but I need the money. I'm stuck." If I had a nickel for every time I heard this. When I first started doing counseling, I'd get sucked into the trap of trying to help people figure it out. I'd do things like asking them to explore the pros and cons of either choice. Or suggesting they check their "gut" for an answer. Well, the pros and cons would always stack up equally for both sides, and the "gut" told them different things on different days. What I had to learn is that some conflicts don't have good solutions. My role is to help the client recognize that any decision involves risk, and when you choose one path in life, you have to mourn the loss of the other path. Understanding that—for my client, and for me—is what growing up is all about.

2. These stages are invariant and sequential.
3. They are both genetically determined and adaptive to the culture and environment.
4. The stages alternate between periods of well-adjusted equilibrium and periods of unstable disequilibrium.
5. Growth may be encouraged by stimulating a person to restore equilibrium at a higher stage of development.
6. Wide differences in development are possible depending on the person's gender and racial and cultural identity.
7. During adulthood, development becomes more cyclical rather than linear as people face life transitions and crises.

During counseling sessions, a practitioner employing a developmental model might be thinking something along the following lines:

This young man is 14 years old. He seems to be functioning at about age level in physical development but is considerably under expected norms in the areas of social and emotional functioning. I wonder when this lag first began to be noticeable? I must remember to check that out later.

I notice my approval seems especially important to him. Hopefully, that should give me some leverage to push him to take more responsibility for his inappropriate behavior. If I can encourage him to take some risks with me here, maybe I could get him to do the same with his parents and teachers. He seems to be perfectly capable, for instance, of controlling his anger when he has advance notice that he will be disappointed; it is surprises that throw him for a loop. I wonder how I can help him to stretch himself a bit in that area?

The work of the counselor is to help the client translate immediate issues of concern into a relevant developmental framework so the necessary growth can be identified and initiated. Pragmatically applying developmental theory, the counselor seeks to stimulate client growth toward successive stages of human maturity.

TEAMWORK

A counselor rarely operates alone; most counselors work in institutional or clinical settings as part of a team that is responsible for a range of activities or services, only one aspect of which is counseling. For example, many counselors work in

VOICE FROM THE FIELD

It was the weirdest thing. This 40-year-old woman before me still had baby fat, or so it seemed. Her face was smooth and round, and there was no evidence of the wrinkles or creases that are the inevitable byproduct of life experience. And that was why she came to counseling. She felt like she had stopped growing at age 15. She still fought with her mom like a teenage girl; her relationships were all crushes on "cute" men; when she didn't get what she wanted, she threw teenage temper tantrums or sulked in her bedroom. The fact was, her father had died suddenly of a heart attack when my client was 15, and the trauma had somehow arrested her development. My job was somehow to get her "unstuck," so she could continue a normal developmental sequence. I still couldn't tell you exactly "how it happened," but as we worked through the buried grief over her father's death, her face changed. I got a call from her just last week, almost a decade after we stopped working. She wanted to tell me that for the first time in her life, she felt her own age.

business and industry settings, helping employees with personal, marriage, career, or substance abuse problems that can affect their work attitudes and productivity. There the counselors frequently consult the employees' managers, as well as supervisors, union representatives, personnel department representatives, and others in the work environment. The counselor is a vital member of a team and strives to work in concert with colleagues to advance institutional goals and provide help to individual employees. Counselors also maintain an active professional liaison with community agencies, mental health clinics, and so on.

The same pattern holds true in most other settings as well. Whether counselors work in school, agency, community, or private practice settings, they function as specialists in resource identification, consultation, and individual counseling.

A DAY IN THE LIFE

See Companion DVD
Settings

One of the goals of this text is to provide you with "voices from the field" that illustrate realistically how counselors apply their knowledge and skills in daily situations that you will face. Perhaps this can best be demonstrated if you have an idea of what a typical day is like for practitioners who operate in a variety of different settings. What follows is a realistic glimpse of counselors in each of several traditional and nontraditional roles, including a sampling of their frustrations and problems as well as their excitement and satisfaction.

These narratives are not intended to represent all practitioners who work within this specialty, or in this setting, but rather to give you a sampling of what life is like for professionals in the trenches. When you conduct your own "field studies" you can augment these stories with your own research. This will help you make some informed decisions about the aspects of the profession that you might like to investigate further.

HIGH SCHOOL

At 7:25 A.M., when the counselor walks into his office, seven students are already waiting. Right away he knows why. There was a glitch in the computer yesterday,

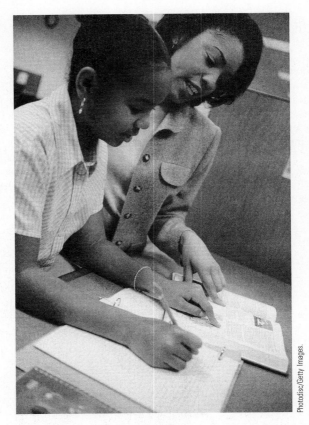

Photodisc/Getty Images.

School counselors are called upon to function in a number of different roles—not only as a therapist, but also a scheduler, administrator, consultant, teacher, and disciplinarian.

and third-hour English was overloaded with twice the number of students the classroom could handle. The teacher about blew her fuse, but at least she has now settled down. As the counselor finishes rescheduling the last student 30 minutes later, he wonders what this activity has to do with counseling.

Scheduling classes not only is boring administrative work, but it also really eats up time, keeping him from getting to what he wants to be doing—working with kids and their problems. He makes a mental note to mention this concern in the afternoon meeting with the principal, knowing he won't even have the full support of the staff. Some of them actually prefer scheduling to counseling; they consider the work less demanding. The thought is depressing.

On the way to the attendance office to check on a student, he suddenly hears shouts and a commotion around the corner. Cringing, he moves toward the disturbance and finds two senior boys wrestling against a locker, each twice his size. Using what he hopes is his most authoritative voice, he pushes between them and manages with the help of another teacher to separate them. His heart sinks when he recognizes one of the offenders as a youngster for whom he went out on a limb two weeks ago—he was in danger of being suspended for fighting. Now this!

An hour later he feels better. The fighting business has been cleared up, and he has just finished a successful interview with a student whose parents have been pushing him toward a military career. It felt good to help him explore what he wants and to become more aware of his tendency to please his parents at all costs. The session seemed to be productive, and he felt confident that the student would make some changes.

His meeting with the principal is grim. Teachers, says she, are complaining because the counseling staff is overloading classes and allowing friends to alter their schedules so they can be together in their mischief. The counselor points out (once again) that class scheduling is administrative work and not the primary responsibility of the counseling department; further, if teachers are having discipline problems in their classes, they should consult with a counselor instead of complaining to the principal.

Lunch provides a needed break. A teacher stops by and suggests that they get together to talk about the teacher's frustrations with his job and hassles with the department chair. The counselor's talk with him seems to help. Sometimes the informal sessions over lunch seem to make more difference than all the appointments during the week.

The counselor tries to keep the afternoons open for working with kids. He has two appointments and will finish the day with a group. But he is worried about the first appointment—a 17-year-old senior who is depressed and extremely worried about smoking too much marijuana. The session is taxing, and he reflects on how difficult it is to work with kids having drug problems. The last individual appointment is a bonus. He has been working with this girl for four months now and can really see the difference. The girl has overcome her shyness, is involved in extracurricular activities, and reports a much improved relationship with her parents. She even has a boyfriend. At the finish of the session, the counselor feels great. As he is leaving for the group, the secretary motions urgently. An irate parent is on the phone demanding an explanation for her son's suspension. She's really upset. The counselor calms her down and makes an appointment to see her after school.

Now for the group: Today's topic is love. As always, he is amazed at how sensitive the kids are and how they really do confront one another as they interact. They know what honesty means.

Hurrying to meet with the irate parent, the counselor reflects on his day. It is the variety of different things he does that most stimulates him. He just can't imagine being stuck in an office all day.

PRIVATE PRACTICE

Through the groggy dream mist, the counselor struggled toward alertness, finally achieving enough to figure out whom she was talking to and what the situation was. She calmed the man down and firmly instructed him to take a hot bath, try to relax, and write his feelings down on paper. She scheduled an appointment for him the next day and then tried to go back to sleep.

The counselor has now arrived at her office, which she shares with other professionals in private practice—a few social workers, a psychologist, and a part-time psychiatrist. Her 9:00 A.M. client already sits in the waiting room, but before going in the counselor returns her telephone messages. One call is from a client who wants to cancel her appointment in the middle of the day. The counselor doesn't

My day as an elementary school counselor starts with three phone messages taped to my door. The first call was from a parent who was worried that her ex-husband was coming to school too much. Usually he comes into my office on the pretense he's there to talk about his son, but then he tells me about all the horrible things his ex-wife does. I'm pretty sure I'm being groomed so he can count on my support in an upcoming custody hearing.

The next call was from the mom of a second grader. She was single too, but only because her husband was killed last Saturday by a drunk driver. She was wondering if she should take her children to the funeral and what she could do to make all this easier for them. I explained that in most cases children need to be part of the grieving process. They might later resent the fact that they weren't allowed to be there. I gave her some information about how children of different ages respond to death and how the younger ones often won't understand the permanence. I assured her that I would include her son in my grief and loss group.

It was time to go to the class where the second grader lost his father. I began by asking the class what they knew. They all started to tell me about how they, too, had lost a family member. Lots of grandparents. Several dogs. A desert tortoise. And a rabbit. A couple of students seemed to feel left out and they said that their great, great grandfathers had died even before they were born.

I was getting a bit frustrated because I was trying to lead them to a point where they would suggest making the grieving boy a welcome-back card. But they just kept adding more and more people to the list of people who died. Then it occurred to me that they might be revealing hurts and that I was the one being honored with their disclosures. You see, I really strive to be available to students by hanging out on the playground, going into classrooms a lot, and being outside before and after school. Students are forever calling to me outside and in the halls, giving me great big genuine smiles when they see me, and wanting to be the one I come to their class for. I almost take it for granted that children are supposed to share personal hurts, big worries, fears, family turmoil, and love with me that I forget how important little bits of information might just be. Kids whose names I don't even remember come and give me a hug as if I were a favorite uncle.

I decided it didn't matter if I made it back to my office to open another pack of donuts or if I missed my afternoon class-guidance lessons. I was right where I needed to be. It took an hour before they finally stumbled on the idea of making cards. I spent the rest of the day reading cards and watching students draw pictures of the people they cared about. The cards turned out to be heartfelt messages of concern—not so much because they were worried about the boy, but because they were expressing their own feelings of loss and healing.

You can tell that I'm extremely proud to be a school counselor. I go to work happy every day because I'm loved by a whole bunch of little children.

know whether to feel disappointed because it is too late to fill that spot or relieved because now she has an unanticipated but needed break to catch up on her paperwork. Next she calls a physician whom she has been trying to reach for months, hoping to arrange a lunch meeting and discuss possible referrals. He is out of his office. Finally, she calls an insurance company that has been refusing to authorize payment for services she has already provided.

The first of six clients for the day then enters her office. The client is relatively easy to work with, is highly motivated, pays her bills on time, and will make rapid progress. The counselor struggles with herself during the session because they have just successfully completed working on the originally stated problem. The client feels great. Her marriage has stabilized. But she wants to continue the sessions. The counselor reinforces the idea that one can never have enough counseling but silently wonders if she is saying that because she means it or because she needs the money. It is such a pain for her to get new referrals.

Yet she feels so proud of her work, her competence, her ability to make a difference in people's lives. In private practice there is the constant pressure to become more skilled at helping; if not, the clients won't return or send their friends. And all over the community she can see the results of her efforts. Her reputation is slowly beginning to build.

Two more clients in the morning, then lunch; she loves the freedom of answering only to herself and decides to do some shopping and visit with a friend. She goes back to the office and an hour of paperwork—progress notes, correspondence, forms. A new referral calls, but the counselor can't persuade her to come in for an appointment because there are financial difficulties. This woman works for a company that uses a managed care system with which the counselor thus far refuses to work: "First, they will only authorize four sessions—and at bargain rates. Then, just maybe, if the client is in the throes of a nervous breakdown, they might grant another four sessions. They've got to be kidding!"

A few colleagues are free, so the counselor has a cup of coffee with them and they chat about their day. One colleague in particular is feeling much stress because he has just had a draining session with a client skilled at playing games.

It's back to work.

The counselor makes a few more calls, including one call seeking referrals from a school system and one offering an in-service program for staff on stress management. The company agrees to let her make a presentation. She feels ecstatic: at last, a breakthrough. Then she makes a follow-up call to an ex-client who is still doing quite well and appreciates the counselor's continuing concern.

The clients file through until early evening. She feels exhausted after so many consecutive sessions. "Is the money worth all the energy it takes?" she wonders as she puts the finishing touches on her case notes. "But it is lucrative, and the freedom is wonderful, at least until the managed care system takes over completely. I like being an important part of so many people's lives, and I especially appreciate not having to answer to a boss."

PRESCHOOL

The counselor arrives at work to find a three-year-old hiding under a picnic table, surrounded by two teachers and his parents, all urging him to come out. Instead he screams "Never!" and continues to cry. The counselor reassures the parents, sends them off to work, and disperses the crowd of children and teachers. She then crawls under the table and sits silently for 10 minutes, until the child halts his tears long enough to ask why the counselor is acting silly by sitting under a table. Without hesitation the counselor replies simply that she is a little scared today, and angry at her parents for dumping her off, and this seems like as good a place as any to hide. The three-year-old understands immediately, nods his head, and tells the counselor that he'll pay extra attention to her today so she won't feel so lonely. He then crawls out and joins the other kids in the sandbox as if this entrance were a natural beginning to a day of school. The counselor, too, crawls out but makes her way to the morning staff meetings that she will direct in planning the day's psychological education.

After the play activities for the day have been discussed, the counselor reviews the past week's discipline problems—how they were managed and how they could have been handled differently. She reports on the outcomes of various conferences

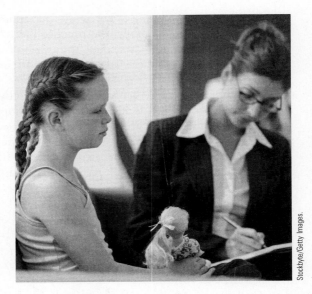

Stockbyte/Getty Images.

A counselor helps a young child talk about her concerns through the use of play therapy techniques.

she conducted with children and their parents, then makes specific recommendations to the teachers about strategies that might be helpful in the future: "When Alice throws a temper tantrum, it is best to isolate her calmly in the 'time-out' room." "Pay special attention to Brian—give him lots of hugs today because his father beat him last night." "Don't let Jennifer test you."

As the art classes begin, the counselor works on test evaluations of the children's aptitude strengths and weaknesses, detailing plans for each child. She then spends some time with the director going over administrative chores before an appointment with parents.

The mother and father of a particularly disturbed child show up 20 minutes late and then proceed to pick at each other about whose fault it was. When the counselor tries to intervene, they turn on her and then launch into an abusive tirade against the school, the teachers, and especially the counselor for being responsible for their child's problems. They decide to pull the child out of the school, and they march up to him while he is occupied on the swings, grab him by the neck, and yell at him all the way to the car. As the child cries for his friends, the parents start arguing again about who is responsible for their having such a screwed-up kid. They spank the child for good measure, throw him into the back seat, and drive off.

Another child sees the counselor fuming, with tears in her eyes, and invites her to play on the slide. They talk about what just happened, and other children ask questions about why parents sometimes get so mad. When the kids resume their play, the counselor excuses herself to break up a fight.

The counselor is exhausted; the children are still literally running circles around her. She mobilizes her energy for the afternoon parent-education class she teaches. Eleven participants attend, almost all of them single parents who have concerns about their effectiveness. She rates the class only "fair" because she feels so

problems that may have an impact on their productivity and efficiency in the workplace. Services provided include (1) individual, group, and family counseling; (2) crisis intervention and conflict management; (3) career guidance and job placement; (4) substance abuse prevention and treatment; (5) retirement planning and counseling; (6) quality-of-work-life seminars; and (7) referral to specialized agencies in the community. The staff also coordinates its activities with those of Human Resources and Affirmative Action.

What the counselors like best about their jobs is that they have the relative freedom to implement a number of new programs that are on the cutting edge of human services. They also enjoy excellent fringe benefits and salary packages, which are the hallmark of corporate settings. And they appreciate working as part of a team of professionals who are overseeing the quality of life for thousands of employees.

On the negative side of the ledger, working for any large organization is frustrating. The work hours are fairly rigid. Most employees tend to be somewhat suspicious of what the counselors do. (Are they really there to help people, or are they spies of management who will report everything they see and hear?) Also, because what they are doing is so new, there is a certain amount of resentment and resistance associated with introducing their programs, especially among the senior employees.

On the whole, though, the counselors feel that they have a great thing going—that is, as long as upper management provides support for their programs. They also realize that, for such a small department, things work smoothly because everyone gets along quite well. As would be the case with any small group, if one member of the staff was obstructive or incompetent, things could be very unpleasant. This group does work well together, however, and its members are able to be supportive and yet confront one another when the need arises.

A number of counselors, working in many different settings, report that this last characteristic is one of the most important in any job—being part of a team in which colleagues are helpful to one another and there is a spirit of cooperation and mutual caring. Counseling is, after all, a stressful job, requiring that we have built-in components to help us function well without feeling burned out. It is for this very reason that beginning counselors look for first jobs that have very supportive environments, such as friendly coworkers and a benevolent supervisor who makes it feel safe to learn and grow as a professional.

THE FUTURE IS NOW: NEW ISSUES IN COUNSELING

In this section we review some of the more current issues impacting the profession of counseling, regardless of the chosen setting or context.

COUNSELING ON THE INTERNET

Perhaps the most significant new setting for conducting counseling is the Internet, which is still in its infancy as a therapeutic modality but has major implications for the future of the profession. Counseling from a distance is certainly not a new phenomenon; suicide hotlines have existed for decades, and some counselors do sessions over the telephone when their clients are temporarily out of town. What

VOICE FROM THE FIELD

I have always been one to embrace technology and would say I'm more computer savvy than most of my friends, so it seemed natural that Internet counseling would be a good research topic for my thesis. I must say that, initially at least, I was pretty skeptical. But once I started interviewing counselors—over the Internet of course—who do this kind of work, I was impressed with some of the benefits they were touting. Perhaps most commonly they talked about how clients, some of whom they had seen previously in face-to-face counseling, were willing to talk about things that they had never broached before. We've all noticed the ways we are willing to say things impulsively and spontaneously in e-mail that we wouldn't say to someone in the room. So, by and large, the results of the study encouraged me to try it myself. So far, I've only been willing to communicate via e-mail with clients with whom I already have an existing relationship, but I know other counselors that have their whole practice on the Web.

makes the Internet different is that (a) it is a medium accessed mainly through written language (as webcams become standard hardware on computers, "Skyping" or "iChatting" may eventually promote a shift from written to face-to-face communication) and (b) sessions can be conducted via e-mail exchanges, creating a time delay between the client's and counselor's responses. Some counselors may use the Internet as an adjunct to traditional face-to-face counseling, but Internet counseling can also be done through Web-based services or a counselor's own Web site, which means it will be possible for counselors to work with clients they have never seen in person.

Some of the advantages of Internet counseling are readily apparent. For example, counselors can reach clients in rural areas, where there may be few or no mental health resources. Clients who are home-bound by a physical disability or agoraphobia can also obtain "e-therapy." For clients whose shame about needing help is so intense that visiting a counselor is prohibitive, Internet counseling provides a safe alternative. However, there are also some striking benefits to this technology that in some ways may make it a more effective counseling setting than face-to-face counseling, even for clients who have access to a mental health agency or counselor's office.

For example, one phenomenon associated with Internet counseling is the "disinhibition effect"—the fact that, because the Web affords anonymity, clients will feel less inhibited about what they self-disclose—perhaps feel safe enough to reveal to the online counselor shameful thoughts or feelings that might be too scary to express in person (Lester, 2008; Suler, 2004). Other benefits relate to the Internet as a written medium. The act of writing is, in itself, a therapeutic experience, both as an opportunity to self-reflect and to verbally express previously unarticulated, amorphous feelings or painful memories. The e-mail exchange between client and counselor means that both have a written record of sessions, a reference tool for the counselor and an opportunity for the client to review sessions and internalize the solutions discussed. The act of writing may eliminate the superficial small talk that can occur in a session, facilitating clients' getting to the core of the matter more quickly. And counselors can supplement their correspondence with online assessment instruments and links to informative Web sites (Rochlen, Zack, & Speyer, 2004; Tate & Zabinski, 2004).

VOICE FROM THE FIELD

I've got all the state-of-the art devices—an iPhone, a heart monitor watch, a GPS in my car, and about a half-dozen different computers of varying sizes and capacities. So I'd say I'm definitely up on the latest technology. But there's still one area that I am very, very skeptical about—VERY doubtful—and that's computer-based counseling. For that matter, I have a lot of concerns about some distance learning programs they have these days as well. They are predicated on the idea that it's all about gaining information, but neglect all the informal interactions that happen when you are hanging out with classmates together. So much of growth and learning takes place within a relationship. I know that can, and does, happen via the Internet, but it's still different.

Another thing that bothers me is how easy it is for people to be deceptive and lie on the Internet. I have friends who have gotten burned repeatedly through online dating services when people exaggerate their appearance or lie about who and what they are. That happens in face-to-face counseling as well but at least there are some ways we can confirm things, or read cues. But if I'm talking to someone on the Internet who is telling me that he has been abused, that he is suffering terribly as a result, how do I know what is real? For that matter, how do I know the person is even a man versus a woman, or that anything he or she says is true?

However, a number of concerns have been raised about Internet counseling. Perhaps the most obvious and salient is that counseling is an interpersonal process, whose efficacy derives not only from client and counselor verbal communication but from the myriad nonverbal signals—facial expressions, tone of voice, physical gestures—inherent in human relating. Someone writes to you in an e-mail message, "I just got home from work. What a day!" If these words were spoken, you could far more easily decode the underlying meaning: Is this person exhilarated or angry or frustrated? But without such cues available, you have to ask for more detail, and then depend on the writing capabilities of the client to describe his or her experience articulately. Meanings can be misconstrued not only by the counselor but also by the client, especially if the client already has social skill deficits in interpreting verbal messages.

Ethical concerns have also been raised about online counseling. As we all know from personal experiences with viruses, spyware, and identity theft, the Internet is not entirely secure, and confidentiality is difficult to ensure. One frequently raised concern is that counselors will be not be able to respond effectively to suicidal or homicidal crises, given both the difficulties in correctly construing client meanings, and the time delay between the client's sending a message and the counselor's reading it. The Internet is also ripe for abuse by both unscrupulous counselors who can easily falsify their credentials and clients who can lie about their age and other important identifying information (Shaw & Shaw, 2006).

Despite these concerns, Internet counseling is here to stay, and preliminary research suggests that its strengths outweigh the negatives. It has, for example, shown to be helpful in treating panic disorder, eating disorders, suicidality, and post-traumatic stress disorder (Lester, 2008; Rochlen, Zack, & Speyer, 2004). Client perceptions regarding their experience with online counseling have so far been positive, and the loss of nonverbal communication has been offset by the comfort level clients report that they experience when self-disclosing personal

VOICE FROM THE FIELD

I'm in a quandary about this whole Internet counseling idea. I'm a strong believer that counseling is and should be an intimate relationship. That's why I wanted to get into the field in the first place. Just the feeling of being there with someone while they cry and release some pain—knowing I've helped them feel less alone. It's such a privilege, and so gratifying. But you can't stop the future. A colleague started using one of these e-therapy Web sites, and he loves it. He says he has more time to think about his counseling responses—and now he makes fewer clinical mistakes. He can work from home, and when he's feeling tired, he just takes a break. I tell myself, that's still not a good way to do effective counseling. But what if that's how the client wants to do it? Do I say, "Sorry, but go find someone else to work with"? Will I end up being a counseling dinosaur?

information in the familiar environment of their own home (Leiber, Archer, Munson, & York, 2006).

If you conduct counseling over the net, either as an adjunct to traditional therapy, or as the primary means of communicating with your clients, the following general principles should be followed:

1. Make sure you are well trained in using computers, including encryption technology. Ethically, you need to take every precaution to protect client confidentiality. One way you can facilitate this is to use a counseling Web service that requires clients to use passwords to connect with you. Professionally, you need to protect yourself from computer crashes and other technological breakdowns. Conducting therapy over the Internet requires the same level of competence as does any counseling modality.

2. Make the limitations of the Internet clear to your clients, including any potential threats to their confidentiality.

3. Remember that you have the same duty to "warn and protect" as you would with face-to-face counseling. Consequently, you need to have thorough identifying information from your clients, including how to reach them in person and how to reach family members or friends in the event of a suicidal/homicidal crisis.

4. Learn to use interventions that work well over the Internet; cathartic exercises, age regression, and other interventions that place clients in highly vulnerable emotional states should be avoided.

5. Use the Internet with clients who are most likely to benefit from it, including clients who desire personal growth, are struggling with normal adjustment issues, or who require primarily psychoeducation. The Internet is not an appropriate medium for clients with serious mental illnesses.

6. Because this is a new medium, ethical codes regarding Internet counseling are likely to be regularly updated. Make sure you keep abreast of American Counseling Association (ACA), American Psychological Association (APA), and other professional counselor association guidelines.

It is always difficult to predict future trends in the counseling profession, or in *any* field for that matter. In the previous six editions of this text, over the course of 25 years, there are many aspects of the profession that have remained stable but many

■ | VOICE FROM THE FIELD

As soon as I completed the introductory course, I knew immediately the things I didn't like, even though I had no idea what I did like. The idea of sitting in an office seemed intolerable to me. I had to find something where I could move around a lot, have variety in my job, and try different things all the time. In the class on career information, I took a lot of those tests we're supposed to give to clients, but they only told me what I already knew. So I visited

five different agencies and interviewed counselors in the field as part of a school project. Then I did two different internships. I tentatively settled on working with small kids because you can help them before they get into too much trouble and you get to see their changes in a matter of weeks instead of years. I also figured that if I don't like that job, I will already be prepared to work with children in any setting I choose.

other things have changed dramatically. Who could have ever imagined that we'd be talking about doing counseling over the Internet, or that something called "managed care" would so rule the lives of practitioners? Who could have thought that it would become standard operating procedure to contain most counseling relationships to a dozen, or even a half-dozen, sessions? Well, school counselors could. But you get the point: Flexibility is the key for survival, if not for flourishing, in this field.

There is one thing we are absolutely certain about: Counseling is a profession in which it is not a luxury, but a requirement, that you remain flexible and fluid in what you do, how you do it, and where you practice. There is one thing that is also highly probable: Things will continue to change; if you want to remain marketable you will have to remain current with regard to advances in research, theory, and practice.

THE VALUE OF A FLEXIBLE SPECIALTY

The days of the counseling generalist are numbered. No longer can the counselor indulge in the luxury of acting like a country doctor who knows a little bit about everything and yet nothing in depth about anything. The technology and knowledge in the field are growing so rapidly that it is impossible to stay current on subjects as diverse as Internet-based resources, genetic predeterminants of emotionally disturbed children, nutritional imbalances in geriatric senility, indirect hypnotic trance inductions, neuroendocrinology related to stress responses, and unionism among school personnel specialists.

Most counselors, by design or by circumstances, find themselves in a flexible specialty. Because of a need in a particular community for family mediation experts, a counselor may choose to affiliate with a court system to fill the gap. A counselor newly hired by an agency may need to adapt to handling drug-abuse cases, sex counseling, or another area in which the counselor has specialized expertise. Sometimes clientele, based on their socioeconomic or geographical background, will present similar problems of economic hardship, bored marriages, or free-floating anxiety. Again the counselor ends up reading and studying more about those particular concerns and thereby becomes an expert in dealing with future cases.

Although you probably should market yourself as a specialist in a few related areas to increase both your employability and your professional mastery, you need not become so narrow in focus that you program yourself for future difficulties. Whether you are a financier, physician, or counselor, the consequences of overspecialization can be equally undesirable, resulting in rigidity, obsolescence, and a narrow field of vision.

It may therefore be advantageous to select a particular field in which to concentrate your study while continuing efforts to survey the wide educational spectrum. Certain specialties even fit well together, depending on your interests and skills.

A survey of broad specialty areas that permit flexibility and the opportunity to develop field expertise is illustrated in the following list:

Child Development	Adolescent Development
elementary school counseling	high school counseling
preschool counseling	youth probation officer
early childhood education	youth work in a residential facility
parent education	career-development specialist
child abuse	college placement

Adult Development	Interpersonal Relationships
adult education	couples counseling
midlife transitions	family counseling
counseling for the aged	sex education and counseling
spiritual/pastoral counseling	personal coaching
criminal justice	divorce mediation

Health	Industry
nutritional counseling	organizational development
exercise and health education	corporate consulting
stress management	staff training and development
physical disabilities	employee assistance programs
weight loss or smoking reduction	public relations

University	Careers
student affairs	lifestyle assessment
residential life	career planning and placement
student counseling	vocational rehabilitation
college administration	occupational therapy

Addictions	Mental Health
substance abuse counseling	private practice
drug education	community mental health centers
crisis intervention	public and nonprofit agencies
primary prevention	hospitals

GUIDELINES FOR SELECTING A COUNSELING SPECIALTY

You should at least consider concentrating in one or more of the categories in the list. The task of considering them is no less overwhelming than any other career decision and needs to be based on a systematic process of solid self-evaluation and the collection of pertinent information about each subspecialty. Beginning this process early in a graduate program allows maximum opportunity for exploration and can guide your classwork and fieldwork so that the eventual decision on a subspecialty can emerge, rather than be forced at the last minute. The choice of some specialties will involve further training beyond your current program level, a factor that may be important for some students.

The following guidelines may be helpful in thinking about specialty areas and creating an innovative personal approach to this important task.

1. *Assess personal strengths and weaknesses.* In thinking about your personal strengths and weaknesses, strive to be extremely honest with yourself and assertively seek feedback from trusted friends, peers, colleagues, and professors. Often a disappointing specialty selection can be traced back to an inaccurate self-assessment. It is important to be scrupulous in all aspects, avoiding any tendency to be overcritical, underplay strengths, or be defensive about weaknesses. Accuracy and honesty are twin hallmarks of an effective self-assessment.

2. *Examine your original motivations for becoming a counselor.* For example, you may have experienced a significant difficulty in your life, and want to help people who are struggling with similar issues. This motivation may quickly illuminate a particular specialty area that will be highly satisfying for you, but can also lead you to overlook other specialties that might be a better fit with your personality and working style. Moreover, choosing a specialty related to your own past and/or current personal issues can lead to loss of objectivity with clients as well as to emotional burnout.

3. *Clarify values related to work.* Personal values exert a substantial impact on work satisfaction and can influence burnout, career development, and professional effectiveness. It is useful to spend some time exploring your personal work values and testing them within possible specialty areas. The counseling field is so large and diverse that it provides ample opportunity for individuals to seek or create work settings and specialties that are consistent with personal values. Nothing is more frustrating than choosing a career or specialty that requires considerable investment, only to discover that it doesn't feel right; for instance, that the job requires evening hours and you hate working after dark. You can avoid, or at least minimize, such disappointments and frustrations by paying careful attention to values early in the specialty-selection process.

4. *Visit as many different specialty settings as possible.* There is no replacement for reality testing in career selection. Although a specialty might sound interesting and comfortable to you, a visit to a site could provide a completely different perspective on what the job is really like. Many counseling students, for example, believe that they would like to work in a hospital setting. However, after visiting a site, they may discover that much of their work

VOICE FROM THE FIELD

It's funny, but I always thought I wanted to be in private practice. That's where the money is—supposedly. So I interviewed several counselors working in a group practice, and what I learned surprised the heck out of me.

Most of them like their work but all said the same thing—being in private practice means being an entrepreneur as well. You just don't get an office and expect clients to show up. Most of the private practice counselors I spoke with said they spend at least one day a week doing nothing but marketing and self-promotion—giving presentations, sending out mailings, attending networking meetings, and writing columns for their local paper. It sounded like a lot of hard work, and I'm not sure I want to do all that. Sure, they were making good money, but when I compared their lifestyles to that of school counselors, I realized that when you add up benefits, retirement, paid vacations, and stuff, it almost came out even. That really opened my eyes to looking at some other jobs I wouldn't have considered.

would be routine and depressing and that counselors are at the bottom of the pecking order. This awareness may cool initial enthusiasm, or it may reinforce a tentative commitment. Regardless of the outcome, decision making will be based more on reality considerations than on fantasy.

5. *Interview as many counselors in the field as possible.* Selecting a specialty depends on awareness of opportunities as well as personal preferences and goals. Interacting with professional counselors allows the student to collect a wealth of valuable information about work situations and opportunities that is rooted in day-to-day reality. A limitation of graduate education is that it is often removed from the experiences of clinicians. You can work to reduce this separation and in the process enrich the basis for choosing your specialty.

6. *Maximize internship and practical experiences.* The heart of a professional training program in counseling is supervised experience. These structures provide an indispensable source of knowledge for specialty selection. Seek as wide a range of experiences as possible. This is a time to experiment and to broaden professional horizons. The field portion of your training is, in a sense, the last "free" opportunity to explore professionally. Once you have graduated, it will be much more difficult to avoid making firm commitments.

7. *Develop a future orientation.* Essayists have repeatedly observed that change is the only stable characteristic of the future. To prepare for a vital and pertinent specialty area, you will need to develop a professional orientation that looks to the future rather than the past for definition and career opportunity. For example, whereas historically school systems have been the largest employer of counselors, we can predict there will be increasing opportunities in the future for those who specialize in working with the aged. To ensure professional relevance, you will have to anticipate settings and opportunities wherein counseling skills and attitudes will be useful and in demand. Creatively forecasting the future will allow you, as a counselor-in-training, to select specialties carefully and to target emerging employment opportunities.

SUMMARY

The selection of a specialty is, in a sense, a sub-goal of counselor training. It is useful to begin the process of specialty selection early in your education but to avoid making rigid or premature commitments. Counselors need to be flexible and open to change as they develop as people and professionals. Specialty selection is really the first step in professional development, which is an ongoing aspect of your work as a counselor.

This chapter has provided an overview of the work of professional counselors in a variety of jobs. Each setting for counseling is vital, dynamic, and filled with both substantial rewards and grinding frustrations. Such is the nature of the profession. Helping people, particularly within an institutional context, is not an easy task—but it does offer a unique and creative opportunity to make a difference in the world.

Professional counselors work in many settings and perform a variety of tasks. Opportunities for employment in the field are extensive and require a proactive orientation. A major task for students in counselor training programs is to begin to think about their careers and to initiate careful research and planning to ensure maximum opportunity. One aspect of this planning is the tentative selection of a specialty area.

PROFESSOR: So much for our overview of the places where counselors work. Are you any more clear on what you can do with your degree?

STUDENT: You're feeling unsure of yourself and your ability to help me deal with a problem so complex.

PROFESSOR: Yes, it is frustrating. All the time I must—ah, yes, I see you have learned something. And I know how it feels to be evaded with active listening.

STUDENT: To answer your question: I learned that it is up to me to market myself for the job I really want. The counseling program provides me with a core of basic skills to apply in any setting I choose.

PROFESSOR: Yes, and it is up to me to help you in your choices by providing honest feedback about your assets and limitations concerning possible specialty areas. In addition, I need to stimulate and challenge your thinking about possibilities.

STUDENT: So I guess it's up to me to use the skills and techniques I'm learning in the program and somehow to combine them with my personal strengths and figure out what I'm going to be when I grow up.

PROFESSOR: You bet—and the process doesn't stop. In fact, right now in my own life I've been doing some thinking and evaluating....

SELF-GUIDED EXPLORATIONS

1. Imagine that it is now three years in the future and you are working in your ideal job. Describe, in detail, what a typical day in your life is like. Include not only what you are doing, but also where and how you are doing it.
2. Describe your plan for making your fantasy described in (1) a reality.
3. Choose a counseling specialty or setting that seems intriguing to you, but not part of your current plans. Pretend that you decided to pursue that career path instead of the one described in the previous fantasy. Describe a day in your life in that setting.
4. Think of three counseling settings where you're fairly certain you do not want to work. Make a list of the reasons why. Now, ask yourself: (a) Which of those reasons are based on unexamined assumptions, rather than on accurate knowledge of the specialty? (b) Which of those reasons are based on fear (e.g., I won't be good at that; I won't make enough money; those kind of clients make me uncomfortable; etc.)?

■ Voice from the Field

I went all the way through my training thinking I wanted to work as a counselor in correctional facilities, or maybe as a probation officer. As long as I can remember, that's what I wanted to do. I studied hard, got good grades, and prepared myself as best I could for my first internship placement.

So there I was, finally, working in a prison. The first day there I sat in on a group of inmates and I was shocked. I mean shocked! They had no interest in God or religion. Every other word out of their mouths was a cussword. They had not the slightest interest in anything I had to say. All they did is stare at me as if I didn't have any clothes on.

I had no idea this is what it would be like. I guess I had a pretty naïve fantasy about how I could "turn people's lives around." So I scrambled for a new internship, and found something at a domestic violence shelter. These women are amazing—they have so much courage, leaving men who said they'd kill them if they ever left. And the thing is, they don't realize how brave they are. They inspire me to want to help them see that. I'm so grateful I ended up here, because I can tell it's where I belong.

For Homework

Write down a list of the places where, ideally, you'd like to work. Make plans to visit each one of these settings. Don't take no for an answer if you find it initially challenging to arrange these field studies. Try to make friends with someone at each site so that you will have a contact person for future internship and job placements.

Then jot down a few notes about what you learned.

Suggested Readings

Broderick, P. C., & Blewitt, P. (2006). *The life span: Human development for helping professionals* (2nd ed.). Upper Saddle River, NJ: Prentice Hall.

Burger, W. E. (2008). *Human services in contemporary America* (7th ed.). Pacific Grove, CA: Brooks/Cole.

Dunbar, A. (2009). *Essential life coaching skills.* New York: Routledge.

Erford, B. (2006). *Transforming the school counseling profession* (2nd ed.). Upper Saddle River, NJ: Prentice Hall.

Evans, J. (2009). *Online counselling and guidance skills: A practical resource for trainees and practitioners.* Thousand Oaks, CA: Sage.

LoPresti, R. L., & Zuckerman, E. L. (2004). *Rewarding specialties for mental health clinicians: Developing your practice niche.* New York: Guilford.

Palmo, A. J., Weikel, W. J., & Borsos, D. P. (2006). *Foundations of mental health counseling* (3rd ed.). Springfield, IL: Charles C. Thomas.

Thompson, R. A. (2009). *Professional school counseling: Best practices for working in schools* (3rd ed.). New York: Routledge.

Wiger, D. E. (2007). *The well-managed mental health practice.* New York: Wiley.

THE THERAPEUTIC RELATIONSHIP | CHAPTER 4

Regardless of the setting in which you practice counseling—whether in a school, university, agency, hospital, clinic, or private practice—the relationships you develop with your clients are crucial to any progress you might make together. For without a high degree of intimacy and trust between two people, very little can be accomplished. It is this idea of safety that is the single organizing principle of counseling, because clients are continually checking out danger signals in the relationship with the counselor—and in all other relationships.

Make a mental list of the important relationships in your life. Include friendships. Add your parents, siblings, and other relatives. Perhaps you might also consider a few teachers, coworkers, or classmates to be influential in your world. Now, what do your best relationships—all those you have ever known—have in common? What are the characteristics you consider to be most crucial in your past, present, and future interactions with other people?

Important relationships in almost any context, except adversarial ones, have certain desirable elements—trust, for one. Mutual respect, openness, acceptance, and honesty are others. Whether we are examining personal relationships or the unique contact between counselor and client, there will be similarities. For in all kinds of relationships, helping or otherwise, we desire intimacy and intensity. The quality we are able to create in these dimensions is directly related to the personal enrichment of our lives. We would argue that the same holds true for helping relationships.

QUALITIES OF COUNSELING RELATIONSHIPS

See Companion DVD
The Counseling
Relationship

Counseling takes place within the context of a very special kind of relationship—one that is similar to other successful alliances but is also distinctly different. In this chapter you will explore the fundamental aspects of the helping relationship, learn how these qualities are developed, and learn how several primary relationship-enhancing skills and interventions may be applied to sessions.

From the outset of the first encounter, the client clearly is in need of some assistance and the counselor is identified as an expert with specialized talent and skills to provide the desired help. The relationship, therefore, involves a contract in which both parties agree to abide by certain rules: the client to show up on time, and to make an effort to be as open as possible; the counselor to be trustworthy, to protect the welfare of the client, and to do everything possible to help the client reach identified goals in the most efficient period of time. The power between the client and the counselor is thus embodied in a unique structure wherein the client is primarily responsible for the content of the relationship, and the counselor has much of the responsibility for directing its style and structure. Although counselors do make an effort to demonstrate complete sincerity and respect to the client, nonetheless an uneven distribution of status and power remains. After all, the relationship takes place on the counselor's home turf. There are diplomas and books on the wall. A warm professional atmosphere pervades, yet the counselor gets the more comfortable chair and, when both speak simultaneously, the counselor usually prevails.

In traditional approaches to counseling developed by Freud and his followers, this power imbalance was conceived as critical to the success of the treatment. Their argument was that when clients perceive the counselor as a person of authority and expertise—in effect, idealizing the counselor as a person of great wisdom who possesses the key to their feeling better—they are more likely to experience hope that the process will help them. This hope and expectation of a positive outcome strengthens their commitment to the counseling process. For some clients, it

VOICE FROM THE FIELD

I had a client who, in the second session, told me that during the week, he had seen me in town driving a brand new BMW. Not only that, I was in the company of a stunningly beautiful blonde. This was completely his fantasy, and my immediate impulse was to correct him and say, "Well, actually, I drive a pretty beaten-up Honda, and my wife is dark-haired and cute, but I wouldn't say, 'stunningly beautiful.'" Instead, I did the usual counselor thing and asked him what he felt about seeing me in town, feeling a little guilty that I was allowing him to hold on to his illusion. That afternoon,

I rushed into my supervisor's office and asked her what I should do. Surely, I thought, I had to dispel this false impression my client had. To my surprise, she said, "Do nothing. This is his fantasy of someone who has the power to help him, and right now, that fantasy is motivating him to come every week. The day will arrive when he will start to realize you're an imperfect human being like everyone else, and you'll have to empathize with his disappointment. And when he's worked through that, he'll really have grown and your therapy with him will probably be over."

even provides immediate relief from some of their emotional distress. You probably have experienced this phenomenon yourself, when you see a medical doctor who gives you a diagnosis and a prescription; if the physician conveys knowledge and confidence, you are likely to feel better even before the medicine takes effect.

Many practitioners, such as Rogers (1957) and followers, Leslie Greenberg (Greenberg, 2002; Greenberg & Pascual-Leone, 2006), and William R. Miller (Miller & Rollnick, 2002; Arkowitz & Miller, 2008); relational theorists, such as Jean Baker Miller and Judith Jordan (Robb, 2006); and more recently, Scott Miller and colleagues (Duncan, Miller, & Sparks, 2004), try to minimize the power dimensions of the relationship, believing that equality is crucial to change. Feminist approaches to counseling (Brown, 2004; Brown, 2009; Worell & Remer, 2003), as well as narrative ones (Monk, Winslade, Crocket, & Epston, 1997; White & Epston, 1990; White, 2008), conceive of relationships that are especially sensitive to those who have been oppressed by the dominant culture. This is in marked contrast to other practitioners, in particular, family therapists (Haley, 1984, 1989; Haley & Richeport-Haley, 2003; Minuchin, 1974; Minuchin, Lee, & Simon, 2006), who made a strong case that the counselor should deliberately and strategically cultivate a powerful position in order to be more influential. In other words, some counselors find downplaying their status to be effective in facilitating change, whereas others wish to emphasize their capability as powerful models.

Regardless of how power is conceived, almost every practitioner would agree that boundaries play a highly important role in the way that the therapeutic relationship is constructed. These limits exist not only to provide a predictable and reliable environment for clients but also to protect the clients' safety from those counselors who use the client-counselor relationship to meet their own needs.

The therapeutic relationship is also different from other interactions in that there are relatively specific objectives and stringent time limitations: The relationship exists to seek solutions, and the discussion ends once the minute hand of the clock reaches a previously agreed-on point. Thus, in addition to many of the characteristics found in other successful human relationships, the therapeutic relationship has several identifying features.

1. Relationships are the forum for change to take place. Regardless of the theoretical orientation that is preferred or the techniques that are employed, it is the connection between client and counselor that is the basis for all further work.
2. The relationship has an explicit goal and purpose—to end the relationship as soon as possible.
3. There is an understanding that one person (the counselor) has more control, responsibility, and expertise in making things go smoothly and helpfully, whereas the other person (the client) is more important.
4. The relationship is essentially one of interpersonal influence in which the counselor seeks to help promote changes in the client through modeling and helping skills.
5. Counseling relationships exist in a cultural context. They are likely to be more helpful when they are constructed in such a way that respects the values, expectations, and needs of clients and their cultural backgrounds, including ethnicity, socioeconomic class, religion, gender, and other relevant factors.
6. The interactions are structured to make the most efficient use of time.
7. The helping relationship can deal with a variety of human behaviors, thoughts, attitudes, and actions—but is often focused on the expression and exploration of issues that are rarely disclosed outside the encounter.

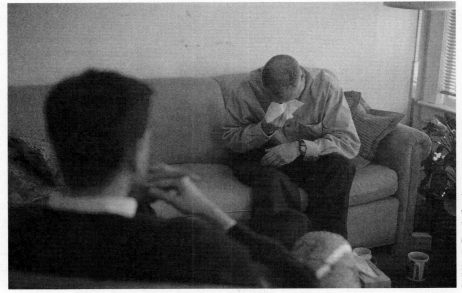

Geoff Manasse/Photodisc/Getty Images.

Counselors develop therapeutic relationships with their clients that are designed to foster trust, openness, mutual respect, and interpersonal influence. Regardless of theoretical orientation, all practitioners are relationship specialists who are highly skilled at creating and fostering the kinds of alliances that best promote lasting change. Ideally, based on this interaction, many clients learn to develop new personal standards of intimacy for all their relationships.

VOICE FROM THE FIELD

Long before I was a counselor, I was first a client. I will never forget what my counselor did for me, even though the ways she helped me were probably different from what she imagined. I can look back and see that she was psychoanalytic, meaning that she was pretty passive and wanted me to talk mostly about my childhood. I was willing to humor her because I just enjoyed having her mother me. Granted, she was a very withholding, coldhearted mother. But that was exactly the kind of relationship I needed at that time in my life.

My guess is that she was basically the same with all her clients. Although I now work very differently than she did with me, using the relationship with my own clients as leverage to push them, I was really grateful for my connection to her. It was probably mostly my own fantasy but it still helped me to regain control of my life. It didn't matter what we talked about in the session, I just really liked that I could count on her to be there for me.

8. Although Rogers's (1969) "core conditions,"—realness, genuineness, freedom, acceptance, trust, prizing, and empathic understanding—are usually found within the relationship, they may not be enough in themselves to promote lasting changes. It is also important to encourage, motivate, structure, and support constructive action.

9. For the relationship to work well, both client and counselor must come to an agreement as to the causes and etiology of the presenting complaints and what must be done to make things better. The most effective relationships are characterized by agreement on goals, consensus on methods, open communication, and a collaborative partnership.

10. The relationship is multidimensional. Most of the features described by various theorists play an important role in the process. Thus, therapeutic relationships are, in part, authentic interactions, as well as "projected" experiences in which both client and counselor distort what is happening between them based on their respective unresolved issues.

11. The relationship is dynamic and changes over time. What is most appropriate in the beginning stages of counseling (authentic engagement) is less important during the working stages when an interactional pattern has developed to accomplish therapeutic tasks. Likewise, as counseling is ending, a return to a more egalitarian relationship is more likely to be helpful than the relationship approach that proved helpful at an earlier stage (Kottler, Sexton, & Whiston, 1994).

What all these points mean is that counselors use research on best practices and combine it with their own experiences, to assess for each client which sort of relationship is going to be optimal for accomplishing stated objectives. Some people in the throes of crisis need a highly supportive relationship in which they can express frightening feelings without fear of judgment and criticism. Other people need a more confrontational relationship to help them translate what they already understand into action. Likewise, relationships can be tailored for each client with an emphasis on things such as:

- Structure or flexibility
- Feelings or thoughts

- Warmth or objective detachment
- Disclosure or planning
- Consistency or novelty
- Exploration or problem solving
- Content or process

There is a beginning stage to all counseling relationships in which the goals are negotiated, and the patterns are established that are most likely to lead a particular client to make needed changes. For some individuals, a highly structured relationship might be best, whereas for others a more flexible pattern is optimal. During the working stage, interactions revolve around attempts to promote alternative ways of functioning, both in the session and in the client's outside world. Finally, in the ending stage, the relationship is designed principally to help the client to generalize results to other areas of life.

PERSPECTIVES ON HELPING RELATIONSHIPS

From whence has come the conception of the therapeutic relationship as we now know it? It is interesting, even if not useful, to understand the origins of how therapeutic relationships evolved to their present forms.

A BIT MORE OF HISTORY

In modern times, helping relationships began within a religious context: Clergy members and other spiritual experts acted as go-betweens in issues between a person and God. The relationship was rigidly defined according to the values of the Middle Ages. At the onset of the Renaissance came Johann Weyer, considered by many to be the world's first psychiatrist. He condemned the archaic witch-purging practices of religious healers and instead extolled the value of a benevolent, kind, and understanding relationship between doctor and patient. A few centuries later, Sigmund Freud also gave considerable attention to the structure of patient-doctor interactions but stressed a more benign, formalized, and unobtrusive relationship. He was, of course, concerned about such things as transference—the fantasy distortions that take place—and warned practitioners of its value and danger.

Historically, the roles within the counseling relationship have not been static. Every theoretical approach you will study in the next chapters has distinct notions about how best to work with clients. Some counselors deliberately encourage dependence in their client relationships, thereby facilitating the transference struggle that Freud found to be so crucial in overcoming unresolved problems with authority. In this type of therapeutic relationship, the counselor remains aloof, dispassionate, and neutral so that the counselor could be a blank slate onto which clients can project their image of a parental authority figure.

From the earliest days of psychoanalysis, it was presumed that a relationship structured around remembering the past is often not enough; it is reexperiencing and reliving prior feelings and impulses that lead to constructive work (Breuer & Freud, 1893). This takes place through a relationship that helps clients access intense, unresolved feelings, express them, and discuss matters nondefensively and objectively (Kahn, 1997).

VOICE FROM THE FIELD

I'm what you'd call a brief therapist, but I've always been uncomfortable with the rather cold and sometimes manipulative aspects of the problem-solving therapies. I'm an old-time humanist from way back when, so when I moved into a job that doesn't give me the time I once had to get to know clients awhile before trying any major interventions, I began to try to preserve my warmth and humanness in sessions even if I saw someone only one or two times.

I've had supervisors tell me that maybe the relationships stuff is more important for meeting my needs than those of my client, and that could be true; I don't deny it. I still think, though, that people are a whole lot more willing to follow through on their homework when they feel some degree of commitment to our relationship. I just don't think you have to choose between being relationship oriented or task oriented. I really think you can do both.

Winnicott (1958), one of the many psychodynamically trained theorists who revised Freud's original prescriptions, spoke of the relationship as a "holding environment" that provides a safe setting with clear boundaries, so that clients feel secure enough to experience their deepest feelings. Winnicott, and later psychodynamic theorists like Gill (1982) and Kernberg (1984), conceptualized the counselor-client relationship as analogous to how a mother holds an upset child in her arms, soothing her with comforting words. In counseling sessions, the boundaries, like a mother's arms, provide a supportive structure, while the counselor's empathy soothes an emotionally overwhelmed client.

CONGRUENCE, POSITIVE REGARD, AND EMPATHY

In marked contrast to this rather structured sort of relationship, Carl Rogers was instrumental in defining a type of alliance with people based on nurturance, warmth, genuineness, respect, and authenticity. This relationship is a mutual involvement, a sharing of feelings in an open, accepting atmosphere; the counselor accepts responsibility not only for creating these fertile conditions but also for communicating his or her own attitudes and feelings within the session. In his personal vision for creating an ideal relationship in counseling, Rogers (1961) explains: "I would like my feelings in this relationship with him to be as clear and transparent as possible, so that they are a discernible reality for him to which he can return again and again" (p. 67).

Rogers (1951) followed his early theorizing about the importance of the counseling relationship with a series of research studies during the 1950s and 1960s in which he attempted to develop some empirical evidence for his ideas. The results of these research efforts led him to conclude that there were several major characteristics of the helping relationship (Rogers, 1957):

1. *Congruence.* Rogers believed that congruence is the most important ingredient in the helping relationship and encouraged counselors to work toward developing more congruence between what they are feeling on the inside and what they are communicating on the outside.
2. *Positive regard.* This means that the counselor does not evaluate and judge clients' actions or statements; behavior is viewed neutrally, and all people are worthy of respect.

VOICE FROM THE FIELD

Hands down, the hardest client I ever had was in my internship, a young male musician with a childhood ruined by physical abuse that had affected his ability to control his emotions. I mean, if you didn't say the right thing to him, he'd go from calm to rage, with no stops in between. He was an imposing man, so when he raged—and he would frequently go off in a session—it was scary. He'd been coming to this agency for years, and had become a legend among the interns, most of whom felt sorry for me. Except for one—his former therapist, a wonderfully talented counselor who was just completing her last internship hours. "Just create a good holding environment for him," she told me. "That's all he needs. Don't do anything fancy. Begin on time, end on time, and when he yells, use your basic listening skills." "That's it?" I said, not believing it could be that simple. But it worked. He'd yell and curse, and I'd say, "You're feeling very angry now … and you want to make sure I understand how upset you are." I'd just do stuff like that, session after session, and gradually he felt safe enough to explore his issues with me without all the fireworks.

3. *Empathy.* This denotes the process of attempting to understand, from the client's frame of reference, the thoughts and feelings underlying behavior—that is, the ability to walk around in the client's shoes and know how he or she feels.

Although there are very few pure Rogerian practitioners today, his legacy emphasizing a caring, respectful, supportive relationship lives on. There are times when almost any counselor will resort to a person-centered relationship, especially when clients most need to feel heard and understood.

WORKING ALLIANCE

A third position is the no-nonsense instructional model of the relationship in cognitive or behavioral or other brief forms of counseling. The practitioner creates a businesslike contract with the client to meet certain specific goals, with an action plan for reaching them. In these circumstances the relationship becomes an encounter between teacher and student. The main purpose of such an affiliation is to ensure compliance with the agreed-on treatment plan. Obviously, clients will be more likely to follow through on their stated objectives when they feel some degree of commitment to the relationship.

Among a number of brief therapists (Ecker & Hulley, 1996; Quick, 1996), attempts at compromise have been undertaken in which issues related to trust and empathy are considered important—but only to the extent that they can be fostered rather quickly and efficiently. Like any other facet of helping, much depends on exactly what clients are looking for and what they need in order to feel safe enough to present themselves honestly.

Researchers have also explored the counseling relationship from other perspectives. Strong and Claiborn (1982), for example, have argued that the interpersonal influence variables of perceived expertness, attractiveness, and trustworthiness all affect the counselor's ability to facilitate change in clients. The relationship is viewed as the vehicle for establishing power and influence (Hackney & Cormier, 2005).

MULTIPLE MODELS OF RELATIONSHIP

In another increasingly popular paradigm, constructivists such as Anderson and Goolishian (1992); Epston, White, and Murray (1992); and Gergen and Kaye (1992) have formulated helping relationships in terms of the language and belief systems that clients bring to the encounter. All social interactions, including those that take place in counseling, are co-constructed by the participants based on their interpretations of their experiences. These internal "narratives" are altered by the dialogues that take place—conversations that are aimed at helping clients to change the ways they interpret their realities. This sort of relationship often evolves into a very active sort of collaboration in which both client and counselor try to educate each other about their respective views.

Feminist theory is also having its impact on the ways we consider gender differences as they affect therapeutic relationships. DeYoung (2003), for example, speaks of the distinctly female way that relationships can be constructed. With a greater commitment to caring and connection rather than to distinctly "male" values of competition and autonomy, quite another kind of relationship develops in the feminist theory–based counseling process, one that emphasizes greater intimacy.

While there is general agreement that regardless of orientation, a strong counselor-client relationship is a necessary foundation for client growth, theorists and researchers continually debate whether the relationship is sufficient as a change agent. The corollary question then becomes what role specific theories and interventions play in effecting change. Given the number of theories in this field, and the even larger number of vociferous proponents of each, this is no small issue; some people's careers are invested in proving that one theory (the theory they like) is better than another. Moreover, trend in the field towards evidence-based practice is exerting an increasing pressure on counselors to use theories proven by research studies to work. Such pressure makes this debate more than an academic exercise; it is a serious matter for all counselors.

At one end of the continuum are those who believe the relationship alone is the primary change-producing element in counseling. First developed by the psychodynamic theorists Alexander and French in the 1940s (Alexander & French, 1980), this line of thinking suggests that a counseling relationship provides for a *corrective emotional experience* that repairs clients' childhood wounds stemming from problematic or hurtful relational interactions with their parents.

Clients are presumed to enter counseling with unconscious expectations that they will be treated in ways similar to the ways they were treated by the first authority figures in their lives, their parents or primary caregivers. For example, if a person grew up with critical parents whom he or she could never please, that client would anticipate that eventually the counselor would also be critical of the client's behaviors. If a client experienced abandonment trauma because of a parental divorce, the client would expect that sooner or later he or she will be abandoned by the counselor, who might abruptly refer the client to another counselor, or tell the client she or he was too difficult to work with. As the counseling progresses, the client becomes increasingly aware that these fears will never be realized; the counselor will be a nonjudgmental, consistently available, compassionate listener regardless of what the client does or says. The counseling relationship is thus said to be a corrective emotional experience, in which clients let go of their ingrained, self-critical expectations and learn more flexible ways of relating both to the counselor and to other people in their lives (Teyber, 2006).

The corrective emotional experience concept is an especially appealing one for novice counselors because it implies that a relationship based on positive regard, empathy, congruence, and a strong working alliance is all you need to help your clients. And there may be some truth to that notion based on our personal experiences as counselors and counselor educators. Well before we mastered a specific theory or technique, during a time when relating effectively to a client was really all we had to offer, we witnessed our clients growing. We see the same phenomenon with our students in their first internship, where they are undeniably making a difference in their clients' lives.

At the same time, we cannot ignore the evidence of numerous studies that demonstrate the efficacy of one theory or intervention over another. In particular the cognitive behavioral theories (which will be discussed in Chapter 6) deemphasize the role of the relationship and yet have an impressive record of success with numerous client concerns, including depression, anxiety, post-traumatic stress, even pain relief. Advocates of these approaches, sometimes referred to as *empirically supported treatments (ESTs)*, would argue that while the relationship may be necessary for eliciting client cooperation with the counselor, it is the counselor's strategies that produce improvement.

The middle ground in this debate is to take the *common factors approach*, which suggests that, though the relationship is one of the curative or growth-enhancing components of all effective counseling (regardless of what theory or strategies are employed), specific interventions also play a role. Research into common factors has found that the relationship accounts for about 30% of client improvement in adults and children; interventions account for 15%; and the rest of the change is due to the placebo effect (i.e., client's expectations of change) and extratherapeutic factors taking place in the client's outside life (Lambert, 1992; Shirk & Karver, 2003). Other research has demonstrated that the quality of the working alliance is the most robust predictor of counseling's effectiveness (Beutler, Machado, & Neufeldt, 1994; Castonguay, Constantino, & Holtforth, 2006; Karver, Handelsman, Fields, & Bickman, 2005; Marmarosh et al., 2009). Regardless of the size of its role, the counseling relationship is a special and necessary aspect of the counseling encounter. At the same time, we believe that although the importance of the relationship is well documented, a helping relationship in and of itself is not a sufficient condition for behavioral change; it is a means to another end. As Egan (2007) has pointed out, putting too much attention on the importance of the therapeutic relationship can be as detrimental as ignoring it altogether. The purpose of all helping is to assist clients in managing their lives better. Certainly this goal is more easily achieved if the client and counselor work well together.

COUNSELORS AS RELATIONSHIP SPECIALISTS

The helping relationship can be defined as a systematic and intentional attempt, using a specified cluster of interpersonal skills, to assist another person to make self-determined improvements in behavior, feelings, or thoughts. Whereas daily

VOICE FROM THE FIELD

I consider myself a relationship-oriented counselor, at least when there is enough time allocated for us to get to know one another. I feel closer to some of the people I see than some of my friends, and I'm a little embarrassed to admit that. But as much as I value the power of a helping relationship to offer support and grounding to a client, I know that sometimes it is not enough. There's a teenager I'm seeing now and we have this fabulous relationship. He confides in me, and tells me everything going on in his life. He trusts me implicitly. He likes me, and I like him as well. Unfortunately, he is still doing the same stupid, crazy things in his life that he was when he first came to me. I keep pleading with his parents to let me keep working with him, and so far they are giving me a little more time, but I know that soon they are going to yank him out of the sessions. It'll be a shame, but I have to admit that while we do relate well together, I still haven't been able to help him change his destructive patterns.

helping encounters such as those between parent and child, teacher and student, or supervisor and employee could also be included, it is primarily counselors who are specialists in developing these nurturing and productive encounters. May (1983) preferred the term *presence* to describe the counselor's real alliance with a client, who is less an object to be analyzed than a being to be understood. Yalom (1980), as well, states that the single most important lesson for a beginning counselor to learn is that "it is the relationship that heals" (p. 401). The therapeutic involvement with the counselor symbolically illuminates other relationships in the client's life, besides providing the opportunity for a real, caring, respectful encounter with someone who is safe. The client feels minimal danger of seduction, manipulation, or betrayal, for the stated bounds of the interaction provide for protection of privacy, confidentiality, trust, and benevolence. It is at once both refreshing and frightening to be involved with a professional who is expert at listening and nonpossessive caring.

The therapeutic relationship helps the client work through feelings of isolation, a condition that the existentialists such as Cooper (2003) and Yalom (2008) consider the "universal symptom" of humanity. The only cure is communication with someone who is sensitive, receptive, neutral, interested, and psychologically healthy. Imagine the deep pleasure, satisfaction, freedom—the complete and total freedom—to be genuinely open with another person who is doing everything within his or her power to subjugate personal needs and focus only on *you*. For one uninterrupted hour you have the absolute attention, full concentration, and vast resources of a specialist in building relationships. This person is caring yet honest, fully capable of perceiving things beyond your awareness and explaining things beyond your understanding. This is a relationship you can truly depend on and use as a model for the kinds of experiences you deserve.

Yalom (1980) further explains that, although the therapeutic relationship is only temporary, the experience of intimacy endures. The key to developing such a meaningful encounter, irrespective of technique, is through the full engagement with the client in the present moment:

> I listen to a woman patient. She rambles on and on. She seems unattractive in every sense of the word—physically, intellectually, emotionally. She is irritating. She has

▮ | VOICE FROM THE FIELD

I'll never forget this couple from India I once saw. They came in, sat down, and waited patiently for me to fix them. I explained what it is that I did in marriage counseling and how I did it. They nodded, then once again told me that they wanted me, as the expert, to tell them what the problem was and then to fix it. Again I explained that I didn't work that way, that my job was to help them to sort out things for themselves. Blah, blah, blah.

They were very polite and understanding but still insisted that I tell them what to do. In their country, that is how healers and helpers operate—they give advice that is expected to be followed to the letter. In exasperation, I finally said, "Okay, here's the deal," and then I proceeded to violate everything I ever learned about doing counseling. They listened carefully. The husband even took notes. Then they thanked me, promised they would do what I asked, and walked out, completely satisfied customers.

I always remember that case when I start out with a new client. It's so important to realize that people have so many different cultural expectations for what helping relationships should be like.

many off-putting gestures. She is not talking to me; she is talking in front of me. Yet how can she talk to me if I am not here? My thoughts wander. My head groans. What time is it? How much longer to go? I suddenly rebuke myself. I give my mind a shake.

Whenever I think of how much time remains in the hour, I know I am failing my patient. I try then to touch her with my thoughts. I try to understand why I avoid her. What is her world like at this moment? How is she experiencing the hour? How is she experiencing me? I ask her these very questions. I tell her that I have felt distant from her for the last several minutes. Has she felt the same way? We talk about that together and try to figure out why we lost contact with one another. Suddenly we are very close. She is no longer unattractive. I have much compassion for her person, for what she is, for what she might yet be. The clock races: the hour ends too soon. (p. 415)

In addition to sharing the attitude implicit in Yalom's moving statement, counselors are quite skilled in their ability to foster helping relationships with a wide diversity of people. Depending on the client's ethnicity, religious and spiritual convictions, gender, cultural and family background, and prior experiences, quite different sorts of relationships are indicated.

Counselors must, of course, be consistent in their ability to create constructive relationships with anyone who walks in the door. This skill and attitude take practice as well as an openness to new people. The place to start, naturally, is in your own personal life. To what extent are you able to relate to people from all walks of life?

In their study of human relationships, a number of writers found that a series of specific skills will allow you to initiate, maintain, and nurture your connections to others. Because this repertoire of behaviors is so crucial to conducting counseling successfully, they recommend that beginning students assess their degree of competence in each of several areas. For each of these categories, a few skills are listed that are considered most significant in creating solid counseling relationships. Read through the list on the next page and consider the degree to which you can improve your effectiveness in each of the broad categories.

As you read through your self-ratings on these items, especially those marked with a 1 or 2, you will see where you most need to improve. It is hardly expected

were better choices. You will feel disappointed in yourself about what you missed, about how awkwardly you phrased something, and about your own sense of competence. Somehow you will have to learn patience—not only with others, but with yourself.

Anxiety/fear. You will fail in your efforts to be helpful. Some of this will occur because of bungling on your part—miscalculations, misdiagnoses, miscues, mistakes, and misjudgments. Other times, you will have to accept that you are not fully responsible for the outcomes in counseling—much depends on the client's efforts as well. It is not only reasonable, but unavoidable, that you will live with a certain fear about screwing up and hurting clients. This is not altogether a bad thing if it keeps you cautious and humble.

Elation/excitement. We saved the best for last. When you are doing counseling during your training and early years, much of the time you will feel utter joy. You will pinch yourself as a reminder of how lucky and privileged you are to share transformative journeys with your clients and to spend time with them. These are sacred moments to be savored. Therapeutic relationships are not only educational encounters but spiritually transcendent ones in which both parties are moved by the experience.

EXPERIENCING THE THERAPEUTIC RELATIONSHIP AS A CLIENT

The best way of all to get a sense of the power of therapeutic relationships, and the corresponding features just mentioned, is to experience it firsthand as a client. Some programs require you to participate in counseling as a condition of admission or graduation. The reasoning is that it is very difficult to get a sense of how counseling works if you have not sat in the client's chair.

Reading about counseling relationships is one thing. Studying the research and literature on their effects is another. Even hearing testimony from practitioners and clients about the therapeutic relationship is educational. But none of these can replace what you could learn as a client yourself.

Apart from whatever personal issues you would have the opportunity to work on, or which interpersonal skills you identified earlier that you are in need of improving, you would be truly amazed at how wonderful it feels to be in counseling as a client. You may have already experienced this before, with a special teacher or mentor, but there is something almost sacred and magical about what happens in counseling.

In order to teach your clients how to get the most from the experience you must be an expert yourself on how to be a good consumer of counseling services. If you have been in counseling yourself, then you know the games that clients play, you know the reluctance they sometimes feel, you know their struggles and inner conflicts. You know what works best and worst. Most of all, you know the power of what can happen in such a relationship.

If you have not yet seen a counselor for any length of time, we would highly recommend that you obtain this experience some time before you graduate. Among all the books we have read (and written) about counseling, all the degrees we've attained, the workshops and seminars attended, the demonstration videos watched,

The first time I went to a counselor it was for career counseling, or so I thought. I wasn't happy in my present job, but wasn't sure what else I wanted to do, and a friend suggested I see this woman—a counselor who was good with career issues. Well, I was in for a surprise. The counselor was a small, red-haired woman in her 40s, sitting comfortably in a rocker with a Navajo shawl around her shoulders—nothing at all like what I expected. After listening patiently to my ramblings about job stuff, she said in this gentle voice I will never forget, "You have this lost look in your eyes, and I suspect you've had it since you were a little boy. What happened to you?" I wept—feeling both seen, and somehow soothed, in a way that seemed astonishing. Years later, when I became a counselor, I realized that the way I used my own voice in a session was just like hers. More than anything else in all my training, learning how therapists speak and sound was the best lesson I ever learned, and I only learned it because of the work I did with her.

the conversations had with colleagues, and the supervision received from mentors, nothing was as valuable to us as the counseling relationships we've known with half a dozen clinicians during our lives.

CREATING A RELATIONSHIP IN THE INITIAL INTERVIEW

Some of the theory and research underlying the counseling relationship has been reviewed. The characteristics, components, and skills essential to these relationships can be identified. Each of these individual aspects, however, must be integrated into the person of the counselor during the interview with the client. The integration process is crucial, because the relationship variables will define the context and texture of the interaction that follows. The initial interview provides the opportunity to operationalize relationship skills and provides the first test of the effectiveness of counseling.

One of the first counseling procedures you will learn is how to conduct an initial interview that will begin building a solid relationship with your clients and to collect relevant information that you will need in formulating a diagnosis and treatment plan. If you have not already had the opportunity to do so, it would be a very good idea for you to begin practicing interview skills. This can be as simple as asking someone what he or she would like to talk about and then probing with a few questions here and there. Or, it can be a far more elaborate and systematic procedure in which you follow a detailed set of guidelines over the course of a 90-minute intake process. Regardless of the setting and clinical situation, your initial contact with a client is likely to cover several important areas.

ESTABLISHING RULES

The relationship between client and counselor is established in the very first encounter. Even before the first words are spoken, the two size each other up, assessing the other's personal competence. The client, usually confused and nervous, will wait for the professional to begin and to define the parameters and tone for the

VOICE FROM THE FIELD

For years, I felt constantly caught in a vortex about my sexual orientation. If I "come out" to people who are close but can't handle my sexuality, then I lose so much. I don't want to be a pariah. I just want what everyone else wants: happiness, partnership, fulfillment, and a chance to contribute. So I went into counseling.

What did I learn from the experience? To face myself, to sit with pain, not to run away from it. Being alone is okay now and I quite enjoy the aloneness and my own discovery. It's certainly better than frantically searching out the next relationship just to fill a void!

Was it useful? Counseling is a good tool for the strong at heart but not for those whose commitment to life wavers. At the end of the day, it's so bloody hard to sit and think about yourself, warts and all, with someone else in the room, with that person determined not to take your pain away from you. That's what I went for. I didn't want life the way it was for me. That's why it's hard. Feeling like an outcast who can't speak about who he loves, except in secret.

sessions. The counselor also bides his or her time, knowing how crucial the first interchange will be to the entire therapeutic process. If ineffective or unsuccessful, the result will be unforgiving: The client will not return for more counseling. Worse yet, the client may return, but with grossly distorted perceptions of what will be involved in the future.

Perhaps the client will view the relationship as unequal, seeing the counselor, an expert, as the authority, the parent, the controller. The client may then adopt behavior appropriate to that situation, showing deference and asking questions. Transference, power, and dependence variables will exert themselves as in other unequal relationships, such as those between parent and child, boss and employee, and, often, doctor and patient.

The client could also perceive the relationship as mostly equal, especially if the counselor introduces himself or herself by first name and does not respond with formal detachment. In this case the client will adapt to the situation and internally define the relationship according to his or her perceptions: "The counselor recognizes that we are equal, that what I have to say is intelligent and important, but we both really understand that I need help and I'm here because the counselor can offer it."

The initial interview, therefore, serves the function of creating and communicating rules for future interactions that are likely to be beneficial to a productive relationship. It establishes the norms for appropriate conduct and capitalizes on the trust, respect, acceptance, and warmth that are so much a part of the therapeutic encounter.

Remember, the client doesn't know how to be a "good" partner in this process; it is your job to teach the person about how to get the most from the experience. This starts with establishing appropriate norms for behavior.

PLANTING HOPE

The client is often motivated to make an appointment out of a sense of helplessness. People rarely pay money, risk embarrassment, or inconvenience themselves

VOICE FROM THE FIELD

I never have an adolescent show up at the door seeking help. It just hasn't happened to me. So if they're there, it's because somebody else is making them come—a parent or teacher or somebody. So now I have to be up front with them in the very first session, and I've got about 15 minutes to grab their attention.

"I know there must be some problem," I tell them, "or you wouldn't be here. It's not my job to change you. I don't even think you need to be fixed. You can make that choice for yourself. At this point, I just want to find out who you are. After we get to know each other, then we can look at some aspects of your life that you might want to change. That's up to you." Saying something like that usually works for me. They appreciate me being honest. They can tell I'm not playing games. That makes whatever else we do together a lot easier.

to visit a professional if there is another way to resolve their concerns. Counseling is usually the last resort, the final step before self-destructive acts are likely to occur.

Clients show up at the first session ambivalent about their behavior and unable to trust their feelings. They want help; they want to change. Yet they have also invested themselves in preserving the status quo and will therefore often resist, on some level, the interventions of the counselor. They want reassurance, easy solutions to their problems, and simple answers to their complicated questions. But most of all they want to believe that they can learn to trust themselves. Clients want to hope that working for the future is worthwhile. They want to believe in their capacity to make needed changes in their lives. They want to hope that, eventually, their pain will diminish and will someday be replaced by something better. Clients have hope that we, as professionals, know what we're doing, that we actually can make a difference. Therefore, favorable expectations for treatment, consistent with what can be delivered, must be quickly established in the initial interview.

This could sound something like the following introduction:

I am so glad that you came to see me at this time. Although I can see how much you are suffering, and what a difficult struggle you are going through right now, I want to assure you that this pain does not have to last much longer. In fact, I am willing to venture that you are already feeling better since you showed up here. It feels good to tell somebody else about what is going on and to know that you have been heard and understood.

Although I can't give you any guarantees about how long it will take to resolve your problems, since much of that depends on you, I can tell you that I have helped a lot of other people who have presented similar issues. I would expect that you will notice some improvement within a very short period of time.

Of course, you don't want to make promises you can't keep, or exaggerate what you can deliver. But it is important to let the client know that relief is on the way. While you are an intern and novice counselor, it will feel disingenuous to say, "I've dealt with this issue many times before." But you can legitimately tell clients, "I'm well trained in helping clients resolve issues like yours."

ASSURING CONFIDENTIALITY

Confidentiality is the verbal contract between two people in which the counselor promises to keep private the communications heard in counseling and the client agrees to believe the promise. Unless such an understanding and basic level of trust can be reached, it is unlikely that the relationship can proceed any further.

For this reason the issue of confidentiality is always discussed early in the initial interview, both to allay fears about how private the sessions will be and to convince the client that the relationship will be safe and sacred, impervious to the questions of a curious parent, spouse, employer, or judge. The counseling relationship thus begins with a mutual commitment—that of the counselor to work ethically and competently in the best interest of the client while safeguarding privacy, and that of the client to be as open, truthful, and self-revealing as possible. These commitments will form the temporary bond of the relationship until real respect and intimacy evolve as a function of working together.

ASSESSING EXPECTATIONS

Often in conjunction with delivering a statement about confidentiality, the counselor further defines the therapeutic relationship to ensure that both parties enter into the verbal contract in ways that will be compatible and satisfying. Clients can come to the first session with fairly outlandish notions about what is possible, probable, or likely to occur. These unrealistic expectations may include any of the following:

- "I talk. You listen. Then you talk. I listen. We take turns until one of us gets too bored."
- "I tell you my problems. Then you tell me yours. Afterward, I can figure out what I should do by what you have done."
- "I tell you my dreams and then you tell me what they mean."
- "You're like a lie detector. Whenever I don't tell the truth or exaggerate a little bit, or go through my standard lines, you interrupt me and tell me I'm full of crap."
- "You give me a tissue and hold my hand and tell me everything will be okay. That's what a helpful person should do."
- "I tell you my problems. You tell me what to do so I can change situations that keep me from getting what I want."
- "You agree with me that it's mostly other people's fault that I don't get what I want."

Then, there will be those clients who have had unsatisfying experiences with previous counselors, and their expectations may have some basis in reality:

- "I'll talk and all you'll do is repeat whatever I say."
- "You'll give me lots of support, but never challenge me."
- "You'll be more interested in telling stories and talking about yourself than in listening to me."
- "I'll ramble on, boring myself and boring you, and you'll never stop me."

Images of a friend, father confessor, nurturing mother, lover, consultant, teacher, and coach all emerge in the client's mind as models for what the therapeutic relationship will be like. Many of the misconceptions and distorted expectations can be cleared up after they are discussed in the interview. As the counselor explains what counseling is and how and why it works, the client's images can be modified to reflect a more accurate portrayal. In this process, client and counselor discuss who will do what, in what order, and what is likely to happen as a result of the fulfillment of these expectations. By the time this component of the initial interview is over, both client and counselor should have negotiated a mutually agreeable set of goals for what will take place.

COLLECTING INFORMATION

Before the counselor can really go to work, some form of data collection usually needs to take place in the first interview. The extent and depth of this activity will depend on the theory to which the practitioner subscribes; a psychoanalytic counselor might spend several entire sessions creating a history, whereas a strategic counselor would devote much less time, limiting the focus to specific information about the presenting problem.

Other models for collecting relevant background information about a client's environment are available, most including some preliminary explorations into the client's development, the evolution of the problem, and a description of self-defeating behaviors. In addition, the counselor should find out which solutions have already been tried and why the client is seeking help at this particular time. Finally, a history is usually collected of relevant medical information, family background, and developmental issues that may be related to the presenting complaints.

Most clinicians have a list of favorite questions for eliciting useful information about how the client characteristically functions. Insightful queries can also create greater intimacy, openness, self-disclosure, and trust in the relationship. The following questions often facilitate the self-examination process and produce valuable data for the counselor. Simultaneously, the client begins to experience the excitement and discomfort of looking inward. Answer these questions for yourself as you review them:

- Who are the most important people in your world, and how do you spend time winning their approval?
- Who else knows that you are having this difficulty, and what will you tell them?
- What is your favorite part of each day?
- When you feel a lot of pressure, what kinds of things do you usually do to calm yourself?
- When are the specific times in your daily life in which you feel most uncomfortable and out of control?

One of the most useful first-session questions, originally developed by the theoretical school known as "solution-focused therapy," is the miracle question, and has become incorporated into the repertoire of many counselors, regardless of

VOICE FROM THE FIELD

Good counselors are nosy. We ask lots of questions, sometimes directly, but most often we just probe to get things going. One of the best ways I learned how to ask effective questions was by trying things out in my personal life. I get bored at parties anyway and I'm impatient with small talk, so at social gatherings I try to get things going by challenging others to ask me any question they want and, within reason, I'll answer it honestly. There are a few exceptions, of course, but I've learned with practice that there is hardly anything that I won't talk about. Then we each take turns trying to come up with better and better questions designed to get people to be revealing. My favorite one of all is: "What is the one question you're most afraid I'll ask?" Then I ask them to answer it.

orientation. The miracle question's effectiveness lies in its insistence on clients' visualizing what it is they are really seeking in their life, rather than on just describing everything that is wrong. It goes like this:

> Suppose you were to go home tonight, and while you were asleep, a miracle happened and this problem was solved. How will you know the miracle happened? What will be different? (De Shazer, 1988, p. 5)

Regardless of the questions or data-collecting model selected, the counselor's intention in the initial interview is to complete a preliminary inventory of the client's complaints, symptoms, and concerns.

IDENTIFYING PROBLEMS

Professional ethics, as well as most agencies, require counselors to develop an initial diagnosis, using the technical terms spoken by all mental health professionals. However, because counselors aren't restricted to a medical model that limits labels to categories of psychopathology, they are also able to concentrate on identifying the specific behavior patterns that may relate to the client's problems. The counselor initially tries to summarize the client's concerns so that the client feels understood. Then, counselor and client collaborate on formulating goals in terms that are specific, realistic, and achievable. Regardless of which diagnostic model is employed (see Chapter 8) the intention is to take inventory of all the areas in which the client may need work and to prioritize which ones will be the focus first.

BEGINNING INTERVENTION

In addition to the traditional uses of the initial interview for beginning the therapeutic relationship and collecting useful information, Kovacs (1982) feels that other goals take even greater precedence. The counselor must intervene in the very first session on some level "to make at least a small dent in the stasis into which the patient has been locked for some time now" (p. 148). Counseling starts immediately in the first session. It is not enough merely to initiate the relationship, fill out forms, set goals, or create structure. These steps are but the means of bringing a sense of commitment to the counseling relationship.

Especially in today's climate of brief therapy and pressure from managed care organizations, it is crucial that some sort of intervention or actual counseling take place in the first session. This can be as simple as a mild confrontation or exploration of the client's thoughts and feelings, or can involve a more elaborate strategy to initiate the treatment plan. Much depends on how much time you have allocated with a client. If you think this may be a relatively long-term case (more than eight sessions), then you have the luxury of using the first session to gather information and then plan interventions in later sessions. If, however, this will be a brief relationship (less than three or four sessions), then you must begin the therapeutic strategy right away. Regardless of the length of treatment, keep in mind that a client will not return for a second appointment if the first one is perceived as less than satisfactory.

FIRST-SESSION AGENDA REVIEW

It's normal for beginning counselors to experience anxiety, if not sheer terror, with their first several clients. While you would not want to bring a "cheat sheet" into a session with a list of everything you want to ask, it is necessary to accomplish certain tasks, including the following:

Opening. Counselors begin the first exchange with a client in different ways, according to the age, gender, and cultural background of the client, and personal style of the counselor. But within the first few minutes, you need to "officially" begin the interview with open-ended questions, like "What's going on?" or "How can I help you?"

Route. Find out through which avenue the client decided to seek help, how the decision was made, and why this particular choice was made.

Reason. Find out why the client is deciding to get help now. This question often elicits important information about a specific event in the client's life that's triggered a feeling of crisis and desperation.

Experience in counseling. Ascertain whether the client has had any previous experience with counseling. If so, ask who she or he has seen and what it was like.

Expectations. Explore what the client's expectations are for treatment. Do they relate to previous counseling experiences? What does the client believe will happen?

Definition. Correct any misconceptions and unrealistic expectations by providing a definition of counseling, detailing how the process works.

Confidentiality. Discuss confidentiality in an effort to establish trust.

Search for content. Identify areas appropriate for counseling content, including problem presentation, self-destructive behavior, and unresolved conflicts.

Important people. Explore the people most important in the client's world, especially those who have a vested interest in the treatment outcome.

■ | VOICE FROM THE FIELD

I used to always begin the first session with a slow, calming voice, designed to show that I was this sensitive, super-compassionate counselor. It got to the point that I was almost doing a parody of what a counselor sounds like. One day I was talking to a friend who was telling me about an experience she had with a new counselor. "I couldn't stand her," she said. "I'd gone to see her because I felt depressed, and all I needed was a little perspective, someone to remind me that my depression was normal and would go away. But she treated me with that serious, heavy, counselor's voice, like I was in agony and she was as depressed as I was. So I'm not going back." From that point forward, I've learned to start sessions more upbeat, with a little energy and excitement about meeting a new person. Misery loves company, but not when the company is your counselor.

Functional levels. Assess the functional level of the client across a broad spectrum of behaviors—intelligence, resilience, confidence, exercise, sleeping and eating routines, dexterity, perceptual and cognitive capacities, life skills, and values.

Structure. Determine a structure for the particular client and counseling situation that will make significant progress likely to occur.

Commitment. Secure a commitment from the client to both change and work toward counseling goals.

Goals. Specifically work with the client to define realistic goals for the counseling that can be reduced to subgoals for and between future sessions.

Summary. Have the client evaluate what his or her perceptions and feelings are about the first session.

Closing. End the first session, solidify the relationship, and set future appointments.

This list may seem comprehensive, and it does include quite a number of elements, but this still doesn't cover all the territory. You would hardly be expected to cover all these features in one session, but they do form a rough structure for how you would proceed. By way of summary, your principal job as a counselor is to create an alliance with your clients in which you establish a degree of trust and intimacy. This must be done efficiently and effectively or your clients will develop unrealistic expectations—or they won't come back.

The steps of an initial interview translate into several core therapeutic tasks: (1) establishing a bond between you and your client, (2) providing preliminary information regarding what counseling is and how it works, (3) assessing client issues and expectations, (4) instilling a sense of hope, and (5) obtaining a commitment to be patient and to work hard in the sessions. From these humble beginnings, the success of all future counseling efforts is firmly established.

■ | VOICE FROM THE FIELD

This woman had come into counseling, referred to me because I'm a male. She needed to decide whether to stay with a husband who was cheating on her. He'd been her high school boyfriend, they got married in college, and had now been together for almost 30 years. And he had been seeing other women during the whole time. So now my client is telling me this story about how her father left her and her mother when my client was nine, and how her mom started smoking pot pretty heavily, and my client had to undress her every night and put her to sleep. And I had this image of this little girl trying so hard to drag her mother into bed, and my eyes watered, and I couldn't hide it.

I asked her, "Did you see me tear up just now?" "Yes," she said, her voice soft, almost inaudible. "What was it like for you?" I asked. "I got it that there are men out there who do care about me," she said. I could feel an initial rush of gratification, a little too much to my ego, probably—and then a frightening sense of responsibility. Followed by humility. And then, just sadness for her. I think that's what it means to be a relational counselor. Techniques are great, but they also keep you at a distance. Being relational means getting close, and, believe me, it can be intense. But do I love it? Yes.

SUMMARY

Considering the energy, motivation, courage, and desperation required for a client to initiate the first appointment, anxiety during the first encounter is usually quite high. This initial interaction in the counseling relationship is marked by fear—fear of what might or might not happen; fear that there is no cure; fear that there is a cure but that it will involve a lot of work; fear that the counselor might tell someone else about the session; fear about what friends, family, even the receptionist might think about the fact that the client needs help; fear of revealing deeply guarded secrets; and perhaps most of all, fear of entering into an intense human relationship.

That the counselor is able, often within the first few minutes, to relieve a client's apprehensions is a testimony to the consummate skill of the professional who is experienced at relationship building. Everything in the easy manner and the calm self-confidence of the counselor indicates that this is a person who is comfortable with intimacy. The soft smile, soothing voice, relaxed posture, and interested eyes all communicate an authenticity that helps the client trust, open up, and feel prized. Rapport is developed not by accident, nor by magic, but by the deliberate efforts of the well-trained counselor who understands the core conditions of nurturance in human relationships and can create them at will.

SELF-GUIDED EXPLORATIONS

1. Describe one of the most influential helping relationships you have ever experienced. What was it about this relationship that was so powerful and influential?
2. One important skill involved in building therapeutic relationships is asking open-ended, exploratory questions. If you could ask a stranger only three questions and had to give a lengthy talk on the essence of what this person is like based on the answers given, what questions would you ask?
3. Answer the questions you just created.
4. Describe the relationship that is most conflicted in your life right now. Then, to work through your difficulty, follow these steps for resolving conflicted relationships:
   a. What most often acts as a trigger for the conflict to begin or escalate?

b. How is this present conflict familiar to you in terms of other difficulties you have experienced in the past?

c. What are the hidden benefits for you in this conflict?

d. In what ways are you disowning responsibility for your share of the problem?

e. What do you vow to do to change the ways you react to the situation?

f. What are some of the creative strategies you might try to break through the impasse?

For Homework

The "Hot Seat" is an exercise in which participants agree to answer any question asked of them as honestly as they can. It is used to build intimacy in groups, but also to train counselors to ask good probing questions that collect valuable information and promote insight. Take the questions you generated in this chapter as a starting point and practice deepening your primary relationships. Take turns with friends or family members asking questions and then answering them.

Write down a few of the favorite questions that you want to remember to use in the future.

Suggested Readings

Brammer, L. M., & MacDonald, G. (2007). *The helping relationship* (9th ed.). Boston: Allyn & Bacon.

Cochran, J. L., & Cochran, N. H. (2005). *The heart of counseling: A guide to developing therapeutic relationships.* Belmont, CA: Wadsworth.

Cowan, E. W. (2005). *Ariadne's thread: Case studies in the therapeutic relationship.* Boston: Lahaska Press.

Egan, G. (2007). *The skilled helper: A problem management and opportunity developmental approach to helping* (8th ed.). Belmont, CA: Brooks/Cole.

Gelso, C. J., & Hayes, J. A. (1998). *The psychotherapy relationship: Theory, research, and practice.* New York: John Wiley & Sons.

Hubble, M. A., Duncan, B. C., & Miller, S. D. (Eds.). (1999). *The heart and soul of change: What works in therapy.* Washington, DC: American Psychological Association.

Keeney, B. (2009). *The creative therapist: The art of awakening a session.* New York: Routledge.

Rogers, C. R. (1980). *A way of being.* Boston: Houghton Mifflin.

Rosenthal, H. (2004). *Before you see your first client: Fifty-five things that counselors, therapists, and human service providers need to know.* New York: Routledge.

Counseling Approaches

INSIGHT-ORIENTED APPROACHES

CHAPTER 5

KEY CONCEPTS

Good theories

Constructivist approach

Feminist approach

Multicultural context

Person-centered

A way of being

Active listening

Existentialism

Presence

Psychodynamic

Defense mechanisms

Transference

Here and now

Unfinished business

Narratives

Feminist theory

INTRODUCTION TO THEORY CONSTRUCTION

Theory has been both a plague and a challenge for students since pre-Socratic times when philosophers would aggressively query their disciples about the meaning of life. Certainly the contemporary student finds little solace in historical precedent for his or her own struggles to understand the differences among the various theoretical systems that are part of the counseling profession. "What good is theory?" students often ask. "I want to be a counselor, not a philosopher."

Yet confusion abounds within the realm of counseling itself, as the differences of opinion on the structure of the therapeutic relationship have shown. Whereas some of the more insight-oriented counseling approaches focus on creating an authentic human encounter for its intrinsic healing properties, the action-oriented approaches use the relationship as a means to another end. And even within a particular orientation there is much disagreement as to style, form, and content. Carl Rogers, for example, proposed that it is the realness and authenticity of the encounter that is important, and so he described an insight theory that encourages naturalness, genuineness, and humanness in the relationship. On the other hand, Sigmund Freud's insight theory postulated that the relationship should be as anonymous and formalized as possible so that the client can work through resistance and transference issues.

A theory, therefore, is a blueprint for action. The counselor's choices of interventions, reactions, analysis, and understanding all flow logically from a theoretical model of what people are like, what is good for them, and what conditions are likely to influence them in a self-determined, desirable direction (Geis, 1973). Some students may be surprised to learn that counselors actually have quite complex and well-developed theories of metaphysics (how the world works), ethics (how people should act), logic (cause-effect relationships), ontology (meaning of human existence), and epistemology (how people know) . It is precisely these theories that guide what a counselor does with a particular client at a particular moment.

Theories are valuable because they organize knowledge and information in an easily retrievable fashion. They are no more or less than models for consistency in action; they permit all practitioners, whether of architecture, medicine, or counseling, to repeat those strategies that have worked previously in similar circumstances (Day, 2008; Prochaska & Norcross, 2010). Theories, of course, have other useful functions, such as attempting to simplify the world and developing rules for explaining, predicting, or guiding behavior.

When you study the various counseling approaches, remember that each is a single attempt to explain the therapeutic process, albeit with emphasis, values, and strengths in some areas and limitations in others. In deciding which ideas have the most personal relevance for you, bear in mind the attributes of good theories set forth by Burks and Steffire (1979) long ago: Good theories are clearly and precisely described, as simply expressed as possible, comprehensive in scope, useful in the real world, and valuable in generating new knowledge and research.

In theory construction, we are indirectly trying to establish a basis for predicting (1) a client prognosis, (2) likely consequences of certain interventions, (3) connections between experiences (and nonexperiences) in a client's life, and (4) the impact of our therapeutic efforts. But because no prediction can ever be

VOICE FROM THE FIELD

There is no more confusing and frustrating thing for me than struggling with all the theories I've been bombarded with over the years. At first, I was a person-centered counselor 'cause that's what almost everyone was where I was trained. I could reflect those feelings with the best of them. Then I was assigned to a new supervisor at work who was real keen on Gestalt therapy; he even grew a beard to make himself look like Fritz Perls. I'm pretty easygoing, so I learned that stuff too—and learned it well.

To make this short, I've been through a half-dozen others and I loved 'em all—Adlerian, Reality, Ericksonian, others I can't even remember. Now I'm at a point where the various theory fads don't faze me anymore. I've been able to take the best parts of each theory I learned and merge it into my own ideas about what is going on with clients. The bottom line for me, and any other counselor worth a damn, is to have a clear plan for how to proceed with my clients.

100% certain, we also use theory to approximate some degree of consistency. Theories are working hypotheses, subject to change and revision as new information about the world, our clients, and ourselves becomes available. We cannot accurately and precisely describe what we see; instead, we filter our experiences through slightly focused images and inadequate language that approximates what we think we perceive. Theory is, in a sense, our beliefs about how to explain reality. Furthermore, this reality is hardly an absolute thing but rather subject to the unique and subjective ways that each of us creates meaning based on our assumptions, language, culture, and social norms (Brown & Augusta-Scott, 2006; Gergen, 1994; Schneider, 1998).

Gregory Bateson (1979), one of the original founders of family systems therapy, described a few of the problems of theory construction in science by listing many of the inherent logical weaknesses in the ways we organize our knowledge:

1. Science can never prove anything, not only because prediction is imperfect and our methods of collecting data are flawed but also because proof occurs only in the realm of abstraction.
2. In human perception, all experience is subjective and hence colored by individual perceptions, as well as by unconscious motives. We can be certain that the reports of our senses will be slightly distorted, viewed through individual prisms that have been shaped by unique genetic structures and cultural experiences.
3. Explanations are the results of descriptions, and these descriptions can be organized in more than one way. Convenience determines how things are classified, and, no matter which model is used, some information will be lost or downplayed.
4. For a theory (and hence its predictive power) to be perfect, it would have to deal with factors that are 100% controllable. Even physical laws, which are far from the whimsical, impulsive nature of the human world, are minutely capricious.
5. Theories are constructed from information. Information is subject not only to inadequate description and arbitrary classification but also to flawed

methods of measurement. Researchers in counseling, for instance, have been debating for decades about whether it can even be reliably demonstrated that therapeutic interventions cure people because we can't agree on definitions of cure, much less figure out a way to measure the degree to which it occurs.

APPROXIMATION OF TRUTH AND REALITY

We advise you, the beginning counseling student, to view each of the theoretical systems represented in these chapters within the aforementioned human context. Each theory is an approximation of truth, one person's or group's attempt at explaining phenomena that are difficult to understand and virtually impossible to describe fully. These theories, as with all other human structures, are imperfect working hypotheses subject to distortions, biases, and limitations. They may be grounded in empirical data and clinical experience, but they are still evolving frameworks that become more refined over time.

We suggest that in this initial exposure to the major theories of the field you don't worry so much about learning all the minute details but instead concentrate on the bigger picture. These two chapters are intended primarily to introduce you to some of the basic terms and language of theory in the counseling profession. This will give you a head start for later courses in which you will be expected to actually apply the concepts to your work with clients.

One other thing to keep in mind is that, historically, most of the popular theories in counseling were invented by white, upper-middle-class older men and so reflect the biases and perceptions of this group (notable exceptions include practitioners of feminist theory, relational theory, indigenous theories, and multiculturally based theories). Yet it is a remarkable fact that this group's innumerable contributions to the field were made in spite of their race, upward mobility, age, and lack of multicultural experience. During more recent times, especially in the last decade, several conceptual forces are having a tremendous impact on expanding the applicability of counseling theory to a much more diverse population.

In a constructivist approach to counseling, any theory is adapted in such a way as to reflect the individual values, culture, gender, language, and perceptions of each client (Berg & White, 2007; Gergen, 2006). Rather than approaching clients with our preconceptions about what their experiences might mean, we work instead to help them create their own meanings based on their cultural and perceptual background. Although later we will look at constructivist thinking and examine its particular approach to counseling, it is important to note that almost all theories are now being looked at through a lens that: (1) recognizes multiple versions of "reality," (2) looks at "truth" as relative to a person's underlying assumptions, (3) considers cultural roots and traditions, and (4) examines how language and social norms shape perceptions of ourselves, others, and the world (D'Andrea, 2000).

The main task of the counselor who takes a constructivist or social constructionist approach (the latter places more emphasis on the ways that language, culture, and social context shape views of reality) is to help people to examine the meaning of their life experiences and recreate alternative narratives that are more

■ | ## Voice from the Field

I have read dozens of books about constructivism and at first I got lost in the language and terms they favor. Stuff like "postmodernism," "deconstruction," and "analogical listening." It felt like I had to learn a foreign language first before I could ever hope to understand what the heck they were talking about. Then again, I'm suspicious anyway about supposedly new theories on the scene that are just old ideas repackaged a bit differently.

After considerable study, and a lot of conversations with colleagues, I now understand how useful constructivist thinking can be for promoting greater humility, flexibility, and sensitivity. It forces me not only to challenge my client's assumptions, but my own beliefs about the way things are. I also really enjoy the collaborative role I play with clients in which we become "co-authors" of new stories in their lives, rather than merely accepting what they think happened as "truth."

empowering. One could also say that, regardless of theoretical allegiances and what one calls oneself, this is what most practitioners do these days.

In a similar vein, feminist approaches to counseling theory (Ballou, West, & Hill, 2007; Brown, 2004; Brown, 2009; Hill & Ballou, 2005) urge practitioners to adapt their theories in such a way that greater emphasis is placed on values other than those emphasized by the dominant male culture. This means that any of the theories that will be reviewed must take into consideration differences in gender roles, as well as the diversity and complexity of human experiences. This is especially the case with regard to individuals who are not members of the dominant cultures that have principally influenced the development of the most popular theories.

Finally, theories are increasingly examined within a multicultural context in which practitioners are encouraged to adapt their methods to fit the needs of a diverse clientele (Frew & Spiegler, 2008; Ivey, D'Andrea, Ivey, & Simek-Morgan, 2007). As we will explore in a later chapter, a client's culture does not just include ethnicity and race but all the different ways that people define their primary identity—including sexual orientation, profession, geographical region, religion, and other factors. Furthermore, it is important to examine critically the inherent biases of each theory, especially as the theory reflects the personal values and cultural assumptions of its inventors.

You will wish to read the following sections openly and critically. Assume that each theory has some merit and value, some practical use and interesting ideas that can help you better understand the process of counseling. It would be helpful to assume, as well, that each of these theoretical orientations has its limitations with some clients, with some practitioners, and in some settings and situations.

The distinction between insight theories (this chapter) and action theories (Chapter 6), although a convenient demarcation for counseling approaches, is hardly a clear-cut one. No longer can we say that any theory is now applied in the "pure" form in which it was invented. Insight practitioners who identify strongly with psychoanalytic or existential frameworks nevertheless make use of behavioral structures to help their clients translate insights into action in their lives. And even the most staunch cognitive and behavioral practitioners will sometimes help their clients understand the source of their suffering.

Nowadays theorists are more likely to collaborate with one another and interact on a regular basis about their ideas, learning from one another and continually updating and refining their ideas. In one sense, it is no longer possible to tell where one theory begins and another ends since their boundaries are far more flexible and permeable. To make matters even more complicated, many theorists admit that they no longer practice the approaches for which they are known (Kottler & Carlson, 2005b).

The theories grouped together in this chapter have one principle in common: It is through the process of self-awareness, self-understanding, and self-revelation that true growth occurs. Whether in a gradual clarification of feelings or in a brief spurt of insight, whether facilitated through open sharing or in-depth interpretations, whether focused on the present, past, or future, the theories treated in this chapter work through the process of self-discovery. Their unifying dimension is the belief that insight into one's problems, along with a grasp of implications, connections, consequences, and perspectives, is a necessary prerequisite before any real and lasting change can occur.

PERSON-CENTERED COUNSELING

ALIASES: NONDIRECTIVE, CLIENT-CENTERED, HUMANISTIC, ROGERIAN, EMOTION-FOCUSED

Before Carl Rogers entered the scene, counseling was largely a directive, prescriptive enterprise consisting of advice, diagnoses, interpretations, and authority. With the publication of his books (Rogers, 1942; 1951), the field was irreversibly pushed in the direction of giving clients more autonomy and responsibility for their treatment. Person-centered counseling caught on quickly because of its optimistic philosophy, which emphasized the wonderful potential of humans to learn, grow, and heal themselves when given the opportunity within a nurturing therapeutic relationship. Further, nondirective counseling became attractive to North Americans as their first native-born approach, one that stressed positive concepts and relatively simple interventions.

Rogers also strongly influenced two other theorists who were later to refine and adapt his ideas, thus allowing his approach to reach a larger audience. Robert Carkhuff and his colleagues ingeniously combined techniques of behavioral analysis into a helping model that presented simplified counselor skills as the essence of constructive intervention. Carkhuff also helped to convert Rogerian philosophy into a system of action. Thomas Gordon is another adapter of person-centered counseling; he created a popular educational system for training parents (Gordon, 2000) and teachers (Gordon, 2003) by applying the skills of "active listening" as a way to clarify a person's feelings.

In more recent times, the person-centered approach has been championed by writers (Kirschenbaum, 2009; Mosher, Goldsmith, Stiles, & Greenberg, 2008; Tudor & Worrall, 2006) who have sought to bring Rogers's concepts of humanism into the mainstream of all counseling practice, or even to apply it to helping neglected children on the streets of Brazil (Freire, Koller, Piason, & da Silva, 2005). Since all counseling is essentially both a relationship and a human activity, Kelly (1997) has proposed that even the most technically oriented practitioners should still make use of humanistic concepts in their work.

Voice from the Field

I'm what you'd call a humanistic counselor in today's climate. That doesn't mean I sit around like Rogers did, nodding my head like a friendly grandfather and concentrating only on reflecting the feelings of my clients. I don't mean to demean the limits of that sort of approach, but I think if Rogers was still alive he would have continued to evolve his thinking to make it more responsive to the demands of what we have to do.

I use a lot of different techniques in my work, actually. I've gone to workshops on just about everything I can. What makes me humanistic, though, isn't so much what I do in my sessions but what I'm after in my work and how I think and feel inside. I truly believe that it is through my relationships with clients that most work is accomplished. I think it's ridiculous even in brief therapy to solve clients' problems without helping them to understand the source of their feelings and to express them in more constructive ways.

BASIC ASSUMPTIONS

Most person-centered counselors are in basic agreement on the following points:

1. Human beings are growth oriented and tend toward self-actualization. This natural process of development toward higher stages of moral, emotional, and behavioral evolution can be facilitated by professional helpers who are able to stimulate the inherent capacity for progress in clients who are temporarily stymied or faltering.

2. "Every individual exists in a continually changing world of experience of which he is the center" (Rogers, 1951, p. 483). This proposition emphasizes the central importance of the individual and the subjective nature of personal experience. No matter how empathic you try to be, you can still never really know the full experiences and perceptions of another person.

3. An important vehicle for change is the therapeutic relationship that exudes qualities of trust, openness, acceptance, permissiveness, and warmth. The degree to which the counselor is able to create this nurturing atmosphere will influence the client's possibilities for growth.

4. The legitimate focus of counseling content is on affect and the exploration of feelings. Both interpersonal relationships and self-conception may be improved by becoming aware of feelings about oneself and others and by learning to express these emotions in sensitive and self-enhancing ways.

5. The universal goals of counseling are to help people to be more free, intentional, ethical, contemplative, and human. This means that time is spent in sessions helping clients to examine their values and personal characteristics so that they may become more humane and caring in their relationship with self and others.

6. The client/student has the primary responsibility for the course of treatment/study—i.e., for what constitutes appropriate content and whether, ultimately, it succeeds. Thus a goal is shared by the client and counselor; they both share a mutual understanding of the client's world.

7. Human beings are intrinsically good and trustworthy. They will instinctively move, in a deliberate way, toward goals that are satisfying and socially

VOICE FROM THE FIELD

I do person-centered play therapy with elementary school kids. People have watched me work and told me they couldn't figure out what the heck I was doing besides playing a board game with a seven-year-old. I get the same question from beginning counselors I supervise: "There's got to be more to it than just play. When does the actual therapy begin?" But there really is an art to doing person-centered play. Letting the child stay in control, accepting the child just where she or he is, reflecting the process of what the child is doing, without probing—it's not as easy as it looks. I admit, there are many times I can't believe myself that all I'm doing is playing a game, and somehow this is helping someone. But what it comes down to is this: There is only one place in the world where my young clients know they won't be judged, interrogated, told to do something better, or told their behavior is a problem and has to change—that place is my office. Doesn't every child deserve that for one hour a week?

responsible. Irresponsible or socially undesirable behavior emerges from a defensiveness that alienates human beings from their own nature. As defensiveness declines and people become more open to their own experiences, they will strive for meaningful and constructive relationships.

In a way, talking about techniques violates the very philosophy of a person-centered approach, because this is more a "way of being" with a client than it is a "way of doing." Nevertheless, beginning students are anxious to translate this elusive but powerful orientation toward helping into something concrete that can be seen, touched, or applied. More recent developments of the person-centered approach, such as *emotion-focused therapy* (Elliott, Watson, Goldman, & Greenberg, 2004; Greenberg, 2002; Greenberg & Watson, 2006; Watson, Goldman, & Greenberg, 2007), have included theories that are far more structured and that respond to the current demands of managed care for increased accountability and specific treatment goals.

FAVORITE TECHNIQUES

Person-centered counseling is hardly technique oriented; it prefers instead to explore curative variables and focus on developing solid relationships with clients. Nevertheless, there are a few standard intervention strategies. The bread-and-butter technique of the person-centered counselor is the reflection of feelings, also referred to as *active listening*. This skill is now so universal and generic that it is used by virtually all practitioners of every theoretical persuasion.

Communicating from a posture of empathic understanding, the counselor intently attends to a client's verbal and nonverbal messages, interprets the surface and underlying meanings, and then formulates a response that demonstrates a deep-level understanding of the client's experience. This technique has several advantages:

1. Although it is the most difficult counseling skill to master, it is relatively simple to learn and fosters an open and honest helping relationship. At its

most basic level, the beginner listens carefully to the underlying feeling that is expressed and then communicates back what is heard:

> **CLIENT:** I don't know what's going on with this situation. The more I think about it, the more ... I just don't know.
>
> **COUNSELOR:** You sound really confused.

2. Even if the reflection of feeling is inaccurate and ignores the client's actual messages, it still encourages further self-exploration.

> **COUNSELOR:** You sound so angry at your brother for not writing you to join him.
>
> **CLIENT:** No. Not really. I'm not so much angry at him as I am frustrated at myself for not telling him it was important that I go.

3. It helps the client to feel reassured that he or she is deeply understood and accepted.

> **STUDENT:** I really think it's stupid to give us an exam in a class like this that emphasizes skills instead of stuff to memorize.
>
> **PROFESSOR:** You feel as though I don't treat you with enough respect, and you also have some real concerns about how well you are doing in this class.

4. It clarifies a client's feelings so that the situation may be viewed more objectively.

> **CLIENT:** My father always butts into my life when he can't take care of his own.
>
> **COUNSELOR:** You are really afraid that, although you love your father very much, you may follow in his footsteps as a disaster in love relationships.

5. It provides an opportunity for emotional catharsis, bringing relief of pent-up tensions and pressure.

> **CLIENT:** I don't know how I feel about it.
>
> **COUNSELOR:** You're afraid to let yourself feel.
>
> **CLIENT:** You're damn right I am! I gave that bastard the best years of my life. I don't know whether to cry, scream, fight, or give up. I'm so confused.

6. It encourages the client to move from superficial concerns to deeper, more significant problems.

> **CLIENT:** I don't know. I've just never had good study habits. You have any tricks for doing better on true-false exams?
>
> **COUNSELOR:** You have some real reservations about your ability to discipline yourself. You sometimes feel as though you aren't smart enough to hack college and are afraid that, even if you do study, you'll flunk out anyway.

Like any of the techniques presented in this book or in your counselor training, in order to make them part of you and your natural style of interacting with others, you *must* practice them in your daily life. Active listening skills can be learned rather quickly even though it takes a lifetime to master them. You can get

VOICE FROM THE FIELD

I remember when I first learned active listening in my counseling program what a difference it meant in so many of my relationships. At first I was so awkward at it that every time I slipped it into a conversation I thought I'd get caught, that a friend or one of my kids would accuse me of acting like a counselor with them. But what I discovered is that adopting this stance helped deepen all my relationships. It taught me to listen more deeply and respond more compassionately. The fact is that in most conversations, people don't listen to one another very well; they are never giving all their attention. Ever since I first learned these skills I made a commitment to myself that I would give the people I love the same kind of quality attention that I give my clients.

a head start by finding as many opportunities as you can—with your friends, family, classmates, coworkers—to really listen and respond actively to what they say. This does *not* mean that you should be counseling family and friends in your personal life, just that you can choose to listen and respond more attentively to the people you love the most.

Remember that when you are applying this approach to helping clients, your job is not to solve problems or offer advice, but rather to reflect back to others the essence of what you heard. It is their job to take this feedback and integrate it in such a way that it makes sense to them, facilitates a deeper level understanding, and motivates them to make needed changes.

CRITICISMS OF PERSON-CENTERED COUNSELING

Although a valuable and—at the time of its inception—radical departure from usual procedures, person-centered counseling can be criticized on several grounds:

1. It may give too much responsibility to the client and reduce the role of the counselor as the trained expert. Clients don't often know what they are feeling.
2. It may be somewhat naive in its view of clients as naturally evolving and able to pursue lofty goals that may not be possible to reach. Counselors, for example, may be unable to create "unconditional positive regard," because everything is ultimately conditional.
3. It does not respond to the difficulties encountered in the process of translating feelings into action.
4. It is narrow in its focus on feelings and tends to ignore thoughts and behavior.
5. It may overemphasize the importance of relationship factors, which may be a necessary but insufficient condition for therapeutic change.
6. It is not useful for clients who are in crisis and require directive intervention.
7. It tends to be more useful for highly verbal clients and less appropriate for those who have difficulty expressing themselves.
8. It may overfocus on issues of freedom, autonomy, and independence—distinctly North American values—and underestimate the importance of sociocultural influences that are prevalent in other cultures and countries.

Similarly, it may ignore the psychological impact of social oppression and marginalization experienced by ethnic minorities and gays and lesbians.

9. Clients from non-European cultures that do not place high value on self-disclosure and insight might be uncomfortable with its nondirective approach and with the counselor's emotional genuineness (Sue & Sue, 2008).

Whereas the person-centered approach has been legitimately criticized for placing too much emphasis on individual issues while neglecting systemic and cultural forces, more contemporary practice has used Rogers's ideas to identify one's own values and biases and the importance of treating each person as unique. This no longer means looking solely at the client's self, but also looking at the cultural context for self-development (MacDougall, 2002).

PERSONAL APPLICATIONS

Principles of person-centered counseling can help you to:

1. Create greater self-awareness, especially with regard to your feelings, and thereby expand growth and congruence. It helps you to create a growth orientation and encourages an active attitude toward life and personal growth.
2. Gain appreciation for the importance of genuineness, unconditional regard, acceptance, and empathy in dealing with other persons. This may help you to stifle or mute the critical voice inside your head.
3. Take more responsibility for your own education and life experiences. The person-centered approach emphasizes self-empowerment.
4. Recognize the importance of exploring your feelings and risking and sharing them with others. You can therefore practice in your own life what you want for your clients.

EXISTENTIAL COUNSELING

ALIASES: HUMANISTIC, PHENOMENOLOGICAL, EXPERIENTIAL

Existentialism is a particularly rich and difficult theory because it intersects so many different fields. It had a long and distinguished career as a philosophy long before it was recruited to the more practical dimensions of reality in counseling. Beginning with Socrates and continuing onward into the 20th century, such well-known philosophers as Kierkegaard, Nietzsche, Heidegger, Husserl, Tillich, and Marcel have led an international search for the ultimate meaning of human existence. These complex philosophies were later absorbed into the world of art (Cezanne, Picasso, Van Gogh, Chagall) and literature (Kafka, Camus, Sartre, Dostoyevsky). Existentialism has now been translated into a style of living, a way of being that encourages a person to use and accept anxiety constructively (May, 1983). Fortunately, it is not necessary to fully comprehend existentialist philosophy in order to make use of its concepts in counseling. For our purposes, we will concentrate our discussion on its practical applications.

Among the several theorists who were responsible for translating existential philosophy to practical reality, Viktor Frankl (1962) adopted this mode of meaning-making thinking as his survival strategy in Nazi concentration camps during World War II. The main determinant, according to Frankl, of an inmate's likelihood of living or giving up and dying was the ability to assign a personal meaning to the experience: "If there is a meaning in life at all, then there must be a meaning in suffering. Suffering is an ineradicable part of life, even as fate and death. Without suffering and death human life cannot be complete" (p. 106).

Whether this is a rationalization or justification of the unjustifiable, Frankl observed the importance of the basic existential hallmarks in the everyday life of anyone who suffers humiliation and pain—in a hospital, death camp, or counselor's office. Freedom, choice, being, responsibility, and meaning are the ideas that helped him to survive and the ideas that help clients to flourish:

> We who lived in concentration camps can remember the men who walked through the huts comforting others, giving away their last piece of bread. They may have been few in number, but they offer sufficient proof that everything can be taken from a man but one thing: the last of the human freedoms—to choose one's attitude in any given set of circumstances, to choose one's own way. (Frankl, 1962, p. 104)

The implications of this brief statement are profound, not only for the counselor who is helping others to find their way, but also for ourselves as counselors. So often people come to us feeling trapped in their lives, without hope, without choices, as if they are in a prison with no escape. Yet the bars are of their own creation because of a refusal, or inability, to accept responsibility for the choices in their lives. Feeling trapped is the result of not recognizing freedom. That is one of our jobs as counselors: to help people find the meaning in their suffering, to help them to make choices that lead to greater freedom.

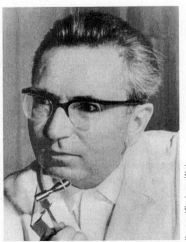

Keystone/ The Image Works.

Victor Frankl, one of the founders of existential therapy, developed his approach while trying to make sense of the pain and suffering he witnessed in the Nazi concentration camps. His book, *Man's Search for Meaning*, is cited by librarians as among the most important works of the last century.

Rollo May (1958) introduced these compelling ideas, previously restricted to the European continent, to North American psychotherapists and counselors. The focus of therapeutic intervention is to help clients become responsible for their choices, to manage their freedom and thereby transcend the meaninglessness of their lives, thereby moving into a more authentic existence. May contributed a series of books on love, power, creativity, anxiety, freedom, and various other issues of existential relevance. His goal was to assist the client to develop insight regarding the life forces that can be mobilized to overcome the existential crises of powerlessness and freedom:

> After many a therapeutic hour which I would call successful, the client leaves with more anxiety than he had when he came in; only now the anxiety is conscious rather than unconscious, constructive rather than destructive. The definition of mental health needs to be changed to living without paralyzing anxiety, but living with normal anxiety is a stimulant to a vital existence, as a source of energy, and as life enhancing. (May, 1981, p. 191)

If anxiety has its usefulness, so too does the concept of death to the existentialist. Yalom (1980, 2001, 2008) writes about the idea of death as the primary savior of humankind because it motivates an intense appreciation of life's value. By confronting our own vulnerability, the ultimate threat to our existence, we are made aware of people and things that are truly important. Death and the companion existential issues of isolation, meaninglessness, and freedom are seen as the legitimate focus of counseling. Yalom was able to translate much of the confusion, complex language, and abstract ideas of existentialism into a system of helping and into an attitude for the helper, complete with methodologies for analyzing and solving human problems.

Existential counseling is richly endowed in its affiliations with Rogers's client-oriented approach, Maslow and Shostrom's self-actualization psychology, and Freud's theory of psychoanalysis. Far from postulating a rigid set of therapeutic procedures, the existentialist offers a way of thinking about clients and their concerns, about humans and their dilemmas, and about life and its puzzles (May & Yalom, 1995). In its more recent forms of evolution (Cooper, 2003; Mahrer, 2008; Watson & Bohart, 2001), existential approaches have become more highly structured and responsive to the demands of managed care.

PREMISES OF EXISTENTIAL COUNSELING

The existential approach has been minimally concerned with the techniques and specific interventions of counseling, concentrating instead on philosophical principles that aid the understanding of the client. As an insight-oriented theory, its main goal is to help people find personal meaning in their actions, their lives, and their suffering. A counselor working from an existential posture would assist people primarily in expanding the range of their choices, and hence their freedom to develop in new ways.

Clients who present the symptoms of existential anxiety (lack of meaning, fear of death, isolation, avoidance of responsibility) can be helped to become more capable of determining the outcome of their daily life. They become aware of their

I'm an existentialist. I think. But then I've never been sure what that means. If it means being fascinated with what we are all doing here on this planet, then count me in. If it means helping clients to sort out what their meaning and purpose in life is all about, then that's what I do. No extra charge either.

I just kinda throw it in with whatever else they have in mind they'd like to accomplish. I just think that human beings are drawn, maybe even driven, to figure out meanings behind things, including their own behavior. And I see it as my job to help them do that.

fears. They understand the significance and personal meaning of their refusal to enjoy freedom. They confront the naked fact that each person, from the moment of birth, stands alone. Yet, far from necessarily condemning the self to loneliness, we may choose to take responsibility for our aloneness, our freedom, our choices, and the consequences of what we choose. "The one who realizes in anguish his condition as being thrown into a responsibility which extends to his very abandonment has no longer either remorse or regret or excuse, he is no longer anything but a freedom which perfectly reveals itself and whose being resides in this very revelation" (Sartre, 1957, p. 59).

Similar to the person-centered counselor (which is often included in this same family), the existential practitioner seeks to enter into the client's world and, remaining in the present, to use the therapeutic alliance—the relationship—as a fulcrum by which to lever more involvement and commitment to living, to being. This process of counseling and change is more than a little ambiguous. The existential approach is a philosophy, an attitude, a way of thinking, analyzing, and experiencing; it is, therefore, difficult to describe specifically how the counselor acts, even though a few techniques reluctantly emerge from the theory.

The basic distinguishing features of an existential approach include the following (van Deurzen-Smith, 2002):

- A focus on issues of freedom, with their accompanying feelings of exhilaration and anxiety
- An examination of the choices you make, as well as their consequences
- A confrontation with fears of death, alienation, and aloneness
- An emphasis on taking responsibility for your actions and your life
- A quest for greater authenticity, honesty, integrity, and identity
- A compatibility with other, more action-oriented theories
- A search for a personal philosophy to guide daily life

Existentialism is basically an attitude toward living and, as such, emphasizes the role of understanding and insight into the human condition. The counselor works toward knowing the client rather than knowing *about* him or her. The process of knowing includes the three separate modes of human existence: the client's natural, biological world; the interpersonal world; and the uncharted territory of the solitary individual in relationship to himself or herself. It is the counselor's *presence* with the client rather than any specific technique that encourages growth to greater autonomy. Presence involves more than being physically together with the

VOICE FROM THE FIELD

I really like the existential idea that we have to take responsibility for who we are and the choices we make. Making choices is hard—with every path we take, there is loss—the road we didn't go down. Would that road have turned out better for us? We'll never know. That's what making a choice is all about, and why we like to avoid doing it. But I also find there is a feeling of ease when you know you have fully, consciously, made a decision. You've done it. You've acted. There is no going back. Second guessing yourself is normal, but basically wastes precious moments of life.

That's why I insist my clients thoroughly think through with me important decisions. I have a woman client, who is considering marrying a guy I know in my heart is wrong for her. But my job is not to dissuade her; it's to help her be fully conscious as she considers whether to marry him. That's all I can ask of anyone. No matter what choice she makes, I'll be proud of her, because she made it from a place of awareness.

client; it means being with the person in body, in spirit, and in every possible way so that you can be perfectly open and accessible to whatever is presented (Bugental, 1991; Sapienza & Bugental, 2000).

CRITICISMS OF EXISTENTIAL COUNSELING

Existentialism is often misunderstood by philosophers and can be obtuse to those who are untrained in this discipline. It has been described as a particularly abstract, ambiguous, mystical theory that is difficult to apply to the circumstances of everyday living. Also, because the philosophy is so intellectually complex, it is not often appropriate for clients who are of low to average intelligence, or for people with severe emotional and cognitive disturbances. Needless to say, other individuals, ones who are in the midst of a crisis or who are barely meeting their basic economic needs, are going to be relatively unconcerned with their "existential angst" or with "phenomenological non-being." They have other, more pressing problems to worry about.

The existential approach is also hard to study because it is nonempirical and doesn't lend itself to scientific scrutiny. Further, although practitioners of this theory are extremely versatile and flexible in their willingness to use a variety of techniques, relatively few specific interventions are available.

PERSONAL APPLICATIONS

Stop reading for a moment. Put your hand on your heart. (We're not kidding. Do it. Now!)

Feel your heart beating. Feel it pumping through your chest. Duh-dum. Duh-dum. Duh-dum. About once every second, 60 times every minute, 360 times every hour, it beats without your awareness. Feel it beating right now, pumping away as if you don't have a care in the world.

Your heart is a muscle, squeezing blood in and out, circulating it throughout your body and brain. It is also a muscle that is wearing out. This very second, as it continues to beat, it is slowing, inevitably, wearing out. Each of us is allocated only a certain number of heartbeats before the heart just stops beating altogether.

Now think about all the heartbeats that you waste every minute, every hour, every day. Think about all the heartbeats you give away when you're bored and wile away time as if you have all the heartbeats in the world. But you don't. Maybe a hundred left. Or a thousand. Or even a million. But the number left is finite.

So the question remains: What do you intend to do with the precious few heartbeats you have left?

If you actually followed this process, if you really paid attention to its implications, your heart is probably beating a little quicker right now. Thinking about death and our eventual demise is terrifying. Yet according to the existentialist, it is actually death that saves us, that motivates us to live life more intensely and passionately. If every heartbeat is a gift, if at any moment your heart could stop beating, or an artery explode in your brain, or a piano fall on your head, what choices are you making to become more intensely involved in living and to accept responsibility for your decisions?

If that doesn't get your attention, you weren't listening.

PSYCHOANALYTIC COUNSELING

ALIASES: PSYCHOANALYSIS, PSYCHODYNAMIC THERAPY, OBJECT RELATIONS, SELF PSYCHOLOGY

We talked earlier about how the profession of counseling can be traced to Sigmund Freud and his prodigious insights regarding the nature of the unconscious, the role of child development in the etiology of adult psychological disorders, defense mechanisms, and the value of talking about childhood memories as a therapeutic intervention. The image of the patient on the couch talking to the bearded psychoanalyst—a caricature of Freud and his followers conducting a session—remains the stereotype of what therapy looks like. Prior to Freud, a few European physicians had successfully cured "hysterics" (an outdated term for patients suffering from such as ills as blindness or paralysis when there was nothing physically wrong with them) by hypnotizing them. Freud experimented with hypnosis, but discovered that a more effective treatment was the "talking cure," in which he allowed patients to recount painful memories as well as reveal their innermost unconscious desires. From the late 19th century until his death in exile from his native Austria at the outbreak of World War II, Freud not only revolutionized our conceptions of human psychology but also single-handedly recruited an army of psychoanalytic thinkers to continue his work. Carl Jung, Otto Rank, Alfred Adler, Wilhelm Reich, Karen Horney, Theodore Reik, Franz Alexander, Harry Stack Sullivan, Erik Erikson, Erich Fromm, Heinz Kohut, and Anna Freud form an impressive list of theorists, brilliant in their own right, who were able to expand, revise, and adapt the psychoanalytic approach to their respective settings, situations, and personalities. As a footnote, even the creators of completely new schools of counseling, such as Fritz Perls, Albert Ellis, Eric Berne, and Rollo May, were once practicing psychoanalysts who grew beyond the confines of traditional psychoanalysis.

An additional point of clarification: There is a difference between *psychoanalysis*—the orthodox application of Freudian theory—and *psychoanalytically oriented therapy*, which makes use of some Freudian concepts but is more flexible in their application (according to the preferences of the practitioner). Some theorists have successfully abbreviated psychoanalytic methods into a short-term psychodynamic approach that can be more efficient, economical, and appropriate for counseling settings (Coughlin, Della Selva, & Malan, 2007; Davanloo, 1992; Fosha, Siegel, & Solomon, 2009; McWilliams, 2007; Stadter, 2009). Our discussion will focus on some of the more universal and practical ideas of psychoanalytic theory—those that are most relevant to the practice of counseling.

BASIC PSYCHOANALYTIC CONCEPTS

Traditional psychoanalysis is quite complex and time consuming. Its practice requires five years of intensive postdoctoral training, which includes undergoing personal treatment as well as seminars in order to have a working knowledge of the theory. Most of its practitioners have doctoral or medical degrees, although private practitioners in social work and other disciplines also have favored this theory historically. In this treatment, clients typically see their "analyst" three or four times a week, lie on a couch, and say whatever comes into their minds, no matter how shameful, banal, or even silly. The responsibility of the client to hold nothing back, and be completely honest, is what Freudians term the fundamental rule of psychoanalysis. The analyst may do nothing but listen for months, but in fact is carefully thinking about everything the client says, searching for hidden meanings and clues as to what may be the client's unconscious fantasies and desires. When the analyst is confident in having figured out these secret impulses and their causal relationship to the client's present problems, he or she will reveal them to the client. These explanations, called, "interpretations," are then repeated over the course of many subsequent sessions until the client no longer fears knowledge of what lies in the unconscious, and the client's symptoms abate.

Many psychoanalytic terms have crept into our everyday language—for example, *ego, catharsis, unconscious, defense mechanisms,* and *rationalization*—making a basic understanding of some important ideas necessary for any practicing counselor. Even for those who have no intention of ever using this particular style of helping, the conceptual vocabulary of psychoanalysis has become crucial as a mode of communication with other professionals, as an orientation toward analyzing the etiology and development of human problems, and as a foundational base for constructing new counseling strategies. The following sections discuss some of the most basic psychoanalytic concepts.

LAYERS OF AWARENESS

Freud introduced the concept of different levels of awareness that motivate behavior. He postulated that there are several regions of the mind: the *conscious mind*, which contains those thoughts and feelings that are always accessible; the *preconscious mind*, which holds elements on the edge of awareness that, with minimal effort, can be made immediately accessible; and the *unconscious mind*, which harbors the secrets of the soul.

Each layer of awareness can be peeled away, providing deeper access into the human psyche, only by permitting unconscious thoughts to surface. This task may be accomplished through analysis of dreams, free association of thoughts, catharsis of feelings, and interpretations that provide a level of insight sufficient to release unconscious, inhibiting desires and facilitate their continued awareness.

STAGES OF PERSONAL DEVELOPMENT

As a medically trained physician, Freud had a particular interest in neurology and the instinctual basis of behavior. He thus viewed the development of human personality as following a series of biologically determined stages, each an expression of the pleasure principle—the child's insatiable urge to reduce tension and maintain psychic equilibrium by self-indulgence in oral, anal, or genital preoccupations. Freud's original conception of psychosexual development is often paired with the theories of Erik Erikson (1950), whose writings still have relevance for counselors seeking to understand the orderly progression of human development. Freud was concerned mostly with early childhood development and its impact on later life; Erikson's stages more accurately reflect growth throughout the life cycle, with a particular emphasis on social influences.

STRUCTURE OF THE PSYCHE

The personality, according to Freud, consists of three separate systems, the id, the ego, and the superego, which are perpetually in conflict with one another. A person's mental health may be defined as the extent to which these conflicts are kept to a minimum and do not disrupt a person's ability to function in the real world.

The *id* is the source of all energy and instinctual drives. It is often referred to as a "seething cauldron," of angry feelings, sexual desires, and infantile wishes. The id, which is unconscious, is constantly trying to push its dark impulses into the person's conscious awareness, ultimately in hopes that the person will act on them.

The *ego* is the contact between the id's uncontrolled desires and the world of reality. The ego either pushes these desires back into the unconscious, or, using its capacity for rationality and logic, thinks about these often frightening impulses and recognizes that so long as the person does not act on them, he or she will not get into trouble. Sometimes the ego realizes that these dangerous impulses can be modified into a productive use of their energy; for example, the client who realizes he is enraged with his father may channel his anger by working to defeat a political candidate he dislikes. In this way, the ego enables a person to find socially acceptable and appropriate ways to fulfill one's needs. On the other hand, when the ego cannot handle the id's powerful desires, the person often feels intense guilt ("I must be a horrible person for hating my father!"). This person, according to the theory, would benefit from psychoanalysis, a process through which the analyst would help the client see that his or her feelings are understandable and not shameful.

The *superego* is concerned primarily with moral issues. All the lessons we learn as a child about the nature of right and wrong become part of the superego. In the best sense, the superego can be our conscience; however, it can also be unnecessarily harsh and punitive, an overly stern parent telling us we should feel guilty for

VOICE FROM THE FIELD

Any counselor, regardless of where she works, had better know the language of psychoanalysis down cold. Everybody in the field uses the jargon. Besides, with all the jokes about Freud and psychoanalysis, you won't know when to laugh unless you know the theory. Just kidding.

The theory does give you a foundation for other stuff you'll learn. I don't know too many people, except a few in private practice, who even use the theory that much any more. Well, lots of people use it but don't necessarily apply it the way Freud intended. Still, it is absolutely a brilliant framework for helping clients understand their past, and especially how that affects their present behavior. When I do family counseling, for example, there are some psychoanalytic ideas I use to look at family-of-origin stuff.

having certain thoughts or feelings. In this three-part system, the ego has the most difficult task, dealing with the impulses of the id, the "critical parent" superego, and the laws and rules of society. Somehow, it must enable the person to function normally while struggling with all of these forces. When the ego fails in its role, and our upsetting unconscious impulses or punitive parental voices become known to us, we experience anxiety. Too much anxiety makes us sick, and in need of therapy. It is no wonder, then, that Freud believed that psychological health was, at best, an exhausting struggle to adjust to all of these pressures without becoming mentally ill. The humanistic ideas of growth and self-actualization are truly utopian and unrealistic within the Freudian worldview.

DEFENSE MECHANISMS

The defense mechanisms are a major contribution of psychoanalysis to practicing counselors. In early psychoanalytic formulations, the ego was said to use defense mechanisms as a way of protecting a person from awareness of the id's negative feelings. Such awareness would cause anxiety, guilt, and shame. However, over the decades, the idea of defense mechanisms has been expanded to mean a psychological maneuver designed to protect us from any feeling, wish, thought, or memory that might be painful to experience consciously. Usually, we associate these feelings, thoughts, and so forth as dangerous to recognize because in our childhoods, we learned that such experiences literally *were* dangerous. Thus, if we were punished as children for expressing angry emotions, we learn to defend ourselves against angry feelings in our present life, keeping those feelings in our unconscious. If we were punished for expressing values different from those of our parents, we learn to use defense mechanisms to keep our true values unknown to us.

Defense mechanisms, then, can be obstacles to our living authentic lives, to recognizing our honest emotions, yearnings, values, and aspirations. Put most simply, the job of today's psychoanalytically oriented counselor is to help us see that the dangers we experienced as children have lost their relevance to our lives; we no longer need to defend ourselves from knowing our true inner experiences, because such knowledge is no longer a threat. However, our defenses can be powerfully entrenched guardians, resisting our attempts to make our inner realities known to us out of a desperate fear that such knowledge will be too painful to bear. Given that insight-oriented counseling succeeds to the extent that clients look honestly and uncompromisingly inside themselves, it is understandable how these unconscious mind–directed defenses make the job of counseling and facilitating change much more difficult. Better we should recognize the opponents that will be resisting our best treatment efforts:

Repression: The selective exclusion of painful experiences of the past from conscious awareness; a form of censorship used to block traumatic episodes.

Projection: The art of putting onto another person those characteristics that are unacceptable to yourself, such as accusing someone of being angry when we are actually feeling the anger.

Denial: The distortion of reality by pretending that undesirable truths about ourselves, uncomfortable feelings, or unacceptable events are not really happening. In contrast to repression, denial occurs on a preconscious rather than unconscious level.

Sublimation: The disguised conversion of forbidden impulses into socially acceptable behaviors. For instance, athletes may unconsciously choose their profession as a way to release aggression. Creative enterprises such as da Vinci's paintings or Shakespeare's sonnets were seen by Freud as sublimated sexual desires.

Reaction formation: Used to counter perceived threats, substituting an opposite reaction for the one that is disturbing. For example, the mother who unconsciously feels angry at her two-year-old daughter puts on a show of always adoring her.

Rationalization: The intellectual misuse of logic to overexplain or justify conflicting messages. For example, "It doesn't matter if I type the paper or not; I'll probably flunk the class anyway."

Displacement: The rechanneling of energy from one object to another, as when we get angry at a friend or partner when we are really angry with a teacher or boss.

Identification: The incorporation, in exaggerated form, of the values, attitudes, standards, and characteristics of persons who are anxiety provoking, as when a child punishes herself or himself for being bad.

Regression: The retreat to an earlier stage of development because of fear. Any flight from controlled and realistic thinking may constitute a regression. When we return home for the holidays and act as though we were children again, we have "regressed."

Fixation: The tendency to remain at one level, interrupting the normal plan of psychological development. It is generally a defense against anxiety and results from the fear of taking the next step in psychological development.

While Freud's ideas have contributed enormously to all forms of contemporary counseling, the practice of Freudian analysis has dwindled considerably, confined mainly to institutes within a few major cities. However, theoretical descendants of the Freudian tradition, such as *object relations* and *self psychology*, are widely practiced, and continue to grow as vital and richly complex

Voice from the Field

I've always been sensitive to what's going on between people—all those little cues people send that say, "I don't want to be too close to you right now" or "I really love you but I'm afraid to say it." It's a gift and a curse—I can tell when my boyfriend is hurting inside and needs to pull away, but I also can feel his pain, almost like it's my own. That may be why I'm attracted to object relations ideas; what goes on in intimate relationships fascinates me.

When I'm doing object relations therapy, I try to stay just as sensitive to how my client feels about me,

to understand when they want to get close or need to back off. Sometimes there are these moments that are like a window to their childhoods, where I can get a vision of how they might have been treated by their parents. It's not that I believe parents are the cause of all our problems. I don't—I'm a big believer in personal responsibility. But I do believe that all of us have wounds from childhood, and that counseling can help to heal them.

---

insight-oriented approaches. Although retaining the Freudian emphasis on exploring the unconscious and connecting childhood developmental experiences to present-day problems, in other ways these theories have departed significantly from their heritage—to the extent that an observer of an object relations or self psychology session would likely see counseling more in common with the ideas of Carl Rogers than with those of Sigmund Freud.

Object relations counselors, rather than focusing on the id's dark impulses, are interested in how clients' difficulties in developing and sustaining fulfilling intimate relationships may have originated in their early childhood experiences with their significant caregivers—usually their mothers. These theorists believe that painful early childhood experiences of not getting our critical needs met by our caregivers become vague memories in the unconscious. These memories influence how we expect intimate partners to treat us in our current relationships. If, when you were a toddler, your mother had to focus her attention on nurturing an ill sibling, you might have memories and attached feelings of being abandoned. As an adult, you might anticipate that a partner who claims to love you will eventually abandon you as well. Consequently, you might protect yourself from this feared pain by distancing yourself, or by leaving the relationship prematurely.

Object relations theorists such as Scharff and Scharff (2005, 2006) and Wallin (2007) believe that counseling is an opportunity for clients to change their expectations of how intimate partners will treat them, because the relationship between client and counselor is also an intimate one. Thus, the client who fears abandonment will anticipate that her counselor will eventually abandon her; the fact that the counselor remains emotionally available and caring throughout treatment proves to the client, on an unconscious level, that her worst fears need not be realized. In sessions, the client and counselor may discuss her fears of being abandoned and the client may experience the painful emotions surrounding this issue. Some of this discussion will focus on the client's childhood experiences, some on her present-day intimate relationships, and some on the in-the-moment relationship with the counselor. The counselor's role, in addition to being an empathic, compassionate listener, is to make interpretations that link together the past, present problems, and the client-counselor relationship.

CRITICISMS OF PSYCHOANALYTIC COUNSELING

Traditional Freudian psychoanalysis has been criticized on a number of grounds, including its deterministic philosophy, the expense and time involved in psychoanalytic treatment, and its pessimistic view of the unconscious as the repository of mainly sexual and aggressive drives. Although some of these concerns are not relevant to contemporary psychoanalytically oriented practice, even therapies that have departed from their Freudian origins are subject to a number of criticisms:

1.   Psychoanalytic theory is extremely complex and dense, requiring years of specialized training.
2.   Because psychoanalytic theory requires that clients participate in counseling for at least a year and usually several years, it is not useful as an approach for treating large numbers of people who require mental health services.
3.   There is an overemphasis on the role of insight and very little emphasis on making life changes.
4.   The approach puts the clinician in a position of power over the client because of its reliance on the clinician's expertise in making sense of the client's unconscious motives and feelings.
5.   The concepts of the various psychoanalytic therapies are difficult to research and support empirically.
6.   The theory tends to ignore the effects of social and cultural factors in the development of clients' concerns.
7.   It is not useful for persons in crisis who require immediate relief of symptoms.
8.   The theory has traditionally been criticized as strongly culturally and gender biased, but that is what you would expect from an approach developed more than a century ago. Just as in every other theory currently practiced, efforts have been made to make the theory more responsive to issues of client diversity.

PERSONAL APPLICATIONS

One of the distinguishing features of psychoanalytic theory is the strong emphasis placed on applying the concepts and techniques to one's own life. In a revealing letter to a friend, Freud remarked on his own painful struggles with self-analysis, which eventually led to further refinements of his ideas:

15.10.97.

IX. Bergasse 19

My dear Wilhelm,

My self-analysis is the most important thing I have in hand, and promises to be of the greatest value to me, when it is finished. When I was in the very midst of it, I suddenly broke down for three days, and I had the feeling of inner binding about which my patients complain so much, and I was inconsolable. . . .

It is no easy matter. Being entirely honest with oneself is a good exercise. Only one idea of general value has occurred to me. I have found love of the mother and jealousy of the father in my own case too, and now believe it to be a general phenomenon of early childhood. (Freud, 1954, pp. 221, 223)

The theory and techniques of psychoanalysis naturally lend themselves to personal experimentation; it was that exact method that Freud employed in their invention. Interpreting dreams is an especially fruitful method of understanding our unconscious desires and avoiding resistance, because even our defense mechanisms sleep at night. Other techniques designed to unlock the secrets of the soul include hypnosis and free association. In applying any of these strategies to ourselves, it is crucial to follow Freud's imperative that we be entirely honest about our desires, wishes, and motives.

GESTALT COUNSELING

ORIGINATORS AND BASIC CONCEPTS

Gestalt counseling has distinguished roots that go back to the very beginning of psychology as a discipline. Scientists interested in the process of learning and perception noted that problem solving is less a gradual phenomenon as it is a critical moment of insight. Kurt Koffka (1935) and Wolfgang Kohler (1929) spent considerable time between the world wars creating certain laws of behavior that could be used to explain the process of learning. For example, they noted that we tend to perceive things grouped together as clusters, according to their proximity to one another, and that we learn to focus our attention selectively on those events, situations, or stimuli that provide internal psychological equilibrium, even though we may thereby distort reality.

The basic goal of Gestalt theory is to describe human existence in terms of awareness. Gestalt counseling has been influenced philosophically by existentialism and psychologically by humanism. Each of these influences has reinforced experience as the central concept on which awareness is built. Gestalt therapy focuses on the *what* and *how* of behavior and on the central role of *unfinished business* from the past that interferes with effective functioning in the present. By helping individuals more fully to experience the present—the "here and now"—Gestalt counselors facilitate greater self-awareness and understanding.

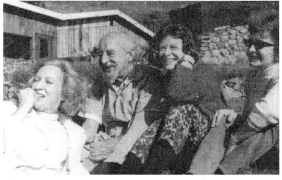

Esalen Institute.

Fritz Perls was the charismatic leader of the Gestalt therapy movement, an approach to counseling that emphasizes direct experience and staying in the present moment.

VOICE FROM THE FIELD

I've always been intrigued by Gestalt stuff but never really got a handle on it. I think I probably do a lot of Gestalt-type work, but I'm never sure what that means. I remember one time I saw a book in which Perls was interviewed and the cover said something like, "Fritz finally reveals the secrets of what his theory is all about," or something like that. I bought the book, got home, and dipped into it right away. The first question was, "So Fritz, tell us what your theory is all about." Not only did Perls not answer the question but within minutes he had the interviewer pretending he was an airplane.

I love this goofy stuff—even if I don't know what it means. Maybe Perls would consider that progress because he was so anti-intellectual. Anyway, sometime soon I intend to experience this theory more since you can't really learn it by studying it from the outside.

Gestalt counseling is most closely associated with Fritz Perls (1969a), who organized the contemporary Gestalt movement in California and was its central figure until his death in 1970. Many writers such as Oaklander (2006), Ginger, Spargo, Colean, & Evans (2007); Lobb & Amendt-Lyon (2004), and Polster (2006) have followed in Perls's tradition by emphasizing creativity, intuition, and spontaneity within the therapeutic relationship. Direct experience in growth and learning is valued, rather than an emphasis on theoretical purity.

Gestalt counseling stresses the role of personal responsibility in the development of awareness and the experiencing of feelings. Unfinished business from the past is brought into the present, and the impasse it represents is dealt with therapeutically. The term *stuck* is used to describe the inability to resolve issues and thereby avoid dealing with the "now." *Polarization* is another key Gestalt concept; it refers to the various parts of the self that are in conflict. In his autobiography, Perls interrupts the flow of his narrative to conduct an internal dialogue between his polarized, conflicted selves:

TOPDOG: Stop, Fritz, what are you doing?

UNDERDOG: What do you mean?

TOPDOG: You know very well what I mean. You're drifting from one thing to another.

UNDERDOG: I still don't see your objection.

TOPDOG: You don't see my objection? Man, who the hell can get a clear picture of your therapy?

UNDERDOG: You mean I should take a blackboard and make tables and categorize every term, every opposite neatly?

TOPDOG: That's not a bad idea. You could do that. . . .

UNDERDOG: So what do you want me to do? Stop letting the river flow? Stop playing my garbage bin game?

TOPDOG: Well, that wouldn't be a bad idea, if you would sit down and discipline yourself. . . .

UNDERDOG: Go to hell. You know me better. If I try to do something deliberate and under pressure, I get spiteful and go on strike. All my life I have been a drifter. (Perls, 1969b, pp. 117–118)

TECHNIQUES OF GESTALT COUNSELING

Gestalt counseling could be seen as the more pragmatic sibling of existential theory. Whereas the latter is heavy on philosophy and light on practical strategies, the former is absolutely loaded with hundreds of techniques. Indeed, the number of counselors who identify themselves as strictly Gestalt practitioners is arguably decreasing, but the interventions Perls and other Gestalt theorists developed have endured, becoming vital tools in many counselors' repertoire, regardless of their orientation.

HOT SEAT This technique requires an individual to be the focus of attention and answer all questions with complete honesty and sincerity. The participant is challenged to be the "here-and-now" self at all times, a task that is quite difficult, considering the intensity of questions that could be posed: "What is your most common fantasy?" "What in your life are you most ashamed of?" "Which person in the group are you most attracted to and why?" This is an exercise that we find particularly interesting to use in classes when demonstrating how to ask good open-ended questions, the kind that generate a lot of reflection and exploration. You will also find that this works equally well in social situations to foster greater intimacy.

RESENTMENT EXPRESSION Perls believed that it was essential to express resentments, which, if unexpressed, are converted to guilt. To take an example: Make a list of all the things about which you consciously feel guilty. Now change the word *guilt* to *resentment*: "I feel guilty because I do not spend enough time with my children" becomes "I resent having to spend time with my children." Exploring and expressing the resentment can help a person become unstuck and work through unfinished business.

DOUBLE CHAIRING This technique is designed to help people to experience the opposite poles of the self. The counselor explores a problem with a client and identifies the opposing feelings. Two chairs are then set up, and the client is instructed to take one and talk to the empty chair from one (specified) pole of the issue. On instruction from the counselor, the client moves to the second chair and talks from the opposite perspective. For example: "I can't stand the way my wife puts me down for everything, and I won't take it. I won't spend another minute in that house. I'm going to ask for a divorce and stick with it. Being alone is better than this misery." From the opposite pole: "Even though I feel very dissatisfied and maybe even angry with my wife, I really need to try harder to make this marriage work. We have a lot of years invested, our kids deserve an intact home, and I really don't like the idea of being alone and starting over. Besides, I'm not the easiest guy to live with." The purpose of this technique is to increase the awareness of feelings, resentments, fears, and issues from each pole of the individual's experience.

OWNING THE PROJECTION In this exercise the client is encouraged to apply his or her projections to himself or herself to demonstrate how we sometimes avoid our negatively perceived qualities and traits by putting them onto others. For example, a client says to a group member, "I think you are manipulative" and then says, "I am manipulative." Or, "I don't think you are trustworthy" and then, "I don't think I am trustworthy."

CRITICISMS OF GESTALT COUNSELING

As is immediately evident from this brief presentation, Gestalt counseling is considerably different from the other insight theories in that little attempt has been made by its creators to explain concepts, and more emphasis has been placed on experiential aspects. Consequently, the Gestalt approach is rich in strategies for helping the client and counselor stay in the "here and now" and work toward greater integration of the self's polarities.

But Gestalt counseling has been soundly criticized for its lack of a clearly articulated theory and its limited empirical base. Among other criticisms are these:

1. There is a tendency for counselors to be overly manipulative and controlling.
2. Gestalt counseling is sometimes viewed as anti-intellectual because cognitive thinking factors are greatly deemphasized.
3. Gestalt counseling is sometimes viewed as gimmicky and as having a high potential for abuse.
4. It sometimes encourages a "do your own thing" attitude, which can create a sense of irresponsibility.
5. There is very little emphasis on acquiring behaviorally useful life skills.
6. The theory often overemphasizes feelings to the exclusion of cognitive aspects of existence.

NARRATIVE THERAPY

Narrative therapy was launched as a distinct counseling model with the publication of the book, *Narrative Means to Therapeutic Ends*, in which author/clinicians Michael White and David Epston introduced a theoretical approach that emphasizes separating clients from their problems and encouraging them to envision their lives and futures from new perspectives (Becvar, 2008; White & Epston, 1990). White was a family counselor in Australia and Epston an anthropologist living in New Zealand when they first met in 1980. Over the next 10 years, the two men developed the central premises of narrative therapy built around the concept of "story": (1) the meaning people give to their lives is shaped by the stories they tell themselves; (2) these stories can constrict their lives and are often influenced by the dominant culture in which they live; (3) the proper focus of counseling should be helping people examine and "re-author" their stories. White and Epston cited a number of influences in developing narrative therapy, including family therapy, feminism, anthropology, and the poststructuralist ideas of Michel Foucault, the French intellectual.

Kathie Crocket, a New Zealand-based narrative therapist, has suggested that a particular movement among family counselors in her country in the 1980s made a strong impact on White and Epston's views of counseling. According to Crocket, counselors working with Maori clients (the indigenous New Zealand population) came to believe that their traditional counseling approaches (e.g., the models we just discussed in this chapter), which were developed by Western, Eurocentric theorists, were oppressing Maori clients in the same way the entire Maori population had been oppressed by the dominant European culture that originally colonized and still politically controlled the country. This line of thinking convinced these counselors that not only were their interventions harming the people they were supposed to help, but that the source of their Maori clients' distress lay not within their internal psychological makeup but in external forces, specifically their mistreatment by the dominant European-influenced New Zealand culture (Crocket, 2008).

Meanwhile, the notion that individual problems may stem from cultural oppression was also gaining strength among feminist-oriented counseling theorists throughout the Western world, who were suggesting that many of the psychological issues that women enter counseling to resolve were actually rooted in a patriarchal society's constriction of women's aspirations and emotional needs. Exposed to both of these influences, White and Epston came to value the social and political contexts in which emotional difficulties develop, and imbued in their theory development an insistence that counselors must not pathologize a client's problematic condition (that is, conceptualize it as a psychological illness) that in fact stems from external social forces.

BASIC PREMISES

POSTMODERNISM AND POSTSTRUCTURALISM   Perhaps the most important philosophical influences on narrative therapy's development are postmodernism and its derivatives, constructivism, social constructionism, and poststructuralism—approaches to understanding human phenomena that we touched on earlier in this chapter. Many counseling students, when first encountering these ideas, especially postmodernism, are thrown by the seeming contradiction in the very term: if "modern" means "contemporary," how can something be "post"? The puzzle becomes clearer if we think of "modernism" as a 19th and 20th century worldview that envisioned scientific, medical, and technological progress as ever-expanding, premised on the belief that the research methods of science would inevitably lead to increased knowledge about biology, physics, chemistry, and other natural phenomena. Freud was the consummate modernist in his belief that science could discover objective truths about human nature by applying the methods of scientific research to the exploration of the unconscious. The postmodernists challenge the assumption that the scientific method is appropriate for the study of human phenomena, and argue that the very notion of objective truth about human experience is flawed. The constructivists believe that people construct their own personal knowledge of reality, while the social constructionists insist that what we call "reality" is particular to the culture in which we live and is created through human discourse and the language used within a particular social context.

While narrative therapy can rightfully be called a postmodern theory, Foucault's poststructuralism is the postmodern school that most influenced White and Epston. This epistemology questioned the notion that people's difficulties are symptoms of deeply-rooted structures in the individual's psyche and that there

VOICE FROM THE FIELD

I began working with this middle-aged woman who in the very first session talked incessantly about how depressed she was and how her whole existence was a failure. She almost had me convinced. Without my prompting, she began telling me the story of her life: that awful moment in her childhood when she brought home a bad report card and the look of disappointment in her parents' eyes. I listened to how she struggled to build a small dry cleaning business that failed because of her incompetence. Her woe was palpable as she described her loveless marriage and how her inability to please her husband ultimately led to his infidelities and the marriage's dissolution.

Narrative therapy saved me from being buying into her hopelessness. First of all, I could tell immediately this was a problem-saturated and thin story; her life had to be so much more complicated, filled with moments that were not nearly as depressing as the one she told me. So I helped her tell a different story, about a woman with the strength to survive emotionally-withholding parents, the persistence to graduate college despite obstacles, and a marriage she stuck out because of her determination to make it work. And we talked about how the whole idea she was responsible for her husband's infidelities came from the women's magazines she was reading and the soaps she watched on TV. Together, we fashioned a whole new narrative, and she began to have a glimmer of hope that the next chapter in her life might be way more satisfying.

was some fixed true, inner self that could be uncovered through psychological exploration. "Poststructuralist therapists do not search for deep structures or a true self, but they are interested in people's stories as they choose to tell them" (Tarragona, 2008, p. 182).

THE ROLE OF STORIES Narrative therapists believe that everyone creates stories, linking together particular events that occur in their lives and organizing these events into a sequence. These narratives help us make sense of and give meaning to our lives. Not only do we all construct stories, but we also tend to create "thin" stories, omitting the many interwoven and complex strands in our histories. For some people, these thin stories are "problem-saturated"; that is, the unifying theme running through their personal narrative is one of emotional pain, personal failures, inadequacies, or the myriad other ways in which we can envision ourselves as doomed to unhappiness. Narrative therapists suggest that as people develop their problem-saturated story line, they filter out the events that might contradict or challenge their narratives, thus giving even more credence to their dominant story.

Our stories are also influenced by the particular social contexts in which we live. Our gender, family, community, socioeconomic class, regional and national cultures help shape these stories in ways we are not aware of. As narrative therapists Freedman and Combs put it,

> We are born into the dominant stories of our local culture, and they shape our perceptions of what is possible from the day of our birth. However, people do not usually think of the stories they are born into as stories. They think of them as "reality" (Freedman & Combs, 2008, p. 230).

Narrative therapy is strongly associated with the concept of social justice, largely premised on the idea that the dominant culture inevitably influences the stories we create, often to our detriment (Morgan, 2000; Winslade & Monk, 2008).

TECHNIQUES OF NARRATIVE THERAPY

Narrative therapy is a highly interactive, egalitarian, and collaborative process. It is a conversation between counselor and clients based on the counselor's belief that clients are the experts on their problems and the counselor's primary role is to facilitate the creation of new stories or perspectives through careful listening and intense curiosity. Consistent with the emphasis on shifting clients from problem-saturated to alternative and richer narratives, the therapy can involve a number of specific interventions. Examples include:

EXTERNALIZING CONVERSATIONS The counseling process often begins with "externalizing the problem." This is perhaps this theory's most controversial method because it is so at odds with other approaches that emphasize accepting responsibility for your troubles. The focus instead is on helping clients to deal with the problem as an enemy to be defeated. Michael White believed that people come to see their problems are a reflection of their identity, of their true nature, and this perception "sinks them further into the problems they are attempting to resolve" (White, 2008, p. 9). To externalize the problem is to see it as something outside of yourself. (As you read this right now, imagine that you're highly anxious about succeeding in your counseling program. You can't sleep, you're fidgety, your mind is racing all the time. And you don't know what to do about your anxiety. Do you feel more hopeful when you think of yourself as an anxious person who needs to change? Or is it more constructive to think of yourself as a normal person who just happens to have "an anxiety difficulty"?) In externalizing conversations, the counselor and client discuss the problem as this outside entity, which enables the client to feel less guilty that they have the problem and more hopeful that it can be gotten rid of, since it is separate from the client rather than something that emanates from within her or him (Tarragona, 2008).

NAMING THE PROBLEM In the very beginning of treatment, counselors help clients come up with a one-word name or short phrase for their complaints, which facilitates clients' experiencing often complicated problems as a single external entity. For example, a set of emotionally distressing symptoms might be labeled as depression, or given a metaphor like, "the dark hole." Preferably, the counselor's questions will help clients discover their own name, but if necessary the counselor will provide one.

PUTTING THE PROBLEM IN A SOCIAL CONTEXT Narrative counselors' sensitivity to the impact of cultural, political, and social factors on peoples' lives plays out in therapy by examining with the client how these forces relate to their issues and self-descriptions. The impact of government economic and social policies on a person's problems might be explored, perhaps alleviating the clients' self-blame for their problems (Payne, 2006).

IDENTIFYING UNIQUE OUTCOMES White and Epston emphasized the importance of listening for times in clients' recounting of their stories when their problems did not exist, or when they had found a way to solve them. These moments are then fully explored, and become the basis for developing alternative, more complex stories, in which the clients see themselves in a more positive and hopeful light.

USE OF THERAPEUTIC DOCUMENTS All of us have a series of documents—certificates, letters, diplomas, psychological reports, etc.—that may add to our sense of something being wrong with us. Narrative counselors sometimes will create new documents for the client, including fake diplomas, letters of recommendation, and non-pathologizing psychological notes that serve as "counter-documents" and facilitate clients' developing alternative stories.

MAINTAINING A COLLABORATIVE RELATIONSHIP In keeping with narrative therapists' insistence that clients, not counselors, guide the therapeutic process, they often engage in discussions on how the treatment is going. Morgan (2000) noted that counselors may ask such questions as:

- How is this conversation going for you?
- Should we keep talking about this or would you be more interested in ..."
- Is this interesting to you? Is this what we should be spending our time talking about?

CRITICISMS OF NARRATIVE COUNSELING

In a world in which evidence-based interventions are becoming increasingly mandated by professional associations and governmental and third-party payers, narrative counseling inevitably runs into the same problem the humanistic therapies encounter. Advocates of a counseling model that rejects logical positivism as a legitimate approach to understanding human behavior are unlikely to test the efficacy of their approach with traditional empirically-designed studies. This makes it difficult for narrative counselors to counter one of its major criticisms: There is scant data-driven research demonstrating that narrative therapy works. There is, on the other hand, much case study research, and an increasing number of qualitative studies that do support its efficacy (Etchinson & Kleist, 2000; Archer & McCarthy, 2007).

Other criticisms have been leveled at this approach as well:

- It tends to use its own unique vocabulary (e.g., "languaging," "re-storying") or common words in unusual ways (e.g., "thin" or "thick" stories). This use of language can make the theory hard to comprehend and makes more difficult an effective exchange of ideas with clinicians who work with other models.
- It can be argued that encouraging people to externalize their problems helps them avoid personal responsibility for them.
- Its insistence on an egalitarian relationship between counselor and client denies a hierarchical relationship that is inherent to the counseling relationship.
- Despite its social justice emphasis, it has yet to demonstrate how it can be culturally sensitive with clients who feel safer with counselors they perceive as experts.

PERSONAL APPLICATIONS

If anyone asks you to tell them about your life, you will tell a story. But it won't be a random series of events; it will have a coherent narrative, with a plot, and a beginning, middle, and end (the point where you are now). If you think about it, you'll discover you even have a title to your story, a phrase that expresses how you see yourself. One of this book's authors (David) used to tell himself the following story to sum up his life (we'll get to the "used to" part after the story):

The Fraud Who Got Lucky

I was never all that smart, but I worked hard, and took school seriously. I happened to go to an elementary school in a poor area of town (just because it was near my home), where most of the kids came from families with no education beyond high school and little expectations that their own children would go further. It was easy to academically shine and have all the teachers admire me, because I was the only kid with parents who could help me with my homework and stay on me when I got lazy.

I then was fortunate enough to go to an expensive private high school, because my mother worked there as the music teacher, and one of her perks was I could attend for free. It just happened to be a new school, with no track record of placing its students in good colleges, and the principal was determined that one of his students would get into a top institution. So he personally made trips to well-known New England universities, finally convincing one of them to take me. Meanwhile, I started doing adolescent rebellious things, and one day I was caught by the vice principal for a serious violation of a school rule, but, again, fortunately, because I had already been accepted into a college and the school had placed their hopes in me, he decided to ignore my behavior, rather than expel or suspend me.

So I went to this very challenging college, and muddled through, but I was terrible at science and there was no way I was going to pass the final exam in the college's required science class. Now, this was the 1970s, and the Vietnam War was in full swing, and college students were demonstrating all over the country, shutting down universities. Wouldn't you know—the day before I was to take the science exam that surely would have ended my college career, President Nixon sent troops into Cambodia, outraging both the faculty and student body. My luck was holding! The entire university went on strike, classes were cancelled for the rest of the semester, and everyone got automatic "B's" for the course, and I never had to take that final exam. So I graduated, and no one knew that it was all a matter of luck.

This was the dominant story David told himself for years, a narrative that implied his achievements were not deserved, he had no reason to feel confident in his abilities, and sooner or later he would be discovered as a fraud. You can imagine how this impacted how he felt about himself and how it constrained him from taking chances in life that might expose him as the imposter he believed he was. It took him years (and some good counseling) to realize his story made no sense; it implied that his successes in life were due to a series of events virtually conspiring together (including the Vietnam War) to make him appear intelligent and academically competent. Left out of the story were the hours he spent studying, the grades he achieved because of effort and ability, the good relationships he had developed with school authorities, and so on. And once he saw how he had written a life-constricting story, he knew the next chapters could be based on an entirely different theme, where he could be the agent of his own achievements.

All of us have stories like David's. Reflecting on our own narratives exposes their "thinness" and gives us both an opportunity to create a richer, more complex story of our lives, and to imagine future chapters in which we achieve our goals and aspirations.

HONORABLE MENTIONS

You have probably heard that there are dozens of counseling theories currently in practice and way more than a handful that may be considered relatively common. We don't mean to slight any particular approach by not including it in this chapter or the next one. Because of space limitations we can only give you a sampling of a few representative approaches. In later courses you will have the chance to study these theories, and many others, in greater depth. Other books devoted exclusively to counseling theory can provide you with greater detail (see, for example, Capuzzi & Gross, 2007; Corey, 2009; Fall, Holden, & Marquis, 2010; Frew & Spiegler, 2008; Lebow, 2008; Wedding & Corsini, 2008). And, of course, you will want to read many of the theorists' original works when you have the chance.

We would, however, like to mention a few other insight-focused therapies that have been influential in the field. The decision not to give them as much space as the ideas discussed previously is based solely on our belief that they *currently* exert less influence on the field than those previously mentioned. These theories are potentially as valuable or useful as the ones that have been presented; a theory's inclusion is a matter of personal opinion about what is most appropriate for beginning students to learn first. We are sure your instructor will point out other theories that we've neglected or underemphasized and will encourage you to examine them in greater depth. Your instructor may also take issue with the way we've classified these theories as "insight" or "action" oriented when, in fact, this simple dichotomy does not do justice to the complexity and flexibility of these approaches.

ADLERIAN COUNSELING

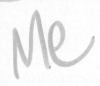

Alfred Adler, one of Freud's disciples who went his own way, developed a remarkably integrative theory for his time—one that combined some of the premises of psychoanalysis with a more pragmatic approach that emphasized such ideas as: (1) the social context for human behavior, (2) the interpersonal nature of client problems, (3) the cognitive organization of a client's style of thinking, and (4) the importance of choice and responsibility in making decisions.

Adlerian counselors, although subscribing to the tenets above, are quite flexible in their style of practice. After all, they hold much in common with some of the existential practitioners (the emphasis on personal responsibility), the cognitive therapists (the focus on the subjective perception of reality), the psychoanalysts (attention to dreams and the unconscious), and even the behaviorists (the focus on specific tasks to be completed).

A resurgence of interest in Adlerian approaches has been evident in recent years, due in part to the systematic organization and explication of Adler's ideas by a number of authors (Carlson & Englar-Carlson, 2007; Carlson, Watts, & Maniacci, 2005; Mosak, 2005; Rule & Bishop, 2005; Sweeney, 2009; Yang, Milliren, & Blagen, 2009). Prior to these contemporary spokespeople, it was primarily Rudolf Dreikurs who popularized Adler's work. Dreikurs (1989) formulated five basic norms of Adlerian theory:

1. *Socially embedded:* All problems are basically social problems and emerge from the need to belong and find a place in the group. A well-adjusted person

is oriented to and behaves in line with the needs of the social situation. A maladjusted person has faulty concepts, feelings of inferiority, and mistaken goals and is overly concerned with what others think of him or her or with what is in it for him or her.

2. *Self-determining and creative:* Adler believed that life is movement and that individuals have the power to change interactions by what they do. The belief that individuals can change and are active participants in their lives is the basis for such optimism.

3. *Goal directed:* Behavior, according to Adler, is directed toward goals that are inferred from the consequences of behavior. Looking for causes of behavior is unproductive because they are unknowable and, even if known, cannot be changed. Goals, once recognized, can be modified and represent a behavioral choice.

4. *Subjective:* Reality is as we perceive it and is not absolute. Adler further believed that it is not what happens to us that matters, but how we feel about it. As a result, Adler emphasized interactions and movement in all relationships as the units of analysis.

5. *Holistic:* Human beings are integrated, whole, and incapable of being reduced to discrete units. One must deal with the entire person.

In Adlerian theory, feelings of inferiority are the basis of anxiety and are destructive to clients. Inferiority feelings are not feelings in the usual sense but are a belief system or a reasoning process about how one should be. One's response to inferiority feelings is the basis for character formation.

Adler (1958) believed that the purpose of counseling is to restore faith in the self to overcome these feelings of inferiority. The process of counseling contains four steps for the individual:

1. *Become aware of prejudices.* Recognize that as children we learned that we were not good enough as we were; thus, we were urged to do better.

2. *Stop being afraid of making a mistake.* Overconcern with error encourages more, not fewer, mistakes. Further, it is human to make mistakes; do we expect ourselves to be superhuman? Mistakes reflect an opportunity to learn if they are accepted and if we avoid becoming discouraged by them.

3. *Cultivate the courage to be imperfect.* Working to resist self-evaluation and to do our best to respond to the needs of a situation is preferable to feeling inadequate because we could improve performance. We don't have to be any better than we are.

4. *Enjoy the pleasure in an activity.* It is important not to reduce pleasure in life by being overly concerned with success, failure, or prestige. Learning to do one's best and accepting the outcome increases the pleasure in life.

The Adlerian approach is concerned with helping individuals develop a lifestyle that is socially responsible and personally fulfilling, one that allows for growth and a holistic integration. A person who is labeled as psychopathological is discouraged and has lost faith in the ability to change. The objects of counseling are to: understand a person's "private logic," offer encouragement and support, explore and reconfigure lifestyle choices and family constellations, challenge faulty thinking, help the person to set realistic personal goals, and encourage involvement in activities that promote social interest (Carlson & Englar-Carlson, 2007). If this sounds like a rather integrative approach that includes features from many other approaches familiar to you, that is because Adlerian counseling was not only the first truly pragmatic theory, but also one that became the stimulus for many other theories (cognitive, existential, family systems, integrative) to follow.

FEMINIST THERAPIES

There is no single feminist therapy but rather a school of thought that also is rather "constructivist" in orientation. Similar to narrative therapy just mentioned, a person's experience of a problem or issue is shaped by forces within our culture, the influence of language, and especially the way that power is exercised.

No doubt you have noticed that most of the theoreticians who have shaped the fields of counseling and therapy were "old, white guys." It has only been in the last few decades that influences from marginalized groups have been integrated into mainstream thinking.

Most feminist approaches to counseling all share certain beliefs that guide clinical practice (Ballou, West, & Hill, 2007; Brown, 2009; Evans, Kincade, Marbley, & Seem, 2005; Worrell & Remer, 2003):

1. Gender and culture are the central organizing principles of people's lives.
2. Males and females develop in unique and sometimes different ways. These differences related to language, worldview, values, and perceptions should be honored and respected in counseling.
3. Women and various minority groups have been marginalized historically. Thus, dealing with issues of power is an integral part of therapeutic work for those who feel powerless.
4. Political/social/cultural influences are often at the core of many presenting complaints. Individual concerns are examined within this broader context.
5. Alternative diagnostic systems are needed that are not so biased against traditional female behavior. Thus, what has been described as "hysterical" (overemotional) or "dependent" (socially considerate) have often been treated as a form of psychopathology.
6. Women's unique "voices" have been underappreciated and disrespected.
7. The assumption that psychological health is characterized by a person's sense of autonomy and self-sufficiency is a male idea: For women, growth is toward connection rather than separation.

The notion that counseling needs to emphasize connection rather than individuation is the hallmark of *relational-cultural theory*, a feminist model that emerged in the 1990s, as theorists like Carol Gilligan and Jean Baker Miller began to challenge long-held beliefs about how children develop. From their perspective, throughout the lifespan, people are naturally motivated to yearn for connection, both to others and to their authentic internal feelings. Psychological problems develop when children learn that suppressing certain feelings and parts of themselves is necessary in order to maintain ties to their parental figures. For example, a child whose expression of angry emotions is met with nonresponsiveness (i.e., lack of empathy) or outright discouragement from parental figures learns to disconnect from her own experience and internalizes self-blame for her angry feelings. As an adult, this person's capacity to enter into an authentic relation with others is compromised by her fear of displaying her disowned feelings; even if she has seemingly good relationships in her life, she experiences feelings of isolation and painful disconnection.

The goal of counseling is to bring clients back into the state of healing connection, to help clients reconnect with themselves and develop more authentic relations with others (Hartling & Sparks, 2008; Jordan, 2001; Miller, 2008). The counseling process contains two main components: (a) exploration of the various disconnections and connections in the client's life; (b) a mutually empathic relationship with the client, in which the counselor is authentic with regard to his or her emotional reactions to the client. The counselor's responsiveness to all of the client's emotions helps her to reconnect with parts of herself cut off in childhood; the counselor's authenticity allows the client to see that she has impact on others, thereby enhancing her relational self-confidence and competence.

Regardless of their specific philosophies and approaches to counseling, feminist therapies have been misunderstood as applying exclusively to women's issues. In fact, these theories are equally liberating for men and women because they define gender roles with more flexibility. Just as women have been trapped in certain norms and roles, so too have men. Feminist therapies seek to help all clients gain insight into the choices they have made, the parts of themselves they have disowned, and how they have been shaped by the gender expectations of their cultures.

THE FUTURE IS NOW: NEW ISSUES IN COUNSELING

INTERPERSONAL NEUROBIOLOGY

Two of the most prominent criticisms of insight-oriented theories have been the value they place on the counseling relationship as a curative factor, and the lack of "hard data" demonstrating these theories' efficacy in producing client change.

This critique might be losing its credibility in the 21st century, thanks to the new brain-imaging technologies like magnetic resonance imaging (MRI) and positron emission topography (PET) scans that allow researchers to view the workings of the brain. The seminal figure in synthesizing brain research and relating the most recent findings to counseling is psychiatrist Daniel Siegel, who has termed this new science *interpersonal neurobiology* (Siegel, 1999; Siegel, 2007).

According to Siegel, brain-imaging studies reveal that representations of our life experiences, including our earliest ones, are stored in various parts of the brain, in the form of connections between neurons. What we learn from experience is best described as a particular pattern of neurons firing throughout the brain's different structures, in what Siegel calls, "a neural network." Siegel uses the example of a traveler to Paris who sees the Eiffel Tower while also feeling hungry. If the traveler was later asked to recall this experience, neurons in both the visual and sensory components of the brain would fire, enabling the travel to remember both the image of the Eiffel Tower and the hunger pangs associated with the memory (Siegel, 1999).

The big news for counselors is that neuronal networks are plastic, continually being altered as individuals gather new life experiences; even the most strongly "hard-wired" networks, those first developed during infancy and relating to expectations for love and nurturing, are amenable to change. Here is how this relates to counseling: A significant number of clients come to us to deal with relationship issues, including fears of abandonment, destructive patterns of interpersonal behaviors, and difficulties in dealing with emotional closeness. These problematic behaviors and emotions may be caused by networks of neurons that connect feelings of intimacy to memories of abandonment and trauma in previous intimate relationships. According to Siegel and other researchers in this field, the empathic, nonjudgmental interpersonal relationship between the client and the counselor actually creates biological changes in the brain, rewiring it so that neurons connected with intimacy now link to the positive experiences of the client-counselor matrix, thus contributing to a resolution of the client's interpersonal difficulties (Atkinson, 2005; Siegel, 1999; Siegel, 2007; Fosha, Siegel, & Solomon, 2009). If Siegel's ideas continue to be validated by brain-imaging technology, insight- and relational-oriented counseling models will have the kind of scientific support not even dreamed of by Freud, Rogers, and most other insight-oriented theory founders. Indeed, given that all of the theories discussed in this chapter emphasize the counseling relationship as an essential healing factor, the implications for beginning counselors are enormous. You will now have one more thing to keep up with throughout your career (as if you didn't have enough!): emerging evidence in neurobiology.

SUMMARY

In this chapter we have looked at some of the more prominent insight-oriented theories that influence counseling. There are, of course, many we have neglected, such as the other psychodynamic approaches of Jung, Alexander, Bordin, Sullivan, Reich, and Fromm; some of the "expressive" therapies (transpersonal, bioenergetics, drama, or dance therapy); approaches from the Far East (Morita or Buddhist approaches); or some more recent innovations that are both insight and action oriented (Eye Movement Desensitization Reprocessing). Part of the task of developing into a mature professional counselor is coming to terms, on a personal and intellectual level, with the many options available. At some point in your training

you will be expected to make some hard choices about which approaches are most suitable to your personality, interpersonal style, work setting, and client needs.

Each of the insight approaches presented offers the counselor a framework for understanding the client's world and a methodology for promoting greater self-awareness and self-understanding. It is assumed that such exploration and knowledge will lead a client toward making desired life changes. It is also believed that the presence of the counselor and the relationship between counselor and client provide nonspecific curative effects that are helpful in the process of being and becoming.

SELF-GUIDED EXPLORATIONS

1. Many approaches to counseling are based on helping clients understand how and why they have developed particular behavioral, emotional, or cognitive patterns. As a result of studying several of the insight-oriented theories (psychoanalytic, existential, Adlerian,

   Gestalt, person-centered, etc.), describe some of the insights you have become aware of about your own characteristic personality style.

2. Describe a time in which some dramatic insight or realization provided a major change

in your life. What was it that helped you translate that awareness into constructive action?

3. Helping clients to identify and explore their feelings constitutes a significant part of insight-oriented counseling work. What are some of the feelings that you struggle with on an ongoing basis (for example, anger, envy, jealousy, frustration, anxiety, shame, depression, sadness, cynicism, fear of failure)?

4. A number of coping mechanisms are used by people to deal with threatening material that might arise in counseling sessions or in life. Which of these do you recognize as part of the characteristic style with which you protect yourself from perceived attacks? Describe specific examples.

Repression	Rationalization
Projection	Displacement
Denial	Identification
Sublimation	Regression

5. Psychoanalytic, person-centered, existential, and relational-cultural theories all emphasize the need for clients to reconnect with emotions they learned to suppress in childhood. Look at each of the emotions listed below, and ask yourself how comfortable you were expressing them in front of your parent(s). If you avoided any of these, reflect on how you learned they were unacceptable.

Pride	Anger
Joy	Self-pity
Excitement	Fear
Affection	Sadness

6. Existential theory is concerned with living more in the present by accepting how precious is each breath we take. Consider how fleeting your own time is on this planet. On one end of this continuum is your birth; the other end represents your death. Place a mark on the line to represent where you are now in your life span. Write down any reactions, thoughts, and feelings that come up for you as you reflect on how much of your life is over and how much time you have left.

Birth _____ Death

7. In small groups, talk to classmates about the ways you have been limited by your gender role. How have you felt your choices restricted and options minimized because you are a man or woman?

8. You can try narrative therapy to shift your perspective on a current problem in your life. Respond to the steps below, which are ordered in the same sequence a narrative counselor would likely follow if you were the client (Payne, 2006). It might be helpful to use a journal in this exercise.

1. Discuss the problem in three or four paragraphs.
2. Name the problem, using a single word if you can (e.g., "procrastination").
3. Say or write a one-sentence description of the problem, using externalizing language (e.g., "I get caught up by procrastination.").
4. Consider social or political influences on your problem. Is this problem caused or exacerbated by the values in any of the cultural contexts in which you live (e.g., national, community, school, family)?
5. Search for unique outcomes. What was a previous time in your life when you successfully addressed the problem?
6. Discuss with as much detail as you can how you solved the problem.
7. Reflect on how you feel about the problem having gone through these steps.

FOR HOMEWORK

Talk to a classmate or partner about an issue you are struggling with and your plans for resolving it. But before you start, ask the other partner to take note of every time you say words and phrases like, "probably," "I guess," and "maybe." When the conversation is over, discuss with the other person how frequently you used this kind of tentative language. Each time you say, "I guess" or "probably," or use similar terms, you are avoiding being truly present with yourself. These words also help you circumvent taking full responsibility for your feelings and insights.

Next, have the same conversation again, this time without using words that help you avoid being present. What was the experience like when you were being real with yourself, and owning everything you said? Ask your listener what he or she noticed about how you were different when you were being present.

SUGGESTED READINGS

Ballou, M., West, C., & Hill, M. (2007). *Feminist therapy theory and practice: A contemporary perspective*. New York: Springer.

Brown, C., & Augusta-Scott, T. (Eds.) (2006). *Narrative therapy: Making meaning, making lives*. Thousand Oaks, CA: Sage.

Brown, L. (2009). *Feminist therapy*. Washington, D.C.: American Psychological Association.

Carlson, J., Watts, R., & Maniacci, M. (2005). *Adlerian therapy: Theory and practice*. Washington, D.C.: American Psychological Association.

Corey, G. (2009). *Theory and practice of counseling and psychotherapy* (8th ed.). Belmont, CA: Brooks/Cole.

Frew, J., & Spengler, M. (Eds.) (2008). *Contemporary psychotherapy for a diverse world*. Boston: Lahaska Press.

Jacobs, M. (2004). *Psychodynamic counseling in action* (3rd ed.). Thousand Oaks, CA: Sage.

Jordan, J. V., Kaplan, A., Miller, J. B., Stiver, I., & Surrey, J. (1991). *Women's growth in connection*. New York: Guilford.

May, R. (1983). *The discovery of being*. New York: W. W. Norton.

McWilliams, N. (2007). *Psychoanalytic therapy*. Washington, D.C.: American Psychological Association.

Mearns, D. (2009). *Person-centered counselling in action*. Thousand Oaks, CA: Sage.

Payne, M. (2006). *Narrative therapy: An introduction for counselors*. Thousand Oaks, CA: Sage.

Perls, F. (1969). *In and out of the garbage pail*. Lafayette, CA: Real People Press.

Rogers, C. (1980). *A way of being*. Boston: Houghton Mifflin.

Rule, W. R., & Bishop, M. (2005). *Adlerian lifestyle counseling: Practice and research*. New York: Routledge.

Scharff, J., & Scharff, D. (2005). *The primer of object relations* (2nd ed.). New York: Jason Aronson.

Siegel, D. (2007). *The mindful brain: Reflection and attunement in the cultivation of well-being*. New York: Norton.

St. Clair, M. (2004). *Object relations and self psychology: An introduction* (4th ed.). Belmont, CA: Thomson Brooks/Cole.

Tudor, K., & Worrall, M. (2006). *Person-centered therapy: A critical philosophy*. New York: Routledge.

Wedding, D., & Corsini, R. J. (2008). *Case studies in psychotherapy* (5th ed.). Belmont, CA: Cengage.

Woldt, A. L., & Toman, S. M. (Eds.) (2005). *Gestalt therapy: History, theory, and practice*. Thousand Oaks, CA: Sage.

Yalom, I. (2009). *Staring at the sun: Overcoming the terror of death*. San Francisco: Wiley.

ACTION-ORIENTED APPROACHES | CHAPTER 6

The theoretical perspectives presented in the previous chapter emphasized the importance of self-awareness and understanding in the counseling process. The primary medium used in insight-based approaches is verbal intervention designed to promote the client's exploration and understanding of presenting complaints. In this chapter, we will examine theories that stress not insight, but interventions that lead more directly to relief of symptoms. These approaches blend an emphasis on action with verbal processing to accomplish specific therapeutic goals. Furthermore, they are designed as brief treatment models.

We would like to mention once again that although, for the purposes of this textbook, we have divided theories into those that primarily focus on understanding versus those that more directly promote action, most practitioners help their clients do both. Of course, the particular treatment plan and approach employed would depend on several factors, such as how much time is available and what the client needs.

Action-oriented approaches to counseling are generally characterized by their reliance on behaviorally specific interventions and outcome measures. The counselor in these approaches works actively to structure sessions so that concrete, observable, and measurable goals can be established and accomplished. The role of the counselor tends to be active and directive, working with the client to structure the sessions. Action-oriented counseling gives less attention than insight theories do to the therapeutic relationship and to process, interpretation, and insight. Instead, its proponents emphasize a more objective and scientific approach to counseling that makes use of a variety of techniques and structures.

The field is currently undergoing dramatic reshaping of its primary mission, not just in the traditional domain of school counseling but in all of the other specialties, including community counseling, mental health counseling, rehabilitation counseling, marriage and family counseling, and pastoral counseling. Increasingly we are being called on to make a difference in clients' lives in briefer periods of times, to prove that our efforts have had an impact, and to be accountable to third parties for our relative successes and failures.

The climate with regard to the community, the popular media, and insurance companies tends to be more and more skeptical that we are indeed being helpful. Consequently, most counselors feel pressure to plan some sort of therapeutic tasks with clients that can be implemented quickly and can be measured as to their effects. Action-oriented theories are becoming increasingly popular as a framework for preparing some sort of intervention, specifying how long the treatment will last, and determining what outcomes can be expected when the counseling is over.

Quite a number of new volumes are being published each year to help all counselors, even those who are insight-oriented, to respond to the demands of the marketplace and the realities of everyday practice. Whether we like it or not, we are being forced by managed care organizations to make adjustments in the ways that we help people, and greater emphasis is being placed on swift, efficient, and measurable methods (Langs, 2009; Parsons, 2007). School counselors are also jumping on the bandwagon of brief counseling models because they have always been required to help children in just a few sessions (Baker & Gerler, 2007; Murphy & Duncan, 2007; Sklare, 2004).

Regardless of the setting and circumstances in which you intend to practice or the clientele you intend to reach, it is highly probable that proficiency will be

VOICE FROM THE FIELD

I think the thing that most surprised me when I got out of my training program was how different my job was from what I learned from role-plays in my classes. I've heard the same thing from friends who work in other places as well. You see, we did so much reading and got so much practice working with clients who supposedly would come for as long as they needed to get better.

Then I got this job as a school counselor where I'm really lucky if I get to see a kid for more than a semester. Which is not to say their problems are easy—I mean, these kids have lots going on. I get cutters, anorexics, suicidal kids, you name it. At first, I was really angry at the whole system—it seemed so unfair to the kids. But once I realized I couldn't change the system, I adapted. There are some short-term interventions you can do that actually make a difference. I don't pretend these kids' problems are going to go away. But I'm frankly amazed at how they feel better after a few sessions when I've put together a solid, short-term treatment plan.

required in at least one brief counseling approach, no matter how much you prefer to work with more in-depth, long-term cases.

BEHAVIORAL COUNSELING

ALIASES: BEHAVIORISM, BEHAVIOR MODIFICATION, BEHAVIOR THERAPY

The influence of behaviorism on counseling has come a long way since B. F. Skinner and his rigid prescriptions for human control and manipulation (Skinner, 1938, 1953). Once viewed as a radical counterpoint to the humanism of Carl Rogers and Abraham Maslow, behavioral principles have been assimilated into the mainstream of counseling to the extent that even insight-oriented counselors regularly use many of the behavioral techniques, such as thought stopping, goal setting, assertiveness training, relaxation training, systematic desensitization, self-management, and other methods of skill acquisition. Ironically, the reverse is true as well: Relationship variables emphasized by client-centered counselors are also part of the ways behavioral counselors operate. One reason for this is that clients are more inclined to follow through on prescriptions if they feel some degree of commitment to the counselor and accountability to the relationship (Cormier, Nurius, & Osborne, 2009). Also, behavioral counselors are discovering the effectiveness of a mutual relationship in which clients routinely give feedback to their counselor regarding the progress of the treatment (Miller, et al., 2006).

So many different kinds of behavioral treatments are currently in practice that it is difficult to lump them all together into a common camp. Some emphasize cognitive features; others stress reinforcement, modeling, self-control, or behavioral analyses. Nevertheless, most behavioral approaches have the following elements in common (Spiegler & Guevremont, 2010):

1. An emphasis on the present rather than on the past
2. Attention to changing specific dysfunctional behaviors
3. Reliance on research as an integral partner for developing and testing interventions
4. A preference for carefully measuring treatment outcomes
5. Matching specific treatments to particular presenting problems

These factors common to behavioral approaches are now being integrated more and more into many other counseling styles.

EARLY BACKGROUND

The term *behavioral counseling* was first introduced by John Krumboltz. He suggested that counselors should remind themselves that the purpose of their activity is to foster behavioral changes in clients; thus all counseling is ultimately behavioral (Krumboltz, 1965). From a behavioristic perspective, counseling can be viewed as the systematic use of procedures to reach mutually established therapeutic goals that will resolve client concerns and conflicts (Thoresen, 1969). The behavioral approach therefore views counseling less as a philosophy of life and more as a set of principles to be used in a targeted and situationally specific manner.

Although the behavioral approach to counseling has many variations, most proponents agree that clients' problems are the result of maladaptive learning patterns; treatment thus takes the form of learning new life skills. Concepts central to the work of a behavioral counselor include: (1) behavioral assessment and identification of target symptoms; (2) reinforcement (both operant and classical); (3) social modeling of skills and desirable behaviors; (4) skills training (that is, assertiveness or stress inoculation); (5) environmental changes that will encourage identified goals; and (6) objective measurement of changes over time. In many ways, behavioral counseling is viewed as an educational process that borrows heavily from learning theory and emphasizes the acquisition of more adaptive ways to act.

The work of Ivan Pavlov, with his salivating dogs and their responses to the ringing of dinner bells, John Watson's discovery that neurosis can be induced by scaring infants, and B. F. Skinner's fascination with teaching pigeons to play table tennis are important milestones in the development of behaviorism. Those early research efforts were translated into action techniques for promoting systematic client change (Kanfer & Goldstein, 1991; Lambert, 2003).

John Dollard and Neil Miller (1950) attempted to combine psychoanalytic insights and practical learning principles into a science of human behavior. Joseph Wolpe (1958, 1969) worked to apply Pavlov's classical conditioning to systematic desensitization. Julian Rotter and Albert Bandura worked independently on a behavioral approach that stressed the impact of social learning and modeling concepts, in which context behavior is shaped by the interactions of an individual personality with significant others. Kanfer and Phillips (1970) used Skinner's operant model as a basis for developing the methods we now know as "behavior modification." Within the counseling literature, significant contributors such as John Krumboltz (1966), Carl Thoresen (1969), and Ray Hosford (1969) have been active in translating learning-theory principles into therapeutic practice.

The theory of behavioral counseling is deceptively simple. We are born into the world basically empty-headed, with a few reflexes. All our values, attitudes, preferences, emotional responses, thinking patterns, personality styles, and problems are the result of learned behavior. We are shaped by our environment, reinforced and molded by the world around us. A systematic and scientific approach is used to (1) identify specific behaviors in need of elimination or acquisition, (2) set objectives that are reasonable and desirable, (3) collect data on the client's functioning levels,

(4) design and engineer initial change efforts, (5) isolate and diminish client resistance, (6) modify distracting variables, (7) monitor and assess the impact of planned interventions, and (8) make alterations as needed in the treatment plan (Spiegler & Guevremont, 2001).

BEHAVIORAL TECHNOLOGY

One valuable tool of the researcher in general—and of behaviorists in particular—is the use of time-series charts for graphic portrayal of client change. This method helps the counselor to study a single case intensively, plotting baseline data and the results of therapeutic interventions. It aids in quantitatively and specifically describing the behaviors targeted for changes, as well as in noting the effects of any action. In Figure 6.1, the counselor has available at a glance a summary of the client's presenting problems and the results of several attempts to change the behavior.

A strength of the behavioral approach consists not only in its assessment procedures but in its wide variety of treatment strategies. Its technology of helping is consistently and reliably applied to produce observable client changes, which the behaviorist is skilled at identifying, measuring, and changing. Many behavioral methodologies are now part of the repertoire of every counselor; some are discussed here.

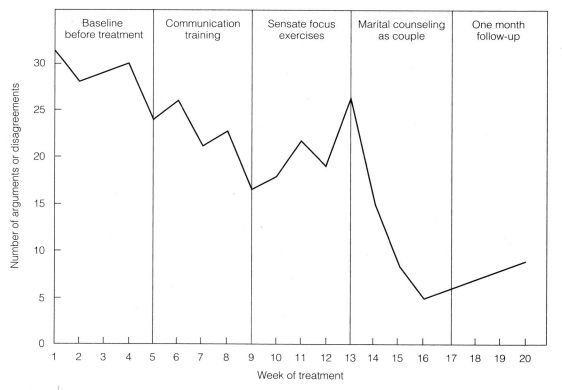

FIGURE 6.1 | EFFECTS OF INTERVENTIONS ON CLIENT'S RELATIONSHIP WITH SPOUSE

Operant-conditioning procedures, including those based on the work of B. F. Skinner (1953) and other researchers, are methods in which the frequency of behavior may be increased or decreased according to the type and timing of stimuli presented. In positive reinforcement strategies the counselor hopes to increase behavior by rewarding the client. Implicitly, the most subtle nods, "uh-huhs," smiles, and twinkling eyes positively reinforce the client's talking, trusting, and opening up. Operationally, this methodology is used in token economies with a variety of normal and maladjusted client populations, often in classroom settings, to spell out and encourage acceptable behavior as it spontaneously or deliberately occurs. Participants receive rewards in the form of points or privileges in exchange for their cooperation and lose points for obstructing progress.

The counselor's task is to (1) identify the specific target behaviors in need of upgrading, (2) discover situation-specific, individually designed rewards that motivate a given client, (3) administer the reinforcement soon after the target behavior is displayed, and (4) slowly wean the client from any dependence on the external motivation in favor of internalized, self-administered reinforcers. These same principles would hold true for any other operant procedure.

Negative reinforcement also produces an increase in desired target behaviors such as assertiveness, but it does so by removing a stimulus that the client perceives as aversive. Resistant clients, for example, can rid themselves of the inconvenience and discomfort of their counseling sessions only by being more cooperative and working faster to change.

Punishment strategies are used to reduce the frequency of a client's behavior by presenting an aversive stimulus. Unfortunately, many parents and teachers rely too heavily on this strategy because of its seeming convenience, even though it usually produces negative side effects in the child such as withdrawal, aggression, and generalized fears. Gershoff (2002) reviewed numerous studies on corporal punishment and found that although it did cause children to immediately comply with the authority figure, as adults they often exhibited antisocial behavior, and many abused their own children or spouses. Another problem with punishment is that its effects are brief and the behavior that is stopped often reappears at a higher level of frequency. Punishment may be used in conjunction with other operant procedures, such as in a weight-loss program in which the client writes a self-contract such as the one shown in Table 6.1.

The behavioral counselor has a variety of other standard techniques that have developed from laboratory research on conditioning processes.

Extinction involves the removal of the reinforcement for a given behavior, such as ignoring a child's temper tantrum. Two factors should be kept in mind when using extinction: (1) During the initial phase, after the reinforcer has been removed, the target behavior increases dramatically; during the second phase, the behavior decreases; and (2) extinction, once implemented, must be applied systematically and consistently.

Covert reinforcement uses mental images that function as reinforcers and can be generated by the client. The client is asked to imagine a situation in which he or she might refrain from an undesirable behavior. The counselor then instructs the client to visualize the reinforcing image.

Contingency contracting is the use of a behavioral contract that defines the necessary contingencies on which a reinforcer will be presented (see Table 6.1). Clients

TABLE 6.1	SAMPLE CONTRACT
Goals:	To lose 15 pounds in 60 days. To change my eating habits to include more fruits and vegetables and less chocolate. To exercise three times per week for no less than 20 minutes.
Procedures:	I will limit myself to 1,500 calories per day and restrict all eating activities to the dinner table. Snacks and in-between meals are strictly forbidden.
Consequences:	Daily reward: For each day I am able to stay within my calorie limit, I am permitted to play my tuba for two uninterrupted hours.
Daily punishment:	For each day I violate my calorie limit, I will set my alarm for 3 A.M., wake up, and vacuum and clean the house from top to bottom.
Contract reward:	If I am successful in losing 15 pounds within two months, I will treat myself to a four-day skiing weekend and buy myself a new outfit in a smaller size.
Contract punishment:	If I am unsuccessful, I will agree to do all housekeeping chores for a month.

Signed _____ Date _____

Witness _____

decide how often and at which levels they desire the reinforcer, thus shaping their own behavior.

Shaping is a process in which complex terminal behaviors are reinforced in approximate successive stages. The client receives consistent reinforcement in small steps as movement is made toward the ultimate goal.

In *classical* or *Pavlovian conditioning*, a presented stimulus elicits automatic responses. *Systematic desensitization*, an example of classical conditioning developed by Joseph Wolpe (1958, 1982), is the most common of these methodologies; clients are taught to substitute relaxation responses for anxiety when confronted by previously frightening situations such as tests or social events.

This method initially involves teaching the client how to relax. Next, a hierarchy of perceived threat is developed in which the client lists minimally stressful scenes (for example, watching a film of someone receiving an injection) and works toward progressively fearful images (receiving a flu shot in the arm). A more recent innovation is to use virtual reality computer technologies as an alternative to mental imagery in order to expose the client to the feared situation (Romano, 2005).

The counselor will usually use a hypnotically calm, relaxing voice, even pacing her words ... to ... the ... rise ... and ... fall ... of ... the ... client's ... breathing. The client is instructed to relax each muscle in the body, to imagine all tension draining away, to visualize a floating, drifting scene on the beach, perhaps feeling the warm sun and cool sand, hearing the waves crash against the surf, seeing birds sailing high above. After the client reaches a state of total relaxation, she or he is asked to work through the fear hierarchy, systematically reducing any tension with learned relaxation responses. After a few practice sessions, almost anyone can learn to inhibit his or her anxiety.

In *flooding,* an opposite strategy is employed to erode the stimulus/response sequence. A phobia, fear, or bad habit can be extinguished by bombarding the person with the stimulus until fatigue sets in or until (in the case of a habit) the stimulus loses its pleasurable value. A colleague of ours who lectures on this subject once was confronted by a disbelieving student who aggressively asked, "If this stuff works, how could I use it to stop smoking?" Our colleague flippantly replied, "Lock yourself in the closet with a pack of Camels, and don't come out until you're done smoking them all," never once considering that the student might actually follow the advice. A week later the student showed up in class again to report his story:

> I wasn't sure if you were kidding or not but I decided to try this behavior stuff anyway. I bought a pack of unfiltered cigarettes, went home, told my mother I was doing an experiment for school, and proceeded to lock myself in the bathroom. Since I usually smoke filtered menthols, I was, at first, a little surprised that I actually enjoyed the first two cigarettes. I even thought to myself, "Not only is this not going to work, but now I'm going to be addicted worse!" By the fifth cigarette I noticed I was feeling a little dizzy, and by the seventh the smoke was starting to burn my eyes. I finally started to get really sick by the tenth. I guess I must have passed out because the next morning I woke up in a pool of vomit with a cigarette burn on my leg. Not only will I never smoke again, but I can't even stand being in the same room with someone else who is.

This student's experience illustrates not only the effectiveness of behavioral strategies but also the importance of carefully monitoring their application so that abuse and harm can be avoided. Because the counselor has a more forceful role in behavioral counseling, the client's rights and freedom of choice are jeopardized unless great caution is taken to ensure that the ends justify the means and that the client is fully informed about the implications, dangers, and limitations of a given procedure.

CRITICISMS OF THE BEHAVIORAL APPROACH

Behaviorism has been criticized most often because of its narrow focus on observable human behavior and its lack of attention to feelings and thoughts, which also make up a significant part of a person's functioning. In addition, the behavioral approach works only with the presenting complaint, which could be a symptom of underlying intrapsychic conflicts. Many insight-oriented theorists therefore believe that symptoms thus cured will inevitably be replaced by others, because the internal condition of the client has not been altered.

As an action-oriented approach, behavioral counseling has also been criticized as mechanistic, manipulative, and impersonal because it downplays the role of the therapeutic relationship and all but ignores the value of self-understanding in the change process. Because it also works toward empiricism (that is, specificity or quantification), prediction, and control, it often sacrifices the values of intuition and artistry in change endeavors. Regardless of a counselor's philosophical concerns with behavioral therapies, they are still one of the accepted treatment modalities for when clients seek relief from phobias and other anxiety disorders, and behavioral interventions need to be at least considered as a component in any comprehensive treatment plan.

COGNITIVE BEHAVIORAL THERAPY AND RATIONAL EMOTIVE BEHAVIOR THERAPY

ALIASES: CBT, COG-B, REBT, RATIONAL BEHAVIOR THERAPY, COGNITIVE RESTRUCTURING

In the 1960s, two men trained as traditional psychoanalysts developed new theories of counseling and of the etiology of emotional distress that have virtually revolutionized the fields of counseling and psychotherapy. Aaron Beck, attempting to validate Freud's contention that depression resulted from anger being turned inward, discovered instead that depressed clients exhibited a negative bias in how they cognitively interpreted life events. Further research led him to theorize that maladaptive thinking patterns lay at the heart of psychological disorders, and counseling's proper goal should be to modify these patterns (Beck & Weishaar, 2005). Albert Ellis, feeling confined and bored by the rigid structures of traditional psychoanalysis, came to similar conclusions and developed a system of counseling based on principles of logic and rational analysis (Ellis, 1994).

Both Beck and Ellis helped promulgate their ideas through numerous publications and scholarly articles. Beck's "cognitive therapy" has been studied for its efficacy in treating such disorders as depression, anxiety, obsessive-compulsive disorder, personality disorders, and substance abuse, as well as physical problems like chronic pain and tinnitus. Ellis, also insistent on establishing a solid empirical base for his Rational Emotive Behavior Therapy (REBT), collaborated with researchers on numerous studies (e.g., Ellis & Grieger, 1986; Ellis & Joffe, 2002; Ellis& Whitely, 1979), and worked with other theorists to develop models integrating his REBT ideas with different frameworks, including constructivist and brief models (Ellis, 1995, 2001, 2005).

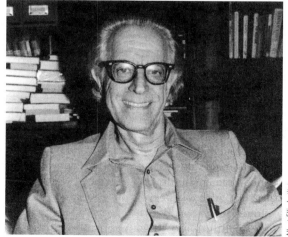

Albert Ellis developed Rational Emotive Behavior Therapy (REBT) in the 1960s, about the same time that Carl Rogers was working on his person-centered approach. Ellis emphasized the importance of identifying and challenging irrational beliefs that interfere with optimal functioning.

It is fair to say that while Ellis has successfully popularized REBT through hundreds of presentations and publications—even songs and coloring books—Beck's cognitive therapy has gained wider acceptance in the counseling field; indeed, it has become the theory of choice for thousands of practitioners and has generated a prodigious amount of research, most of which empirically supports its efficacy for numerous conditions (Butler, Chapman, Forman, & Beck, 2006; Stathopoulu et al., 2006). Although Beck calls his model "cognitive therapy," it is generally referred to as *cognitive behavioral therapy* (CBT) because of the theory's utilization of behavioral interventions in addition to techniques for modifying distress-causing thinking patterns.

CBT begins with the premise that we all learn in childhood a set of assumptions and beliefs, called *schemas*, that throughout life influence our interpretations of daily situations and incidents. We experience these interpretations or inferences as the thoughts (Beck called them *automatic thoughts*) that instinctively flit across our conscious minds right after the event itself and when we later ruminate about the meaning of the event. Self-critical belief systems learned in childhood can be activated by certain life situations and can generate distorted, unrealistic, automatic thoughts, which in turn negatively affect our mood. Thus, CBT was initially proposed as a theoretical model designed to address disturbances of mood, specifically depression (Beck, Rush, Shaw, & Emery, 1979).

Here is an example: Frank is a 35-year-old engineer who grew up with highly critical parents. He was scolded severely by his parents for every grade less than an "A" (*Frank's childhood experiences*). Frank had excellent math skills, but English and writing classes were difficult for him, and no matter how hard he tried, he could not meet his parents' expectations. Frank gradually developed the core belief, "I am not good enough" (*Frank's schema*). Frank compensated for his lack of confidence by relentlessly pushing himself, which enabled him to succeed in college and later as an engineer in a large computer company.

Then, the roof caved in; Frank, as well as his whole department, were informed they were going to be laid off because of corporate downsizing. When Frank heard the news, he thought to himself, "It's my fault—if I had worked harder, this wouldn't have happened. I'm responsible for my whole team losing their jobs. My wife will never forgive me for this. I'll never get as good a job as this again—hey, I may never get hired as an engineer again. Everyone will see me as a failure" (*Frank's automatic thoughts, generated by his schema*). Other employees, without this schema, responded differently, with thoughts like, "Well, maybe this will be a good opportunity to make some changes in my life," or, "Oh well, this stinks, but that's life—I'll be OK."

Frank's thoughts started him on the road to a deep depression (*mood disturbance caused by his thoughts*); he moped around the house, sometimes not bothering to get out of bed. He didn't have the energy to even read the want ads, and he became irritable to his wife and children. As Frank lay in bed, he kept thinking to himself, "I'm such a loser. I should have seen this coming. I can't do anything right. Pretty soon, we'll all be homeless, and it's my fault." Frank badly needed the help of a counselor, and was a good candidate for either CBT or REBT.

Both CBT and REBT are "top-down" counseling approaches, because they work at the level of the client's unrealistic and irrational thoughts, which are more accessible to the client than deep-seated schemas; this is an important point, because a common misunderstanding of cognitive behavioral therapies is that they ignore feelings and underlying issues. Cognitive behavioral counselors would argue that they are most definitely interested in hearing the client's feelings, and conceptualizing core issues; however, their best leverage for *helping* the client is by getting at the client's conscious thoughts. Thus, an REBT counselor might confront Frank, pointing out the ways in which his thoughts are irrational and self-destructive. "It's not the loss of your job that is making you depressed," an REBT counselor might say. "It's your beliefs, your negative interpretations of what happened, that's created your depression. I'm going to show you how these thoughts like 'It's all my fault' and 'I should have seen this coming' are completely illogical, and when you start talking to yourself more rationally, you're going to start feeling better." As Ellis put it,

> My approach to psychotherapy is to zero in, as quickly as possible, on the client's basic philosophy of life; to get him to see exactly what this is, and how it is inevitably self-defeating; and to persuade him to work his ass off, cognitively, emotively, and behaviorally, to profoundly change it. My basic assumption is that virtually all "emotionally disturbed" individuals actually think crookedly, magically, dogmatically, and unrealistically. (Ellis, 1988, p. 581)

Ellis developed an "ABC Theory" of emotions that helped explain the ways that irrational beliefs lead people to negative emotional outcomes. In Table 6.2 you can see how an upsetting situation leads one to focus on upsetting interpretations that produce correspondingly negative consequences. Also note the ways that these irrational beliefs can be challenged, with quite different results.

Beck's CBT model emphasizes a more collaborative approach with clients in which the primary goal would be to help clients carefully examine their thoughts, holding them to the light of day: In a process Beck called *collaborative empiricism,* the counselor facilitates the clients' own discovery that their thoughts are unrealistic (Beck & Weishaar, 2005). Rather than directly disputing thoughts as irrational, the counselor reframes them as hypotheses that can be tested. "OK, Frank, I see you think you're responsible for your entire team's getting fired. Let's check this out. Let's make a list of everyone on your team, and figure out how it was you, not corporate downsizing, that caused them to lose their job." As you might expect, when Frank puts his belief to the test, it doesn't hold up, which not only improves his mood, but also forces Frank to challenge his core schema.

BASIC POINTS OF CBT

CBT counselors use a variety of interventions, both cognitive and behavioral, developing a treatment plan that can be completed in 10 to 12 sessions (making CBT a brief therapy model). Like any effective approach, CBT is embedded in a particular kind of relationship that builds an alliance and that is flexible according to the needs of a client in a particular moment in time (Gilbert & Leahy, 2007). The specific interventions used are tailored to the needs of each client, and counselors can choose from a long list of interventions, or even create their own. Nevertheless, certain techniques have become staples of CBT counseling (Murdock, 2008). Regardless of the techniques used, the primary goal is relief of the client's emotional distress; while basic counseling skills like reflection and empathy are important to establishing a working

TABLE 6.2 | ABC THEORY OF EMOTIONS

A

Activating Emotional Experience

Reading chapters on counseling approaches that present a dozen complex theories

B

Belief or Interpretation of Experience

"I feel so stupid that I can't understand all of this stuff."

"This is terrible. I'll never be a good counselor since I already feel lost."

"I should be able to pick this stuff up faster."

C

Consequences

Anxiety

Fear

Confusion

Frustration

Anger

D

Disputing Irrational Beliefs

"Of course I feel overwhelmed—that is what an introductory student is supposed to feel when presented with an overview of the field in just a few weeks."

"Just because I don't understand everything about these theories doesn't make me a stupid person—just a person who will have to work a little harder and have more patience."

"This isn't a terrible situation—it's only difficult and slightly uncomfortable."

E

Emotional Effect

Relief

Mild tension

Mild annoyance

Excitement

---

alliance, the counselor's focus is on implementing strategies that will alleviate symptoms as quickly and efficiently as possible.

1. *Teach the client the categories of cognitive distortions.* Beck and his colleagues developed a list of the typical kinds of unrealistic, distorted thoughts clients experience. This list was subsequently modified by other cognitive theorists, the most popular of which was developed by Burns (1999) and often given to clients to learn. (See Table 6.3).

2. *Create a thought diary.* Clients record in a chart their irrational thoughts following a mood-affecting situation, the category the thoughts belong to, and

TABLE 6.3 | CATEGORIES OF DISTORTED THINKING

All or nothing thinking. Life is seen in black or white terms. "Either I get perfect grades, or I am a failure."

Emotional reasoning. A feeling is wrongly assumed to be a fact. "I feel hopeless about passing this course, even though my grades are OK so far. There's no way the teacher will pass me."

Mind reading. Assuming you know what others are thinking about you. "I'm sure my teacher is thinking I don't have any potential as a counselor."

Should statements. Saying I "should," "I must," or "I ought to," statements that are common attempts to motivate ourselves, are more likely to make us feel anxious or depressed. Ellis's REBT makes a similar point, calling this tendency *Musterbating.*

Catastrophizing. Making a mistake or having a bad experience, and assuming that it will lead to the worst possible outcome. "I got a 'C' on this paper. I'll fail this course, and never get to be a counselor." REBT counselors call this *Awfulizing.*

Labeling. Calling ourselves a derogatory name, something we all do from time to time, inevitably making us feel worse. "I'm such a jerk for not studying harder."

Personalization. Unrealistically taking responsibility for other people's moods and behaviors. "Jane is really upset today. It must be something I did."

Disqualifying the positive. Ignoring our positive qualities and achievements, and only seeing our negative characteristics or mistakes. "I'm really unhappy about that paper I wrote. That last paragraph was very confusing" (even though the rest of the paper was fine).

Magnification. Overemphasizing the importance of one negative event. "I forgot to study for the pop quiz. I'm a terrible student."

Fortune telling. Assuming we know what's going to happen down the line. "By the time I finish this program, there will be no jobs left for counselors." (Burns, 1999)

more realistic alternative thoughts. They rate on a scale of 1–100 how they first felt when they responded to the event, and then how they feel after recognizing their cognitive distortions and writing down a more rational response to the same situation. For example, Frank experienced the thought, "I may never get hired as an engineer again," which understandably made him feel depressed, and which he scored as 80 (100 would be the worst he's ever felt in his life). In his thought diary, Frank would recognize this as the "fortune telling" cognitive error, and then would come up with an alternative thought, such as, "I can't predict what the future holds, but there's no reason I can't get another engineering job when people see my résumé." As he generates this alternative, Frank notices his mood lifting a bit, which he now scores as 40.

3. *Engage in a Socratic dialogue.* The counselor questions the client's thinking processes, persistently challenges illogical ideas, and gradually leads the client to appreciate that his or her negative cognitive response to an event does not make rational sense.

4. *Test the evidence.* The counselor assigns the client the task of testing the validity of a negative belief. For example, someone who believes no one likes

VOICE FROM THE FIELD

I was trained as a humanistic counselor, and I still believe in the idea that counseling is a great opportunity for people to really examine themselves. I learned all those important values humanists hold so dearly—letting the client set the pace, trusting the client's inner wisdom; counseling is supposed to be about growth, not fixing things. It all really sounds good. Easy ideas to embrace. Except I had one problem—I'm not sure that deep inside I really believed it. Clients would come to see me wanting help with their depression or anxiety or other problems, and I felt guilty that I wasn't really trying to help them. "Growth" and "fulfilling their human potential" was something I wanted for them, sure, but it wasn't what they wanted from me. They were feeling awful, life was no fun, and they wanted to feel better. It was as simple as that. Why wasn't I doing the best I could to help alleviate their pain?

Because the research is clear—that CBT does help clients feel better, and works pretty quickly, too—I couldn't keep ignoring study after study showing how effective CBT can be. I was beginning to question whether it was unethical of me not to use CBT. But I'll tell you what really sold me on this theory. I'd start to slip CBT ideas into one of my client-centered sessions. Like I said to one man, "What you're doing is catastrophizing and predicting the future. I know life is tough for you right now, but there's no evidence it has to stay this way." And you know what? Next session, he said he felt better for the first time, and the one thing he remembered from the session was the little CBT intervention I threw in there. And for the first time in a long time, I felt good about doing counseling. I had actually helped someone, and the proof was right there in front of me.

her might be given the assignment of making a list of everyone she has known, and checking off all the people who liked her and all those who didn't. Chances are good the client will discover that the belief, "no one" likes me, will be proven incorrect.

5. *Break big problems down into smaller ones*. A staple of CBT is the idea that overwhelming problems feel more manageable when broken down into smaller tasks to accomplish. Telling yourself that you must stop drinking is unlikely to be of much help. On the other hand, making a task list, including seeing your doctor, investigating local 12-step programs, identifying the situations that cause you to drink, and getting counseling are all achievable goals framed one step at a time, which increases the chances of success.

6. *Use behavioral exercises*. Relaxation techniques, physical exercise, practicing new social skills, role-plays in sessions, assertiveness training, and behavioral desensitization are all used by CBT counselors as part of an overall treatment approach. Exercise, for example, consistently has been demonstrated by research as helpful in relieving depression (Stathopoulou, Powers, Berry, Smits, & Otto, 2006).

CRITICISMS OF COGNITIVE-BASED THERAPIES

1. Human beings are multifaceted, with feelings as well as thoughts. Critics suggest that CBT and REBT put undue emphasis on thought processes to the exclusion of many legitimate feelings, thereby contributing to repression and denial of feelings.

■ | VOICE FROM THE FIELD

Of all the theories I've used—and believe me, I've used a bunch—REBT is the one I found most useful in my own life. I don't even practice it that much anymore with my clients, but I still use it every day inside my own head. So often, I get down on myself because I feel like I'm failing my clients or not doing as good a job as I should. Then I hear Ellis's voice in my head, confronting me about my "shoulds" and absolute judgments. It really does work miracles.

Why don't I use it anymore with my clients? I don't know. I guess I just got bored with it after a while. It's not that it stopped working; really, it's powerful stuff. It's just that I got tired disputing the same old irrational beliefs over and over. I moved on to something new and more dynamic. But I still use it sometimes with clients who really seem like good candidates for a more confrontational, thinking approach.

2. CBT and REBT are probably less effective with some kinds of clients—those who already have problems with overintellectualizing or who don't have the capacity to reason logically (young children, schizophrenics, some clients with personality disorders, or clients with minimal intelligence).
3. Many cognitive-behavioral counselors complain of boredom and burnout from continuously repeating the same arguments and processes with all clients.
4. CBT and REBT are difficult for some professionals to practice if they are not outgoing and assertive and don't enjoy vigorous debate and confrontation.
5. Because the counselor's role is so verbal, active, and directive, the client may feel overpowered, dominated, and not responsible for the outcome.

PERSONAL APPLICATIONS

Among counseling approaches, CBT and REBT lend themselves particularly well to personal adoption by the professional. Ellis has said repeatedly that, by talking our clients out of their crazy beliefs, we cannot help changing our own in the process. Other REBT practitioners report that they have noticed themselves becoming more psychologically healthy as they become more experienced clinicians. Ellis and Wilde (2002) describe how this approach can be applied to a series of cases, demonstrating the kind of parallel process that can occur in which practitioners confront their own issues with perfectionism and low frustration tolerance as they challenge these beliefs in their clients.

Personally useful ideas from CBT and REBT include the following:

1. The idea that, because we create our own emotional misery through distorted thinking, we can potentially change these negative feelings by changing the way we think about our situations. A highway accident, critical comment, and missed appointment can all be viewed as inconveniences or disasters, depending on our point of view.
2. The technique of carefully monitoring our language for words such as should, must, and ought, which may imply irrational beliefs. As we become more aware of illogical language, we start to hear faulty phrases in others and ourselves: "She makes me so angry" (how can anyone make you feel anything

without your consent?); "This weather is so depressing" (rain is just rain—it's your interpretation that makes it seem depressing); "It just frustrates me so much" (don't you mean, "I frustrate myself over what I perceive is happening"?).

3. The structure of mentally rehearsing difficult tasks for the future or painful events of the past in order to relieve anxiety and work through unsolved irrational beliefs. These imagery techniques are helpful, for instance, in allaying fears about an upcoming interview. For such a situation, penetrating questions could be asked: "What's the worst that could happen? Even if I mess up the interview and perform less than perfectly, does that mean I'm not a good counselor and will never be competent? And even if that were so, what does that have to do with my 'goodness' as a human being?"

SOLUTION-FOCUSED COUNSELING

ALIASES: SOLUTION-ORIENTED COUNSELING, SINGLE-SESSION THERAPY, PROBLEM-SOLVING THERAPY, BRIEF THERAPY

CLIENT (First session): Every time my husband and I talk about money, I start getting angry. I think it has to do with when I was a kid; my father ...

COUNSELOR (Gently): Instead of talking about the past, let's focus on your goal. What would it look like if this problem didn't exist?

CLIENT: Well, that's the thing. I can't help myself. I have this problem with anger ...

COUNSELOR: Talking about the problem is not going to solve it. Talking about a solution will. If I were watching a movie about you and your husband talking about money, and the two of you had a great conversation, what would I see?

CLIENT: Well ... I guess you'd see me laughing, and he'd be laughing, too. You know, joking around when we were paying bills. Turning it into a fun thing.

COUNSELOR: Interesting. When was a time when something like this actually happened, when you talked about money and you had fun doing it?

CLIENT: Well, there was this one time a couple of years ago, I think.

COUNSELOR: Try to remember exactly what you were doing when this problem didn't exist.

CLIENT: We were both drinking some wine. And we had the oldies radio station on. And it was on a Sunday night, instead of a weekday, when we usually deal with bills.

COUNSELOR: That makes things much clearer. Okay, here's what I would like you to do. Only pay bills on a Sunday. Have some wine, and turn on the oldies station. Don't even talk about money any other day of the week.

CLIENT: That's it?

COUNSELOR: That's it.

CLIENT: Oh, one more thing, how many sessions do you think we need?

COUNSELOR: You already know what works. You have the ability to laugh about difficult subjects. That's your strength. It's worked for you in the past. So use it! You'll notice the problem start to go away immediately, even if you have a few setbacks. The solution was always within your grasp.

This excerpt from a solution-focused counseling session, however simplified and abbreviated, demonstrates what makes this model one of the most exciting and dramatic approaches to counseling to occur in many years. Every theory discussed so far in this book—insight- or action-oriented—hypothesizes that problems have a cause, and client change occurs when counselor and client collaboratively address that cause. Psychoanalytically-oriented counselors illuminate unresolved childhood conflicts; humanistic counselors respond to client mechanisms for avoiding being present and authentic; cognitive behaviorists hone in on irrational thoughts and beliefs. What solution-focused counselors propose is that looking at the causes of a problem is irrelevant to client change; in fact, talking about the problem itself mires the counselor and client in unnecessary conversation, resulting in client discouragement and feelings of hopelessness (Berg & DeJong, 2005). Problem-focused thinking also can extend the length of counseling well beyond what is necessary for achieving client goals. Understandably, with its emphasis on making the counseling process as brief as necessary (only a single session in some cases), a solution-focused orientation is well suited to our era of managed care and efficient clinical practice.

The solution-focused theory, developed primarily by Steve de Shazer, William O'Hanlon, Insoo Kim Berg, and Michele Weiner-Davis (De Jong & Berg, 2008), is strongly influenced by the work of Milton Erickson, a psychiatrist and hypnotherapist noted for his extraordinary talents in entering clients' world view, recognizing their strengths, and helping them see how they can utilize their strengths and inner resources to solve their problems. O'Hanlon, for example, so admired Erickson's genius that he worked as his gardener for a year because he wanted to learn from Erickson but didn't have the money to pay for training (O'Hanlon, 1986). The solution-focused theorists—inspired both by Erickson's success in using language and metaphor to help clients shift their perspective on problems and by his focus on tapping already-existing client strengths—worked separately and together to create an approach based on five assumptions. These are summarized by Cepeda and Davenport (2006):

1. If it doesn't work, do something different, and if it works, do more of it.
2. Clients have the strengths and resources to change.
3. Client problems result from not recognizing alternatives, rather than from underlying pathology.
4. A small change in any aspect of a problem begins the process of solving it.
5. Change comes from focusing on future possibilities and solutions. (Cepeda & Davenport, 2006, p. 3)

Clients in this model are often called *customers, complainants*, or *visitors* (Murdock, 2008). Customers are able to describe their problem and are motivated to change it; complainants are just like the word sounds—people able to describe the problem but not ready to do anything about it. Visitors come to counseling because a family member told them to go, not because they see their role in the problem or solution. As you might expect, customers are the kind of clients most likely to experience successful outcomes. But a skilled solution-focused counselor can help a complainant and visitor shift their attitude toward becoming a customer. Notice also that the use of the word *customer* implies a therapeutic relationship where the client has literally hired a counselor to facilitate solution finding as efficiently as possible—usually in several sessions, and rarely in more than 10.

The underlying premise to solution-focused counseling is a disarmingly simple one: Clients already have solved their problems at some point in their lives (see the dialogue that began this section); the resources they drew upon and strategies they used in the previous situations can be applied to the current problem. The goal of the counselor, then, is to assist the client in discovering those relevant resources and strategies through a collaborative counselor-client conversation; the art of this process is to keep the client from backtracking into "problem talk" and remain oriented toward "solution talk." While there are a number of techniques available to solution-focused counseling, core interventions include the following:

THE MIRACLE QUESTION Solution-focused counseling almost always begins with the counselor asking in some form, "If a miracle occurred and the problem no longer existed, what would be different and how would I know?" (de Shazer, 1988). Notice the last phrase; it insists that the client imagine with clarity and concreteness what it would look and sound like if the problem had been solved. It asks the client to tell a story of life without the problem, and contained within that story will be specific details suggesting to the counselor and the client possible solutions to the presenting issue.

PRETENDING This is a strategy that Madanes (1984) preferred when working with children who have disruptive symptoms irritating to their parents. After the child has been deliberately directed to engage in the symptoms, they lose their controlling power. Other forms of directive intervention involve shifting the power in a family, changing the family members' style of interaction, and posing paradoxical tasks: The client is given instructions that the counselor hopes he will disobey. With clients who wished to lose weight, for example, Milton Erickson was fond of ordering them to gain five pounds before the next session. If they complied, they demonstrated the potential control they had over their weight—the ability to increase (and, by implication, decrease) it at will. More likely, however, they would think Erickson crazy, deliberately disobey the order, and lose weight, thereby following the road to recovery.

EXCEPTION FINDING The counselor and client play detective, searching for times in the client's life when the problem did not occur. It's presumed that in that particular situation, the client had employed an effective solution. The counselor facilitates the client's examining exactly what he or she did that allowed the exception to occur. Exception finding is another technique for tapping into the client's repertoire of preexisting strengths and effective strategies.

SCALING QUESTIONS Throughout the course of treatment, solution-focused counselors like to ask clients to rate their progress in achieving their goals. Assigning a 1–10 number not only provides evaluative information to both counselor and client, but also enables the counselor to ask, "What one or two things could you do this week to bring you up 2 points?" (Murdock, 2008, p. 422).

Questions take on a particularly important role in solution-focused counseling. They are not only used to collect meaningful data about the nature of the problem, but they are also critical as interventions to encourage clients to take different actions.

TABLE 6.4	SOLUTION-FOCUSED QUESTIONS USED IN AN INITIAL INTERVIEW

- What's the trouble?
- Why are you here and what do you expect?
- How is that a problem for you?
- When, where, and with whom does the problem occur?
- What are some exceptions to the times when you experience this as a problem?
- If you woke up tomorrow without the problem, what would be different?
- If your problem was solved by a miracle, what form might that take?
- What have you already tried to do to solve the problem that doesn't work?
- What have you tried that does work sometimes?
- When is the problem not a problem?
- When is the problem the worst?
- How did you manage to overcome your problem in the exceptions you described previously?

Table 6.4 provides examples of how questions might be introduced into an initial interview.

TASK ASSIGNMENTS Ultimately, the success of this theory relies on the counselor's assigning clients to perform specific tasks in between sessions. Often, the counselor will ask clients to repeat the strategies unearthed in the "exception finding" intervention; another task would be to have them recreate in their daily life details of the story they articulated in response to the miracle question. For example, a wife complaining about her husband's emotional unavailability might have imagined a scene in which both partners greet each other with kisses after coming home from work. The counselor would assign the woman the task of kissing her husband, just as she imagined; her husband may or may not respond in kind, but the wife's new behavior may still initiate a solution-oriented, positive spiral in the relationship. Whatever the task, the emphasis is on formulating goals tailored specifically to match the client's personal strengths and problem-solving capabilities.

CRITICISMS OF SOLUTION-FOCUSED COUNSELING

Like all theories, solution-focused counseling has earned its fair share of criticism, some perhaps from counselors who fear it legitimizes arguments voiced by managed care supporters that counseling takes too long. There are other criticisms, however, that may have more validity.

1. It's helpful only because of the placebo effect. Most clients feel better after a few sessions regardless of the theory used. The real test of any theory is its utility after the initial feelings of hopefulness fade, and the client must face the challenge of changing. It's hard to know if solution-focused counseling is more than a placebo, because it is so brief.

VOICE FROM THE FIELD

I have no doubt that solution-focused counseling helps people—at least helps them solve their immediate problem. And in my experience, usually solving one problem has a kind of domino effect—it starts a whole sequence of things getting better. Its basic principles seem pretty humanistic, building on people's own resources—I like that part of it, too. And I'll be the first to admit that introducing the miracle question into the way I do counseling has improved my work.

But I have one problem with it (well, two, I guess, if you count the fact that I can't make a living seeing people for just a couple of sessions). Here's my big concern: Every client I've had, at some point, has wanted to reveal to me something they were ashamed of—just to get it off their chest. Whoever said that counseling was "confession without absolution" was right on the money, because I do think that a big part of what we do is make it safe for people to confess something, knowing they won't be judged. It doesn't matter if it's something they should feel guilty about, like actually hurting people—or something really minor and harmless, but important to the client. An unkind word spoken to a family member. A tactless break-up with a lover. An embarrassing sexual fantasy. I'll never forget a middle-aged client who said to me one session, "I'm going to tell you something I've never said to anyone before. This is really hard for me." I held my breath, expecting to hear some shocking, sordid tale, and hoping I wouldn't accidentally show criticism on my face. The client leaned forward, and quietly said, "I screen my mother's calls. If I see it's her number calling me, I don't always pick up. Sometimes, I won't even get back to her until the next day. I know I'm a horrible person. But it's a relief just to admit it." To you or me, that may not have been much of a crime, but it was to her. And if we had been doing brief counseling focused entirely on solutions, she would never have felt the wonderful release of tension that happens when you confess.

2. Clients may not grow from the experience or learn new skills.
3. Some clients need the opportunity, at least initially, to talk about their problems and explore their meaning.
4. Insight is unnecessarily downgraded or totally ignored as a distracting variable, even though self-understanding is an important goal of many clients.
5. Because the focus of this approach is on solving problems, it could rely largely on a male-oriented, control-based methodology that is inconsistent with the values of some cultures.
6. Many of the strategies are intuitively constructed and are therefore difficult to learn and apply reliably. Many of the successful cases presented in the literature and in training workshops were constructed by teams of experts working from behind one-way mirrors, an option not available to most practitioners in the field.
7. There is a limited empirical base for these approaches, and by their nature they prove difficult to research. (Murdock, 2008)

PERSONAL APPLICATIONS

Solution-focused counseling emphasizes a flexible, pragmatic approach to solving problems. Many of the therapeutic principles applied to client issues are equally helpful in working through conflicts of your own, especially when following a few rules:

1. At some point in your life, you have found a way to solve even the most daunting of challenges. Recall as carefully as you can how you solved a

problem in the past, and you will discover your personal repertoire of effective strategies.

2. When you try something and it doesn't work, don't do the same thing; try anything else other than what you are doing. For example, if you repeatedly push on a door to get out of a room, and nothing happens, pushing harder is not likely to work either. Try pulling. Although there is no guarantee that this will be any more successful, at least it gets you out of a situation in which you are stuck repeating the same thing over and over.

3. When you are facing a problem that feels insurmountable, reframe it in a way that makes it more manageable. Imagine, for example, that you are feeling discouraged because you keep "failing" at something that is important to you. Morale can be substantially improved by casting the term failure in a different light: Not succeeding at something is simply a means of gaining greater experience and practice.

4. Typical of the innovative ways that strategic counselors tackle difficult problems, O'Hanlon and Weiner-Davis (2003) describe a dramatic method of change called "time travel." Assume that you are a client who feels stuck. First, you are asked to practice traveling into the past and future through the use of fantasy. Once you can easily move forward or backward at will, you are asked to travel into the future to a time when your problem is resolved. Are you there yet? Okay, then—what did you do to fix your problem? You can then retrospectively "look back" from your perch in the future and tell yourself what you need to do.

HONORABLE MENTIONS

We mentioned in the previous chapter that limited space requires that you are exposed to only a few theories representative of those that are action-oriented. Your instructors, your coworkers, and other authors could easily suggest that models other than those described be included. The good news is that you will most likely have at least one other course devoted exclusively to studying theories in greater depth. Nevertheless, here are a few others that deserve honorable mention.

MULTIMODAL COUNSELING

Among several other action-oriented practitioners, Arnold Lazarus has sought to combine features from several theories into a flexible system for analyzing and treating clients' problems. Originally a behaviorist, Lazarus was influenced by the behavioral therapy of Joseph Wolpe and, later, by the cognitive therapy of Albert Ellis. He has endeavored to create an approach to counseling that is behavioral in its systematic analysis, comprehensive in its scope of exploring the total person, and pragmatic in its selection of techniques (Lazarus, 1981, 1993, 1995, 2006, 2008).

This theory is called *multimodal* because it seeks to understand and intervene at the levels of all seven modalities of the human personality. People are capable of experiencing sensations, feelings, thoughts, images, observable behavior, interpersonal responses, and biochemical and neurophysiological reactions. These human

VOICE FROM THE FIELD

I've always found reality therapy to be my preferred theory because it kind of gives you a road map. You have an idea of where you are with a client—and where you need to go next—at any moment. I really like that structure.

I don't think I'll hurt anyone with it either. Basically, what I'm doing is helping people to evaluate for themselves the consequences of their behavior. I don't have to be the expert.

components are conveniently organized into the acronym BASIC ID, in which each letter represents a different modality that can be used to explore and change behavior. Multimodal assessment thus permits the practitioner to understand at a glance (1) how the client characteristically functions; (2) how, where, and why the presenting problem manifests itself; and (3) how specifically to use the profile as a blueprint for promoting change.

One distinct contribution of this approach is that it avoids the use of formal diagnostic labels and psychological jargon in favor of more down-to-earth terms. It encourages the counselor to design individualized treatment strategies for each client and can often accomplish specifically defined goals relatively briefly (Palmer, 2006).

REALITY THERAPY

William Glasser (1965, 1990, 1998, 2000, 2001; Wubbolding, 2008) is credited as the founder of reality therapy, which reflected his dissatisfaction with contemporary psychoanalytic theory. It is an essentially didactic approach that stresses problem solving, personal responsibility, and the need to cope with the demands of a person's "reality." Reality theory is based on the assumption that all individuals need to develop an identity, which can be either a "success identity" or a "failure identity."

Reality therapy has been enjoying a resurgence of interest in the past few years due in part to renewed focus on the role of personal responsibility in life problems and to the application of "choice theory" to a variety of settings, including schools, agencies, and medical facilities (Glasser, 1990, 1998, 2001; Loyd, 2005; Wubbolding, 1990, 2000; Wubbolding, 2008).

The counselor's job is to become highly involved with the client and to encourage motivation toward a plan of responsible action that will lead to constructive behavior change and a "success identity." The reality-therapy approach is active, directive, and cognitive, with a strong behavioral emphasis that makes use of contingency contracting. The counselor assumes simultaneous supportive and confrontational roles with clients.

Reality therapy is a short-term treatment that has been widely used in schools, institutions, and correctional settings. It is a fairly simple therapeutic approach, at least as to the basics, and can be mastered without lengthy training and supervision. The disadvantages of reality therapy include its tendency to reward conforming behavior, the danger of the therapist's imposing personal values of reality, and its tendency to treat symptoms rather than possible underlying causes.

EXPRESSIVE THERAPIES

Expressive therapies include a variety of therapeutic approaches that, although loosely integrated, all rest on the assumption that primarily nonverbal media are effective in the release and resolution of clients' problems. Whereas most of the other theories presented in this chapter rely primarily on cognitive and behavioral factors, expressive therapies tend not to rely on language and thus are able to bypass much resistance and to intensively explore underlying conflicts and dysfunctional issues.

Frequently the use of expressive therapy is not theoretically isolated but occurs as an adjunct to other theoretical modalities. To balance the more traditional modalities that we have previously explored, we offer several examples of these alternative approaches.

ART THERAPY   Art therapy has long been a form of treatment for children, helping them to express feelings actively as well as to talk through images represented in their drawings (Case & Dalley, 2006; Waller, 2006). The *Journal of Art Therapy* contains suggestions for using materials for promoting better cooperation in children, for gathering data for diagnoses, and especially for helping people become more creative and emotionally expressive. When verbal strategies are ineffective, practitioners resort to such alternative therapeutic media as musical instruments, games, sculpture, photography, drawing, cartooning, poetry, journal writing, puppetry, and drama (Gladding, 2005). Resistances and emotional blocks can therefore be bypassed through these treatment strategies and through other therapies that are primarily nonverbal.

MUSIC AND DANCE THERAPY   Movement is a popular form of expressive therapy, used with music or without. There is even the American Dance Therapy Association, which seeks to guide practitioners who employ such methods in their work. As with most of the other nonverbally mediated treatments, this strategy has the advantage of bypassing intellectualization and verbal defenses with the intent of helping people to become more self-expressive, more in touch with their bodies and minds, and more inclined to explore their potential in creative ways.

BIOFEEDBACK   Another action method that can be used to improve client control, biofeedback gives clients accurate information about their psychophysiological responses. Readings can be taken of bodily functions such as brain activity, heart rate, muscle movement, blood pressure, and skin responses in order to improve muscular and neurological control. Biofeedback has been used to reduce general tension, control headaches, modify vascular disorders such as hypertension, better tolerate chronic pain, relieve sexual dysfunction, control seizure disorders, or prevent stress-related problems (Moss, 2002; Nestoriuc, Rief, & Martin, 2008). A similar, more recent feedback technology is EEG neurofeedback, which enables clients to manipulate their brain's electrical waves by interacting with specially designed computer games. Clients are connected to the computer via electrodes attached to the skull and forehead; the neurofeedback counselor measures clients' maladaptive brainwave status on a computer readout, and designs a protocol allowing clients to adjust their wave patterns. Neurofeedback, though still in its infancy, may be a promising treatment for attention deficit disorders, anxiety, and cognitive impairments resulting from brain injuries (Demos, 2005).

PLAY THERAPY   Most counseling with children employs some kind of play, whether it involves drawing, playing cards or games, building structures, dressing up in costumes, or playing catch with a ball. Beginning from about age two until the teen years, but especially during the early childhood and elementary school years, play is the primary form of expression for children. The counselor seeks to establish trust with the child, as well as to facilitate communication and even solve problems, through the interactive nature of play. There is a wide spectrum of different counseling theories, and each has its own approach to play therapy. Some theories emphasize play only and others integrate play with talking about the issues (Drewes, 2009; Giordano, Landreth, & Jones, 2005).

HYPNOTHERAPY   Another area that requires additional training and certification for counselors is hypnotherapy. Hypnosis has been applied widely in therapeutic situations since Freud's day—by behavioral counselors who wish to intensify systematic desensitization techniques; by psychoanalysts in order to access the unconscious; and by many other clinicians who use imagery, rehearsal, and fantasy techniques. Whereas hypnosis has most commonly been integrated into weight-loss and smoking-cessation programs, its methods of inducing relaxation and hypersuggestibility are also used in working through many forms of client resistance.

EXERCISE   Other more natural forms of handling stress have evolved through the popularity of structured exercise programs. Many people have discovered the therapeutic benefits of activities such as running, walking, bicycling, rowing, aerobic dance, swimming, weight lifting, and the martial arts.

It is only recently that mental health and medical experts have begun to recognize the potential benefits of exercise (such as running) for improving creativity, confidence, self-control, and well-being, as well as for reducing negative addictions, boredom, anxiety, and depression (Annesi, 2005; Stathopoulu et al., 2006; Strohle, 2009). Running and similar activities have thus become integrated into many therapeutic programs as adjuncts to treatment, as transitional support systems for after counseling has ended, and even as a sole means of psychological and spiritual rejuvenation. Some therapists, such as Glasser (1976), recognized a while ago that positive addictions such as running can combat self-destructive patterns and be a form of self-medication for stress.

BIBLIOTHERAPY   Perhaps it is fitting that we end this chapter on action approaches by talking about the importance of supplementary reading assignments, not unlike the suggested readings at the end of each chapter. Routinely, quite a number of therapists who come from different theoretical orientations recommend to their clients that they read certain books that complement or reinforce the ideas that come up in sessions. Clinicians have a long and honored tradition of suggesting self-help or psychology books, or even novels, that deal with relevant themes (Joshua & DeMenna, 2000; Lampropoulos & Spengler, 2005; Redding, Herbert, Forman, & Guadiano, 2008). Some bibliotherapy approaches use therapeutic books that target particular client populations, such as children (Heath, Sheen, Leavy, Young, & Money, 2005) or women (Chrisler & Ulsh, 2001). For example, Pardeck and Pardeck (1993) did a survey of feminist therapists to determine which books they would most frequently recommend to female clients. Although the list is now somewhat dated, the most commonly cited book was *The Courage to Heal* (Bass, 1994).

Bibliotherapy has also become a frequently used intervention in cognitive behavioral therapy treatment plans; in particular, the book *Feeling Good: The New Mood Therapy* (Burns, 1999) is typically assigned to clients in the beginning of treatment in order to educate them on the basic components of CBT (Gregory, Canning, Lee, & Wise, 2004).

As you develop experience, and broaden your own reading interests, you will collect your own favorite sources to recommend to people. Those books that we recommend the most include fiction like Michael Dorris's *The Yellow Raft in Blue Water*, which is a story of abuse told from the perspective of a child, mother, and grandmother, each of whom believes the others are at fault; or Barbara Kingsolver's *Poisonwood Bible*, about a family's struggle to understand one another in the midst of their immersion in a foreign culture. There are also dozens of excellent self-help books on the market that you might use to supplement the work you do with people. For example, Harville Hendrix's *Getting the Love You Want* (1988; 2007) is well received by the couples we work with, and inevitably stimulates partners to examine their motivations for initially getting together.

Lest you think that adjunct structures must be limited to books, quite a number of counselors also make use of films to supplement their sessions (Lampropoulos, Kazantzis, & Deane, 2004; Solomon, 2001). The use of *cinematherapy* can serve a variety of therapeutic services (Dole & McMahan, 2005; Wedding & Niemec, 2003). It can introduce clients and family members to mental disorders; for example, clients with obsessive-compulsive disorder might be asked to watch *As Good as It Gets*, clients who have alcohol problems might watch *Leaving Las Vegas*, families dealing with schizophrenia might view *The Soloist*, or families struggling with bipolar illness could see *Michael Clayton*. According to Hesley and Hesley (2001), films can offer clients hope and encouragement, provide role models, reframe problems, help clients prioritize values, and intensify clients' emotions.

Films can also help to normalize clients' distress by depicting characters facing similar difficulties; the triumph of the central characters in overcoming their challenges can inspire and motivate clients, as well as provide a corrective emotional experience (Lampropoulos & Spengler, 2005). We have also found that films can help unlock vulnerable emotions by making it safe for clients to experience feelings vicariously. For example, male clients who may never cry in counseling will allow themselves to tear up when watching Kevin Costner cry in *Field of Dreams*. At the very least, films can facilitate clients' discussion of uncomfortable subjects. Wedding and Niemec (2003) suggested that *Boys Don't Cry* can stimulate a dialogue on gender identity issues; *Philadelphia* may initiate a conversation on HIV-AIDS and discrimination based on sexual orientation; and *Kramer vs. Kramer* can spark discussion of fathering and divorce issues.

Despite the potential benefits of cinematherapy, this intervention must be used with the same care and caution as any counseling technique: The client needs to be someone who enjoys watching movies; cinematherapy must be timed appropriately

VOICE FROM THE FIELD

I personally love movies, and find the idea of talking about movies with clients very appealing. In fact, whenever I see a film, in the back of my mind I'm thinking about whether it might be useful for a specific client to watch. But I've also learned the hard way that there are risks to cinematherapy.

One winter, during the holiday season, I assigned a depressed client the movie *It's a Wonderful Life*. If you don't know the story of this classic, it's about a depressed man who believes he's let down his family and friends, and thinks they'd be better off if he'd never been born. By the end of the film, he's discovered that his life has had value in ways he'd never imagined.

Anyway, I was sure my client would get the message of the story, and I looked forward to talking with him about the movie. So I was really taken aback when he came into the next session furious with me. "That movie sucked!" he said, "I believed it when the guy was really depressed, but that phony, sappy Hollywood ending was pure bull. How could you possibly think this would help me?" I lost a lot of credibility with this client, and our work was significantly set back. As I think about it now, I should have realized he might have a negative reaction. He was seeing the film through the eyes of a depressed person—I was seeing it through my own subjective filter.

You know, my husband and I constantly disagree about movies. Why should it be any different with clients?

within the course of treatment; clients' cultural background and values need to be considered; counselors need to make sure they have screened the film prior to assigning it (preferably using a film recommended in the cinematherapy literature); and subsequent counseling sessions need to be used to process the clients' emotional and intellectual responses to the film (Lampropoulos, Kazantzis, & Deane, 2004).

The main point we'd like to make is that it is never too early in your career to start collecting good books, films, and other media that might supplement and strengthen the work that you intend to do. Remember the key to action-oriented methods is that talk is not enough; people have to go out in the world in order to do things that make the changes last.

THE FUTURE IS NOW: NEW ISSUES IN COUNSELING

MINDFULNESS

You know a counseling intervention is "hot" in our field when you go to Amazon.com and discover over 40 books on the subject of mindfulness. Do a Google search and you'll find a slew of continuing education courses for counselors about mindfulness, plus a number of institutes devoted to the study of mindfulness as a therapeutic approach.

Although there is a lack of consensus on a definition of mindfulness, the concept is generally understood to have two components: (1) a person strives for focused attention on whatever he or she is experiencing (i.e., thoughts, emotions, physical sensations) in the present moment; (2) a person maintains a stance of nonjudgmental acceptance towards whatever he or she experiences in the present moment (Vujanovic et al., 2009). There are a variety of methods to achieving a mindful state of attention and acceptance, but a simple one might go like this (and you can practice this yourself):

> Sit in a comfortable position, with your arms on your thighs. Close your eyes, and pay attention to your breathing. Note whatever sensation you experience as you feel yourself inhale and exhale. You might notice the sensation of your chest rising up and down, or the air that you take in and let go as you breathe. It doesn't matter what you experience: just observe the sensation. As you do so, you will find your mind drifting away to various thoughts. They can be any thoughts at all. That's OK. Just take note of your drifting thoughts, and gently bring your attention back to the sensation of breathing.

This exercise is known as *mindful meditation* and derives from age-old Buddhist practices. "Mindfulness," as the term is used in counseling, is a secular approach used not only as a relaxation technique but as a method for dealing with psychological distress. The premise is a simple but powerful one: pain, whether emotional or physical, gets worse when we try to either avoid it, ignore it, or fight it. Pain actually reduces when we accept it by simply taking note of it with no attempt to do anything about it. This "acceptance way of being" gives us some distance from our distress, so we are not "in our pain" but rather in a state of observing it—that is, being mindful of it.

Mindfulness has become the core component of four different counseling modalities (Baer & Huss, 2008; Turner, 2009):

1. *Mindfulness-Based Stress Reduction (MBSR)* was originally developed by John Kabat-Zinn as a pain-reduction treatment for chronically ill patients and has been expanded to apply to clients with psychological as well as physical problems. MBSR is a relatively simple modality, in which clients are taught a variety of mindfulness meditation techniques, similar to the breathing exercise we described above (Kabat-Zinn, 1996).
2. *Mindfulness-Based Cognitive Therapy* (MBCT) is used primarily to help chronically depressed clients avoid relapse (Segal, 2002). In traditional CBT, clients are taught first how to identify their irrational thoughts, and then how to counter them with more realistic ones, with the ultimate goal of reducing illogical thinking. In MBCT, clients are asked to accept their irrational thoughts without trying to change or stop them.
3. *Dialectical Behavior Therapy (DBT)* was developed by Marsha Linehan (Crowell, Beauchaine, & Linehan, 2009; Heard & Linehan, 2005; Linehan, 1993) as a treatment approach to borderline personality disorder, a notoriously difficult-to-treat disorder in which individuals can experience intense emotional pain and engage in self-mutilating or suicidal behaviors. Linehan theorized that this condition results to some extent when children who are prone to experiencing especially strong and confusing emotions have their feelings invalidated by adults. These children thus learn to be harshly self-critical of their feelings, and by adolescence, have developed desperate behaviors to avoid them. Practitioners of DBT teach their clients mindfulness so they can achieve a state of nonjudgmental acceptance of their feelings, rather than resort to self-destructive avoidance maneuvers.

4. *Acceptance and Commitment Therapy (ACT)* is similar to the above mindfulness therapies, emphasizing the value of accepting one's painful thoughts and feelings rather than escaping from them (Hayes et al., 1999). ACT counselors teach clients how to see their internal experiences as transitory events rather than harmful emotions that need to be eliminated (Baer & Huss, 2008).

Mindfulness is not only a skill we can teach our clients, it is a state of mind that we as counselors can strive for as we listen to our clients. By being mindful of our own feelings and thoughts as they emerge in our interactions with clients, we can better maintain a state of attention, empathy, and calm (Turner, 2009).

Mindfulness approaches have been demonstrated to be therapeutically effective in the treatment of depression, PTSD, borderline personality disorder, anxiety, and substance abuse, and counselors of varying theoretical orientations are finding ways to integrate it into their work (Vujanovic et al., 2009). Any counselor who works with so-called "borderline" clients, whether the person leans towards psychodynamic, humanistic, cognitive, or postmodern thinking, needs at least to be familiar with DBT. Even Leslie Greenberg, a noted theorist, clinician, and researcher whose Emotion-Focused Therapy helps clients express their strongest emotions, suggests that mindfulness may be appropriate for those clients who are overwhelmed by their feelings and who would benefit from gaining a measure of distance from them (Greenberg, 2002). In short, while mindfulness may be a "hot" intervention at the moment, it is probably here to stay.

SUMMARY

The previous chapters on counseling theory have reviewed some of the most popular therapeutic systems currently in use. Action-oriented approaches mentioned in this chapter place more emphasis on the technique and technology of change.

At this juncture, your state of confusion is probably unavoidable, if not desirable. It is overwhelming to study so many different explanations of how best to do counseling, especially when each system appears to have attractive components.

On an unconscious if not deliberate level, your mind is already sifting through the vast array of new ideas and making decisions about what to reserve for further study and what to throw out because of apparent clashes with your values, personality, skills, and interests. In the next chapter you can carry on with the task of building a tentative personal theory of counseling; this is a process that will continue throughout the balance of your life.

Self-Guided Explorations

1. Describe a time in your life in which insight was not enough: You understood what the problem was all about, you even had some idea of how it evolved, but you felt powerless to make needed changes. What would it (or did it) take to help you make needed changes?

2. Use a behavioral contract to commit yourself to making some desired change in your life. Make sure your goals are specific, measurable, and, most of all, realistic—given your time parameters and track record.

Goals:

Procedure to reach goals:

Consequences:

Daily reward:

Contract reward:

3. Use a CBT thought diary to help you with a situation that's stressing you out. Start by making a three-column grid on a blank sheet. In the first column, briefly describe the situation that's bothering you. Now, recall the situation as vividly as you can, until you feel some of the anxiety again. What thoughts do you have as you feel the stress? Write them down in the second column. In the third column, try to write a more rational thought for every irrational one you recorded. One way to do this is to imagine how someone else, a person who was not upset by the same situation, would respond cognitively. (By the way, this last technique is another intervention used by CBT counselors.)

4. Consider a problem in your life that you're having trouble resolving. Apply a solution-oriented strategy, starting by asking yourself the miracle question. Assuming the problem has vanished, imagine as vividly as possible a scene in your life. What are you wearing in the scene? What are you doing? What is the expression on your face? Now try to actually recreate that scene in your real life, wearing the same clothes, doing the same things, with the same expression.

FOR HOMEWORK

Hollywood has depicted counselors in films throughout cinema history, and, unfortunately, most of these portrayals range from the inaccurate (clients are cured immediately upon recalling a repressed memory from childhood) to the grossly unethical (counselors become romantically involved with clients). The following films and television shows portray counselors in a good light, bad light, and sometimes a bit of both. Rent or purchase three of these. What do you think of the way the counselor is portrayed?

What do you like about the way these counselors work, and what concerns you?

Analyze This

Antwone Fisher

Good Will Hunting

In Treatment

Ordinary People

The Prince of Tides

The Sopranos

SUGGESTED READINGS

Beck, J. S. (2005). *Cognitive therapy for challenging problems*. New York: Guilford.

Carmichael, K. D. (2006). *Play therapy: An introduction*. Upper Saddle River, NJ: Prentice Hall.

Case, C., & Dalley, T. (2006). *The handbook of art therapy* (2nd ed.). New York: Taylor and Francis.

Ellis, A., & MacLaren, C. (2005). *Rational emotive behavior therapy* (2nd ed.). Atascadero, CA: Impact.

Gilbert, P., & Leahy, R. (Eds.) (2007). *The therapeutic relationship in the cognitive behavioral psychotherapies*. New York: Routledge.

Gladding, S. T. (2006). *Counseling as an art: Creative arts in counseling* (3rd ed.). Alexandria, VA: American Counseling Association.

Glasser, W. (2001). *Counseling with choice theory*. New York: Harper.

Graziano, A. M. (Ed.) (2006). *Behavior therapy with children*. Somerset, NJ: Aldine.

Guterman, J. T. (2005). *Mastering the art of solution-focused counseling*. Alexandria, VA: American Counseling Association.

Hesley, J. W., & Hesley, J. G. (2001). *Rent two films and let's talk in the morning: Using popular movies in psychotherapy* (2nd ed.). New York: John Wiley & Sons.

Kaduson, H. G., & Schaefer, C. E. (2006). *Short-term play therapy for children* (2nd ed.). New York: Guilford.

Lazarus, A. A. (2006). *Brief but comprehensive psychotherapy: The multimodal way*. New York: Springer.

Ledley, D. R., Heimberg, R. G., & Marx, B. P. (2005). *Making cognitive-behavioral therapy work: Clinical process for new practitioners*. New York: Guilford.

McMahon, L. (2009). *The handbook of play therapy and therapeutic play* (2nd ed.) New York: Routledge.

Nardone, G., & Porter, C. (2005). *Knowing through changing: The evolution of brief strategic therapy*. Norwalk, CT: Crown House.

O'Connell, B. (2005). *Solution-focused therapy*. Thousand Oaks, CA: Sage.

O'Hanlon, B., & Weiner-Davis, M. (2003). *In search of solutions: A new direction in psychotherapy*. New York: W. W. Norton & Company.

Palmer, S. (2006). *Brief multimodal therapy*. Thousand Oaks, CA: Sage.

Rubin, J. A. (2009). *An introduction to art therapy: Sources and resources*. New York: Routledge.

Simmons, J., & Conlon, R. (2010). *CBT for beginners*. Thousand Oaks, CA: Sage.

Simmons, L. L. (2006). *Interactive art therapy: No talent required projects*. New York: Haworth.

Spiegler, M. D., & Guevremont, D. C. (2010). *Contemporary behavior therapy* (5th ed.). Pacific Grove, CA: Brooks/Cole.

Ulus, F. (2003). *Movie therapy, moving therapy: The healing power of film clips in therapeutic settings*. Vancouver, British Columbia, Canada: Trafford.

from two major sources of knowledge: the techniques and theories of counseling and the richness and realities of life itself. Minuchin and Fishman (1981), two leading family therapists, admonish the beginner to "disengage from the techniques of therapy and engage with the difficulties of life" (p. 10). Developing a valid and useful personal theory of counseling depends on knowing yourself well and participating in the experience of life. Such evolution in your thinking may follow a series of progressive stages (see Figure 7.1).

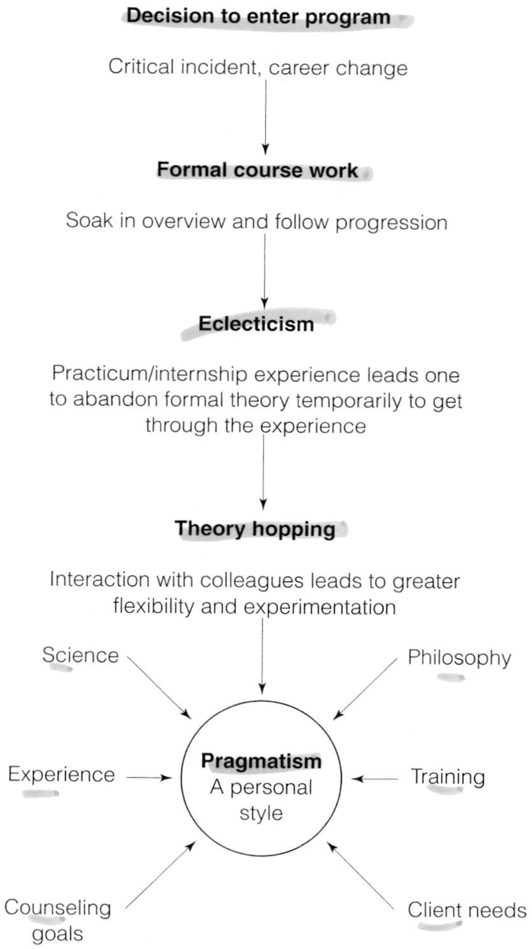

Decision to enter program

Critical incident, career change

Formal course work

Soak in overview and follow progression

Eclecticism

Practicum/internship experience leads one to abandon formal theory temporarily to get through the experience

Theory hopping

Interaction with colleagues leads to greater flexibility and experimentation

Science   Philosophy

Experience →   **Pragmatism**
A personal
style   ← Training

Counseling goals   Client needs

FIGURE 7.1

Increased flexibility, variability, and work demands encourage many counselors to integrate their training, supervision, and personal experiences with their clients' needs and goals. The result is often a personal style of practice that is solidly grounded in theory and research but reflects one's own personality, beliefs, and style in such a way that client individual and cultural differences are honored and respected.

ENTRY

The counseling student begins the task of theory building by learning an overview of theories. Even those students with substantial practical experience choose a formal counselor education program to legitimate their status, as well as to refine skills and acquire additional knowledge. The course of study normally begins with an introductory course, using a text similar to the one you are reading.

The first stage of professional theory development is usually confusing. Within a short period of time the beginning student is exposed to a variety of approaches to counseling. The theories' conflicting points of view can be disorienting enough, but the student is also learning about relevant theories in other courses. Just when the names and terms of basic theories are beginning to make sense, additional input from these other courses renews the confusion. It is no wonder, then, that the first stage in a beginning counselor's attempts to construct a personal blueprint for guiding behavior is marked by swings from enlightenment to frustration. Eventually most new students, out of a sense of self-preservation, decide to suspend judgment temporarily and try to understand all the theories, deferring evaluation until later. It is difficult, if not impossible, to organize information at this point because all the information is so new that it is hard to know what questions to ask.

The slightly stressful job of the learner is occasionally interrupted by an inevitable question from colleagues that will push the student onward to the next stage of theory building. The query is, "What *are* you?" Students' responses reveal the first of their many alliances to a particular theory.

MENTORHOOD

When you attempt to answer that deceptively simple question, consider the consequences of declaring your primary theoretical affiliation. Because "I don't know," "What do you mean?" and similar responses may make you appear unstudious or less mature than your classmates, you will probably prefer to name a particular theory that sounds good and that you understand to some degree. Now you have catapulted yourself into the second stage of theory construction and will experience added pressure to find a label to describe the way you think (even though you are not yet certain about your choice).

During this phase a student is sometimes impressionable and susceptible to hero worship. Professors or supervisors who are good at their work and skilled at helping others learn are good candidates for this hero role. These mentors and modeling influences are particularly important to later student development, for they provide guidance and a behavioral model. It becomes relatively easy to affiliate yourself with the point of view of a model that you admire, and even to convince yourself that this is the model that will work best for you.

You now have reason to study one theory thoroughly and intensively. An unfortunate side effect of concentrated interest can be a mental block against examining other theories that increase cognitive dissonance. Some practitioners never progress beyond their allegiance to one counseling approach. Many of them become extraordinarily knowledgeable and skilled at applying its concepts; they can devote time and energy toward improving themselves as specialists in a particular style. With such a commitment comes an increased acceptance of your mentor and of the support system of other like-minded practitioners. There are special books, journals, meetings, and conventions, all intended to help counselors grow in their chosen affiliation. The result can be immunization against others from outside the "club" who could lead a confused counselor astray.

For many students, participation in the practicum or internship helps to shatter the illusion that only one theory works. Taking a class in technique also helps because it is there you learn the generic skills practiced by almost all counselors. The temporary sanctuary of the mentor is left behind as the student continues on to the next stage.

ECLECTICISM

Held (1984) distinguishes between *technical* and *prescriptive* eclecticism. In the former, the counselor is a technician, a skilled master of technique who may be successful on a practical level but who doesn't have a well-articulated guiding philosophy. Prescriptive eclecticism rests more firmly on a solid theoretical base and places more emphasis on prediction and explanation of phenomena. Flexibility is the hallmark of both eclectic approaches, in which professionals subscribe to parts of many different theories.

Renewed flexibility is the logical result of your first actual experience as a counselor. You soon realize that imitating a mentor is hollow without an integrated understanding of the theory. You may have temporarily abandoned organized theory in your attempts to get through the practicum experience, experimenting with a variety of ideas to alleviate the personal anxiety that occurs while helping a client. Adventurous students will even try out a few of their own ideas, but such behavior may be risky unless it is successful. You are wise to be conservative and cautious in trying out the range of theories the way that you have personally interpreted and integrated them. When in doubt, you can always fall back on the ideas of your mentors—who, after all, have spent decades developing and practicing the techniques— or revert back to a previous theory of your own. When not under pressure, you can find another favorite to study. Ever so slowly, your own personality and preferences begin to demonstrate a unique style.

EXPERIMENTATION

School is over. As an employed professional, you now have the opportunity to test the theories and techniques that were presented in the classroom. Refinement of theory is encouraged by colleagues and supervisors who have firm ideas of their own regarding the best ways to help clients. The fundamental concepts favored in the textbooks and classroom are sometimes downplayed by the seasoned professionals, who warn: "Forget relying on theory. Around here we do things our own way." Of course, the supervisors are really presenting theories of their own choice.

This particular stage of professional development is often marked by experimental theory hopping, trying out attractive concepts, listening to more experienced peers, and remembering the wise words of mentors. Books play an influential role as the ex-student revels in new freedom while feeling eager for the excitement of

VOICE FROM THE FIELD

Early on, I really found that narrative counseling fit me like a glove. Perhaps even better, it seemed to fit my clients, who are mostly members of oppressed minority groups. I like the way it can be applied so efficiently. I like the way it looks at the world. I just like it! Maybe sometime I may move on to other things, but for now I like the comfort of learning this one approach as well as I can. And there is so much more to learn! I just can't imagine trying to juggle several different theories. And what's the point? People a lot smarter and more experienced than I am have gone to a lot of trouble to develop this stuff. That's good enough for me.

new ideas. Because there is so little time and structure for reinforcing learning, classic books become the mainstay of further theory development.

PRAGMATISM

Not all counselors reach the stage of pragmatic flexibility—nor do they want to. Many practitioners remain satisfied and quite effective at applying the concepts of their favorite theory. The principal advantage of this is a sense of comfort and familiarity with the theory and its accompanying techniques. The counselor becomes increasingly more experienced and eloquent at personalizing and adapting the preferred theory in his or her work with clients.

For others, single-theory allegiance feels conforming, limiting, boring, and routine. Some choose to move beyond mere eclecticism—a stance of technical proficiency in many techniques—to a philosophy of pragmatism.

As originally conceived by the first psychologist, William James, "Pragmatism unstiffens all our theories, limbers them up, and sets each one at work" (James, 1907, p. 46). The pragmatic counselor is concerned with integrating the body of knowledge from all relevant disciplines into a personalized and pluralistic philosophy that is empirically based and can be practically applied to specific situations.

One of the hallmarks of a pragmatic approach is that prior to any therapeutic action, a counselor asks several internal questions:

1. What appears to be happening?
2. What do I wish to accomplish?
3. How will this intervention meet the desired goal?

If the counselor is unable to answer these questions in a clear and cogent manner, depending instead on intuitive hunches such as, "I have a gut feeling that this will work," then it may be necessary to examine personal motives. A detailed analysis of "gut feelings" will aid the counselor in understanding more precisely the underlying rationale for intervention choices and will also help to stifle counselor self-indulgence. Before using confrontation, for example, the counselor can ask internally: "Am I confronting this client because he is genuinely disrupting the process or because he is irritating to me?" Beyond eliminating inappropriate verbalizations, defining the rationale for actions helps the counselor to develop for future use a repertoire of strategies that have been found to be effective in similar circumstances.

Pragmatism is a useful philosophical stance for counselors because it encourages them to view the profession in a broad interdisciplinary context, integrating approaches and techniques from a variety of theoretical perspectives. It also encourages the counselor to avoid an overdependence on a single theoretical construct as heir to truth and facilitates the mechanisms of personal theory building so that relevant principles may be systematically collected from the universe of available knowledge. Perhaps Pablo Picasso best summarized the simplicity of a pragmatic philosophy: "When I haven't any blue, I use red."

EVIDENCE-BASED PRACTICE

Whether a counselor identifies closely with a single theory or develops a personal, integrated approach, one question every counselor needs to reflect upon is whether empirical support for a treatment approach is a necessary criterion for using it with clients. Applying treatments that have been well documented as effective in statistically based research studies is known as *evidence-based practice (EBP)*, although there is some confusion in the field about what exactly constitutes "evidence-based." There are some who simply equate it with empirically supported treatments (ESTs); that is, treatments that have been subjected to the same kind of rigorously designed, randomly controlled research studies that the medical profession requires. Others hold a more expansive definition, emphasizing a counselor's mandate to continuously search objectively and efficiently for the best evidence available on how to help a client, and to base counseling interventions on that evidence (Gibbs, 2003; Levant & Hasin, 2008). Although at the moment there is some disagreement about a precise definition, what is clear is that the whole idea of using only evidence-based therapies has aroused an intense, even angry, debate in the counseling profession, and no counselor should avoid examining his or her own views on this contentious issue. Deciding where one comes down on the issue is a critical part of developing a personal theory and approach to counseling.

On the face of it, the arguments for evidence-based practice appear to be both reasonable and compelling: (a) Clients have a right to be given treatments that have proven efficacy and it is unethical for counselors to diverge from this principle (Drake et al., 2001; Hunsley, 2007); (b) managed care companies, government programs (e.g., Medicare), and the marketplace require that counselors be held accountable for using the best-possible approach (Sue & Sue, 2008); and (c) the counseling profession is enhanced in the eyes of the public when counselors, regardless of settings, are consistent in their methods (Sanderson, 1998).

However, for some insight-oriented counselors, the movement toward evidence-based practice is a serious concern, perhaps because it is the action-oriented approaches, in particular cognitive behavioral treatments, which have received the strongest empirical support. Nevertheless, critics of the EBP movement marshal several arguments on their behalf that counselors need to consider:

- Cognitive behavioral counseling performs well in research studies because the researchers themselves prefer this approach; this is known as the "allegiance effect" and it biases studies (Messer, 2001; Sparks, Duncan, & Miller, 2008).
- Regardless of the treatment used, it is the counseling relationship and working alliance that are the most powerful agents of client change, a fact that has

been repeatedly demonstrated in research (Andrews, 2007; Duncan & Miller, 2006; Wampold & Bahti, 2004).

- Clients, not treatments, are ultimately responsible for client change; clients grow when they are active self-healers. Moreover, clients should have the right to choose between a growth-oriented treatment and a short-term symptom-relief approach (Bohart, 2005).

- Empirical research studies only tell us what clients report on a psychological test, which may have little relationship to how clients experience their daily life. For example, a client may show improvement on a statistical measurement of depression, apparently proving the efficacy of the treatment used; however, the client may still *feel* depressed and behave like a depressed person (Kazden, 2006).

While this debate is particularly heated at the moment (at conferences we have seen arguments break out between well-known counselors), it is quite possible that a middle ground will be reached, perhaps a compromise where qualitative case studies are considered as valid as empirical research in demonstrating a treatment's effectiveness. Regardless, the evidence-based practice issue may be conceptualized as the last step in a counselor's decision-making process with regard to the basis for choosing theories, designing treatments and implementing specific interventions with clients. Whether you become a single-theory adherent, or develop a pragmatic, flexible approach, sound consideration of these issues means continually revisiting your core values and philosophical beliefs regarding the nature of counseling and the counseling relationship. As you engage in this often-challenging reflective process, you can take some comfort in knowing you are participating in one of the most important, and oldest, debates in this field—a debate that seeks to conceptualize the basis upon which we say, "This approach works."

In Table 7.1 on the following page, we have listed some of the psychological disorders you are likely to encounter if you conduct mental health counseling, followed by the most current evidence-based treatments (Society of Clinical Psychology, 2009). Notice how approaches with very different theoretical philosophies and interventions have all proven to be helpful, a finding that continues to puzzle researchers and gives support to the notion that ultimately, it is not the specific intervention so much as it is the counseling relationship that facilitates change.

HOW ARE YOU DOING SO FAR?

In spite of feeling a degree of confusion, or even being overwhelmed, by the sheer volume of information contained in the theories presented in these chapters (and the ones to follow), you have already been sorting and organizing things to the point where your options are becoming more manageable. Some theories you've read about you feel immediately drawn to, just as others are not quite your cup of tea. This attraction you feel toward certain theories, and your rejection of others, is not based solely on the pure intellectual and logical analysis of merits and limitations. Your personal values and core views of the world also play an important role, although many of these are likely to change as your counselor education unfolds.

Halbur and Halbur (2006) suggest that the process of choosing a theory should *begin* with identification of your values, worldview, and life philosophy. You may, for example, place high value on independence and self-reliance,

TABLE 7.1 | RESEARCH-SUPPORTED THERAPIES FOR EMOTIONAL DISORDERS

Disorder	Treatment
Attention Deficit	**Stimulant Medication** Behavioral Parent Training
Bipolar	**Medication** **Psychoeducation** Cognitive Behavioral Therapy
Borderline Personality	**Dialectical Behavioral Therapy** Schema Therapy (integration of CBT and Emotion-Focused Therapy)
Depression	**Cognitive Behavioral Therapy** Mindfulness-Based Therapy Emotion-Focused Therapy Brief Psychodynamic Therapy
Generalized Anxiety	**Cognitive Behavioral Therapy**
Obsessive-Compulsive Disorder	**Behavior Therapy** **Cognitive Behavioral Therapy**
Panic	**Cognitive Behavioral Therapy** Relaxation Exercises Psychoanalytic Therapy
Post-Traumatic Stress	**Behavior Therapy** **Eye-Movement Desensitization Reprocessing (EMDR)**
Social Phobia and Public Speaking	**Cognitive Behavioral Therapy**

or instead have a more communal, mutually interdependent orientation toward life. Certainly, your cultural background will play a significant role in how you view the world, and what constitutes an emotionally healthy, meaningful life. The next step would be to choose one of the schools of thought (e.g., psychodynamic, humanistic, behavioral, cognitive, feminist, etc.) that best reflects your philosophy; then, you can choose a specific theory within the broader schools (e.g., object relations, client-centered, cognitive behavioral).

In a sense, you allow a theory to choose *you*. Reflect upon what you believe in, and then see which best matches your values. You might find it interesting to take an inventory at this point as to where you stand in terms of the basic questions every theory needs to address. For each of the following 10 categories, you are presented with three possible positions that might be taken legitimately. There are no correct answers. In fact, among successful practitioners, there are those who feel quite strongly about each of these points of view. We encourage you at this point to go through each of the items and select the choice that most closely fits with the way you think about the world, about other people, about yourself, and about the ways that people change.

You will find at the end of this exercise that a pattern will emerge for you in terms of what it is that you think, feel, and believe about counseling. Many of your opinions will be supported by some of the theories you have read about, perhaps even one or two of them that most closely parallel your own beliefs. As you continue your study of the literature in the field, you will probably discover that other opinions you hold are not supported by research that has been completed to date. In fact, there may be more quantitative and qualitative evidence to support one position over others, but those debates are better left for another time. This Theoretical Dilemmas Inventory is only a starting point.

THEORETICAL DILEMMAS INVENTORY

Directions: For each of the following items, select the one position that most clearly articulates your own beliefs. Be prepared to defend your position with some evidence based on your experience.

VIEWS OF PEOPLE

_____ People are born basically good.
_____ People are born basically evil.
_____ People are born basically neutral.

RESPONSIBILITY FOR OUTCOMES

_____ Clients have primary responsibility for counseling outcomes.
_____ Counselors have primary responsibility for counseling outcomes.
_____ Responsibility is shared equally.

LEGITIMATE FOCUS

_____ Counseling should focus primarily on feelings.
_____ Counseling should focus primarily on thinking.
_____ Counseling should focus primarily on behavior.

CONTENT

_____ Counseling content should deal with the past.
_____ Counseling content should deal with the present.
_____ Counseling content should deal with the future.

SCOPE

_____ Counseling should concentrate on specific goals.
_____ Counseling should concentrate on broad themes.
_____ Counseling should concentrate on the process of what takes place.

SKILLS

_____ The most important counselor skill is structuring.
_____ The most important counselor skill is interpreting.
_____ The most important counselor skill is reflecting.

COUNSELOR DIRECTIVENESS

___✓___ Counselors should be active.

_____ Counselors should be nondirective.

_____ Counselors should allow the client to decide what is best.

COUNSELOR ROLE

___✓___ The counselor should be an expert.

_____ The counselor should be a friend.

___✓___ The counselor should be a consultant.

THEORY

_____ Counselors should become experts in one theory.

___✓___ Counselors should become proficient in several theories. •

___✓___ Counselors should combine several theories.

CRITERIA FOR SUCCESS

_____ The most important predictor of good counseling is knowledge of theory.

___✓___ The most important predictor of good counseling is mastery of core skills.

_____ The most important predictor of good counseling is a healthy personality.

To compute your score, just take the number of items and multiply by your age, add the number of years you've experienced counseling, then divide by the course number … just kidding! There is no score—but there is a result that may be meaningful to you. As you look over your responses, you will note that you do indeed have some strong opinions about some of these issues, whereas others you are hesitant about until you collect more information and accumulate more experience. That is exactly as it should be.

In asking you how you are doing so far, we hope you recognize that it is normal and appropriate to feel a degree of confusion. It is also useful to realize that you do have some well-articulated beliefs that are already becoming part of a theory of your own that you are in the process of creating at this moment.

GENERIC COUNSELING SKILLS

In this chapter we have chosen to tackle two important subjects that are interconnected. The first had to do with making sense of counseling theories, especially with regard to integrating them into a model that is best suited to your approach, setting, and client needs. Now we wish to briefly introduce you to the core counseling skills that are considered atheoretical, meaning that they transcend any single theory.

While it is true that there is considerable debate about the best theoretical approach for helping people, there is a reasonable consensus about which skills you need to learn in order to be helpful to someone. Many of these skills emerged from specific theories. For example, reflecting feelings is originally associated with client-centered counseling, disputing beliefs is associated with cognitive therapy, and goal setting is associated with a behavioral approach. Nevertheless, in spite of their origins, many helping skills are now in such wide use across the spectrum of specialties and settings that they are virtually universal. The same can be said for the general stages of counseling.

STAGES OF THE COUNSELING PROCESS

Just at a time when you may be feeling somewhat anxious because of the lack of agreement about which counseling theory is best, you should be relieved to know that most practitioners share a similar view of the process involved, if not of the progressive stages that should be followed. Most counselors, whether they are insight- or action-oriented—whether they favor theories that focus on the past or present, on cognitions or affect—still subscribe to a five-stage model that relies on several skills for moving forward (Hackney & Cormier, 2009; Okun & Kantrowitz, 2008; Patterson & Welfel, 2005).

ASSESSMENT In the first stage, counselors use both written instruments and clinical observation skills to formulate ideas about the client's presenting complaint. A working diagnosis is usually created that helps the practitioner to make some decisions with the client as to what treatment plan might be best—individual, group, or family counseling, short- or long-term sessions—and how things will be structured. During this initial stage, counselors make use of attending, listening, focusing, and observation skills to help them decide exactly how they will proceed. Some clients, for example, respond better to some approaches than others. A kind of contractual arrangement is negotiated in which both parties are satisfied with the intention and means to reach those goals.

EXPLORATION During the exploration stage, reflections of feeling and content, as well as questioning and probing, are used to help clients clarify issues in the present and from the past. Efforts are also devoted to building a solid therapeutic relationship. Clients are helped to tell their story; in other words, to describe the circumstances that led them to their current predicament. There is a catharsis, or release of tension, in being able to explore more deeply what is going on. Typically, exploration is also undertaken to collect background information related to family-of-origin issues, health and emotional history, and other relevant areas that may be helpful in the case.

UNDERSTANDING Whereas not all practitioners believe that promoting insight is sufficient for producing lasting changes in behavior, most agree that there is some benefit to helping clients understand how their troubles developed and how they are connected to other issues in their lives. Through the use of empathic listening, interpretation, confrontation, and other helping skills mentioned later, the counselor works to promote in the client some degree of insight that can serve as a bridge to taking constructive action.

Insights can take a number of forms, depending on the theoretical orientation of the counselor. Promoting understanding can focus on issues from the past, current family interactions, dysfunctional thinking, behavioral inconsistencies, or even the functional aspects of continuing to act self-destructively. Regardless of the emphasis, the intent in this stage is to help clients understand what they have been doing and why they have been acting in those particular ways, and to explore other options that may be available to them.

ACTION Just as some counselors prefer to spend most of their time working in the previous stage, others are more action-oriented and like to help clients work toward observable changes. Nevertheless, most counselors would agree that some form of action is helpful, whether it involves having the client complete specific homework assignments or, more subtly, simply asking what the client intends to do with regard to the insights that have been generated.

Skills that are most often a part of this stage include goal setting, role-playing, paradoxical interventions, and other strategies that help clients translate what they have been working on in sessions to their lives outside of sessions. Typically, this may be communicated to clients with the following statement: "It isn't what you do with me that matters most; rather, what really counts is how you apply what you've learned to your own life."

EVALUATION As with any planned activity, it is helpful to assess the degree to which efforts have reached desired goals. Counselors use all the previously mentioned skills, as well as their knowledge of assessment, evaluation, and research methods, to help clients determine the extent to which they have reached desired goals. Adjustments may need to be made to recycle the process back to previous stages as needed.

PIVOTAL COUNSELING SKILLS

Many things influence what a counselor does in a session with a client. Certainly many of the previously presented theories on the practitioner's personal philosophy and style of practice play a significant role. The counselor's personality or mood on any given day, as well as the client's concerns and goals, influence the choice of interventions. Nevertheless, most counselors have a core of skills that they use on a regular basis, and a fairly solid research base exists to support the effectiveness of those skills. Because of the research support for the core skills, educators of counselors at different institutions across the world teach basically the same skills. Increasingly, however, it is being recognized that these skills must be adapted to fit the cultural, ethnic, and gender differences of each client.

This section will introduce a group of pivotal skills that describe what counselors do during the counseling process and the various stages previously described. First, you are reminded that the overall goal of counseling is the development of new behavior that is more adaptive, self-enhancing, and personally fulfilling. Self-exploration is the first goal of helping, and subsequent steps follow a pattern that employs the skills of attending, responding, initiating, and communicating, eventually leading to constructive action.

The process of exploration, understanding, and action is continuously recycled in the helping process. Action provokes feedback, which provides a stimulus for further self-exploration, which in turn facilitates increased and more accurate self-understanding. Real understanding is often the result of learning that follows action. Finally, action is further modified in accordance with a more accurate understanding of self.

Until now, we have focused on how counselors think. We will now examine what counselors *do* in their sessions—the specific interventions that are often used to facilitate client self-exploration, self-understanding, and desired changes in behavior, feelings, and thoughts.

Being Intentional and Reliable

Developing skills, techniques, and procedures that are valid and tend to influence clients to experience constructive change is a primary concern of counselors. The discussion of validity is complex. Everyone claims validity for his or her chosen approach—and to some extent, each is right. Everything is valid. All techniques, approaches, and styles (even the most bizarre) work—with some clients at some times. Because validity is a measure of whether the technique or process does what it claims to do, most practitioners and theorists can demonstrate validity. The debate over whether or not something works can often be better replaced with an exploration of *when* it works. Kagan (1973) has stated it succinctly: "The most important issue for our field is not if counseling works but rather what methods work consistently" (p. 234). Reliability is a measure of the consistency of valid treatment effects with a wide range of client types. In other words, do your basic counseling/human relations skills influence positive change in most clients with whom you have professional contact? Consistency of effects is the trademark of the intentional counselor. Achieving reliability in counseling is a function of several factors: selection of valid and appropriate techniques, careful training, and integration of one's personal style into a systematic counseling approach. In a sense, being intentional and reducing the impact of chance effects maximize the potential for delivering valid and reliable counseling services. Such is the essence of professionalism and integrity.

Achieving reliability in counseling—that is, reducing the impact of chance on counseling relationships—is often related to the counselor's being consistent. Intentionality refers to the development of a cognitive flexibility integrated into an open and dynamic worldview. An intentional person will clarify choices, focus priorities, and implement goals and action. In a sense, an intentional person is the opposite of those who come for assistance or counseling. Often clients lack direction in their lives, evidencing immobility and the inability to see choices.

As a counselor, your goal, naturally, is to help clients create more options and to do so with methods demonstrated to be reliable and valid. This task is more difficult than it seems, for many counselors can feel successful without really being able to prove they have made an impact. This problem has, not surprisingly, received some attention in the literature and is often an unspoken client concern. Counselors have a responsibility to answer the question for themselves and their clients and to know how and why they believe counseling actually works—and works consistently.

Significance of Attending Skills

See Companion DVD
Listing Skills

Perhaps the basis for all therapeutic interventions is physically and psychologically attending to persons in need of help (Cormier, Nurius, & Osborn, 2008; Ivey & Ivey, 2007). It is through posture, body position, head nods, facial expressions, eye contact, gestures, and verbal encouragements that the counselor communicates intense interest in everything a client says and feels. And it is through such active attending that the counselor can also observe the nonverbal cues evident in the client's behavior. A quivering lip, clenched hand, or furrowed brow provide evidence that is helpful for understanding what the client is experiencing. This focused attention is highly important in all stages of the counseling process, but it is especially critical during the assessment and exploration stages when you are first establishing a relationship.

Effective listening, the core of attending skills, involves the following elements:

1. *Have a reason for listening.* Know what to listen for and how it will be important to the client's exploration, understanding, and action.
2. *Be nonjudgmental.* To listen effectively, you must suspend temporarily the things you say to yourself. Let the client's message sink in without making decisions about it.
3. *Resist distractions.* Resist both internal and external distractions so that your attention and listening focus will not be disturbed.
4. *Wait to respond.* Give yourself time to respond fully and deeply to the client's statements, avoiding hasty and possibly superficial responses.
5. *Reflect content.* Reflecting back to the client what you hear him or her saying communicates understanding and provides an opportunity to check out the accuracy of your perceptions.
6. *Look for themes.* Be selective about all the stimuli presented, and attend only to the content that is relevant and meaningful. Identifying themes will help you to understand where the client is coming from and how the client perceives his or her relationship to the world.

LISTENING SKILLS Several response options tend to promote verbal expression and convey interest:

1. *Passive listening:* The use of verbal encouragement and nonverbal attending in order to acknowledge messages communicated by the client.

   EXAMPLES:

   "I see."

   "Uh-huh."

   "Go on."

   "Yes."

2. *Parroting:* Repetition of the client's words to indicate interest, demonstrate accuracy of listening, or stall for time until a more elegant response can be formulated.

   EXAMPLE:

   CLIENT: Boy, am I upset.

   COUNSELOR: You're really upset.

3. *Paraphrasing:* Restatement of a message's content to clarify or to focus the client's attention.

   EXAMPLE:

   CLIENT: My life feels useless. My job is a dead end. I don't have any friends. And my parents are always on my case.

   COUNSELOR: You are isolated, trapped, badgered, and don't see a way out.

VOICE FROM THE FIELD

I remember when I first learned reflective listening skills. I came home that first night all pumped up, just dying to try out what I learned with my family. It just blew me away how powerful this stuff was. At the time, I was so awkward. I probably just repeated whatever anyone said to me. The thing is, though, that it's just so rare that people feel really listened to that when I started to give my full attention to whomever was talking, they just loved it. At first, they weren't even aware of what I was doing; they were just so delighted to be getting my attention. Nowadays, though, they tell me to cut out that counseling crap if they think I'm trying to manipulate them or something.

---

4. *Clarification:* Confirmation of a message's accuracy to encourage elaboration.

    EXAMPLE:

    COUNSELOR: You are saying that this issue of feeling vulnerable and getting hurt when you trust others has been a lifelong theme.

5. *Reflection of feeling:* Focus on affect to promote catharsis and self-expression.

    EXAMPLE:

    CLIENT: I don't know. Maybe this marriage isn't worth holding together any longer. We've already tried just about every option.

    COUNSELOR: You feel so frustrated and overwhelmed trying to resolve your conflicts without help from your wife. It's as if she had already given up on your relationship and now you are feeling hopeless and helpless.

6. *Summary:* The linking of several ideas together in a condensed way to promote insight, cut off rambling, identify significant themes, or draw closure.

    EXAMPLE:

    COUNSELOR: So far you have talked a lot about the ways you keep people at a distance. You tend to hang back whenever you feel a potential for a friendship, and those who approach you are quickly discouraged by your reluctance. You have also mentioned that you might have learned your aloofness from your parents, who never seemed to have much time for you.

EXPLORATION SKILLS   There is a set of counselor behaviors that can be especially helpful in drawing out client concerns, facilitating insight, and exploring thoughts and feelings. Most use these skills as the staple of their therapeutic efforts during the first few stages of the process:

1. *Probe:* Questioning in an open-ended manner to gather relevant information or to encourage self-examination.

    EXAMPLE:

    "What are the things you've tried to do throughout your life when you have faced similar struggles?"

VOICE FROM THE FIELD

I've been doing counseling for 20 years, and I still find that just listening and reflecting is hard. There's this voice in my head whispering over and over, "You should be doing more, you should be doing more …" I remember this one client who was really anxious about a career change she was thinking about making. There were so many tools I wanted to use—tests to give her, charts to fill out, guided visualizations to see what her unconscious was telling her. I tried them all, but none of it did anything for her anxiety.

Then, one session I was coming down with a cold, my throat was hurting, and I felt really tired. All I had the energy to do was sit and listen and nod my head and say "Hmmm" from time to time. The next week she came in looking more relaxed than I'd seen her for some time. She told me that whatever it was I did last session, it was great. Could I do more of that? So—three years of school, two more years of an internship, my head stuffed to the gills with theories and strategies—and I did my best work when I was too exhausted to talk!

2. *Immediacy*: Attempting to bring the focus to the present, to comment on the style of interaction in the session, or to give feedback.

EXAMPLE:

"Right this very moment you are deferring to me in just the same way you back down from your boss."

3. *Self-disclosure*: Sharing personal examples from your life to build trust, model personal effectiveness, or capitalize on identification processes.

EXAMPLE:

"I can recall the time in my life, at about your age, when I would see someone I liked. I finally swallowed hard and started taking risks. Although I felt rejected a lot, eventually I started meeting new people."

4. *Interpretation*: Promoting insight by pointing out the underlying meaning of a behavior or pattern.

EXAMPLE:

"So to compensate for the lack of attention you got from your father, you have constantly searched out relationships with men who are nurturing and dependent."

5. *Confrontation*: Diplomatically identifying discrepancies among (a) what a client has said in the past and is saying now, (b) what a client says versus what she or he does, and (c) what a client describes about herself or himself and what you actually observe.

EXAMPLE:

"Whereas you have repeatedly called yourself shy, withdrawn, boring, and a loser, I notice that in our sessions you are usually quite animated, outgoing, and assertive in getting what you want."

Voice from the Field

I love listening to shrinks on talk radio and watching them on afternoon television. They have this way of cutting to the chase, just nailing people where they live. And the way they can reduce people to tears within seconds—these are the skills I always wanted to have. I had the hardest time learning in my counseling program that confrontation means something different—honest, helpful feedback delivered without any hint of judgment.

Now that I'm in my internship, there are still moments when I feel that urge to clobber my client with a spot-on confrontation. I don't know what I think would really happen—I guess I expect the client to have this shocked look and say, "Oh, geez, I never thought of it like that, but you are so right … and now my life will be changed forever." If only it were that easy. Truth is, I've learned the hard way that whenever I feel the urge to confront, that's the warning sign I shouldn't be confrontational. It usually means I'm feeling critical of my client. On the one hand, well-timed confrontations are one of the most powerful tools I have as a counselor; on the other hand, when I use them for the wrong reasons, my clients just get defensive or, worse, feel wounded.

ACTION SKILLS Most counselors rely on several action responses to move the client beyond self-understanding to constructive life changes:

1. *Information giving*: Providing concise, accurate, and factual information to dispel myths, pique client interest, or create structure.

   EXAMPLE:

   "One of the reasons why you may be having difficulty initiating sex with your girlfriend is that you are not beginning a series of pleasurable activities called 'foreplay' that slowly lead to lovemaking. Instead, you just rip off your clothes and jump into bed.

2. *Advice giving*: Offering interventions designed to provide practical suggestions or motivate the client to action.

   EXAMPLE:

   "Perhaps the next time you go out on a job interview you might want to give more attention to your appearance and the impression you give."

3. *Goal setting*: Structuring a direction, planning for the future, providing a basis for measuring progress, and obtaining the client's commitment to make needed changes.

   EXAMPLE:

   "You are saying, then, that in the next week you would like to concentrate on being more open with your friends and that, on at least three occasions, you will tell people something that they don't already know about you."

4. *Reinforcement*: Giving support and encouragement to increase the likelihood that desirable behaviors will continue.

   EXAMPLE:

   "The more risks you take, the more courageous and confident you feel. After the great week you have had, I can hardly believe you are the same person."

| VOICE FROM THE FIELD

Goal setting is a dynamite skill. And so easy to learn and apply in many situations. When I first learned it, it was from a behaviorist guy who was just in love with defining, specifying, and measuring things. He taught us this mnemonic device, SPAMMO, in which each letter stands for a different criterion of effectively set goals. So good goals should be specific, pertinent, attainable, mutual, and, of course, measurable and observable. He just loved that part. Ever since I learned this years ago, I've tried to apply it to my own life. Clients just eat it up too, because they can see progressive steps they are taking toward their ultimate goals.

---

5. *Directives*: Giving instructions designed to change by specific means the structural patterns of interaction or communication.

   EXAMPLE:

   "Since you aren't having much success urging your husband to come in for counseling, I think it would be best if you tried a different approach and let him know you'd prefer he didn't come in."

   The listening, exploration, and action skills just described will be covered in great depth throughout other courses. You have plenty of opportunity to practice these skills, at first with classmates, and later with clients. They form the foundation of what many counselors do in their sessions, regardless of their espoused beliefs and theories.

   In addition to these behaviors that occur mostly in individual sessions, there are also skills that are part of counselors' other roles as negotiators (McRae, 1998), consultants (Parsons, 2007), group leaders (Johnson & Johnson, 2006), and family specialists (Carlson, Sperry, & Lewis, 2005). Other chapters and future courses will prepare you for these varied tasks, even though the bread and butter of what you will do in most settings and situations is to rely on basic listening, exploration, and action strategies within the context of your own preferred theoretical framework.

SUMMARY

Theory is not the enemy. It should not constrict your freedom and movement. In the words of Leona Tyler, one of our profession's most eminent theoreticians, "If by theory one means a tightly organized set of postulates from which rigorous inferences can be drawn, I certainly do not have one. Furthermore, I do not even want one.... If by theory, however, one means simply the organized set of concepts by means of which one attempts to fit experience into a meaningful pattern, then I may call myself a theorist" (Tyler, 1970, pp. 298–299). To Tyler, theory is no more and no less than the organization of ideas and a search for personal meaning.

The preceding chapters on theory have given you a foundation for understanding the variety of approaches to counseling. Study the concepts you are exposed to in class and in books, practice the new skills you see demonstrated, and learn the techniques described in the various theoretical orientations. But only after you have mastered, summarized, and mimicked these approaches should you then strive to personalize them.

SELF-GUIDED EXPLORATIONS

1. You have been briefly exposed to a number of counseling theories such as the following:

Client-centered	Cognitive behavioral
Behavioral	Psychoanalytic
Existential	Adlerian
Gestalt	Multimodal
Reality	Solution-focused
Narrative	Feminist

You may already feel yourself gravitating toward some of these approaches, while eliminating others. Of the theories that are listed above, circle a few that you especially like and cross out a few that you have rejected. Talk to yourself about why you feel drawn to the choices you have circled. What is it about your personality, values, and experiences that has influenced your choices?

2. Critically evaluating, developing, integrating, and applying theories is crucial to the work of counseling practitioners, especially with regard to how people learn, grow, and change. Based on your limited experiences thus far, what is your theory to explain how you have made changes in your life?

3. Here is a brief vignette:

> A woman comes into your office, clearly agitated. Her knees shaking, she tells you, "I just don't know what to do about my marriage. I feel so hopeless. I'm sure my marriage is doomed to failure. And it's all my fault. I'm so embarrassed … I knew from our wedding day I'd made the wrong choice. Should I leave? Should I stay? Can you help me decide?" Her face brightens a bit. "You know, I'm really glad I've come for help. I hear you're a great counselor."
>
> Suddenly, her shoulders sag; a defeated look comes over her face. "Forget it. I don't know why I should think you'd be able to help me. No one can help me. I chose to marry him, so I have to pay the price. You make your own bed and lie in it. That's the way the world works."

Make a list of the following: (a) every feeling the woman experienced; (b) every belief the woman seemed to have; (c) her expectations regarding how authority figures (in this case, you, as her counselor) will treat her and possibly help her. Time yourself on how long it takes to make your lists.

How long did it take you? If you were the actual counselor, how many of these three kinds of client "phenomena" do you think you could have noticed and responded to in this one-minute session excerpt? (Trick question. You know the answer. Not much. In fact, the only way you could have been effective in this session is if you had limited yourself to focusing on one of the three categories. In a nutshell, that's why counselors have to have a theory—you just can't pay attention to everything, and so many different things are happening at once.)

The feelings you listed are what humanistic counselors would pay most attention to.

The beliefs you listed are what cognitive behavioral and REBT counselors would pay most attention to.

Expectations regarding authority figures are what psychoanalytic counselors would pay most attention to.

4. Use the following self-assessment instrument to rate your current functioning in several areas:

RELATIONSHIP SKILLS RATING SCALE

(5) All of the time (4) Most of the time (3) Sometimes (2) Rarely (1) Never

SELF-AWARENESS

____ I am in touch with my inner feelings.

____ I am comfortable with myself.

____ I am aware of my fears, anxieties, and unresolved conflicts.

SELF-DISCLOSURE

____ I express my feelings honestly and clearly.

_____ I am concise and expressive in my communications.

_____ I am open in sharing what I think and feel.

ACTIVE LISTENING

_____ I can focus intently on what others are saying and recall the essence of their communications.

_____ I show attention and interest when I listen.

_____ I am able to resist internal and external distractions that may impede my concentration.

RESPONDING

_____ I am perceived by others as safe to talk to.

_____ I can demonstrate my understanding of what I hear.

_____ I reflect accurately other people's underlying thoughts and feelings.

INITIATING

_____ I have the ability to put people at ease.

_____ I am able to get people to open up.

_____ I am smooth and natural in facilitating the flow of conversation.

ATTITUDES

_____ I am nonjudgmental and accepting of other people, even when they have different values and opinions than I do.

_____ I am trustworthy and respectful of other people.

_____ I am caring and compassionate.

MANAGING CONFLICT

_____ I can confront people without them feeling defensive.

_____ I accept responsibility for my role in creating difficulties.

_____ I am able to defuse explosive situations.

Based on this honest self-inventory, as well as consultation with instructors and peers, what would you describe as your current strengths and weaknesses? Describe your plan for improving the areas that you wish to upgrade.

For Homework

1. Team up with two or three partners. Each of you take on the role of passionately arguing one of the theoretical positions presented in the chapter. Afterward, discuss your respective opinions, supporting them with your own experience.
2. Ask someone you know who has an infant if you can take photographs. Try to capture as many different expressions as you can. Get some of the baby playing with a parent, observing a toy, being diapered, feeding. Or any other situation that interests you. When you can look at your photos, list every different emotion the baby experienced. These are the innate emotions all humans experience, and the primary emotions counselors observe and reflect in clients, regardless of age.

Suggested Readings

Clarkson, P. (2005). _The transpersonal relationship in psychotherapy._ New York: John Wiley & Sons.

Corey, G. (2009). _Theories of counseling and psychotherapy_ (8th ed.). Pacific Grove, CA: Brooks/Cole.

Cormier, S., Nurius, P. S., & Osborn, C. J. (2009). _Interviewing and change strategies for helpers_ (6th ed.). Pacific Grove, CA: Brooks/Cole.

Egan, G. (2007). _The skilled helper_ (8th ed.). Pacific Grove, CA: Brooks/Cole.

Evans, D. R., Hearn, M. T., Uhlemann, M. R., & Ivey, A. E. (2008). *Essential interviewing: A programmed approach to effective communication* (7th ed.). Pacific Grove, CA: Brooks/Cole.

Halbur, D. A., & Halbur, K. V. (2006). *Developing your theoretical orientation in counseling and psychotherapy*. Boston: Allyn & Bacon.

Okun, B. F. & Kantrowitz, R. E. (2008). *Effective helping: Interviewing and counseling techniques* (7th ed.). Pacific Grove, CA: Brooks/Cole.

O'Leary, O., & Murphy, M. (2006). *New approaches to integration in psychotherapy*. New York: Routledge.

Prochaska, J. O., & Norcross, J. (2010). *Systems of psychotherapy: A transtheoretical approach* (7th ed.). Belmont, CA: Brooks/Cole.

Teyber, E. (2006). *Interpersonal process in therapy: An integrative model* (5th ed.). Belmont, CA: Wadsworth.

Young, M. E. (2009). *Learning the art of helping: Building blocks and techniques* (4th ed.). Upper Saddle River, NJ: Merrill.

ASSESSMENT, TESTING, AND THE DIAGNOSTIC PROCESS

CHAPTER 8

KEY CONCEPTS

Assessment process

Standardized measures

Nonstandardized measures

Test reliability

Test validity

Norms

Stanford-Binet

Wechsler scales

Aptitude tests

Achievement tests

Personality tests

Interest inventories

MMPI clinical scales

Projective tests

Test usability

Observational assessment

Self-assessment

Functional diagnosis

Medical model

Developmental model

Behavioral model

Phenomenological model

Systemic model

DSM-IV-TR

Whether counselors subscribe to insight-oriented theories, action-oriented approaches, or individually designed personal models, there is virtually universal endorsement for an assessment process in helping. This can take the form of an elaborate set of testing instruments and procedures, or it may simply involve an informal conversation about what is going on (and has been occurring) in the client's life.

How, after all, could you expect to help someone if you don't have some idea about what is going on? Assessment, testing, and the subsequent diagnostic process allow both client and counselor to proceed in a relatively organized, systematic way. Imagine, for example, that a young woman tells you that she is feeling depressed and would like your assistance in regaining her composure. Before you could jump in and expect to be useful, a number of questions would come to mind.

- What does she mean by "depressed?" Depression to one person could mean incapacitating despondency; to another, it could mean simply a sad feeling; and to someone else, thoughts of suicide.
- If she has had suicidal thoughts, does she have a plan and the means to carry it out?
- What else is going on in her life? What is the context for her present predicament? Was there a precipitant to this particular episode? If so, what are the contributions of her family situation, developmental stages, social adjustment, and other relevant variables? What is the cultural context for her reported experience?
- What would it mean for her to regain her "composure"? What was she like before this current predicament? What is her usual state of functioning?
- What are her expectations about what you can do for her? What would it take for her to feel as though counseling was successful?
- What has worked for her before when she has experienced similar symptoms?
- What sorts of interventions have proven to be most and least effective in the past?

This is just the merest sampling of the questions that might run through your mind as you first listen to her tell you about her struggle. Many others may also come to mind: Why is she is seeking help now? What was she like before this problem began? What effects is the problem having on other aspects of her life? What benefits is she enjoying as a result of having this problem? What would be the consequences of solving the problem? Who else is invested in having her change in a particular direction? What is her support system like?

And then there is the suicide issue; if she answered "Yes" to the question about considering self-destructive behavior you would have to shift from a treatment

VOICE FROM THE FIELD

There's always this moment of panic I feel when a new client walks in the door. Will I be able to help this person? Will I even know what the heck is going on? As I sit there trying to listen during the first few minutes, I feel such urgency to get a handle on the "problem." I know that as soon as this person walks out the door, I'm expected to fill out a treatment plan in which I specify what are the presenting complaints, the therapeutic goals, and the diagnosis. It strikes me as so stupid that I'm supposed to know all this after a single interview. No matter how much experience I gain and how much I practice doing intakes, I am still humbled by the complexity of each and every human being.

I know that whatever assessment I do—and whatever diagnosis I come up with—is just a starting point. As I get to know the person better, I will have a much better idea of what is going on. The hard part, though, is taking a deep breath and reminding myself to be patient.

mode to conducting a full suicide assessment. You would have a whole new set of questions to ask, and, depending on your assessment, you might have to initiate a highly directive suicide prevention plan.

It is not that you are procrastinating when you hesitate to answer the client's query about how you will help her; it is just that you would be foolish to attempt any intervention without some understanding of what you are attempting to accomplish. It would be as if you went to see a doctor complaining of a stomachache and she immediately scheduled you for surgery without running appropriate tests to determine what might be wrong.

LISTENING VERSUS ASSESSING

In whatever form it is structured—as paper-and-pencil tests, detailed background questionnaires, structured interviews, or lengthy conversations—an assessment process is crucial to accomplishing several important tasks:

- Familiarizing yourself with the client's world and characteristic functioning.
- Learning about past events and developmental issues that have been significant.
- Studying family history, cultural background, and the current living situation.
- Assessing the client's strengths and weaknesses with regard to intellectual, academic, emotional, interpersonal, moral, spiritual, and behavioral functioning.
- Checking out risk factors related to substance abuse, suicide, or harm to others.
- Learning about the client's expectations, goals, and aspirations.
- Identifying presenting problems and their related issues.
- Formulating a working diagnostic impression.
- Developing a flexible treatment plan to reach mutually agreed-upon therapeutic goals.

Within any counseling relationship, you must conduct a thorough investigation of the present situation, its current context, and its past history. You are not only thinking in terms of "problems" and "symptoms" that might require attention, but also "core issues" that represent reoccurring themes in a client's life (Halstead, 2007). Care must be taken not to jump to conclusions with too little information, because we often have a tendency to seek data that support our preexisting notions about clients. And most important, you must follow the usual standards of care for someone who may be acutely suicidal or dangerous to others (McGlothlin, 2008; Simon & Hales, 2006).

What can make the need for assessment so confusing for novice counselors is its conflict with another "rule" that is often introduced: Early sessions should be devoted to relationship building, with the counselor practicing active listening skills and letting clients set the pace at which they feel most comfortable. This can indeed be at odds with the need to gather a fairly extensive amount of knowledge about clients, their presenting complaints, and the nature of their worlds. The differing approaches to assessment associated with the various counseling approaches further complicate the issue of what information to seek. For example, psychodynamic counselors want to know about childhood experiences; person-centered counselors are assessing clients' capacity to be emotionally congruent; cognitive behaviorists are looking for signs of distorted thinking; and solution-focused counselors need clues about clients' repertoire of problem-solving strategies.

Finding a balance between conducting a thorough assessment and practicing good listening skills is indeed a challenge, but actually not beyond your ability. For example, an early session might go something like this:

COUNSELOR: So, Consuela, when did you first start to have this feeling of your heart pounding in your chest?

CLIENT: Well, it was when I read the syllabus in my very first counseling class, and saw all the reading I had to do.

COUNSELOR: Sounds like you got kind of scared.

CLIENT: You got it. Not just scared. I'd say, terrified.

COUNSELOR: Have you ever experienced symptoms like this before?

CLIENT: Nope. This was the first time. I don't think of myself as an anxious person.

COUNSELOR: So this was a new experience for you. You felt sensations in your chest that you had never had before. I can imagine how that might be terrifying for you.

CLIENT: Yes, and I don't want them to happen again! What can I do to stop them?

COUNSELOR: Well, that's what we're here to work on.

In this brief excerpt you can recognize that the counselor is doing two different things that you might have imagined are contradictory. On the one hand, there is a lot of active listening and reflecting going on—communicating that the counselor understands the client's experience. Yet the counselor is also guiding the conversation in order to assess the specific nature of the symptoms and determine whether they are chronic or situational. These dual tasks will be present in most initial interviews you do.

VOICE FROM THE FIELD

I can't tell you how many times my instructors would tell me, "Stop asking questions and just reflect, reflect, reflect." I mean, they were really on top of me about this, almost like drill sergeants, pounding it into my head until I finally got the message. So what happens on my first day in my fieldwork placement? My supervisor gives me this list of all this information I need to collect about my clients. It was like I was in a no-win situation—do what I was taught in school, or do what I was told by my supervisor. Sure, I'd taken a class in assessment and diagnosis, but nothing prepared me for this, and, frankly, I felt a little pissed off at my instructors.

Here's how I resolved my frustration. Good listening is still my number one job—I want my client to feel counseling is safe. If I think the client is in crisis, and at risk, I most definitely go into a questioning mode. There's information I simply have to get. But if it wasn't an emergency, and I just listened, adding the right open-ended question at certain points, this interesting thing happened—I found myself getting the information I needed without interrogating the client. It just would kind of happen naturally.

WHAT IS ASSESSMENT?

Assessment is a multifaceted process that involves a variety of functions to determine an individual's characteristics, aptitudes, achievements, and personal qualities. Assessment can be viewed as an integrative process that combines a variety of information into a meaningful pattern reflecting relevant aspects of an individual. It never depends on a single measure, nor does it emphasize one dimension at the expense of another. For an assessment profile to be meaningful and useful, it must provide a means for understanding the individual from as broad and integrative a perspective as possible.

Only with the most accurate information can an assessment be appropriately used in counseling. Consider the challenge, for example, of evaluating a candidate's suitability for entrance into a counselor training program. Let's say we are looking for people who have shown a degree of academic success in the past, who are reasonably intelligent, who write and speak well, and who are highly motivated to help people. Furthermore, we might be looking for those who present themselves well in human interactions and who are perceived as likable and compassionate. We also wish to search for people of high moral character, who take feedback well, and who are inclined to be both introspective and analytic about others' behavior. Finally, we want people who are reasonably healthy emotionally, who will not harm others because of their own unresolved issues that may get in the way.

We are also faced with some practical concerns. We have limited time and resources to screen a number of applicants. In an ideal world, we could spend weeks investigating each of several hundred applicants; in actuality, we need a shortcut method that might at least give us a rough indication as to which applicant might be predicted to achieve success in our program and in a career as a counselor.

We might wish to include a standardized test score—a measure of past academic performance—in our assessment process. With this score, we might weight those aspects that seem most relevant to our purposes—say, verbal over quantitative

VOICE FROM THE FIELD

When I first started using assessments with children in the school system, I was very rigid and focused a lot of energy on making sure that I administered tests exactly as per the standardized protocol. I looked exclusively at the numbers and the standard deviations of the child's scores and paid little attention to other important aspects of test administration such as rapport, motivation, attention level, and other stuff. But, after I became more experienced in using tests, I began to understand the merit of observation during the assessment process. I began to document in my reports more information regarding how the children responded, their affect, their general demeanor, and their level of interest. I found that these bits and pieces of information were as important as simply looking at the numbers.

I also found that using more than just one instrument helped immensely in painting a more vivid portrait of who the person really is. I believe fully that for this very reason, many agencies and schools rely on a battery of tests and assessments rather than on just a single instrument to gain a clearer understanding of the client's personality, achievement, aptitude, strengths and weaknesses, and overall functioning. I also believe that the assessment process in itself can be therapeutic as well, because the clients learn so much about themselves. This new information gives clients an additional mirror to reflect on and evaluate themselves.

ability. We would probably wish to review past experiences most similar to the present challenges, that is, performance in school and previous jobs. Recommendations from knowledgeable observers, certainly previous supervisors, would be helpful in this regard. We would wish to see a writing sample, perhaps one that discusses personal and professional goals. Finally, if all these data seem to fit with what we are looking for, a structured interview would provide additional information that might be useful.

Each of these segments would provide information from which to construct an integrated portrait. Assessment thus attempts to build a comprehensive composite of an individual's characteristics, qualities, or aptitudes from as broad a vantage point as possible, sampling several pertinent sources of information.

Conducting an assessment requires that a wide range of information be gathered to illuminate as many relevant aspects of the person as possible. Information sources can be divided into two general categories. *Standardized measures* include tests that have been designed to ensure uniformity of administration and scoring and for which norms are generally available. *Nonstandardized measures*, which do not ensure uniformity of measurement and tend to be subjective, take a more general and diverse approach to gathering information.

THE ROLE OF TESTING IN THE ASSESSMENT PROCESS

Although it certainly is not the only way to collect useful information and assess client functioning, testing is one of the most common methods that counselors employ. The history of our profession is very much interwoven with the parallel evolution of the testing movement.

At the beginning of the 20th century, James Cattell, one of the first experimental psychologists, coined the term *mental test* to describe his attempts to measure the intellectual ability of students. Building on the work of Sir Francis Galton and his development of rating scales, questionnaires, and statistical methods, Cattell

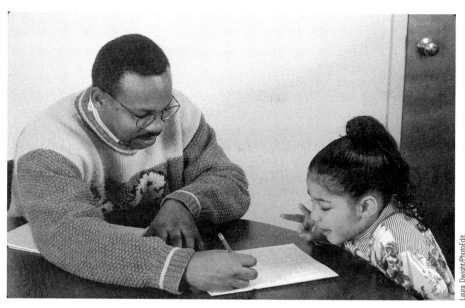

Laura Dwight/PhotoEdit.

Psychological testing instruments, such as those that measure aptitude, achievement, personality traits, and interests, provide a variety of information for counselors and clients that cannot be accessed through interviews alone.

began the science and industry of testing, along with researchers in Europe—Kraepelin, who made assessments of the mentally ill, and Alfred Binet, whose scales measured children's mental abilities. Although Binet's intelligence tests for screening schoolchildren were the first widely accepted tests, it was the development of group intelligence testing during World War I that gave real impetus to psychological and educational testing as we know it today. The U.S. Army Alpha and Beta were the first group intelligence tests used to screen out those who might be unfit to serve. Army psychologists also worked to develop group personality tests to screen recruits for potential problems.

The army's experience with group intelligence and personality testing provided the basis for a significant expansion of the assessment process in the 1920s. Between 1920 and 1940, many other tests were developed to measure a wide range of characteristics, including intelligence, aptitude, ability, attitude, personality, and interests. The number of tests expanded to the point at which a catalog of instruments was needed just to familiarize the practitioner with all the options that were available. Originally published by Oskar Buros, this publication still exists today as the *Mental Measurements Yearbook* (Geisenger, Spies, Carlson, & Plake, 2007).

The second major acceleration in the development and use of testing occurred in the years around World War II for many of the same reasons mentioned earlier—to find more efficient ways to screen personnel and thereby make use of their talents in optimal ways. Tests such as the Wechsler Adult Intelligence Scale (WAIS) and the Minnesota Multiphasic Personality Inventory (MMPI-2) were first developed and extensively used during this time.

In spite of whatever advantages testing might offer, it has come under increased criticism, primarily because of concerns that the instruments are culturally and ethnically biased, reflecting the values of the majority culture to the disadvantage of others who are exposed to a different set of educational experiences growing up. These problems have led to a number of restrictions on the use of tests and to some professionals' disenchantment with them. In spite of these concerns, recently there has been an increased use of testing for a variety of purposes because of its economical way of helping decision makers predict future behavior (Hood & Johnson, 2007; Neukrug & Fawcett, 2010).

TECHNOLOGY AND ASSESSMENT

Computers have greatly simplified the general process of assessment, as well as test development, scoring, and interpretation. Counselors now routinely use the Internet, specialized diagnostic software packages, videoconferencing, and Web-based sites to conduct their client assessments and to consult with various sources during this procedure (Hohenshil, 2000; Naus, Phillipp, & Samsi, 2009). Computer generated reports are playing an increasingly significant role, not so much as a substitute for clinical judgment but rather as an aid to help counselors make sense of client experiences and plan effective treatments (Butcher, Perry, & Hahn, 2004; Lichtenberger, 2006; Trull, 2007).

These recent developments and innovations certainly enhance counselors' ability to select appropriate instruments, score and interpret them, and make sense of the data—but also at some cost. Concerns continue to be raised about compromised privacy and confidentiality (Koocher, 2007). How safe do you feel, for example, when any government agency—or even a meddling computer hack—can access the most personal data about your life without you even knowing about the invasion of privacy?

WHY STUDY TESTING?

Perhaps a useful way to begin a study of testing and assessment is to explore why it is important in the first place. The process of counseling involves decision making at many levels to help the client resolve concerns, effect change, and plan for contingencies and opportunities. For decision making to be maximally effective, it must be based on self-understanding, awareness of various options and alternatives, and a fund of relevant information. We have already examined a number of widely accepted techniques used in counseling to provide information for decision making.

Verbal and nonverbal techniques, in particular, have been presented as basic counselor-offered conditions that facilitate counseling and help the client integrate a variety of information about self and relevant counseling issues. Testing, as part of an appraisal process, is an additional source of useful information about clients that can affect the decision-making process. In fact, tests offer a type of information not readily available through nontest methods: They gather information that highlights the ways in which clients are alike and different. The results of a test or series of tests can provide clients with information about themselves and illustrate how they compare with others who are similar to them. This information can help

VOICE FROM THE FIELD

I'm a humanistic, person-centered counselor, and quite honestly, I balk at the idea of starting treatment with a battery of tests. Sure, I need to know if my client is inappropriate for the way I do counseling—in which case I refer out. Otherwise, I think this whole testing thing gets in the way of forming a relationship, which in my mind is the most important thing.

I know there are counselors who like the way tests tell you how depressed or anxious or crazy clients are. But I do wonder if tests really can tell you something meaningful—let's face it, most tests don't tell you what the client is feeling inside. They just give you numbers. I know I'm not alone in feeling this way—a lot of my colleagues never give tests. Are we being unprofessional? I really don't know.

clients understand themselves and can be an asset in exploring alternatives during decision making.

The information provided by testing is not always consistent; therefore, the counselor must be skilled in appraisal technology so that discrepancies in test data can be resolved in an exploration of the information. To help clients have the broadest possible source of information about self, the counselor must be knowledgeable about the selection, use, and interpretation of tests. To be uninformed about testing and assessment is to arbitrarily delete a potentially valuable source of data that could improve the quality of decisions about change of lifestyle, work, or behavior patterns. It is fascinating, even if not downright useful, to know how well we perform in a particular area when compared with others who have attempted the same task.

Your clients may have experienced some type of trauma as a result of test abuse. Without the ability to make sense of the raw data to judge the suitability of the particular test, you will never be able to challenge its appropriateness in a given situation. Thus, even if you were never going to administer tests yourself (a highly unlikely situation), you must be familiar with norms, reliability, validity, clinical versus statistical significance, and other relevant concepts so that you can help your clients make sense of their own testing experiences. This knowledge is not only crucial to collecting meaningful information from the client but also helpful in formulating a plan with which to begin therapeutic efforts.

STANDARDIZED MEASURES

A test is nothing more or less mysterious than an attempt to measure a sample of behavior objectively and consistently. Whether the issue is a client's career preferences, mathematical skill, verbal reasoning ability, personality characteristics, or potential for success, tests are a convenient basis for judging the strength, utility, or desirability of various human qualities.

Tests are used to match the most capable and well-suited individuals with a particular program, position, or job. They have value as predictive devices for hypothesizing about a person's future performance or action. And certainly tests help counselors in their overwhelming task of understanding clients—their characteristic behavior patterns; their strengths, deficiencies, values, aptitudes, and mastered skills; and, most important, their potential and capacity for growth.

For a test to be useful, it must be a *reliable* and *valid* measure of behavior. *Reliability* refers to the consistency or accuracy of a test score, whereas *validity* refers to the extent to which tests actually measure what they purport. Although no test is perfectly reliable or absolutely valid, any assessment instrument or methodology that a counselor uses must meet these criteria for the specific group and context in which it is employed. One other consideration is that certain personality and intelligence tests may only be administered and interpreted by professionals who hold particular licenses in that discipline.

Despite being scientifically designed to be fair, objective, reliable, and appropriate, test content, testing procedures, and test interpretation may still be biased against nonwhite middle class clients. Hood and Johnson (2007) note three ways in which biases may occur: (1) The questions and norming procedures of many standardized tests may reflect the language and customs of the white majority; (2) clients from minority groups who historically have experienced barriers to success may not be as motivated to do as well as test takers from the dominant culture; (3) test results used for employment or academic admissions reflect bias when they lead to findings that vary significantly among groups and cultures. Indeed, the professional codes of ethics for all the helping professions mandate that counselors be knowledgeable about the impact of diversity on testing accuracy, including age, gender, ethnicity, race, disability, and linguistic differences.

There are several other criticisms and cautionary factors involved in testing procedures:

1. Tests create classificatory categories that are potentially harmful to clients. Application of labels such as "retarded," "mentally ill," "underachieving," and "passive-dependent" often follows test interpretations. And even though sticks and stones will break your bones, names will also hurt you.
2. Test construction is an imperfect science leading to results not necessarily accurate or useful. Test validity and reliability statistics are not impressive. For instance, when a mother brags that her son has an IQ of 116, she is certainly exaggerating appropriate levels of confidence in that magical number. To be honest, she would actually have to state the result in a considerably more cautious way: "There is a 68.4 percent probability that my son's real IQ falls somewhere between 112 and 120."
3. Despite the growing number of bilingual clients, the research is scant on how to administer and interpret tests with non-English-speaking populations (Confresi & Gorman, 2004).
4. Testing is often used as an excuse to guide clients in specific directions, often limiting their future vision and potential. A fifth grader who shows early promise as a math wizard may never have the opportunity to develop latent artistic and writing talents.
5. Tests often reveal hidden and disguised information (one of their functions) and therefore may be construed as an invasion of privacy. They reveal aspects of the self that a client may not wish others to know.

Their limitations and ethical problems notwithstanding, standardized tests have several useful functions that cannot be duplicated by alternative assessment strategies, such as the clinical interview and other nonstandardized procedures. First, the fact that tests are standardized means that attempts are made to ensure uniformity of administration and evaluation for all clients. No matter where the test is being administered, at what time, by whom, or to whom, subjective factors will tend to be minimized. Therefore, it is very important that counselors are trained in the use of these standardized tests before actually administering them. Credentials such as licenses to provide counseling services do not necessarily ensure competence in administering these tests. The concept of standardization also refers to the common practice of providing "norms," or measures of normal performance, so that any individual's sample behavior may be compared with that of a large group of others.

Standardized assessment procedures provide a database for making predictions about a client's future behavior. In making clinical judgments about whether a client is a likely candidate for suicide, a good prospect for a particular job opening, or a potentially responsive client for counseling, the interpretation of results from tests is invaluable. Tests can also be used to evaluate the effects of various counseling methods to determine whether supplemental interventions are necessary. They are often used as selection and classification tools as well, helping in the complex process of matching the right jobs with the best people. Finally, tests are simply an additional source of information for clinicians, a concise summary of the client's typical behavior.

Whether administered in groups for the sake of efficiency and economy or given individually, tests come in every conceivable size, shape, and purpose. There are instruments for measuring ability, aptitude, achievement, personality, and interests. Other tests can be used for assessing relationship conflict, marital satisfactions, and a host of other areas in human behavior.

TESTS OF ABILITY

Defining intelligence has been a difficult task, surrounded by controversy and strong debate. Although the dialogue is likely to continue for some time among experts, it is now generally agreed that intelligence consists of several factors: (1) abstract thinking, (2) problem solving, (3) capacity to acquire knowledge, (4) adjustment to new situations, and (5) sustaining of abilities in order to achieve desired goals.

In spite of the difficulty in defining intelligence, a number of instruments attempt to assess an individual's general mental ability or stable intellectual capacity for reasoning and applying knowledge. Tests that attempt to measure intelligence are most likely to reflect a person's scholastic/academic learning potential, especially with conceptually difficult or abstract material. Most of these tests also include a set of tasks that require a client to demonstrate memory, pattern recognition, decision making, verbal and analytic skills, general knowledge, and the ability to manipulate the environment.

Two of the most popular intelligence tests are the Stanford-Binet, probably the most well-known test, and the Wechsler scales, which are the most widely used intelligence tests (Neukrug & Fawcett, 2010). The Weschler tests include specific instruments designed for adults (Wechsler Adult Intelligence Scale), children (Wechsler Intelligence Scale for Children), and preschoolers (Wechsler Preschool and Primary Scale of Intelligence). Both the Wechsler scales and the Stanford-Binet are examples of individually administered intelligence tests that attempt to measure

VOICE FROM THE FIELD

As an educational diagnostician for a smaller community college, I have tested many college students for learning disabilities. I enjoy testing a great deal and find that the real challenge in assessing intelligence is not how to administer the Wechsler or the Stanford-Binet but what we actually do with the results of such testing. Understanding how each subscale score affects clients in their daily life and how to help them overcome their weaknesses and build on their strengths is the true key in testing of this nature.

I've also learned that discussing the results with the client at follow-up is a very sensitive issue and many times the client is very apprehensive and anxious to find out their results, especially when there are significant weakness areas. It's hard to present the results in such a way that the client doesn't leave discouraged or feeling like a failure.

IQ (intelligence quotient) as a general underlying composite of intelligence, often with an emphasis on verbal and nonverbal problem solving. Administering these tests requires special training and often a state license as a psychologist or other mental health professional.

There are also group ability tests, such as the Cognitive Ability Test and the Otis-Lennon Scholastic Ability Test, that tend to measure intelligence as scholastic aptitude and are more dependent on previous learning experiences. These group tests, however, do not have the same administrative requirements as the individual tests and are often used in educational settings.

TESTS OF APTITUDE

Aptitude tests are concerned primarily with prediction of a person's performance in the future. All of us have, at one time or another, run the gauntlet of tests to determine whether we are good candidates for an available slot. It is likely that you have had experience with the Scholastic Aptitude Test (SAT) or the American College Test (ACT) for admission to college, or with the Graduate Record Exam (GRE) for entrance to a graduate program. You may also have some rather strong opinions about the validity of these instruments for predicting academic success.

The Law School Admission Test (LSAT) is another example of a test used to predict success in programs of advanced study. At the level of state employment agencies, aptitude tests such as the General Aptitude Test Battery (GATB) are used for job placement, and school systems rely on instruments such as the Differential Aptitude Test (DAT) for assessing academic aptitude and educational placement of children.

TESTS OF ACHIEVEMENT

Often called proficiency tests, achievement tests are used to measure learning, acquired capabilities, or developed skills. They are widely used and can be adapted to almost any type of task from measuring course content (a typical exam) to administering the road test for a driver's license. Results can be used as diagnostic tools, as demonstrators of accountability, and, because past performance is the best measure of future performance, as predictors. Commonly used tests in this category are the California Achievement Test and the Metropolitan Achievement Test.

TESTS OF TYPICAL PERFORMANCE

Tests designed to measure an individual's day-to-day behavior or performance are interested not in what a person can do (ability) but in what a person does. Although motivation is important in this type of test, it is less so than in ability testing. Two common categories of typical performance testing are personality inventories and interest inventories.

PERSONALITY INVENTORIES   These tests are designed to gather information on an individual's preferences, attitudes, personality patterns, or problems. Results are expressed by comparison with a specific reference group. A concern with personality inventories is the possibility of faking responses, but most instruments of this type have a "lie scale" to detect a tendency to present an overly favorable profile. Examples of personality inventories include the Meyers-Briggs Type Indicator MBTI), the California Psychological Inventory (CPI), the Sixteen Personality Factor Questionnaire (16 PF), the Minnesota Multiphasic Personality Inventory (MMPI-II—see Table 8.1), and the Beck Depression Inventory-II (BDI-II).

TABLE 8.1 | MMPI-II SCALES AND SIMULATED ITEMS

State licensing codes vary in permitting non-psychologists to administer MMPI tests. Nevertheless, it is quite possible you will be called upon to interpret a client's scores; at the least, you should have some working knowledge of the various clinical scales:

1 or Hs (Hypochondriasis) Items derived from patients showing abnormal concern with bodily functions such as reporting chest pain several times per week.

2 or D (Depression) Items derived from patients showing extreme pessimism, feelings of hopelessness, and slowing of thought and action.

3 or Hy (Conversion Hysteria) Items from neurotic patients using physical or mental symptoms as a way of unconsciously avoiding difficult conflicts and responsibilities.

4 or Pd (Psychopathic Deviate) Items from patients who show a repeated and flagrant disregard for social customs, an emotional shallowness, and an inability to learn from punishing experiences.

5 or Mf (Masculinity-Femininity) Items that distinguish gender differences.

6 or Pa (Paranoia) Items showing abnormal suspiciousness and delusions of grandeur or persecution.

7 or Pt (Psychasthenia) Items based on neurotic patients showing obsessions, compulsions, abnormal fears, and guilt and indecisiveness.

8 or Sc (Schizophrenia) Items from patients showing bizarre or unusual thoughts or behavior, who are often withdrawn and experiencing delusions and hallucinations.

9 or Ma (Hypomania) Items from patients characterized by emotional excitement, overactivity, and flight of ideas.

0 or Si (Social introversion) Items from persons showing little interest in people and insecurity in social situations.

VOICE FROM THE FIELD

The MMPI amazes me. I've watched psychologists interpret it, and they can tell me an astonishing amount of information about my client, stuff it took me weeks to diagnose. And the fact that you can tell right away if someone is trying to lie is really impressive. One thing that became clear is that it takes a lot of expertise to use the MMPI correctly. It looks pretty simple—clients who score above or below the normal range have an emotional disorder, and clients who score within the normal range, don't. But it's actually a lot more complicated to evaluate the meaning of MMPI results.

Although my knowledge of the MMPI is limited, I have found it to be very helpful to know what the various numbers stand for. Like the fact that an elevated 2 is depressed, or an elevated 2, 4, 6, and 8 suggests a personality disorder. Of course, the downside is, the first thing I think of when I see some clients for the first time is that "she's a 2, 4, 6, 8" and I've given her a poor prognosis before I've even started working with her. It sometimes takes extra work to keep tests in perspective and not let them bias me.

Of all of these, counselors are most likely to have some involvement with the BDI-II; many agencies give new clients the BDI-II as part of their intake procedures, and it is a staple intervention in a cognitive behavioral course of treatment. The instrument consists of 21 questions, with each question asking clients to rate on a 1 to 3 scale the intensity at which they are experiencing a specific symptom of depression. The higher the score, the more intense the depression, whereas scores under 13 usually signify the absence of depression (Beck, Steer, & Brown, 2004). Counselors often use the Beck Depression Inventory to track a depressed client's progress throughout the therapeutic process, knowing that when the scores become consistently low, the treatment can be brought to a close.

Personality inventories, regardless of what they measure, are known as paper-and-pencil tests (for self-evident reasons), and also as self-report instruments. This latter characteristic is an important one for counselors to appreciate, because what clients report about themselves may not be an accurate representation of what they actually feel or believe. While it is difficult to fake an MMPI exam, it is fairly easy to exaggerate or minimize self-reports of depression or anxiety. For example, some clients may consider depression to be shameful or a sign of weakness, and may be reluctant to answer truthfully on a BDI. Other clients may have a vested interest in appearing to be in worse shape than they actually are (e.g., a client who is afraid to leave counseling, despite clear improvement). Finally, self-report tests tend to measure what the clients are experiencing at the time they take the test; someone who is having a particularly difficult day may report high levels of emotional distress that are not reflective of his or her typical functioning and mood. Prudent counselors use self-report information as just one piece of an overall picture of a client; other tests, observations, even intuitive responses to a client need to be considered as well in order to develop an accurate assessment.

Another type of personality measure is the projective type, which does not use a pencil-and-paper format but is individually administered (usually by a psychologist). This type of test requires a client to respond to unstructured stimuli such as an inkblot or an incomplete sentence. A qualified examiner then interprets these responses as reflective of underlying personality organization and structure. Examples include the Rorschach and the Thematic Apperception Test (TAT). Counselors who work with

| VOICE FROM THE FIELD

I know a lot about teenagers. Having been a high school teacher in the past, I have seen the best of times and the worst of times in kids. But as a vocational counselor for the past three years, I find my new role in the lives of these kids to be very exciting. I am able to help them through certain aspects of their identity confusion by helping them to find a sense of direction for their future careers.

I find that using interest inventories with them such as the Strong-Campbell or Holland's Self-Directed Search can be a really valuable and enlightening experience for them. Some of them seemed reluctant to sit down and go through all the questions on these inventories. However, once they are scored, most of the students are very glad for such an experience and seem to have a fresh sense of direction.

You shouldn't place too much emphasis on the results of interest inventories but should simply use them as a tool to empower the student with another piece of information about who they are. I have also seen many families drawn closer together from such a testing experience since many of these students take their results home and discuss them with their moms and dads. Sometimes their parents become more involved in their lives as they realize that their children are starting to become adults and are in need of support to make the next transition from school to work or college.

children sometimes use the House-Tree-Person drawing test, which may reveal how a child feels more accurately than do the child's spoken words.

INTEREST INVENTORIES Interest inventories attempt to develop a profile of an individual's career interest areas through a series of questions about preferences, jobs, hobbies, and other activities. The pattern of responses is then compared to the responses of persons successfully engaged in a variety of occupational areas. Profiles are constructed by matching high and low scores in occupational clusters. A limitation of these inventories is that, because interest does not reflect ability, it is possible for a person to dislike a career area in which he or she has earned a high score. Commonly used interest inventories are the Strong-Campbell Interest Inventory and the Kuder Preference Record.

SELECTING TESTS

One of a counselor's important responsibilities is to select tests from myriad choices. The selection of a test is complex because a number of competing factors must be analyzed and evaluated. Neukrug and Fawcett (2010) suggest the counselor follow five steps in order to make the best possible choices.

1. *Determine the goals of your client.* Before you even consider what tests to use, gather information from interviewing the client in order to define the client's goals for counseling.
2. *Choose instruments to reach client goals.* Once you have become clear on what the client is seeking from counseling, you can begin considering the kinds of tests that might assist the counseling process.
3. *Access information about possible instruments.* There are a number of sources you can turn to that will help you choose the best possible instruments. For example, Buros's *Mental Measurements Yearbook* (Geisenger, Spies, Carlson, &

Plake, 2007) contains reviews of major tests by experts in the field who evaluate them critically, emphasizing shortcomings and strengths. It is a reasonably objective source of information about tests and should be consulted in the process of making selections. Test manuals accompanying published tests compile relevant data on the theoretical base, development, standardization, validity, reliability, and other technical features. This information can assist the potential test user in evaluating a test's suitability for a target population. Finally, test reviews often appear in professional journals and on Web sites, which also publish articles reporting technical data. The test's publishers also offer information about their tests on their sites.

4. *Examine validity, reliability, cross-cultural fairness, and practicality of the possible instruments.* All of these factors need to be taken into account; if the publisher's own data on a specific test does not provide information on cultural fairness, you can do a journal search to find articles that have assessed whether an instrument is in compliance with multicultural assessment standards.

5. *Choose an instrument wisely.* After you have narrowed down your selection to a few choices, consider such issues as convenience, cost, ease of administration, ease of interpretation—and finally, your own comfort level.

When selecting tests, remember that no one test will be ideal for a given task; there are *always* trade-offs. It is the counselor's responsibility to select tests that have the highest possible relevance for the purposes at hand, recognizing their limitations and imperfections.

NONSTANDARIZED MEASURES

Nonstandard assessment tools are widely used to gather information about clients. They represent a "nontest" approach and are especially useful in gathering data that do not lend themselves to numerical reduction. Combining the results of standardized and nonstandardized measures often creates an optimal base for developing a truly multifaceted assessment process. Some of the more common types of nonstandardized measures are discussed here.

OBSERVATIONAL ASSESSMENT

Observational measures are commonly used to gather information that is often unavailable through other means. Observational procedures can be classified in a number of different ways, according to type (systematic, controlled, or informal), the setting in which they take place (natural or contrived), or methods used (interview, direct observation). For example, one direct and systematic means of observation in a natural setting might involve counting the number of times a client averts his or her eyes whenever an emotional topic is introduced in counseling. Another more contrived and controlled method of observation would be to use a standardized interview technique to ask a series of questions and note responses.

The interview is the most commonly used observational technique in counseling; however, other methods are also used. Anecdotal data, for example, often form the basis for progress notes, and role-playing structures might be seen as situational tests. Observational methods, however, lack the normative data available from well-defined populations, a characteristic of standardized assessment tools, and are therefore more susceptible to biases. They have also been criticized because subjects can change their behavior if they know they are being observed, and the relatively limited range of situations available for observation may not produce an adequate sample of behavior.

Nevertheless, among all the assessment tools available, you will be using your eyes, your ears, your intuition, and all your senses to observe carefully what your clients are experiencing and communicating. You will attempt to decode these cues and make sense of their behavior. And you will coordinate these observations with other data at your disposal.

Rating Scales

Rating systems provide a common basis for collecting certain types of observational data. They differ from observation in that observation is only the recording of behavior, whereas rating involves both recording behavior and simultaneously making an evaluation of specified characteristics, which are usually tabulated on a scale. The value of ratings depends primarily on the care taken in the development of the rating form and the appropriateness with which it is employed.

When doing a simple observation you note that a client appears anxious. You make this assessment based on several nonverbal cues—a repetitious tapping of the foot, averted glance, and wringing hands. You check out your assumption by reflecting the feeling you observe: "You are feeling anxious because you aren't sure where to go next." If you attempted to actually measure the degree of anxiety that is experienced, you could ask the person to rate on a 1 to 10 scale just how nervous he really is. Such rating scales, whether administered in verbal or written form, are often useful in getting a more accurate assessment of not only what someone is feeling or thinking, but to what degree.

Self-Assessment

Self-assessment is a valuable nonstandardized assessment tool that is often underused in appraisal programs. Self-assessment reinforces self-determination and recognizes that the individual is truly the expert on himself or herself. It further enhances the participatory aspect of assessment. Person-centered approaches to assessment particularly emphasize the importance of the client's self-authority in identifying and using assessment information. Portfolios are often used as supporting documentation in which a number of items—including journal entries, videotapes, photographs, and drawings—are included.

There is actually a parallel process involved in assessing the self. While you are asking your clients to check out how they are doing, what they are feeling and thinking, and then asking them to reflect on these self-observations, you are doing the same thing. This becomes the source of your intuition that develops from experience but also your way of monitoring how you are doing at each stage of the process. How are you reacting to this person at this moment in time? What is being triggered inside you by this interaction? Who does this person remind you of?

VOICE FROM THE FIELD

The thing I have learned to rely on most during difficult or confusing times with clients is my own intuition about the situation. What does my heart tell me? I listen to my head as well, of course, but it is in my heart that I often find answers—or at least clues— that elude me when I am solely in a thinking mode. I analyze what is going on. I use logic and systematic reviews to try and unravel what is happening, especially with a very challenging, difficult case. Yet when this strategy fails me, or comes up short, I try to listen carefully to whispers inside me.

In order to access the intuitive part of me, I try to disengage as much as I can at the time from what is going on. The client might just see me as quiet and reserved but what I am tapping inside are the hunches, the wonderings, the most subtle guesses about what I sense and what I feel. I am not always right; I may not even be on target most of the time. But I find that approaching a case or situation like this often frees me up to see and hear things that I might ordinarily miss.

What fantasies are elicited as a result of what is going on? What is your felt sense about what this means? A host of such questions are often reviewed as part of your supervision, but also as an ongoing part of your work during sessions.

USING ASSESSMENT METHODS IN COUNSELING

Ideally, in conducting an assessment, a counselor would choose options among both standardized and nonstandardized measures to ensure the broadest possible base of information upon which to plan intervention techniques. Although developing a comprehensive base for each client assessment is not always possible, counselors should strive for the fullest range of information and acknowledge the limitations of overly relying on any single measure.

TEST INTERPRETATION

A prerequisite of effective interpretation of tests and other assessment results is a thorough understanding of their technical aspects, including limitations of the assessment data. Further, the ability to integrate information into meaningful patterns, as in the case-study method, is a crucial skill. Under-girding these skills, however, is the necessity of applying counseling methods in both individual and group interpretations. Computer technology is helpful as an aid to the counselor in the process, but it is unlikely to replace the need for trained counselors to work in face-to-face situations with clients exploring assessment results.

The interpretation of assessment data should fully engage the client in thinking about the implications of the assessment results for his or her own problem solving and self-awareness. Clients should not have interpretations done of them but must be directly involved in the process. The following factors should be considered when interpreting test results for clients (Hood & Johnson, 2007; Welfel, 2006):

1. Engage the client in a discussion of reactions to the test experience.
2. Use simple, clear language, rather than technical jargon, when talking about tests.

VOICE FROM THE FIELD

I think of testing as a kind of consultation—just a way to check out my own hunches and impressions. For instance, if I'm seeing a new client who strikes me as unusually manipulative and gamey, I might use an MMPI—not even so much for the clinical scales as just to see how the person comes out on the "lie scales." Or with a client who seems confused and inarticulate about career preferences, I might use a career inventory to help pin things down. In any of these cases, I use testing as just another source of information to combine with what I already know—or think I know.

One of my favorites is to ask clients to draw themselves with their families. That can say a real lot about relationships and self-image and even give information about alignments in the family. It provides a wonderful stimulus for things to talk about, too.

3. Review the purpose of the testing procedures and discuss how the results will be presented. Ensure that the client understands concepts such as norms, percentiles, stanines, ranks, and other relevant measures, including the use of profiles.
4. Present the test scores and examine the actual test. Discuss what the scores actually mean to the client.
5. Remind the client that test scores are fallible, and that the results are just hypotheses rather than facts.
6. Integrate the test results with the client's other self-knowledge, helping the client to see the relationship between the scores and the self.

SUMMARY OF ASSESSMENT PRINCIPLES

1. Never use an assessment device without having a specific purpose and use for the results.
2. The results belong to the test taker, who has a right to have them explained in understandable terms.
3. The test user is responsible for preparing clients to take the test under optimal conditions (pretest orientation).
4. No set of numerical test results captures the essence of a human being.
   a. It's possible and desirable to describe things nonnumerically.
   b. Numbers have no meaning in themselves; only people experience meaning. Thus there is no such thing as objectivity.
   c. Numbers as labels imply static beings. Humans are dynamic.
5. Things that can be measured precisely tend to be relatively unimportant.
6. Assessment must be carried out with techniques that
   a. are suitable for the test taker.
   b. are of high validity and reliability.
   c. engage the participation of the assessed person as much as possible.
   d. are supported by multiple observations.
7. Interpretation should focus on strengths, on possibilities, and on remedies. Healthy optimism is a key to helpful interpretation.

CRITICAL APPLICATIONS OF ASSESSMENT PRINCIPLES: RECOGNIZING RED FLAGS

For many counselors, the process of assessment can be very different from the ideal of integrating information from a variety of sources that are standardized, observational, and intuitive. A number of factors influence the methodologies counselors utilize, including the setting where they work, the availability of instruments, "turf battles" over which professional license entitles one to administer tests, and counselors' theoretical orientation. In some states, for example, only school psychologists can administer psychological and intelligence tests; school counselors need the ability to make sense of test results, but are limited to consulting on which tests would be appropriate for a particular client. Community mental health agencies may not have the resources to purchase standardized measures, which can be expensive. Finally, certain tests tend to be associated with particular theories: Psychodynamic counselors tend to use projective instruments because of their ability to tap into clients' unconscious feelings and perceptions; cognitive behavioral therapists prefer paper-and-pencil instruments that provide numerical indicators of clients' moods and level of functioning; and some humanistic, feminist, and narrative counselors eschew the whole concept of testing on philosophical grounds, arguing that tests are by definition reductionist and therefore inappropriate for gathering information about the complex experiences of human beings.

Regardless of setting and theory, all counselors need to begin their work with every new client by assessing whether "red flags" exist—signals to the counselor that certain issues must be addressed immediately, before the actual "counseling" can proceed. These issues are the following:

1. Is there evidence of abuse—physical, emotional, or sexual when the client is a child; physical or emotional when the client is an elderly person or a dependent person (i.e., unable to care for himself or herself)? If so, further assessment and a report to authorities will likely be necessary.

2. Is there evidence that the client is a danger to self (suicidal) or to others (homicidal)? Suspicions of suicidal or homicidal tendencies are triggers for initiating specific assessment procedures.

3. Does the client need to be examined by a physician in order to rule out the possibility that the presenting issue is caused by a medical problem? Depression, anxiety, indecisiveness, anger issues, and interpersonal conflicts can all be rooted in physical disease; all too often, counselors fail to consider a physical explanation, not only wasting a client's time, energy, and money, but possibly delaying appropriate medical care. This does not mean counselors need to spend a semester in medical school, but rather to be aware that when a client's symptoms cannot be related to a specific stressful event in his or her life, a referral to a physician may be appropriate. Some helpful tips: Almost any psychological symptom can be the side effect of a medication a client is taking; additionally, depression can result from hormonal disturbances, anxiety from heart malfunctions, and changes in personality from brain-related maladies.

4. Is there an issue of diversity that the counselor needs to consider? Counselors must orient themselves to the values and needs of clients from marginalized

populations and/or ethnic and cultural backgrounds different from that of the counselor.

5. Is there a legal or ethical issue that needs to be considered? Legal and ethical issues are particularly salient when counselors work with couples and families, where issues of confidentiality are often complex and confusing.

Diversity issues will be addressed in Chapter 13 and ethical issues in Chapter 14. We will discuss here the two most important "red flags," abuse and danger to self, because the counselor's ethical and clinical duty is to take certain steps to protect the safety of clients.

Reporting Child Abuse

If there is one clear area that demonstrates the need for reliable, consistent, and appropriate assessment procedures, it is in protecting the welfare of children. Regardless of your professional affiliation, state of residence, or clinical setting, almost all licensing jurisdictions require practitioners to report suspected child abuse or neglect. This awesome mantle of responsibility does not solely fall on your shoulders, because many other professionals—including medical personnel, child care workers, teachers, clergy, even animal control officers and film developers—are also required to report such suspicions. Nevertheless, you are almost certainly going to face situations in which you will have to assess the possibility of abuse. We mention this critical application of assessment skills not only because it is so important to protect children against harm, but also because it represents a fairly uniform and consistent procedure.

Basically, if you have any reasonable suspicion that a child has been (or is currently being) harmed physically, emotionally, or sexually, you *must* report this to authorities. Failure to do so not only continues to put the child in harm's way but also subjects you to possible prosecution for failing to do your duty. You are not, by the way, held responsible for being absolutely correct in your assessment of the situation; you are merely required to report whenever you have some reasonable evidence that abuse *may* be taking place.

So, how do you know that child abuse may be going on? You don't. You can only make your best professional judgment based on the evidence that you have examined. It is then up to the authorities (child protective services and law enforcement) to investigate and make a determination. Nevertheless, this assessment challenge is a very good example of how to apply your clinical skills, knowledge about laws and standards of care, and training in recognizing possible symptoms of abuse.

What would you look for as evidence of possible neglect or abuse? A number of signs may suggest physical abuse and parental neglect: Emotional indicators include nervousness and hyperactivity, disruptive aggressiveness, passivity and shyness, and unusual fear of other children. Physical indicators can be unexplained injuries (e.g., bruises on the arms and legs, missing hair); difficulty going to the bathroom; emaciation; and inappropriate clothing (e.g., underdressed for winter; long-sleeved shirts in summer that can cover bruises on the arms). Signs of sexual abuse can be emotional, including depression, fear and distrust of authorities, and

Voice from the Field

I hate dealing with child abuse. So many intense feelings come up. My heart breaks for the children, because no matter how helpful I am, I can't take away the trauma they've been through. I can hardly stand the frightened look in their eyes when I explain I have to report abuse to the authorities; they know right away what that means—the county is going to step in and maybe remove the children from the home. What can I say to them that might bring them some solace? And then the rage I feel at the parents—I'm sorry, but I just can't stay emotionally neutral about this.

And then, what if I'm wrong in my assessment? I remind myself that I'm just a reporter; child welfare services makes the decision whether to act on my report. I feel a little better knowing that, but still, I have this image of a social worker and a cop knocking on the door, this terrified little girl inside—my client, fearing she's done something terrible simply by telling me the truth. So I keep reminding myself about what I know in my heart to be true—any child is better off when an abuser is removed from the home. What it comes down to is simply this: A child's safety is way more important than my guilty feelings.

shame about one's body image. Behavioral indicators can be precocious sexual interest, pregnancy, and—never to be overlooked—the direct reports of a child (Kanel, 2007).

Within a remarkably brief period of time, you may be called on to form a judgment about whether a client is at risk for some form of harm. Applying a decision pathway model to assessing domestic violence, Miller, Veltkamp, Lane, Bilyeu, and Elzie (2002) provide a framework that is useful in making other sorts of clinical decisions that involve clients at risk.

1. The first step is always that you see some sign or symptom of abuse, whether that is physical evidence (bruises, lacerations), anecdotal evidence, or emotional effects.
2. Next, you screen for a history of abuse by reviewing the situation with the client and the family, as well as informing the client of reporting requirements in your jurisdiction.
3. Next, you *must* comply with all reporting laws and requirements by contacting the appropriate agency.
4. Assess safety considerations of your client, and any others who might be at risk.
5. Make appropriate referrals for medical evaluation and care if needed.
6. Provide support and counseling as needed to focus on the incidents and the consequences of the abuse. Bring in other family members as needed.

Clients at Risk of Harming Themselves or Others

While we used the assessment of child abuse as one example, there are several other areas that you will also be expected to identify accurately, starting with the risk of self-harm. Client suicide is without doubt counselors' biggest fear, and counselors working in schools, community mental health, and private practice are almost assured of having to deal with a client at risk of suicide at some point in their career. Later in your training you will learn the specific steps involved in assessing for and preventing suicide. There are, however, some essential points that you should be familiar with even as you are becoming introduced to the field. You will hear these again throughout your program and internship, because there may be virtually nothing more important for you to learn.

First, any sign of depression (e.g., feelings of hopelessness or loss of interest in life; behaviors like giving away important possessions or driving unusually recklessly) should trigger a suicide assessment. The assessment begins with your asking, straight out and in unadorned language, "Have you had any thoughts of harming yourself?" When in doubt, ask. The idea that you can plant the idea of suicide in a client's head is a myth, and in fact, the opposite is true; clients are relieved you asked, even if they were not considering killing themselves (Cavioloa & Colford, 2006). Second, you cannot stop a client determined to take his or her own life; your job is to act professionally, which means conduct a suicide assessment and implement a prevention plan consistent with the standards of the counseling profession. Third, always get help from a supervisor or consultant. Fourth, always document everything you do. Fifth, keep in mind that most clients do not commit suicide, and are looking to you to remain calm in the face of their personal crisis. (Yes, you are allowed to fake it—clients do not need to know your mind is racing and stomach is in knots). These five points are just the backdrop to your continued study of assessment, counseling skills, and crisis prevention, but will stand you in good stead when you sit face-to-face with your first client or family.

Less likely in your career, but just as important to learn, is how to assess clients' potential threats of and inclinations toward violence, which means being able to determine if someone is likely to engage in violent behavior toward others. This determination is made by assessing, among other factors, the person's motivation, previous patterns, mental condition, and specificity of plan (Daniels, 2002; James & Gilliland, 2008). This issue will come up again when you study ethics and legal issues for counselors, because in certain circumstances, counselors have a legal responsibility to warn potential victims and the police.

A final point: Keep in mind that in spite of our latest technology, advances in training, and best intentions, we aren't all that great at predicting when clients are going to do harm to themselves or others. It is better to be safe than sorry, and to seek consultation with a supervisor whenever you are in doubt.

Now, you can see clearly that while assessment is a general process of checking out both what is going on with your clients and what they need most, it is also a procedure that can be applied to a number of clinical situations. This is especially the case with people who are at risk for harming themselves, harming others, or suffering the effects of others' violence or abuse.

FORMAL AND FUNCTIONAL DIAGNOSIS

A new female client enters the office, furtively glances around for a place to sit, briefly locks eyes with the counselor, and finally, with an inward sigh, burrows deeply into the couch. The mutual assessment process has already begun. While she nervously checks out the furniture, books, and framed diplomas and wonders what sort of image she is projecting, the counselor casually yet systematically makes careful observations. The client's dress, posture, and bearing are noted, as well as where and how she has chosen to sit. Facial expressions, gestures, body language, and other nonverbal behavior also give valuable cues regarding her style.

The interview progresses. Information about the presenting complaint, the solutions that have already been tried, and the current life situation are gathered. The counselor is searching for a summary statement of her problem, a formal diagnosis to describe the general pattern of behavior, and a behavioral label to describe meaningfully and individually what the client is doing, feeling, and thinking. Making these distinctions is important. In the assessment process, diagnoses are significant because they have implications for selecting a treatment strategy and because they are often required by the system. For example, the diagnosis of "cyclothymic disorder" might imply a condition involving dramatic mood swings that have been chronic throughout the client's life and may be biochemically triggered, thus suggesting the importance of medical consultations on the case. The diagnosis, however, gives us very little meaningful information about what the client is like as a person. Although useful for the general understanding of a behavioral syndrome, as well as for formulating goals, predictions, and prognoses for the case, a diagnosis alone is not enough information to begin treatment with (Seligman, 2004; Sommers-Flanagan & Sommers-Flanagan, 2009).

There are many diagnostic decisions that counselors must continuously make, revising them as they gather more information. Imagine, for example, that a severely depressed teenager enters your office. Dozens of diagnostic questions will likely flash through your mind:

- Is he a good candidate for counseling?
- Is he most suitable for individual, group, or family treatment?
- Which counseling interventions are likely to be most helpful?
- Is medication indicated in this situation? Should I ask for a psychiatric consultation?
- Is he actively suicidal?

During an assessment process such as this, there rarely is a single correct diagnosis that accurately summarizes what is happening for a client. That is one reason why you should not rush to judgment but take your time weighing all the complex factors involved (Hill & Ridley, 2001). The question, more appropriately, should be not whether your diagnostic impression is correct but whether it is useful. "A useful diagnosis is one that offers us a treatment plan that is (1) easy, (2) efficient, and (3) effective" (Weltner, 1988, p. 54). By this Weltner means that, when assessing where clients are, what their problems are, and what is causing them, it is important to be pragmatic and flexible. Because there is probably no single correct diagnosis of a situation, Weltner believes, the best counselors can do is generate as many definitions as possible. For each one you can then develop a different treatment plan, systematically trying them all until you get desired results.

For example, suppose you are called on to help a nine-year-old girl who is referred to you by her teacher because she appears withdrawn. Although she is a cooperative and likable young girl, as well as a good student, the teacher has expressed some concerns because she doesn't interact much with other children. She stays pretty much to herself or clings to the teacher.

The girl, who has only recently moved to the school district, is an only child. After meeting with her for a very brief period of time, you readily agree that she does indeed appear to be unhappy. How, then, would you proceed in your counseling efforts?

There are, of course, a number of directions in which you might head, depending on which part of the problem draws your attention. Although you would certainly want to collect quite a bit more background information before you formulated a reasonable plan, this case illustrates that a number of diagnoses and corresponding treatments are possible. Each of the definitions of the problem and courses of action shown in Table 8.2 is based on reasonable assumptions drawn from the limited clinical data provided and the various theoretical approaches presented in the previous chapters.

The point of this summary is not to overwhelm you with all the options that are possible but rather to acquaint you with the intrinsically elastic properties of the assessment process. Before we move into some of the more traditional forms of diagnosis and assessment that are part of the helping professions, you should understand how subjective this process can sometimes be.

Five major diagnostic models are used by practitioners in the various helping professions. Depending on their professional identity, training, and treatment philosophy, counselors or therapists may rely on a medical, developmental, phenomenological, behavioral, or systemic model. Each of these diagnostic systems is based on different structures, assumptions, and research data and has distinct advantages and disadvantages (see Table 8.3). Although you should become familiar with each of these models so that you may converse intelligently about your cases with a variety of helping professionals, the developmental and medical/psychiatric models are the ones most commonly used by those in the counseling profession. The developmental model has been used traditionally in educational settings and is part of our identity as counselors. As opposed to a medical model (described in the next

TABLE 8.2 | Definitions of the Problem and Possible Courses of Action

Diagnosis	Treatment Plan
She is lonely and isolated because of a deficiency in social skills.	Provide structured practice for initiating relationships.
She is holding in feelings that she has been unable to express.	Reflect her underlying feelings of fear and inadequacy.
She is discouraging herself by repeating self-defeating thoughts.	Use cognitive restructuring to help her think differently.
She is emotionally underdeveloped due to unresolved issues in the past.	Use play therapy to help her come to terms with unexpressed rage and resentment.
She is depressed in response to unresolved conflicts between her parents.	Begin family counseling or parallel marital counseling to help the parents.
She is going through a normal adjustment and grieving process that is part of a major life transition.	Offer reassurance and support until she acclimates herself to her new situation.

TABLE 8.3 | DIAGNOSTIC MODELS

Models	Primary Structure	Source of Information	Advantages	Disadvantages	Treatment Implications
Medical	Discrete categories of psychopathology	Data based on quantitative research	Organization of etiology, symptom clusters, and prognoses	Categories not as discrete and reliable as desired; individual reduced to label	Application of treatment to diminish symptoms and cure underlying illness
Developmental	Predictable stages of normal development	Case studies; qualitative and quantitative research	Ease of prediction; emphasis on healthy functioning	Stages overlap and are difficult to assess; system not universal	Identification of current level of functioning so as to stimulate growth to next stage
Phenomenological	Complex descriptions of the person with minimal use of labels	Qualitative research and personal experience	Focus on capturing essences	Model is subjective, subject to biases and distortion	Use of self as instrument to establish relationship and understand client's world
Behavioral	Specific description and identification of behaviors and reinforcers	Direct observation and quantitative measurement	Ability to be very specific and descriptive	Misses complexity of human experience	Establishment of specific goals to increase or decrease target behaviors
Systemic	Contextual descriptions	Direct observation; family history	Ability to see bigger picture of presenting issues	Negates autonomy and individuality	Works within family dynamics and structures

VOICE FROM THE FIELD

Having been a clinician for many years for a mental health agency, it becomes very easy to label and diagnose an individual with very little information. After asking a short series of questions with each response guiding the next question, I can arrive at a diagnosis in a very short amount of time. However, I have to constantly remind myself that this person sitting across the table from me is a human being with real concerns and should not be treated as a "schizophrenic" or a "bipolar" but rather as a person with symptoms of schizophrenia or with bipolar features.

I have often seen instances in which a fresh new counselor is more sensitive and empathetic than the more well-seasoned clinician that is supervising the newcomer. I suppose that the moral of the story is to continue to work with people and not focus so much on constructed labels. These clients that I diagnose usually have some understanding of their issues and often feel inadequate in certain ways. To brandish a DSM and throw labels at them can leave them feeling even more inadequate.

section), a developmentally based diagnosis describes client symptoms and behavior in terms of their adaptive functions and focuses primarily on levels and stages of present functioning. This is also the case with the systemic model favored by marriage and family counselors (see Chapter 10). This is a quite different way of thinking about assessment than the diagnostic system favored by psychiatrists and many psychologists.

DIAGNOSIS

See Companion DVD
Diagnosing & the DSM

Counselors in community agency settings are expected to have a working knowledge of a diagnostic system. Two models in wide use today are the *Diagnostic and Statistical Manual of Mental Disorders*, fourth edition, with text revisions (DSM-IV-TR); and the *International Classification of Diseases, Clinical Modification*, ninth edition (ICD-9-CM). Both of these diagnostic systems have been developed primarily by psychiatrists employing a "medical model" of conceptualizing mental illness. If you look at the list of consultants and contributors who were involved in the creation of these manuals you will notice that the vast majority hold medical degrees.

Currently the DSM-IV-TR (the fourth edition was put out in 1994; the "TR" stands for text revisions published in a 2000 edition; the DSM-V is set to be published in 2012) is considered to be the "bible" of the mental health professions, containing authoritative information and "official opinions" about the range of mental problems. The DSM-IV and IV-TR editions include a number of changes from their predecessors: They are supposed to be more sensitive to gender and cultural differences, they are more logically organized, and they include 13 new mental disorders while eliminating 8 that are considered obsolete. Counselors rely on the DSM-IV-TR: (1) as a source of standardized terminology in which to communicate with other mental health specialists; (2) for satisfying the record-keeping requirements of insurance companies or credentialing agencies such as the Joint Commission on Accreditation of Hospitals; (3) for classifying clientele in statistical categories, as is necessary for research and accountability;

(4) for predicting the course of a disorder and the progress of treatment based on available evidence; and (5) for constructing a treatment plan that will guide interventions (Seligman, 2004; Sommers-Flanagan & Sommers-Flanagan, 2009).

The actual process of differential diagnosis with the DSM-IV-TR is complex, and mastery of the system requires considerable study and supervised clinical experience. Such a task is very important for counselors entering the field. Wylie (1995) sums up the need for a thorough understanding of the diagnostic process in today's era of managed care: "In short, therapists are expected, as never before, to pass a DSM litmus test for diagnostic legitimacy, to show cause to a stranger sitting in a large corporate office checking off notches on a symptomatic yardstick, exactly why, by what measure and in what way their clients need treatment at all" (p. 24).

Diagnostic information is obtained during a clinical interview that is primarily symptom oriented, focusing on significant behavioral and psychological patterns associated with a presenting complaint. It is therefore very important that the counselor choose a clinical interview (structured or more informal) that provides the most meaningful information for guiding treatment.

One example of the criteria used in the DSM-IV-TR for making diagnostic decisions is illustrated in Table 8.4. You can see from examining this chart that each psychological disorder (in this case, "Generalized Anxiety Disorder") is described in terms of specific symptoms that can be compared to a client's presenting complaints and behavior.

In addition, information is provided about the disorder's essential characteristics, frequency of occurrence, predisposing factors, and suggestions of other problems that have similar features.

The process by which the interviewer uses the DSM-IV-TR involves making a series of decisions about the client's functioning in five different areas called *axes*. These are described as follows:

Axis I: Clinical Disorders

Axis II: Personality Disorders

Axis III: General Medical Conditions

Axis IV: Psychosocial and Environmental Problems

Axis V: Global Assessment of Functioning

The major strength of this diagnostic system is that it captures the essence of the client's symptomatology, personality style, and functioning in a brief descriptive summary. It allows the counselor to communicate information about clients in a standardized format. For example, in a case suggested by Spitzer, Skodol, Gibbon, and Williams (1994), we look at how the diagnostic process would be applied to a young woman.

Misty is a 17-year-old high school junior who became agitated during the funeral of her father, who had died suddenly of a heart attack. She complained of stomach problems that turned out to be stress-related gastritis. She also developed bizarre delusions that the devil was coming to get her and spent hours each day rocking in the corner of her room. She had no previous psychiatric history, and Misty was well adjusted before her father's death and a good student in school. Sometimes she was described as "overreacting" to things in her life.

TABLE 8.4 | DIAGNOSTIC CRITERIA FOR 300.02 GENERALIZED ANXIETY DISORDER

A. Excessive anxiety and worry (apprehensive expectation), occurring more days than not for at least six months, about a number of events or activities (such as work or school performance).

B. The person finds it difficult to control the worry.

C. The anxiety and worry are associated with three (or more) of the following six symptoms (with at least some symptoms present for more days than not for the past six months).
   Note: Only one item is required in children.

   1. restlessness or feeling keyed up or on edge

   2. being easily fatigued

   3. difficulty concentrating or mind going blank

   4. irritability

   5. muscle tension

   6. sleep disturbance (difficulty falling or staying asleep, or restless unsatisfying sleep)

D. The focus of the anxiety and worry is not confined to features of an Axis I disorder; For example, the anxiety or worry is not about having a Panic Attack (as in Panic Disorder), being embarrassed in public (as in Social Phobia), being contaminated (as in Obsessive-Compulsive Disorder), being away from home or close relatives (as in Separation Anxiety Disorder), gaining weight (as in Anorexia Nervosa), having multiple physical complaints (as in Somatization Disorder), or having a serious illness (as in hypochondriasis), and the anxiety and worry do not occur exclusively during Post-Traumatic Stress Disorder.

E. The anxiety, worry, or physical symptoms cause clinically significant distress or impairment in social, occupational, or other important areas of functioning.

F. The disturbance is not due to the direct physiological effects of a substance (for example, a drug of abuse, a medication) or a general medical condition (as in hyperthyroidism) and does not occur exclusively during a Mood Disorder, a Psychotic Disorder, or a Pervasive Developmental Disorder.

Source: From the *Diagnostic and Statistical Manual of Mental Disorders* (4th ed., Text Revision), 2000, Washington D.C.: American Psychiatric Association. Copyright 2000 by the American Psychiatric Association. Reprinted with permission.

DSM-IV DIAGNOSIS FOR MISTY:

Axis I: *Brief psychotic disorder*
Psychotic symptoms of less than two weeks in reaction to father's death.

Axis II: *Histrionic traits*
Her personality style is prone to "overreacting."

Axis III: *Gastritis*
She developed physical symptoms in response to her father's death.

Axis IV: *Severity of stress*: 5, Extreme
A father's death is a fairly severe incident in an adolescent's life.

Axis V: *Highest level of functioning during the past year*: 80, Very Good
Prior to this episode, Misty was generally high functioning.

Voice from the Field

Okay, true confession time. I love the DSM. I love its illusions of truth, as if these conditions described really do exist. I love pretending that I really can figure out which little box fits which client. I like holding my own with doctors and psychologists. I can talk DSM stuff with the best of them. But best of all, I really enjoy the logical process involved in constructing a treatment plan from beginning to end. It all appeals to my own sense of logic in a world that is essentially pretty chaotic. There it is before me: which personality attributes, organic contributors, clinical syndromes, behavioral indices, and family influences might be involved. All of this helps me to figure out the best way to approach a case and which elements I should include.

There is a thinking process that accompanies the use of the DSM-IV-TR in which a client's symptoms are clearly defined and described, compared to and differentiated from other similar kinds of disturbances, and then progressively narrowed in focus from the general to more specific diagnostic categories. In an appendix to the manual, flowcharts are presented that illustrate the process of diagnostic decision making. In the case of Misty, for example, the following questions might be asked:

Diagnostic Questions	Behavioral Evidence
Is there evidence of psychotic symptoms?	Yes, bizarre delusions.
Are there organic factors operating?	No, symptoms appear reactive.
Duration of symptoms?	Less than one week.
Recurrent episodes?	No, first episode.
Major mood disorder present?	No.
Ongoing personality disturbance?	A dramatic style but no disturbance.

This series of questions would then allow the diagnostician to differentiate Misty's brief psychotic episode from other possibilities such as schizophrenia, a schizoaffective disorder, or a mood disorder. Although you may not be called on (or trained) to work with severe emotional disturbances, it is important for you to understand the diagnostic process and procedures that other mental health professionals use in their work.

Counselors also find it valuable to apply differential diagnostic thinking when working with less severe presenting problems such as adjustment disorders. For example, if a client were to come to you complaining about feeling anxious, you should be able to distinguish among an anxiety disorder, an adjustment disorder with anxious mood, a panic disorder, or agoraphobia. There are features common to all these diagnoses, yet the treatment strategy would probably vary with each one. One of the hallmarks of effective practice is adapting what you do with clients depending on their presenting complaints and individual needs.

ETHICAL CONCERNS

Diagnosis, in and of itself, creates its own ethical problems, not through its use but through its abuse and imperfections. First, it has less-than-perfect reliability: When several clinicians view the same client in action, they may be unable to agree on the proper category. Diagnoses are often inconsistently applied and err in the direction of pathology rather than health. Counselors often find this last point to be particularly restricting, because much of their orientation views client symptomatology from a developmental rather than a psychopathological perspective; that is, rather than trying exclusively to find out what is wrong with clients, they attempt to focus on clients' internal strengths, capacity for self-healing, and resources for resolving normal life crises.

Other sources of error that affect the accuracy and validity of a psychiatric diagnosis include the counselor's expectations, theoretical orientation, and observational skills, as well as the client's inconsistent behavior, attitudes toward treatment, similarity to the counselor in basic values, and socioeconomic background.

It is now almost universally recognized that the DSM has failed to account for the role of culture in its diagnostic system. For example, cultural, racial, and gender differences can be sources of diagnostic error. Poor people are more often diagnosed as crazy, whereas rich people are labeled eccentric. Other authors have argued that emotional distress must be understood within the context of such social forces as racial discrimination, patriarchy, homophobia, and poverty; the impact of these larger forces on human suffering may be lost in the DSM's focus on the individual (Kress, Eriksen, Rayle, & Ford, 2005).

In one study of extraordinarily creative individuals such as novelists Ernest Hemingway and Virginia Woolf, jazz musician Charles Mingus, poet Sylvia Plath, dancer Vaslav Nijinsky, artist Mark Rothko, composer Brian Wilson, actress and singer Judy Garland, and comedian Lenny Bruce, their therapists were more likely to label their clients as psychotic because they had little understanding of the creative cultures to which they belonged (Kottler, 2006). In almost all the cases, the clients never felt understood by their therapists, resulting in tragic outcomes (most of them committed suicide).

There is nothing magical about the classification scheme currently in use. There is no overwhelming evidence or research data to support the discrete categories that make up the various DSM-IV diagnoses (Widiger & Samuel, 2005). Kroll (1988) has pointed out that this is especially true with the "personality disorders," which are supposed to be stable, relatively permanent traits that are part of a person's characteristic style of functioning. Although there are an even dozen of such diagnostic classifications—paranoid, schizoid, schizotypal, histrionic, narcissistic, antisocial, borderline, avoidant, dependent, compulsive, passive-aggressive, and atypical—they are not necessarily mutually discrete groups, nor do they represent an exhaustive list. Kroll points out that, although there is no diagnosis for "macho" or "pedantic" personality disorder, he certainly knows people who would fit. Likewise, although borderline, narcissistic, and histrionic personalities are supposed

VOICE FROM THE FIELD

Here's the dirty little secret every working counselor knows. When it comes to using the DSM-IV, we tend to stretch the truth. We diagnose our clients with "adjustment disorder" or "dysthymia," conditions that just about everyone has at some point in their lives, and which have minimal stigmatizing potential. Sure, our clients are having difficulties adjusting to something, or are a little depressed, but they don't always meet the DSM criteria for a disorder. Basically, we are giving diagnoses to clients so that the insurance companies or the government will reimburse them. No insurer will reimburse for "personal growth" or "relationship difficulties" or even feeling mildly depressed. They've got to have something wrong with them.

Another secret. I never give a client a "Borderline Personality Disorder" diagnosis, because I don't know who's going to see it. Her employer? His health insurance company? Someone working for the government? Even another counselor who might work with my client will be negatively affected if they read "Borderline" in a chart. I know, because I've been there. I see the borderline label on a new client's chart, and immediately I think, "This client is going to be a headache to work with." And I haven't even met the person!

Things are different, of course, when you do counseling in an agency funded by taxpayer sources; you have to be absolutely scrupulous about your diagnosis. This is one area in our society where the government really does hold you accountable.

to be different entities, some clients meet the criteria for all three. To complicate matters further, traditional diagnostic systems such as the DSM-IV-TR can be easily abused in that they encourage practitioners to look at people as labels. In one review of the literature on the subject of so-called difficult clients—meaning those who do not meet the counselor's usual expectations—they were called "character disordered," "stressful," "hateful," "abrasive," and even "bogeymen":

> Difficult clients are frightened. Their behavior, which we call resistance, is normally something that we try to prevent or circumvent—an enemy to be defeated. These people are certainly not ferocious barracudas seeking to eat us alive. Difficult clients are often just people with problems that are more complex than those we usually confront, and with an interactive style that is different from what we might prefer. Calling them names only disguises the reality that resistant clients are attempting to tell us about their pain, even if their method of communication is sometimes indirect and annoying. (Kottler, 1992, p. 391)

Application of the medical model to counseling has been eloquently and passionately denounced as morally unacceptable by such influential writers as Thomas Szasz, R. D. Laing, Erving Goffman, Theodore Sarbin, and even the late Chief Justice of the U.S. Supreme Court, Warren Burger (Edwards, 1982). Critics warn that the diagnostic scheme developed from the medical model is not useful for therapeutic practice because its concepts are descriptive rather than normative, exhibit physical symptoms instead of behaviors, rely on known physical causes, use physical treatment interventions, and define the client as "sick" or "diseased." Other authors remind us that the DSM was developed by psychiatrists, not counselors; inevitably, it reflects the worldview of its creators who were trained in medical school to be scientists. They bring to their categorization system the notion that emotional distress can be categorized as an objective truth (Duffy, Gillig, Tureen, & Ybarra, 2002). Humanistic and postmodern counselors would argue that the idea of an objective reality independent of human subjective experience represents a particular philosophy of knowledge, appropriate for categorizing medical disorders that can be observed under a microscope or in an MRI exam but not suited to the assessment of human suffering.

Moreover, diagnoses can be dehumanizing in that they pigeonhole human beings into slots that can be difficult to escape. Some clinicians are especially concerned with the overuse of terms such as *minimal brain dysfunction, hyperkinetic,* and *retarded* to describe children who are disruptive, active, or easily distracted. Although in some cases these labels denoting disturbances of conduct or organic problems may be justified, in other instances, the child's behavior is the logical response to a teacher's or parent's confusing messages. Meanwhile, the labels remain forever imprinted in the minds of others and in the records that follow the child wherever he or she may go. It is for this very reason that it is so important to use the least stigmatizing label possible that is consistent with accurate reporting. Furthermore, counselors and school counselors alike should collaborate efforts whenever possible with primary care physicians and other appropriate mental health professionals when dealing with clients with severe mental disorders.

There are alternatives to diagnostic systems based on the medical model, which equates client problems with pathological processes. Boy (1989), for example, describes a diagnostic method based on a person-centered model that emphasizes a person's individuality and uniqueness rather than trying to put her or him into a particular box. You have also read about how strategic counselors prefer to use diagnoses that are descriptive and phrased in such a way that they imply that a solution is likely. A developmental model of diagnosis is another alternative that allows counselors to assess a client's current functioning levels in terms of cognitive, language, physical, self-perception, social relations, moral, and personality factors (Capuzzi & Gross, 2007). Finally, constructivist/narrative models of diagnosis are less interested in classifying and labeling any disorder than they are helping clients to understand their own struggles within a larger context of their culture and history.

BEHAVIORAL DIAGNOSIS

Functional behavioral labeling is another alternative assessment and diagnostic strategy. In this process, a client's specific behaviors are described in meaningful, illustrative, individualized language, not only to help the counselor to understand exactly which concerns are to be addressed but also to aid the client's understanding of how, when, where, and with whom the self-defeating patterns are exhibited. There are thus therapeutic advantages to functional behavioral labeling:

1. Clients learn the methods of identifying and describing complex, abstract, ambiguous processes in specific, useful terms.

   BEFORE: "Ah, I don't know exactly. I just can't seem to concentrate anymore."

   AFTER: "I have difficulty structuring my study time on the weekends I spend at home, particularly when I allow the distractions of my brother and girlfriend to interfere."

2. Clients understand that they are unique individuals with their own characteristic concerns.

> BEFORE: "I've been told that I'm a drug addict."
>
> AFTER: "I'm a person who tends to overindulge in cocaine and marijuana when I feel school pressures building up."

3. Clients describe their behavior in such a way that it can be changed. Whereas a personality characteristic is stable, invariant, and permanent, a behavior can be changed.

> BEFORE: "I'm shy. That's the way I've always been."
>
> AFTER: "I sometimes act shy when I meet a new guy I find attractive."

4. Clients label their behavior in the specific situations in which they have difficulty.

> BEFORE: "I'm depressed."
>
> AFTER: "I feel depressed in situations like my job and marriage, in which I feel powerless to do anything to change."

5. Clients accept responsibility for their destructive behaviors rather than blaming them on something beyond their control, such as bad genes.

> BEFORE: "I'm passive. Everyone in my family is. What do you expect?"
>
> AFTER: "I act passively in some novel situations because I have learned to let others take charge. Yet in other situations, in which I feel more comfortable, I don't act passively at all."

Within the context of the assessment process are several methodologies that may be used to collect valuable data, formulate workable diagnoses, and create specific behavioral assignments. Standardized testing is certainly helpful in that regard. However, all assessment efforts and testing practices are effective only in the context of the therapeutic relationship.

SUMMARY

In this chapter we have presented a brief overview of the major themes involved in testing and assessment. The field is broad, the focus controversial, and the need for technical expertise and cogent thinking great. Assessment cannot ethically be avoided by counselors; it's their job to observe, evaluate, diagnose, and intervene. It is our contention, and we hope your growing awareness, that using as broad a range as possible of relevant assessment devices, including standardized instruments, provides to both client and counselor the maximum amount of potentially useful information. Assessment will be done; the only question is: Will it rest on a defensible base?

SELF-GUIDED EXPLORATIONS

1. In what ways have particular tests or assessment instruments had an influence in some major choices and decisions you have made in your life?

2. Recount an episode in which you were assessed and evaluated by someone. What was that experience like for you? How do you wish the experience had been handled

differently? When you are in a position to assess others, what do you intend to do that is different from your experiences?

3. From what you know and understand about the various diagnostic labels that counselors and therapists use, write a diagnostic assessment of yourself. Include as much professional jargon as you can, as if you were writing up a case report of a client.

4. Think of times when you have been depressed or anxious. Make a numerical list of every symptom that you experience when you feel this way (e.g., sadness, didn't feel like doing anything, upset with yourself, worried a lot, heart beating faster, etc.). How many symptoms can you come up with? Reflect on how well your list describes what depression or anxiety feels like for you. What is it about depression or anxiety that a list of symptoms fails to capture?

5. In addition to the medical model described in the previous question, there are several other diagnostic models (developmental, phenomenological, behavioral, systemic) that are sometimes employed. Describe some aspect of your life in the language of each of these alternative models.

Developmental—current functioning in terms of stage- and age-related norms

Phenomenological—essence of your experience while minimizing labels

Behavioral—specific description of your observable behavior

Systemic—attention to interactive factors in your family and peer group

6. Write three sample test questions that you believe measure accurately what you learned in this chapter about the assessment process. Describe the challenges you experienced in developing some means of evaluating your performance.

For Homework

1. Make plans at the career center, counseling center, or some other agency to take a series of tests including an interest inventory, an aptitude test, a projective test, and an objective personality instrument. Review with the counselor the limitations and most useful information derived from this experience.

2. Below is a list of movies that depict people with DSM disorders. View each film and, without consulting the DSM, see if you can identify symptoms that suggest to you a character might be experiencing a disorder.

Depressive Disorder—*The Hours*

Post-Traumatic Stress Disorder—*Flags of Our Fathers*

Borderline Personality Disorder—*Girl, Interrupted*

Obsessive-Compulsive Disorder—*As Good as It Gets*

Narcissistic Personality Disorder—*Wall Street*

Schizophrenia—*A Beautiful Mind*

Suggested Readings

American Psychiatric Association (2000). *Diagnostic and statistical manual of mental disorders* (4th ed., Text Revision). Washington, D.C.: American Psychiatric Association.

Bongar, B. (2002). *The suicidal patient: Clinical and legal standards of care.* Washington, D.C.: American Psychological Association.

Drummond, R., & Jones, K. D. (2006). *Assessment procedures for counselors and helping professionals* (6th ed.). Upper Saddle River, NJ: Prentice Hall.

Echterling, L., Presbury, J., & McKee, E. (2004). *Crisis intervention: Promoting resilience and resolution.* Upper Saddle River, NJ: Prentice Hall.

Halstead, R. W. (2007). *Assessment of client core issues*. Alexandria, VA: American Counseling Association.

Hood, A. B., & Johnson, R. W. (2007). *Assessment in counseling: A guide to the use of psychological assessment procedures* (4th ed.). Alexandria, VA: American Counseling Association.

Kanel, K. (2007). *A guide to crisis intervention* (3rd ed.). Belmont, CA: Brooks/Cole.

Kottler, J. A. (2006). *Divine madness: Ten stories of creative struggle*. San Francisco: Jossey-Bass.

Murphy, K. R., & Davidshofer, C. O. (2006). *Psychological testing: Principles and applications* (6th ed.). Upper Saddle River, NJ: Prentice Hall.

Neukrug, E. S., & Fawcett, R. C. (2010). *Essentials of testing and assessment: A practical guide for counselors, social workers, and psychologists*. Belmont, CA: Brooks/Cole.

Seligman, L. (2004). *Diagnosis and treatment planning in counseling* (3rd ed.). New York: Springer.

Spitzer, R. L. (2002). *DSM-IV-TR casebook*. Washington, D.C.: American Psychiatric Press.

COUNSELING APPLICATIONS

PART | 3

GROUP COUNSELING

KEY CONCEPTS

Group norms

Group modalities

Screening procedures

Spectator effects

Curative factors

Cohesion

Rehearsal

Process stages

High-functioning groups

Intervention cues

Leadership skills

In some ways group counseling is not unlike individual sessions. In both settings, a systematic helping procedure is used to further the work of individual clients toward improving their personal functioning: identifying specific behaviors or issues that clients wish to change, understanding the underlying sources of problems, and designing strategies for making constructive changes. Although individual and group counseling modalities share similar theoretical heritages, basic strategies, and desired outcomes, some fundamental differences between them warrant closer inspection. There is no doubt that counseling in groups is more complex, requires more leader training, and has the potential to do more good or harm than similar helping efforts in individual counseling. It is for these reasons that students are given additional training in group modalities, as well as cautioned in their judicious use.

SURVEY OF GROUPS

We live in a world of groups: social groups, family groups, ethnic groups, athletic groups, fraternities and sororities, neighborhood groups, professional groups, religious groups. The only time we are ever really alone is in the car or the bathroom, and even then we are often invaded by intrusions. Most of us feel an ambivalence about the groups of our lives: On the one hand, we are resentful of the pressures we feel to conform to others' expectations; yet on the other hand, we appreciate all the support we receive being part of something bigger than ourselves.

One group member describes this all-too-familiar feeling:

> I really do appreciate all of you here in this group. When I'm with you I don't feel so alone. Even when I'm not with you, I carry a part of you inside me. I know that you care about me. I don't exactly like it when you confront me and make me look at ugly stuff, but without your efforts I would forever be stuck where I am.
>
> Sometimes, though, I feel so stifled by this group. There are things I want to say or do but, somehow, it feels like I would be letting some of you down. I get confused as to whose expectations I am really living up to—yours or mine. There have been many times when I've thought how free I would feel not to come here again.

The composition of any group, whether for social, business, or therapeutic purposes, involves a collection of persons gathered together for compatible goals. Although they may (and usually do) have personal motives and objectives that they wish to satisfy as a result of their participation, group members agree on a set of basic governing principles to guide their collective behavior. These norms and rules implicitly or explicitly specify leader actions as well as appropriate member behaviors.

Groups have many different labels that have been somewhat arbitrarily used, leaving the public as well as some professionals a bit confused. Some of the most common types are illustrated in Table 9.1.

Differences exist not only in the various modes of group work, but also in the myriad of leadership styles that can be applied, each with its own set of goals (see Table 9.2). Corey (2008) asks whether group leaders should best function as facilitators, teachers, therapists, catalysts, directors, or perhaps just as other more experienced members.

Whereas some approaches focus on the group goal of building greater trust, intimacy, and interpersonal openness, other approaches deemphasize group goals altogether, instead helping each individual member to commit to reaching personal objectives. Just like the varied approaches to individual counseling covered in previous chapters, many theories guide the behavior of group leaders. Some counselors lean toward more directive teaching models favored by cognitive/behavioral theories; others prefer experientially based groups that are patterned after Gestalt, existential, or person-centered philosophy. Recent innovations in social constructivist, feminist, and cultural-relational approaches to group work are also changing the professional landscape in such a way to be more sensitive to issues of power, language, social discourse, and a more humble way of listening to people.

At some later time, you may wish to consult sources (Corey, 2008; Day, 2007; Jacobs, Masson, & Harvill, 2009; Gladding, 2007) that introduce you to group

TABLE 9.1 | CONTINUUM OF GROUP WORK STYLES

Discussion Group	Group Guidance	Human Potential Group	Counseling Group	Group Therapy with Neurotics	Group Therapy with Psychotics
EDUCATIONAL MODEL					MEDICAL MODEL
Cognitively oriented					Affectively oriented
Task oriented					Process oriented
Short term					Long term
For normal functioning persons					For those with problems in reality testing
Identification of goals					Use of differential diagnosis
Focus on upgrading skills or knowledge					Focus on personality restructuring
Use of readings and homework as adjuncts					Use of medication and individual therapy as adjuncts

Source: Kotler, J. A., & Englar-Carlson, M. (2009). *Learning group leadership.* Thousand Oaks, CA: Sage.

TABLE 9.2 | COMPARATIVE OVERVIEW OF GROUP GOALS

Psychoanalytic	To provide a climate that helps clients reexperience early family relationships. To uncover buried feelings associated with past events that carry over into current behavior.
Adlerian	To create a therapeutic relationship that encourages clients to explore their basic life assumptions and to achieve a broader understanding of lifestyles.
Psychodrama	To facilitate release of pent-up feelings, to provide insight, and to help clients develop new and more effective behaviors.
Existential	To provide conditions that maximize self-awareness and reduce blocks to growth. To help clients discover and use freedom of choice and assume responsibility for their own choices.
Person-centered	To provide a safe climate wherein clients can explore the full range of their feelings. To develop openness, honesty, and spontaneity.
Gestalt	To enable clients to pay close attention to their moment-to-moment experiences so they can recognize and integrate disowned aspects of themselves.
Transactional	To assist clients in becoming free of scripts and games in their interactions. To challenge clients to reexamine early decisions and make new ones based on awareness.
Behavioral	To help clients eliminate maladaptive behaviors and learn new and more effective behavioral patterns.
Cognitive	To teach clients that they are responsible for their own emotional disturbances and to help them identify and abandon the ways they keep their disturbances alive.
Reality	To guide clients toward learning realistic and responsible behavior and developing a "success identity." To assist clients in evaluating their behavior and in deciding on a plan of action for change.

Source: Corey, G. (2008). *Theory and practice of group counseling* (7th ed.). Belmont, CA: Brooks/Cole.

counseling theories in greater depth. You may also wish to focus on a more integrative model (Donigian & Malnati, 2005; Johnson & Johnson, 2006; Kottler & Englar-Carlson, 2009; Yalom & Leszcz, 2005), as well as resources that provide ideas for practical group leadership (DeLucia-Waack, Bridbord, Kleiner, & Nitza, 2006; Keene & Erford, 2007).

In addition to the confusion surrounding the different styles of group leadership, each of the different kinds of groups has particular goals, structures, and compositions. Among these various formats, you may be expected to play a variety of consulting or leadership roles.

ENCOUNTER GROUPS

The most ambiguous category of groups includes names such as Human Relations Group, Human Potential Group, T-Group, Training Group, Encounter Group, and Growth Group. All of these groups developed from the early work of the National Training Laboratory (NTL), the Esalen Institute, and the writings of Carl Rogers

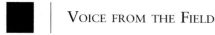

VOICE FROM THE FIELD

There are so many different roles you play when you're leading a group. Initially, you try to be a model for group members, demonstrating as many of the important skills and behaviors as you can. I'm usually the one who does most of the confronting in the beginning, until others catch on to how to do it without being insensitive or offensive. Then I switch to a more supportive role, cuing other members to do the work whenever I can. For example, if I'm feeling bored or irritated with what's going on, rather than being the one to say something I usually look around the group and find someone else who appears to be feeling what I am. Then I'll say to that person, "What's going on with you? You seem to be feeling a bit antsy right now."

I think in general the best way to lead a group is by playing a supportive role and getting the members to do most of the work. In this working stage, you just kind of act like a referee, making sure that people don't get hurt and that things keep moving along.

and Kurt Lewin. These groups were very popular in the 1960s and 1970s because of their emphasis on creating a learning community built on trust and honesty. They were extremely powerful in their impact on participants; the problem is that they often produced casualties as well as fans because of their uneven quality of leadership (Yalom & Leszcz, 2005).

Although today encounter groups have become virtually extinct , there are still a number of personal-growth types in existence, in some of which you may play a leadership role. They are designed for relatively normal persons and usually have a fairly loose structure. According to Rogers's (1970) original conception, the leader is viewed primarily as a facilitator/participant rather than as an expert.

A PERSONAL GROWTH GROUP IN ACTION

The silence has lasted four minutes by the clock, but it feels like an hour. Everyone looks to the leader, who merely smiles and waits. Finally, one woman screams out in exasperation, "I'm tired of this crap! When are we going to do something?"

"This is your group," the leader says softly, meeting her eyes. "What do you want to do?"

Another participant chimes in, then another, all voicing their frustration at the aimless direction in which they have been moving: "What are we supposed to be doing here?"

"I feel frustrated too," the leader answers, nodding his head. "But isn't this a bit like our lives? It's up to us to create structure."

The leader looks around the room and notices some puzzled faces; others are nodding thoughtfully. "Maybe a good place to start," he suggests, "would be for us to tell one another how we are feeling about being here right now. Who would like to start?"

PSYCHOEDUCATIONAL GROUPS

In contrast to the relatively unstructured format of many growth groups, psychoeducational groups usually have a definite agenda. Furthermore, they tend to

I gotta tell you: I do groups as much for me as my clients. There is nothing more exciting in my job, more stimulating, more unpredictable. I've been doing groups for a long time and they're always different, every one of them. You just never know what's gonna happen, even when you think you've seen it all before.

The energy in a group is simply amazing. There is so much to track, to watch, listen to, sense, feel. It's exhausting trying to follow it all. One person speaks and you try and give full attention but there's about a dozen other things going on at the same time, each one potentially meaningful. It's like a roller coaster—you just sort of hang on and enjoy the ride. Well, maybe that's not strictly true—as the leader, I'm supposed to be the one driving the thing, but the truth is that sometimes groups just seem to have a life of their own. That's not usually a problem if you've set things up right and created the right norms. But you've still got to pay very close attention so things don't get out of hand.

be didactic and instructional rather than experiential and focused on feelings. They often have planned, structured activities and fairly definite goals that are identified by the leader, who operates in an instructor/facilitator role. These are the sort of groups that used to be called "guidance" groups in the past in that they were designed in school settings to help students make career decisions.

Among those groups that are organized in school settings, some leaders have combined the features of growth groups described earlier with more structure in order to teach children adaptive skills (Clark, Severy, & Sawyer, 2004; Shechtman, 2006). Whether offered in schools or other settings, group leaders attempt to provide relevant information on careers, sex, parenting skills, job possibilities, colleges, and other topics that might be of interest. Generally, they focus on preventing problems in the future by encouraging developmental growth, aiding the decision-making process, teaching valuable life skills, and providing useful information. Psychoeducational groups are particularly well-suited for many structured interpretations that facilitate self-awareness and values clarification. School, rehabilitation, and substance abuse specialists, in particular, will be called on to lead these types of groups.

A PSYCHOEDUCATIONAL GROUP IN ACTION

"You have all had time to study various careers, visit job sites directly, and hear some interesting talks by representatives of various professions. Still, many of you are confused as to which direction to move in and are even more uncertain as to what you are uniquely suited to do. Although just beginning your lives, you already are aware of things you like and dislike as well as those things you can easily do or not do. Perhaps it might be helpful for you to get some honest feedback from your friends in this group who know you so well. Tina, you had mentioned earlier that you could never be in a medical profession because you can't stand sick people. Based on what the rest of you know about her, what careers do you think she'd be good at?"

COUNSELING GROUPS

See Companion DVD
Counseling Groups

Group counseling is the modality most similar in its goals to those of individual counseling. The techniques and strategies are all designed to help resolve interpersonal conflict, promote greater self-awareness and insight, and help individual members work to eliminate their self-defeating behaviors. Most often, the clientele have few manifestations of psychopathology; they simply wish to work on personal concerns in daily living. In addition, counseling groups are also designed to be rather brief treatments, often focusing on resolving specific problems within a time-limited format.

Group counseling is usually focused in the present rather than on the past. It is relatively short term, spanning a period of weeks or months, and stresses relationship support factors for resolving stated conflicts. For an example, an elementary school counselor might organize a counseling group for kids with learning disabilities who want to talk about their frustrations (Shechtman & Pastor, 2005), or a university counseling center might design a counseling group for students struggling with heavy drinking (Fromme & Corbin, 2004), or mental health counselors might organize groups for people trying to cope with the residual effects of childhood sexual abuse (Gerrity & Mathews, 2006).

In contrast to some growth and psychoeducational groups led by lay-people, and in contrast to self-help groups, counseling groups are always led by a trained expert who is prepared to protect the individual client's rights while stimulating constructive interpersonal action. Clients are usually helped to work toward individually designed goals, although there is a common interest in becoming more intimate, trusting, accepting, empathic, and interpersonally effective.

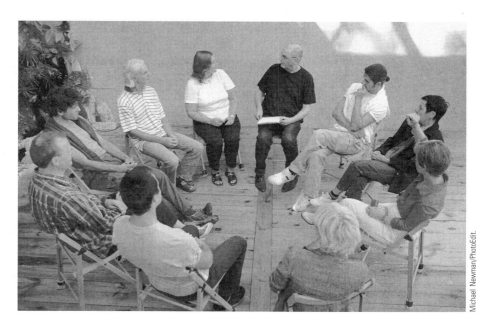

Groups provide support, resources, and opportunities to practice new skills that are not possible in individual counseling.

A Counseling Group in Action

COUNSELOR: Who wants to use group time today? We've cleared up some loose ends from last week and got progress reports on what has happened during the week, so let's move on.

KILE: Well, if nobody else wants—

SARAH: Damn it, Kile! You talk too much. Why don't you give someone else a chance?

KILE: But I was only—

COUNSELOR: Sarah, you seem unusually frisky today. I don't think you're as angry at Kile as at yourself for letting things slide so long. But there's plenty of time for both of you. And I remember that you, Paolo, had a concern you wanted to work on as well. Let's budget our time accordingly.

KILE: Sarah, I know you're not angry at me and I'm glad you finally want to work on something. I only need about 10 minutes anyway. A few weeks ago all of you helped me a lot, and things are much better with my girlfriend. The only thing is that I'm having second thoughts about getting married. I just wanted to get some feedback from the rest of you as to how you felt before you got married and how you feel across your situations now.

Therapy Groups

In practice, there is often very little difference between group counseling and group therapy, whereas in theory the goals and purposes are somewhat different. Psychotherapy in groups most often takes place in hospital, medical, or clinic settings with patients who are diagnosed as having some form of diagnosable mental disorder. These severe disorders require longer treatment, intensive analysis, and structural personality changes. In addition, therapy groups frequently have participants who act out in dramatic ways (Dublin & Ulman, 2005).

The content of most counseling programs does not adequately prepare students to deliver group psychotherapy services because of their emphasis on longer-term, more intensive treatment with more disturbed populations. However, often counseling practitioners may find themselves, by choice or circumstances, functioning as group therapists and so often seek to supplement their expertise with further training.

A Therapy Group in Action

The therapy group has been meeting weekly for two years. The support has been crucial for many of the participants, who include an alcoholic, a spouse abuser, a man with severe depressive episodes, a woman with an eating disorder who indulges in periodic binges, another woman fearful of crossing bridges, a man with chronic anxiety and insomnia, and a man who won't admit he has any problems, although his behavior is passive-aggressive. There are two leaders: a psychiatrist who monitors medication and a psychologist who works with them in testing. Both have a psychoanalytic perspective and have been working to help each patient minimize his or her symptoms, understand past actions, and function more normally in his or her world. The sessions are usually quite emotionally charged, requiring all the skills and training of the two leaders to reduce manipulation, resistance, and game playing and to

■ VOICE FROM THE FIELD

What you learn in school is just the beginning, just the barest basics. In a beginning group class, you learn about curative factors, stages in the process and all. You may even get the chance to be part of a group so you can really feel what it's all about. But like so many aspects of learning this job, once you get into the real world, you have to work like crazy to catch up to what more experienced folks are doing.

In school, I learned this one model for doing groups that probably works pretty well with relatively high-functioning counseling students. Then I get this job working with dual-diagnosed inpatients—that means they're not only pretty crazy but also drug addicted—and I've got to tell you, I had to start all over again. Just imagine trying to lead a group with people who are hallucinating.

avoid casualties. The group has acted as a buffer, a transitional step between the members' intensive individual therapy sessions and a gradual tapering off of treatment that will eventually lead to a monthly checkup and support system.

SELF-HELP AND SUPPORT GROUPS

The self-help movement has become a dynamic force for change over the past 30 years. Self-help books have become huge best-sellers, and self-help authors are commonly visible in the media. The self-help movement touches on a strong chord of independence within the North American character coupled with a desire to improve life conditions. Self-help groups have also proliferated widely and are an essential aspect of this self-help movement.

Self-help groups often do not have a professionally trained leader and, instead, use a more experienced member who has hopefully resolved the issues with which others are struggling. The purpose of self-help groups is to provide emotional and social support, to develop new ideas about coping with a common issue, and to provide constructive direction for members. The membership of self-help groups is open and fluctuates from meeting to meeting. Examples of self-help groups might include: Alcoholics Anonymous, an eating disorders group, a Heart-Smart group for individuals with cardiac problems, a group for people diagnosed with HIV, and many others on almost any conceivable topic or issue.

Support groups are closely related to self-help groups; in fact, the terms are sometimes used interchangeably. Support groups are often developed and sponsored by professional organizations or professional individuals, and they rely on the resources of the sponsoring organization/individual to a greater extent than self-help groups. Examples of support groups might include breast cancer survivors, Parents Anonymous, Parents of Children with Attention Deficit Disorders, and spouse loss/grief groups.

Historically, mental health professionals have had ambivalent or guarded reactions to self-help/support groups; however, these attitudes have become more positive recently. The change has to do with the positive personal experiences on the part of many professionals and the recognition that self-help/support groups will continue to play a crucial role in mental health services (Posthuma, 2001).

Self-help groups are not therapy or counseling groups; they differ in several important ways (Corey, 2008):

1. The goals of a self-help group focus on a single issue, whereas therapeutic groups focus on improving mental health and overall interpersonal functioning.
2. Self-help groups often have a political as well as individual focus. Therapeutic groups tend to deemphasize political and social issues and focus on individual change.
3. The leaders of self-help groups are not assigned and tend to emerge from the group. The leaders themselves are dealing with the focus issue. Leaders of therapeutic groups are designated and are generally not personally involved with the focus issue.
4. The problem focus of therapeutic groups tends to be broader and inclusive of more pervasive mental health issues, whereas the focus of self-help groups is less pathological and more targeted.

Self-help and support groups can be a viable resource for professional counselors and their clients. You'd be well advised to educate yourself with all the kinds of groups available in your community so that you can make appropriate referrals for your clients and work cooperatively with those who are attending such groups.

SOME CONSIDERATIONS IN THE USE OF GROUP MODALITIES

There has been considerable debate in the literature about whether group counseling is essentially safe and successful as a treatment modality or whether it produces too many casualties and is a waste of time. Historically, some critics believed that group therapies were faddish and possibly detrimental. Still other writers question whether group counseling is really any different from individual or family counseling because all the treatments make use of essentially the same therapeutic variables (Hill, 1990).

It may therefore be helpful to review some considerations in the use of groups so that you, as a student, may realistically assess the potential and dangers of this helping procedure. If you choose to work in groups—as a leader of a counseling group, as an administrator conducting meetings, as an instructor in the classroom, as a public figure in the media, or as a consultant in the field—study the contraindications of group methods carefully. This will allow you to prepare adequate safeguards, as well as deal with potential criticism. Similarly, you can capitalize on the therapeutic variables that operate in groups only if you are well aware of what can and cannot be effectively accomplished.

The history of group work is checkered with the contributions of many distinguished professionals, as well as with the practices of charlatans and witch doctors. Recall that, throughout human history, group hysteria has accounted for more havoc and death than all contagious diseases. After all, what is war but an organized form of group work, in which one team, led by leaders who are masters of group dynamics, attempts to obliterate the other team in the name of abstractions such as territorial boundaries? In recent history, we have witnessed the dramatic influencing capabilities of self-serving group leaders who could induce murder or suicide with their persuasive tongues and intricate knowledge of the power of group forces. Adolf Hitler and Saddam Hussein are but two of the more skilled group tacticians of the last century who could warp group dynamics to suit their own needs.

It is no wonder that counseling groups are often viewed with suspicion by the public and by some clinicians. It has only been in the last few decades that standards for acceptable practice have been developed and systematic training programs implemented (Association for Specialists in Group Work, 2007). For these reasons, new graduates sometimes experience frustration when trying to begin group work in their schools or agencies. They get opposition from their clients, who resent the pressure to participate in an uncomfortable setting and who thus resist the coercion. Further, clients are often more inhibited in groups, less willing to disclose because of fears—some of which are justified. How, after all, can confidentiality ever be enforced and guaranteed in a group? Who can promise never to let secrets slip out inadvertently or never to talk about private things outside the group? And who would believe such promises?

There are also complaints from parents and spouses: "What's this? I heard that you stuck my son in one of those touchy-feely groups. I'll not have a child of mine in one of your orgies!" Or, "I notice my wife is different since she's been hanging around with those dingbats in that group. How dare you people interfere in my life!"

Some senior colleagues in administration or counseling who never received much group training may resist implementing group strategies. Many counselor/therapist education programs added their first course in the techniques of group work only in recent years, and the lack of depth and intensity in group work training is a limitation of many counselor education programs. Students may have concerns about dual relationships since they may be expected to share intensely personal issues in classes where instructors are also evaluating them. Many of these issues can be addressed by providing students with informed consent, separating what goes on in class from products that are evaluated, and giving them the opportunity to go only as far as they feel comfortable.

It is very difficult to learn to be a group leader without logging considerable experience as a member. Moreover, it is somewhat hypocritical to expect clients to take risks and share personal concerns when the counselor has been unwilling to do so.

In group work, clients receive less time than they would in individual sessions and have less privacy. Groups require more sophisticated training on the part of leaders and are generally not suited for people who are easily intimidated or manipulative or who talk incessantly.

Why, then, would we ever choose to work in group settings? Why indeed?

COUNTERACTING POTENTIAL LIMITATIONS

Many of the disadvantages previously mentioned can be controlled, or at least minimized, through sufficient caution and training. Issues such as the suitability of certain personality types (passive-dependent, sociopathic), appropriateness of the group for individual problems, and level of psychological functioning (borderline personality, psychotic) can be handled through screening procedures that would permit participation only by those who are reasonably respectful of others' rights and who seem to be good candidates for groups (however that may be operationally defined).

Other issues may not be so readily dismissed. Confidentiality cannot be strictly guaranteed, and this presents a number of ethical and legal problems for the participants. One other reality is that clients receive less attention than in private counseling. With these limitations in mind, the leader must take extra care to ensure that time is spent equitably and that adequate safeguards are planned to prevent anticipated problems. Taking these conditions as givens, we can more realistically survey some of the powerful advantages implicit in counseling groups.

ADVANTAGES OF GROUP WORK

COST-EFFICIENCY

A counselor would need two full working days to see a dozen clients in individual sessions; the same number could meet in a single group session for two hours. The counselor is thereby able to reach more prospective clients in a considerably shorter period of time—and at significant savings to the institution and clientele. Most counselors and agencies are already so overburdened with work demands that group modalities allow for the most cost-efficient means to help the largest needy population.

SPECTATOR EFFECTS

While one person is receiving help in a therapeutic group—struggling, confronting, exploring, growing—a dozen other clients are carefully observing the process. They are internalizing the therapeutic messages, personalizing and adapting the content to their own lives. As one client complains about conflicts with a roommate, all others in the group (and those who are now reading these words) must ask themselves: How am I getting along with my spouse/friend/roommate? What things in this relationship am I willing to fight for, and which freedoms am I prepared to sacrifice? How much do I value my privacy? Do I want to live alone? How could we better settle our arguments?

Group work has the distinct advantage of permitting others to learn by observation. Clients are able to monitor the leader's behavior, imitating the actions that they admire: how to speak with confidence, how to create metaphoric language, how to take risks. The clients also scrutinize one another. When one member experiences success, the rest will live it vicariously. When a member is censured for monopolizing too much time, the others note the lesson as well.

The learning effects become contagious as an active participant is silently or not so silently cheered by the enthusiastic spectators. Each time a client opens up, takes a risk, or tries out a new behavior and doesn't die as a consequence, the other clients will feel more ready to test themselves.

STIMULATION VALUE

The atmosphere of a counseling group is a virtual utopia of emotional and cognitive stimulation, with its emphasis on freedom of expression, honest feedback, interchange of novel ideas, acceptance of individual differences, prizing of creativity and spontaneity, experimentation without fear of failure, and focus on risk taking, sharing, and giving. In such an environment it is impossible to be bored or to repeat an experience in exactly the same way.

Group sessions provide an exciting and fertile atmosphere for change because of the collective energy available. The whole is greater than the sum of its parts. Giggles quickly become contagious. As new ideas are passed around, they grow with each input, contribution, refinement. You can feel the hearts beating in a group. You can smell the sweat and sense the nervous shuffling. You can hear the pounding in your brain as it tries so hard to understand. And the sights are a visual Disneyland—nonverbal behavior to monitor, facial expressions, territorial imperatives, positioning and status hierarchies, insight in action, gestures of defiance, respect, or affection. A group is alive with ideas and emotion and change. It is stimulation itself. It is a dozen people struggling to understand themselves and one another.

Counseling groups not only prevent burnout in the counselor, who must constantly stay on top of things, but also energize the clients through lively interactions, spontaneous humor, and abundance of stimulation. Many practitioners with hectic schedules often deliberately plan group sessions to help both their clientele and themselves. The groups are often so professionally rewarding that the leader—although carefully monitoring his or her own behavior to avoid self-indulgence or the temptation to use the session to meet his or her own needs—nevertheless cannot help growing.

OPPORTUNITIES FOR FEEDBACK

Where can you go for truth? Ask your mother or your best friend for an opinion on your new shoes or what you should change about yourself. They will lie, or at least hedge, to water down an unpleasant truth. Where can you go to find out what people really think of you?

A counseling group provides the opportunity for participants to receive straightforward, honest, and constructive reactions to their behaviors, both attractive and unattractive. After role-playing or risk taking, a client gains feedback from astute observers that helps in making needed adjustments, identifies areas that could be upgraded, and provides reinforcement by acknowledging progress. When feedback is diplomatically confrontational, honest without being destructive, expressive but devoid of clichés, sensitive but not overly evasive, and concise in boiling down the essence of a person's behavior into a memorable image, it becomes one of the most powerful of therapeutic devices for promoting change.

In one introductory exercise used to open groups, for example, the leader encourages an exchange of first impressions among participants. Early in the therapeutic experience, the exercise helps them to give one another the gift of honest reactions. After members are instructed about the purposes of such an exercise—to encounter one another in a personal way, to collect information on possible areas of needed growth, to hear (perhaps for the first time) of the effect they have on others—they are then educated in the requirements of effective feedback. They are reminded to avoid stereotypes and clichés, to be brief rather than long-winded, and to be honest, helpful, and constructive by including both effective and

VOICE FROM THE FIELD

I tell kids in my groups to avoid giving "yearbook" feedback. You know, the kind where they write in your yearbook: "You're so sweet. Don't ever change." That feels good for about two minutes, but then what have you got? There's nothing there you can learn from. The best kind of feedback is far more direct and honest.

It might hurt for a little bit, but with a lot of support, it can change your whole life.

Just imagine being able to hear from others what they really think of you. Just think how amazing that would be to hear people tell the things they would usually never say out loud.

ineffective behaviors. To give the exercise structure and direction, which are often necessary in initial sessions until members learn rules and roles, the leader asks the members to write down the name of the animal that each person in the group brings to mind. Using their observations of each person's gestures and appearances, their own intuition, and any other data available—and trying to be creative in their thinking—clients send feedback to one another by disclosing the animals of which they are most reminded and the reasons why.

Angela, a shy, withdrawn girl, learns that some of the others see her as a turtle (because "she loves to swim beneath the surface where no one can see") or as a golden retriever ("because she appears loyal, affectionate, and maternal"). One group member even sees her as an Opaline Gourami (the speaker is a fish expert) "because she's cautious when people are around but prances when alone; she has a beautiful display of colors and grace, yet she hides behind the plants even if she sees a tasty morsel to eat; she prefers to wait for things to come to her." Other members learn from the feedback on first impressions that they resemble a Colorado River mule—because they are survivors, are self-sufficient, and have a flexible diet; or that they resemble a Hobbit—because of their playfulness, innocence, perceptiveness, and love of adventure; or that they seem like a queen bee—because they are good organizers but manipulative and overdemanding.

Any and all feedback in a group is aimed at providing experiences that are rarely available in the "outside world"—direct, honest, and sensitive statements describing exactly how one person feels and thinks about another.

SUPPORT

The tarpon, among the world's greatest sport fishes, will fight for hours longer against the hook and line when accompanied by others of its school than when alone. It is as if it couldn't give in with its peers watching, urging, goading it to fight a little longer. Humans also need to give and receive support in groups. Our ancestors huddled together in their caves for security and division of labor. In the evolutionary scheme of things, the PTA, fraternity, and neighborhood club have inherited many of the social and protective functions of the bonds we originally formed as hunter-gatherers. Groups supply the nurturing elements of intimacy and psychological bonding—the cohesion that results from close proximity over time. A therapeutic group can develop into a surrogate family, without the rigid, authoritarian hierarchies of some natural families. Such an experience can even be sampled within the relative artificiality of your classroom. Although the physical environment, seating arrangement, competition, professional authority, and threat of grading are something less than ideal circumstances for promoting a sense of true cohesion, nevertheless a feeling of belongingness often develops among classmates. Students can draw support from one another, pool their emotional and cognitive energies to get through the hard times, and savor the enlightening experiences.

Yalom and Leszcz (2005) identified the curative factors that are believed to be crucial to the healing and growth process of groups. Many of them have already been alluded to—such things as instilling hope, developing social skills, and facilitating the catharsis of emotion. Support is certainly at the top of the list, as is group cohesiveness (Marmarosh, Holtz, & Schottenbauer, 2005); however, Bemak and Epp (1996) more unabashedly claim that love should be considered the 12th agent of healing in groups. More than mere support in groups, they believe that a kind of "group love" operates in high-functioning groups in which members genuinely and authentically care for one another and that this deep regard is indeed a healing force beyond anything else that transpires.

STRUCTURED PRACTICE

Within a group, not only can we receive feedback, but we can also experience the support and encouragement necessary for practicing new behaviors. Often individuals undergo stress and frustration in their daily lives because they lack needed skills. Shyness prevents them from initiating new relationships, or frustration keeps them hostile and defensive, or low self-esteem triggers procrastination; each of these limitations can be viewed as a skill deficit, and the group becomes a place to develop and refine useful life skills. A man who is passive with his wife, for instance, can practice assertiveness skills. Group members provide feedback and help him to monitor the development of those skills. Laboratory experiences such as these help group members to put insights to use and to rehearse new behaviors in a nonthreatening setting.

The group, as a learning laboratory, can also be used for reality testing. Fears, anxieties, and inhibitions can be examined and explored, permitting the member to test out the validity of those feelings. Commonly a person will hold feelings in to avoid "hurting" someone else. This concern can be tested in the group by checking out others' reactions and by practicing giving both constructive and critical feedback to determine the recipient's reaction. Often the person will learn that being protective and withholding honesty are more hurtful than disclosing it, and he or she can then work toward a personal awareness of what *hurting* means.

BASIC ASSUMPTIONS ABOUT GROUPS

One human life is so complex in its origins, history, functioning, and consciousness as to defy the complete understanding of all the social and physical scientists in the universe. Yet when this solitary life is combined with a group of other lives, the network of ideas and interactions that could be generated is staggering. A single action by an individual group member—rearranging his position on the chair, for example—could signify restlessness, agitation, back pain, hemorrhoids, a desire for attention, postural difficulties, a need for increased blood flow, or an itch. If that same person were to communicate with another in the group, with his eyes or gestures, not to mention the possible variations of his voice, the effects would ripple like waves through the minds of all those present. Each person would seek a personal interpretation of the action and would respond to the stimulus both internally and externally. And it is the leader's task to sift through the confusing assortment of often conflicting stimuli, to attend to those that have relevance to the present situation and goals, to make sense of and give meaning to the behavior, to predict likely consequences, and, finally, to act therapeutically in the best interests of those who are present.

The group leader must not only have mastered basic counseling technology but must also understand dynamics and assumptions as they are applied to group behavior. Initially, each client comes to the group with different expectations, interests, and goals. The most basic assumption about groups, therefore, is that there are often discrepancies among the participants' hopes and expectations and even between those of the leaders and the members. Coalitions are formed on the basis of these common interests and backgrounds and often on the basis of perceived similarities in attitudes, abilities, or attractiveness. The leader may be viewed as the "outsider," as a function of his or her expert role, or possibly as the only "insider," because the counselor alone really knows what is going on during the beginning sessions.

Assuming a diversity of expectations helps the group leader to plan for and permit the realization of individual goals that are compatible with the flexible structure. Individual members are thus helped to clarify their reasons for attending the group and encouraged to set specific goals that may be realistically attained during the time allotted.

LEADER: Before I discuss some ideas regarding what options are available for you in this group and how we can spend our time, let's hear from some of you as to why you decided to come.

ELKA: I didn't decide to come. My parents threatened to ground me for the semester unless I agreed to try this a few times. They think I'm too young to get married; I don't.

NANDO: I heard that this was a good place to meet girls. I could always use a few new ladies in my life.

BETH: I've got some problems at work—I don't know what to do. I was hoping to get some advice.

FRED: Too much booze. Every day. I want to stop. Maybe y'all can help me.

Another assumption about counseling groups to which most (but not all) practitioners would subscribe is that the leader is not a participant of the group but a trained expert. Efforts are thus devoted to keeping the focus on the members, avoiding self-indulgent excesses, and generally staying in the role of paid professional who does not deliberately use group time for self-serving purposes.

CASSANDRA: Oh wise one, you always sit here so omnipotent like you know everything about anything. You are leading us, helping us. What are some of your problems? Why don't we help you?

LEADER: I do have lots of things I could work on in this group—my impatience, my overdriving ambition—and I know that you are all skilled enough to help me; but I don't feel comfortable using your time to work on my concerns. I'm being paid to help you. I can go to another group (and I do occasionally) where I get help. Thanks for your concern, Cassandra. But did I hear you resenting the control you feel I have? Is that something you would like to work on, since your lack of control has been an issue before?

For group work to be successful, or even to get off the ground, there must be an atmosphere of trust. Even more so than in individual sessions, the issue of confidentiality must be directly addressed so that it is clearly understood that all communication within the group is to be private and secure. Actually, there is no way confidentiality can ever be guaranteed or enforced in a group setting, for members are not legally bound to comply with any particular codes. Inadvertent breaches of trust can also occur, destroying the hard-won confidence. It is for these reasons that the leader openly, forcefully, and explicitly discusses the issue.

HECTOR: Why should I ever spill my guts here? I don't know you people. How can I believe anyone is trustworthy if I don't know them?

LEADER: Your point is a good one. There is a risk involved in being open, in this group or anywhere else. You should therefore pace yourself so that you disclose only what you feel ready to share. You will have to trust your own instincts on this. But remember, the degree to which you risk is related to how much you grow. Let's work on some situations that could test your confidential oath and discuss how they might be handled. What would you say, for instance, if your best friend asked what's going on in your group? What are you permitted to talk about outside the group? And what are some of your fears about what would occur if someone in here did tell others what you said?

In counseling groups, perhaps even more than in individual sessions, client discomfort is often associated with change. The very structure of a group environment, with its active audience, stimulates approval seeking, fear of failure, peer pressure, and other forces that do little to help the client feel at ease. This phenomenon isn't necessarily undesirable. A "healthy" amount of discomfort can motivate a person to get off dead center, to reduce dissonance, to make changes, and to restore equilibrium. As risk taking in a group accelerates, with members sharing their feelings, admitting inadequacies, and confronting themselves and one another, there are direct pressures from other members (which are usually held in check by the leader to protect individual rights) and subtle pressures from within to conform to the risky norm. Some begin to squirm as they watch others grow, because they feel left behind. The more they hang back and remain passive, the more dissatisfied they become with their present ineffective functioning. The only way to reduce their discomfort is to leave the group (which sometimes happens if the leader doesn't carefully monitor readiness levels of each participant) or to make needed changes in themselves.

MONICA: This is the eighth session and I know I haven't said much, but I'm just not all that good at talking in front of groups.

STEPHEN: As long as you believe that crap, you don't have to do anything else. Just sit there and watch us sweat. I'm tired of you getting a free ride.

LEADER: [Interrupting Monica before she can defend herself] Back off, Steve. Your point is well taken, even if you put it so harshly. Monica, before you answer him, what's going on inside your head?

MONICA: Just that maybe he's right. I wish I could get involved, but I'm too scared. And yet I hate coming here because I can't open up. I tried to stay home. But I can't do that either. Then I'd really feel like a chicken. I'm so confused; I just don't know what to do.

LEADER: How did you feel about what Steve said?

MONICA: I think he—

LEADER: [Points toward Steve] Talk to him.

MONICA: Ah, I don't know.... OK, Steve, I think you're a bastard and you tried to hurt me. You didn't have to be so cruel about it. I heard what you said, but I didn't like the way you said it.

LEADER: Now we're off and running.

Much of the growth in groups occurs through observation, identification, modeling, imitation, and other social-learning processes that are often not found in individual sessions. There are opportunities to watch the leader in action, who is presumably an expert in social-interactive skills, a model of the fully functioning person. The leader disperses wisdom or settles disputes with Solomon-like grace. The leader articulates metaphors and speeches worthy of a Shakespearean soliloquy. The leader orchestrates behavior, structures situations, organizes, takes charge. The leader radiates warmth and kindness and enthusiasm. And, all the while, the others watch carefully, nodding to themselves when they see something they like, consciously selecting behaviors for their own repertoire, captive to the power and force of the leader's personality.

A client also learns while watching peers struggle with their concerns. Every presented problem is internalized by the attentive audience, adapted to their particular lives. Clients learn from one another's successes and failures.

ORLANDO: Last week, Gianina, when you were talking about how bored you were being a housewife, I was at first bored listening to you. I mean, what could I get out of your situation? My problem is that I'm too busy. I have too much work to do. Then I realized that, although our styles are different, we are both hiding from the same thing.

GIANINA: I don't understand. Your life is far from boring. I stayed a housewife, until last week anyway, because I was afraid to venture out.

ORLANDO: Exactly. And I keep myself so occupied so I don't have to deal with myself and confront how boring I feel I really am.

LEADER: Who else identified with Gianina's concerns last week?

Groups provide many opportunities for realistic rehearsal of new behaviors. Much of what constitutes the permanent acquisition of new learning involves not only the observation of desired behaviors but also the opportunity to practice skills under supervision. Clients spend a good portion of their time applying what they have learned in the laboratory. They can experiment and refine interaction skills and social behaviors. They can take risks or confront others and, afterward, receive constructive feedback. Before they venture out into the world to wrestle with a problem, they can first use other group members to help rehearse their performance.

LEADER: OK, Jerry, who in the group most reminds you of your family members? Let's role-play the disaster you expect to occur when you get home tonight. Maybe we can even give you some ideas on how to handle it.

JERRY: Well, Brenda for sure reminds me of my mother. No, Brenda—I mean you both are so calm and relaxed.

LEADER: Don't apologize—just choose your characters.

VOICE FROM THE FIELD

It sometimes seems so magical to me the way a group transforms itself. You walk in the first day and everyone is so cautious and nervous. You wonder to yourself how you're ever going to get these people to trust one another. The whole task seems overwhelming.

I think to myself how many times I've been through this before. I've run hundreds of groups and I can't think of a single one—OK, maybe only one or two—in which something amazing didn't happen.

It starts out so awkwardly. Everyone is careful and polite, or in some cases, really insensitive. I'm the leader, the one supposed to be running the show, but I often feel like it's out of my hands, too. The group process itself, especially if it's structured right, seems to act with a life of its own to build the kind of safety that everyone needs in order to get some work done. I watch this with wonder. I try to make it happen—I even think I'm the one who is making it happen. But that is delusional. The group members make it happen, if I've set things up in a way that trust becomes possible.

JERRY: OK. I guess Joe would be good to play my Dad. But act real gruff. Grunt a lot and don't look at me when you talk. That's right. Also fidget more. Perfect. Patty, you can be my older sister. But you have to act confident but aloof. And, Louis, you're crazy enough to be my older brother. I guess that's it. Unless someone wants to be my dog.

LEADER: All right, now set the stage and program everyone the way they would normally act. Then you enter the scene and we'll see what happens. We will periodically stop the action, analyze what you did or didn't do, and give you some helpful suggestions. Perhaps we should even add a helper: Nancy will be your alter ego. Every time you are evasive or wishy-washy or back down, she will say aloud what you really want to say. Ready? Lights, camera, action!

The structure and ambience of therapeutic groups are well suited to working on interpersonal conflicts. The arrangement of chairs in a circle encourages direct communication among all as equals. If particular members make eye contact only with the leader while talking, that behavior is quickly extinguished. Constructive confrontations are stressed by encouraging the open and honest expression of feelings toward one another. Members are also helped to communicate and offer feedback sensitively and empathetically while they are taught to hear and interpret personal messages nondefensively.

GROUP PROCESS STAGES

Each group goes through four or five distinct process stages that require a specific focus and agenda beyond the individual goals of each member (Corey & Corey, 2006; Kottler & Englar-Carlson, 2009; Yalom & Leszcz, 2005). Even with minimal group training, you will find it instructive, if not amusing, to watch the underlying dynamics and stages of any group unfold, whether that takes place at a family dinner, party, committee meeting, or counseling group. It is important to keep in mind, however, that like in any developmental process, stages are often not linear and as predictable as we might hope. Under conditions of stress or transition, a group, like an individual, may regress or experience oscillations in patterns (Rubenfeld, 2001).

FORMING STAGE A group begins before its first session. Recruitment and screening take place in which members are often prepared for the group, informed of what to expect, and helped to get ready for the first meeting. Whether this orientation takes place during a pregroup meeting, individual consultations, or in an introductory letter, members still begin thinking and anticipating what to expect.

If a few group members know one another prior to the first meeting, then they are likely to have discussions sharing their perceptions and anticipatory feelings. The leader or leaders (when possible, coleading is certainly preferred), as well, spend considerable time talking about what they want to do, how they want to proceed, what problems they expect, and how they imagine various group members will get along.

The point to remember, whether in group work or in any form of counseling, is that the treatment actually begins long before clients walk in the door. For most people, the decision to join a group involves a long struggle before action is finally taken. Lots of internal dialogue probably takes place, as well as conversations with loved ones. By the time clients actually show up for the first group meeting, they have already been doing quite a bit of work, some of it constructive, some of it more anxiety provoking. Keep this in mind before you make assumptions about where people are before you have checked them out.

INITIAL STAGE The beginning stage is the time when introductions are made, the purpose is determined, ground rules are established, and trust issues are initially explored. The beginning stage can be as short as a few minutes—when the agenda is clear and trust is high—or as long as two or three sessions when more material regarding trust and comfort needs to be resolved.

The initial stage is about not only building trust but also establishing norms that are likely to be helpful throughout the tenure of the group. Participants have some ideas about what is expected, but many of these beliefs are misguided. They may engage in a lot of approval seeking and vie for attention. They may think that being a good group member means being "nice" all the time, but avoiding being honest or confrontational. At this stage it is important for group members to establish and enforce group norms that they believe are optimal for accomplishing desired goals. The leader must provide the right amount of structure at this stage so the group can accomplish process goals and move to the next stage.

TRANSITION STAGE There are a number of critical incidents and predictable problems that come up in most groups—mostly signs of resistance or confusion (Donigian & Malnati, 2005; Jacobs, Masson, & Harvill, 2009). Between the time when members are first getting to know one another and getting down to some serious work, there is a period of transition. You can recognize this stage by a number of signs: long silences, demands for leader structure, expressions of discomfort or anxiety, someone acting out as a distraction, prolonged conflict, or even attacks on the leader (Gladding, 2007).

If these critical incidents are processed in a constructive manner and members are helped to own, express, and deal with their fears, wonderful things often follow. The mood of the group changes from one in which people only pat one another on the back to one in which it is safer to disagree respectfully, confront constructively, and experiment with more freedom and flexibility—that is, all the behaviors needed for the real work to take place.

VOICE FROM THE FIELD

It was awesome what I learned about groups as part of my training. And I'm not talking about job-related stuff, although that was certainly important. I'm talking about the dynamics of groups—you know, the way people behave predictably in certain situations.

I used to hate going to family get-togethers. At best they were boring and at worst I'd go home with a stomachache from all the tension. Dysfunctional family and all that. Then when I learned about group behavior and process, I became a student of the way my family—and all groups for that matter—act. I'd watch people at staff meetings. I especially loved watching my classes. It was amazing to me that the same stages and dynamics I was reading about I could actually see unfolding before my various eyes. You know, you look around the room and you see the same group member roles that are talked about in the books—the monopolizer, the ass kisser, the one who is distracting and off-the-wall. It's all there if you just pay attention to what's going on.

WORKING STAGE In a healthy, high-functioning group it is safe to focus on deeper issues and to interact in new ways. During this stage, members work on specific issues, confront inconsistencies, explore issues, and share personal material. The leader must attend to the individual member on whom the group is focused as well as to the overall interaction patterns and attitudes within the group. This is a most challenging assignment and one that two leaders are often required to do best, especially when you are first learning to do group work (Hazler, Stanard, Conkey, & Granello, 1997; Kottler, 2001).

A number of signs and symptoms tell you that you are well into the working stage:

- When there is good movement from one member to another with almost everyone participating
- When there is less reliance on the leader(s) to direct and structure things
- When individuals are accomplishing their stated goals
- When cohesion, intimacy, and trust are operating at consistently high levels
- When game playing, conflicts, and acting-out behaviors are labeled, confronted, and worked through successfully
- When self-disclosure, constructive risk taking, and sharing are high
- When it appears as if people are making consistent progress in their sensitivity and responsiveness to one another

Of course, these particular behavioral signs are indicative not only of a group in the working stage but really of any group at any stage that is high functioning in terms of its process and productivity.

CLOSING STAGE The final stage allows the group members to assess what they have learned, discuss plans for change, and explore their feelings about the experience. In this stage, members attempt to resolve unfinished issues within the group, evaluate the performance of the group, and say good-bye and deal with ending issues. This stage generally takes anywhere from one to several sessions. Its primary purpose is to help members to keep their momentum going after the group ends.

Counselors should be familiar with the stages and group process issues so they can structure sessions to facilitate movement through each stage. Although group process is important, the group counselor should remember that the one primary purpose of the group is individual work and growth so as not to allow process variables to dominate group time. In many groups members have a good time, do lots of process work with one another, but don't necessarily change the target behaviors that landed them in treatment in the first place. The smooth movement through each stage will maximize individual opportunity for growth within the group.

HIGH-FUNCTIONING GROUPS

Successful groups are those that make their way through the various stages in such a way that their needs are met and distinct and consistent progress is made. Furthermore, it is important not only that the content objectives and desired goals are met but also that the process is relatively smooth and constructive. You have attended meetings in your life, or participated in certain groups, which may have been very efficient gatherings that quickly reached the declared goals. Yet you (and others) left the experience feeling badly about what happened. Perhaps people's rights were trampled, or individuals were not fully heard and respected, or the discussion felt unfinished.

On the other hand, you have attended groups in which the process was lovely. Everyone had a good time. Each person felt honored and understood. There was goodwill among all. The problem, however, was that very little work was completed and very few items on the agenda were worked through. In some cases, it may very well be the process that is far more important than the content or formal objectives. But in other situations, a balance must be reached between the two. High-functioning groups are often both process- and content-oriented. They can be efficient in meeting stated goals, and yet still attend to the participants' experience in such a way that interactions are satisfying and constructive.

Several other indications are important for evaluating whether a group experience is high functioning or not:

1. Do members feel safe? Are people supported? Has trust been established to the point where people are willing to take constructive risks?
2. To what extent are differences respected and honored? Each group will include a great variety of cultural, value, gender, political, and personal beliefs. Yet there is often pressure to conform to the majority. Are people's different worldviews respected?
3. Have constructive norms been established and clear boundaries enforced? Good groups need rules around appropriate behavior (coming late, missing sessions, interrupting, etc.). People have to know what is expected and they have to count on that the rules will be enforced consistently.
4. How is conflict acknowledged and worked through? High-functioning groups do not avoid conflict but seek to deal with the underlying issues. Such disagreements can be helpful if dealt with in therapeutic ways.
5. How are resources shared? Is there reasonable distribution of contributions or are sessions dominated by only a few members? The best groups are those in which everyone feels a part of what is going on.

6. How are distractions, digressions, and acting out handled? It is a certainty that some members will say and do things that may not fit with what is going on. Chaos will ensue if these behaviors are not redirected. Good leaders know how to redirect the focus in such a way that things remain on task—yet without humiliating the person(s) who need feedback.

7. Is there follow-up and follow-through? It is not nearly enough to have a high-functioning session unless it results in some sort of action. It is crucial to follow up on every participant to make sure they are doing what they say they will do, and what they need to do.

CUES FOR INTERVENTION

Although a group leader's behavior involves a degree of intuition, artistry, and feeling for the situation, there are some fairly specific instances in which therapeutic intervention is almost always necessary. In individual sessions the counselor relies heavily on "gut wisdom" but also knows that, when a client becomes self-deprecating or self-deceptive or drifts from reality, an intervention is called for. Group situations contain a virtual overload of stimuli to attend to. The most difficult task, therefore, is to describe not just how and when to intervene but with whom. A leader's behavior can be at best distracting or at worst destructive if ill timed or inappropriately directed. For these reasons, even the beginning student ought to become familiar with the minimally prescribed instances that signal therapeutic action.

ABUSIVE BEHAVIOR

Without exception or qualification, in the event that it can be determined that the physical safety or emotional welfare of any participant is in danger, the leader must intervene. Much of the research on casualties in group work supports the idea that the leader should take responsibility for protecting client safety (Jacobs, Masson, & Harvill, 2009; Yalom & Leszcz, 2005). This can be done only by carefully monitoring each member for cues of internal distress, as well as by keeping a close eye on group interactions to ensure that verbal abuse is minimized.

Usually, interactions that are hostile in their intent are quickly dissipated, or at least brought into the open to be dealt with in a relatively controlled manner. When a member is unaware of or insensitive to the negative effects generated by a comment or outburst, the leader also steps in to repair any damage. However, the vast majority of therapeutic efforts are directed toward heading off potential abuse before it occurs. With some experience, a leader can detect the signs of imminent explosive behavior and can therefore intervene before a fight or screaming match breaks out, in much the way that a skilled classroom teacher always knows when trouble is about to erupt.

RAMBLING AND DIGRESSIONS

For any number of reasons—to avoid meaningful dialogue, to resist treatment, to play games, or often simply because a client is verbally disorganized—the flow of conversation will stray from anything of therapeutic value. Perhaps someone will tell a long-winded story with no direct relevance. Or another might interrupt pro-ceedings to prove some obscure point. Or there is a client (as inevitably there has been in every group we have ever known) who is just scatterbrained. His or her in-terjections can be maddening, interrupting a meaningful silence, badgering the leader with questions intended to win approval, or breaking into every interaction with the preface, "That reminds me of the time…"

Whether the group member's ramblings are mildly inconvenient or downright pathological, the leader will usually establish some norm for appropriate input. Ini-tially, interventions are used subtly to play down digressive comments and reinforce those that are on target. Sometimes the interventions must be more direct. For Cindy, a client who is particularly prone to digressions, the leader may finally cue feedback to indicate when comments aren't appropriate: "Jacob, was it helpful to hear what Cindy just said when she interrupted you? Oh. It wasn't? You wished she would wait until you were through?" and then, "Cindy, what feedback did you just hear?"

Providing such focused input and reactions can be among the most powerful and useful things that can happen in a group. So often in our lives we do and say things that are off-putting to others, but we rarely hear about it in direct ways. We are left to guess how people respond to us rather than relying on honest data. Yet groups can be invaluable for providing honest feedback, especially to those who so desperately need it the most and don't even know it.

WITHDRAWAL AND PASSIVITY

Often the effects of verbal abuse, needless rambling, or other factors internal to the client will result in withdrawal in one or more members. This is a situation that is particularly difficult to deal with: The leader wants to safeguard the right to pri-vacy yet does not want clients to slip into complete passivity. Furthermore, with-drawal is not obvious; it is recognized only by an absence of behavior. The leader must identify individual patterns for each client in order to read signs of with-drawal in averting one's eyes, scooting back one's chair, answering in monosylla-bles, or acting in some other uncharacteristic manner. The counselor may decide to draw the person into the group directly ("You're not saying much today. What's going on inside your head?"), consult with the person after the group in a private conference, or even wait and let other members bring up the issue.

LETHARGY AND BOREDOM

One function of the group leader is to spice up the learning experience to maintain participants' interest. After only a few sessions, a routine sets in that can become predictable or boring. The leader uses humor, spontaneous actions, dramatic ges-tures, and a playful spirit to keep things stimulating. Whenever yawning becomes prevalent, or monotonous voices, or behavior in which clients appear only to be going through the motions (which happens frequently), the leader intervenes.

It is up to each one of you to accept responsibility for your own growth in this group. Usually when you are confronted with a repetitive episode or when you feel lazy, you are content to daydream or doodle, biding your time until the ordeal is over. However, when you feel your mind drifting away in here, as many of you were doing just now, you are cheating yourself of a potentially valuable experience. It is too easy to write off the times you aren't intensely involved in what is happening. You are in this group because you wish to learn to be more focused in the present, to enjoy each moment to its fullest. Why not begin now? Throughout the rest of this session, and those thereafter, when you catch yourself feeling restless or bored, force yourself to focus on what is going on. There is always so much to attend to, even if you find a particular discussion uninteresting. Watch the reactions of the others—how they are responding nonverbally to what they are hearing. Notice what I am doing or not doing and what my rationale might be. And closely scrutinize your own internal behavior. When you drift away, what are you hiding from? There is never a legitimate excuse for feeling bored in this group.

SEMANTIC ERRORS

Depending on theoretical preferences and linguistic sensitivity, every counselor has a list of favorite semantic errors to pounce on. Language is the principal evidence we have of a client's thought patterns; how a person speaks aloud and expresses ideas— the choice and arrangement of words—accurately indicate how that person thinks and feels about his or her situation. Group leaders will intervene when clients distort reality, exaggerate, or use illogical communications. A facilitator versed in the person-centered approach may correct participants by asking them to change "I think" to "I feel." Cognitive counselors would interrupt members when they express themselves with "I must" or "I should," asking them instead to substitute more accurate verbalizations such as "I may" or "I could." And a follower of narrative group work might ask clients to use the language of externalization ("The mistrust and suspicion has been sneaking up on our group when we aren't vigilant"). The leader of a group has the responsibility to understand, to relate, to facilitate, and to structure the interaction of the group members in a way that maximizes the therapeutic potential of the experience for all participants. This is a challenging and, at times, overwhelming task that demands the total energy and concentration of the group leader, who must be trained and skilled in individual and group-focused counseling skills.

SPECIALIZED SKILLS OF GROUP WORK

Working with groups requires the use of numerous techniques in addition to those used in individual counseling. Some practitioners are reluctant to lead counseling groups because of their anxiety over the responsibilities and techniques needed to function effectively. To some extent, inadequate preparation is the result of limited training in group leadership that has been rectified in recent years with the addition of one more group courses, including supervision of groups in internships.

Another area of difficulty has to do with the kinds of group leadership skills that must be mastered in order to work effectively in this setting. While many of these skills are similar to what you would do in individual sessions (reflective listening, confronting, interpreting, questioning, goal setting, giving feedback, and so on), other skills are somewhat unique to group practice. At the very least, generic therapeutic skills must be adapted considerably for group settings and the multiple participants involved. In fact, one of the interesting things that happens is that, over time, group members begin using the same skills as they interact with others both in session and in their lives.

An overview of some common group leadership skills may be summarized as follows:

Active listening. Just as you would in individual sessions, you must attend to verbal and nonverbal communications that arise in sessions and help other participants to do the same. This is what helps to build trust, facilitate deeper exploration, and encourage greater self-disclosure.

Paraphrasing. Again, not unlike what you would do with an individual client, you frequently let group members know that they have been heard and understood accurately. Whereas the previous skill focuses on affective dimensions, this skill attends to content of communication. If you are successful in modeling these behaviors, you will notice other group members begin to use them as well.

Summarizing. Periodically, throughout any session, you will want to help members to take stock of where they are. This also gives greater focus and direction to how things proceed.

Questioning. This involves drawing out additional material and data that is needed to understand a situation. Ideally, "open" questions are asked, or the kind that don't come across as interrogating. At times you will have to step in and stop members from using this skill too much as there may be an overreliance on probing too much.

Interpreting. This is where you offer alternative explanations for what might be going on. The intent is to expand group members' perceptions and understanding.

Confronting. This skill is especially important in groups but must be handled in different ways so that people do not feel humiliated or censured. The best sorts of confrontations are those that come from other members, rather than the leader, so this is another skill you want to teach to others. Basically, you are challenging people to look at themselves and at discrepancies in their behavior.

Supporting. This involves providing encouragement as it is needed. There are times when members begin struggling and may need help to work through the impasses. You want to communicate consistently in groups that the atmosphere is safe, that people will not be left to struggle on their own.

Facilitating. In order to promote open communication between members, it is your job to encourage people to talk to one another. One way you do this is by directing people to talk to one another instead of just to you.

Initiating. Groups need more structure and direction than individual sessions. You must intervene to increase or decrease the pace of what is going on, to introduce new directions, or to prevent a waste of time.

Setting goals. More so than in individual counseling, you must focus on helping each member work on personally declared goals. Otherwise, it is easy for people to get lost in the crowd.

Giving feedback. As with the other skills, it is preferable to get other members to do the work rather than you having to be the one to initiate things. This is where you help people to hear honest reactions to how they are perceived.

Suggesting. You may have situations when you will offer advice, information, or directions for new behavior. Be careful not to do this too much or members will follow your lead and start telling people what to do.

Protecting. Remember your job is to keep members safe from harm. This skill involves protecting people against attacks and against unnecessary risks.

Disclosing. In order to encourage group members to reveal personal material you may model this behavior. Be careful not to be excessive or self-indulgent, as this skill is often overused.

√*Linking.* This skill involves making connections between group members—building further cohesion and shared intimacy.

Blocking. You must intervene during times when someone is being hurtful, disrespectful, or inappropriate.

SPECIAL TRAINING

The skills just described are absolutely critical for helping groups proceed effectively and for dealing with critical incidents that will inevitably arise (Donigian & Malnati, 2005). This would include situations when members gang up to attack the leader, when there is mass denial or a mutual conspiracy among members to avoid real issues, when a member abruptly decides to leave the group, when a member withdraws, or when any of the other cues for intervention mentioned in the previous section occur. In addition, group leaders need a thorough understanding of individual counseling methods and theory, a solid grounding in group dynamics and behavior, and good planning, organizational, and conflict-resolution skills (Jacobs, 2006; Kline, 2003). Perhaps more than any other treatment approach, group leadership requires an extraordinarily high degree of intuition and creativity in order to go with the flow and respond quickly to the ever-changing circumstances (Forester-Miller & Gressard, 1997; Gladding, 2007; Kottler & Markos, 1997). This means adapting the concepts and skills you have already learned to fit the specialized needs of various client populations and group contexts (Capuzzi, Gross, & Staffer, 2009).

It is for all these reasons that you will receive specialized training in group leadership as part of your counselor education. Ideally, you will have the opportunity to study the various approaches to group dynamics and leadership, to experience a therapeutic group as a client in order to work on personal issues, and, finally, to receive supervised experience as a co-leader of a group. After you have completed this sequence of training, you will likely find group leadership among the most invigorating, powerful, and satisfying professional experiences possible—not only for your clients but for yourself as well.

SUMMARY

Counseling in groups represents a powerful and economical strategy for delivering counseling services in a variety of settings. Group work is especially effective because it more closely simulates social interactions and interpersonal communication patterns than does individual counseling. At the same time, group work is more demanding of the counselor, who has a much more complex task in both structuring the effective development of the group and accepting the responsibility for the growth of multiple clients. Specialized training and supervision are essential so that counselors can learn to use group-focused skills effectively and include group work as a part of their professional activities.

SELF-GUIDED EXPLORATIONS

1. Describe an experience you have had as a member of a group of some kind in which you felt some attachment (encounter group, study group, discussion group, counseling group, etc.). What factors are you aware of that operated in that group that made it especially helpful to you?

2. Think of a group in your life that you are currently part of. Describe the characteristic roles you play in this group (rescuer, placater, consensus seeker, rebel, leader, etc.).

3. Look at your behavior in one of your classes right now. How do you imagine that you are perceived by your peers and instructor? Ask two or three other students for honest feedback regarding your interpersonal style. Ask them specifically for one thing you do that they especially appreciate and one thing that pushes them away. Discuss your reactions to the feedback, including how it coincides with your self-perceptions.

4. What are the group dynamics, stages, and processes that you observe unfolding in this class?

5. Imagine that you are leading some type of counseling group. What are some aspects of that prospect that frighten you the most? What are some of your personal strengths that you hope to bring to the group experience?

FOR HOMEWORK

1. Make plans to join some type of growth group as a participant. If that's not feasible for you at this time, then arrange to observe a group in action. If you should have difficulty obtaining permission to view groups (observers *are* obtrusive), then find alternative opportunities to view group dynamics within human organizations, movies, television shows, families, or work settings. Pay particular attention to leadership style— what you notice works best and least. If possible, talk to the group leaders afterward to get their reactions and impressions of what took place. Write down what you learned from the experience.

2. View the following films that depict group counseling and identify the techniques used by the group leaders. What did you like about how the groups were led? What did you not like? (Hint: The first film is generally considered a caricature of group therapy; the second has been lauded as one of Hollywood's more accurate portrayals of an addiction group; the third is a documentary—the group scenes really did occur.)
One Flew Over the Cuckoo's Nest
28 Days
Some Kind of Monster

SUGGESTED READINGS

Berg, R. C., Landreth, G. J., & Fall, K. A. (2006). *Group counseling: Concepts and procedures* (4th ed.). New York: Routledge.

Corey, G. (2008). *Theory and practice of group counseling* (7th ed.). Belmont, CA: Brooks/Cole.

Corey, M. S., & Corey, G. (2006). *Groups: Process and practice* (7th ed.). Belmont, CA: Brooks/Cole.

Donigan, J., & DeLucia-Waack, J. L. (2004). *The practice of multicultural group work: Visions and perspectives from the field*. Belmont, CA: Brooks/Cole.

Donigan, J., & Malnati, R. (2005). *Systematic group therapy: A triadic model*. Belmont, CA: Wadsworth.

Jacobs, E. E., Masson, R. L., & Harvill, R. (2009). *Group counseling: Strategies and skills* (6th ed.). Pacific Grove, CA: Brooks/Cole.

Johnson, D. W., & Johnson, F. P. (2006). *Joining together: Group theory and group skills* (9th ed.). Boston: Allyn & Bacon.

Keene, M., & Erford, B. T. (2006). *Group activities: Fired up for performance*. Upper Saddle River, NJ: Prentice Hall.

Kline, W. B. (2003). *Interactive group counseling and therapy*. Upper Saddle River, NJ: Prentice Hall.

Kottler, J. A., & Englar-Carlson, M. (2009). *Learning group leadership*. Thousand Oaks, CA: Sage.

Shechtman, Z. (2006). *Group counseling and psychotherapy with children and adolescents: Theory, research, and practice*. Mahway, NJ: Lawrence Erlbaum Associates.

Trotzer, J. P. (2006). *The counselor and the group* (4th ed.). New York: Routledge.

Yalom, I., & Leszcz, M. (2005). *The theory and practice of group psychotherapy* (5th ed.). New York: Basic Books.

10 | Marital, Family, and Sex Counseling

KEY CONCEPTS

Family system

Circular causality

Differentiation of self

Joining

Structural approach

Strategic approach

Symmetrical relationship

Complementary relationship

Boundaries

Hierarchy of power

Structural map

Identified client

Symptoms as solutions

Symptoms as metaphors

Genogram

Reframing

Externalizing

Forcing the spontaneous

Pretending

The goal of neutrality

Three-point anger reduction statements

Acceptance models

Maintaining balance

Secrets policies

Sensate focus exercises

Imagine the following scenario: A school nurse refers a painfully thin 15-year-old girl to a counselor. As the girl tells her story, the counselor finds out that prior to her developing this eating disorder, her parents were fighting continually. Interestingly, when she stopped eating normally, the fighting also stopped as both parents joined together to help their daughter. Once in this crisis mode, the father began spending more time at home instead of the office and the mother demonstrated more overt signs of affection.

You are probably thinking as you read this that it seems rather obvious that the family situation has something to do with the girl's eating problem. Even with your beginning knowledge of counseling, it's clear that it would be useless to treat the girl without somehow addressing the underlying family issues. Here are some preliminary thoughts that may have occurred to you:

- The eating disorder serves a function. It has temporarily put a stop to the discord between the parents and earned the girl more attention.
- The eating disorder has given the girl power in the family, as she has changed the behaviors of her parents.
- As long as the parents' marriage is unstable, and the father is emotionally unavailable, the girl has no motivation to solve her problem.
- In order to help the girl, the counselor will have to work with the parents on their issues as well.

Fortunately, in the 1970s, a small group of practitioners began to develop theories and treatment plans based on the notion that an individual's problems often reflected family dysfunctions; the only meaningful way to help clients was to include the family in the treatment process. Concepts like *homeostasis* emerged—the idea that families experience strong pressures to maintain their typical pattern of functioning, no matter how dysfunctional they are. Another key term was the *identified patient*, a client like the girl with the eating disorder who took on the role of expressing psychological symptoms that actually reflected distress of the entire family. Indeed, the very term *dysfunctional family* was developed by this new school of family system thinkers; the term has become such a part of our everyday language that we forget that it didn't exist until the latter years of the 20th century.

If there was a singular critical idea that emerged from family counseling theory, it was this: The behavior of one individual inevitably affects the actions of every member of a family; likewise, the behavior of other family members inevitably affects the actions of one individual. Simply put, *all* behaviors are interrelated. This is a revolutionary concept, because the implication is that there is no psychologically "sick" person in a family and no one person to blame for family problems.

It is the family itself that requires help, often in the form of realigning power imbalances, changing dynamics, and reforming new alliances and structures.

Once family dynamics and processes were understood, family counseling theorists next turned their attention to developing effective treatments. For instance, in the case of the girl with the eating disorder, while she might be treated with individual counseling to help her self-esteem and explore underlying issues, couples counseling for the parents might also be recommended to help them resolve their own interpersonal conflicts. In addition, family counseling might be recommended for the whole group to help them readjust the balance of power and facilitate interfamily communication.

What was once an obscure specialty for radical family theorists and practitioners has become mainstream counseling for practitioners of all disciplines who seek to initiate changes through the involvement of those persons who wield a significant influence in the client's life. The American Association for Marital and Family Therapy (AAMFT) and the International Association of Marriage and Family Counselors (IAMFC) have become established, highly respected organizations, promoting research on family counseling, hosting conferences, contributing specialized training, credentialing graduate programs, and developing ethical codes for family practitioners. Family systems thinking has so permeated our field that it is expected that any counselor who works in schools or community agencies has a working knowledge of family systems thinking and can conceptualize individual problems from a family perspective.

FAMILY VERSUS INDIVIDUAL COUNSELING

Family counseling bears some similarity to group counseling in that the systemic dynamics are as important as individual behavior. The field, however, has carved out a unique niche in its theory, research, practice, and distinct way of approaching a helping relationship (see Table 10.1). When compared to individual counseling, family work is different in a number of significant ways (Nichols & Schwartz, 2007):

1. Family practitioners view problems as located not within the individual but within the larger context of interactions between people.
2. Clinicians must generally be more active, directive, and controlling than they would be in individual sessions.
3. Rarely can the counselor afford the luxury of operating from one theoretical approach. Family practitioners tend to be very pragmatic and flexible.
4. Focus is directed toward organizational structures and natural developmental processes that are part of all family systems. This includes attention to family rules, norms, and coalitions.
5. A model of circular rather than linear causality is favored. This means that when determining the causes of events or behaviors, it is important to look at the bigger picture of how each person's actions become causes and effects of everyone else's behavior.
6. Developmental models are employed that describe the family life cycle, including predictable and natural transitions, crises, and conflicts.

| TABLE 10.1 | DIFFERENCES BETWEEN INDIVIDUAL AND FAMILY COUNSELING |

Individual Counseling	Family Counseling
Asks "why" questions	Asks "what" questions
Linear cause-effect	Reciprocal causality
Subject-object dualism	Holistic
Either/or dichotomies	Dialectical
Value-free science	Subjective
Deterministic	Freedom of choice
Historical focus	Present-oriented
Individualistic	Relational
Reductionistic	Contextual
Absolutistic	Relativistic

Source: Becvar, D. S., & Becvar, R. J. (2008). *Family therapy: A systemic integration* (7th ed.). Boston: Allyn & Bacon.

7. Rather than a single notion of "family" structure, counselors recognize that multiple versions are common, depending on the dominant culture. More often than not, any clients will be members of a nontraditional structure: a blended family of stepparents and children, a single-parent household, a dual-career family, a cohabiting heterosexual or homosexual couple.

What should be clear is that family counseling involves additional training and specialization. Many of the skills and theories that you learned previously about doing individual counseling also fit when doing family counseling, just as they do with all group work. You would probably not be surprised to learn, for example, that all the disagreements among counselors about the best way to do counseling in general also apply to family specialists as well. Nevertheless, in spite of the disagreements about whether to do insight- or action-oriented family work, whether to stay in the present or the past, whether to focus on feelings, thoughts, or behavior, whether to concentrate on the presenting symptoms or underlying issues, and whether to work with one or two members or the whole extended family, there is some consensus about the needed knowledge and skills to master.

Almost all family practitioners would agree, for example, that in order to attain a degree of competence in this type of work you must have specialized training in family systems dynamics, family theories, family interventions, couples counseling, sex counseling, and professional/ethical issues unique to this practice. Given the popularity of this modality, it is likely you will have at least one and probably more courses dedicated to family counseling practice. You will also wish to supplement this basic education with additional training and supervision, because family counseling has all the challenges of individual and group counseling—*plus* you have the added burden of dealing with the fact that everyone is related to one another; each case, therefore, comes with a history of interactions you have not been privy

Voice from the Field

One idea I've used over and over is the notion of developmental struggles; that every family, no matter how healthy, still will face certain challenges. When I see a couple, for instance, and they are agonizing because their adolescent is acting out, it is just so useful to explain how, developmentally, this is perfectly normal. I have favorite stories I tell about how important it is for adolescents to rebel. That's how they become individuals with their own values. They need to create disturbances in order to separate. At least that's true in white, middle-class homes. I know with other cultures, it's often a different story altogether.

to. As if this doesn't seem daunting enough, consider that one or more family members are often working actively to sabotage any of your therapeutic efforts. It is for this reason you need a solid grounding in family theory, research, and practice.

FAMILY COUNSELING THEORIES

Like everything else in this field, there is a tremendous diversity in the ways in which family counselors operate. Similarly to the approaches we explored in the chapters on counseling theory, various counseling systems can be organized according to their basic perspectives (Gehart & Tuttle, 2003; Goldenberg & Goldenberg, 2008; Nichols & Schwartz, 2007). Thus, some approaches examine underlying family structures or patterns of communication, while others focus more on dysfunctional thinking or behavior, and still others concentrate on the individual issues with which family members struggle.

As you would expect, some family counselors (Nathan Ackerman, James Framo, David Scharff) employ a psychoanalytic model. They deal with unresolved conflicts of the past, looking especially at family-of-origin issues. Also expected are some approaches (Virginia Satir, Carl Whitaker) that are humanistic in their orientation. They remain in the present as much as possible and examine issues of freedom and choices. Likewise, cognitive approaches to family counseling (Robert Liberman, Richard Stuart) emphasize the same kinds of maladaptive behaviors that are present in individual counseling.

In addition to these familiar models that have been adapted to family settings, several unique theories were designed only for family work. Family systems theory (Murray Bowen) introduced the concepts of differentiation of self from the family. Structural family theory (Salvador Minuchin) looks at the ways that families become enmeshed and disengaged. Strategic approaches (Jay Haley, Cloe Madanes) look at alignments of power and communication in families. Milan theory (Mara Selvini-Palazzoli, Luigi Boscolo) introduced the paradoxes and games that families get caught in. Narrative approaches (Michael White, David Epston) look at the ways that family stories determine perceived reality. Solution-focused counseling (Steve de Shazer, Insoo Berg, Michele Weiner-Davis) focuses on locating a family's preexisting repertoire of solutions to their presenting problem. Finally, as you would expect, integrative models (Richard Schwartz, William Pinsoff) combine features of several other theories into a more encompassing framework.

VOICE FROM THE FIELD

Family counseling makes sense to me—I even call myself, "a family counselor" to colleagues and clients. In lots of ways, there are some very powerful things you can do with everyone together. But on the other hand, I've had some bad experiences too.

I remember one time I got the whole family in my office—the kids, the parents, even one of the grandparents—and it was total chaos. One kid was drawing on the wall. Another was punching her brother, who kept crying the whole time. The parents were screaming at one another. And grandma, she was gettin' in the act too. I just sat there with my mouth open, not knowing what to do.

Finally, I was able to regain some control but not for long. I resolved, then and there, that if I was going to do this sort of work again, I was going to have to exert a lot more control on the proceedings. Now, whenever possible, I like to work with a co-therapist. Sometimes, though, that just isn't feasible and you've got to do it all yourself.

The intent here is not to overwhelm you with a bunch of new names and concepts. At this point, we wouldn't worry too much about remembering anything other than the realization that family counseling is a very complicated field with a lot of interesting ideas that are helpful in unraveling the interactions that occur among people living together. As with each of the chapters in this book, which are intended to merely introduce you to the basic concepts, there will be plenty of time in later courses to master this material.

After studying the various family theories, you will be struck not only by how different they all seem, but also by the fact that they share some universal features. For beginners to the field in particular, it is useful at this point to understand that most family counselors agree on several areas:

1. Most family counselors rely on the same set of skills, such as "joining the family" or building rapport, assessing power hierarchies within the family system, restructuring coalitions among family members, reframing problems to make them more solvable, and engaging all members in resolving their difficulties.

2. All family counselors think in terms of social systems. Rather than viewing problems in terms of simple cause-effect relationships—that Mother causes Child to act out—they are seen in terms of circular causality: Chain reactions influence each family member, who in turn influences everyone else. For example, a mother becomes impatient because her daughter is slow getting dressed in the morning, making everyone late for work. The child feels pressured and resists the mother's efforts to control her. The father feels jealous because his wife is devoting so much attention to their child while ignoring him. He sabotages his wife's efforts to motivate the child. The mother feels angry at her husband for siding against her, withdrawing further. The child becomes even more obstinate, with more pressure applied by the increasingly exasperated mother. So who is causing the problem?

3. Family counselors, by and large, are more flexible, more active, and more structuring than practitioners of other treatment modalities. Because sessions can become so emotionally charged, things can rapidly get out of hand if the counselor allows family members to become abusive, violent, or out of

VOICE FROM THE FIELD

I can't tell you how many times a child is sent to my office for disturbing the classroom, and as soon as I can make it safe for the kid to open up, I hear such sad stories of what the child's home life is like. It's not that I don't feel for the parents, also—usually, they're overwhelmed with problems of their own, truly frustrated by their difficult child, and trying the best they can. Their child is acting out the parents' conflicts, but the only way they know how to control their child's behavior problems is by punishment—which just makes matters worse. The child's bad behaviors increase, making the parents even more frustrated—etc., etc., etc.

If I can only get the parents to come in for some family work—even just a few meetings will be helpful—I know I can make a big difference. The trick is convincing a mother or father that the child's behavior is related to their own issues. Some get it right away, but some want to blame everything on their child. When that happens, I have to shift my focus from a family approach to an individual strategy, helping the child express her anger and frustrations to me, instead of disrupting the classroom. But it's like bailing out a boat with a big leak. No matter what I do, that child is going home every day to the same set of problems.

control. In addition, family practitioners focus more on the present than on the past, tend to be more didactic in their style, and are concerned primarily with patterns of communication.

Despite their similarities, each approach has distinctive features that permit the counselor to switch from one to the other according to the requirements of the situation. It is often desirable to begin structurally in order to diagnose, analyze, and test boundaries and rules, because this approach is more direct and comprehensible. The counselor can move to strategic intervention once he or she encounters resistance, defensiveness, or confusion. Then it may be effective to revert back to structural theory to pull together any loose ends. In this methodology, therefore, it is possible to think structurally and work strategically. By thinking structurally, the counselor is aware of various predictable patterns and styles that will commonly arise.

Of course, as with any form of counseling, whether in group, individual, or family contexts, success is often related to the quality of the alliance that has been developed with the participants. What has been emphasized previously applies equally well to family counseling: Any interventions and structural realignments take place only after a solid bond has been established where there is a sufficient degree of safety and trust.

POWER IN RELATIONSHIPS

Relationships among family members can be *symmetrical* or *complementary*. The former, according to Haley (1976), has much competition, whereas the latter emphasizes reciprocal exchange as people maneuver for position and power. Minuchin (1974) introduces the notion of *boundaries* to describe how the various coalitions in family relationships tend to intersect. Sometimes, for example, the boundaries between parents and children are clearly defined and at other times an alignment may develop between mother and son, with a disengaged boundary between them and the father. Matters become considerably more complicated as the counselor joins the family system, creates different boundaries by manipulating the various coalitions, and finally restructures the system so that more constructive lines of affiliation develop.

Power within the family must also be carefully understood and balanced. Each family has a regimented hierarchy, within which each person has a specified amount of control and responsibility. Counseling often takes the form of reestablishing a single hierarchical organization in which the boundaries are more clearly delineated so that the parents are in charge and the children have less power.

The locus of power in a family can be deceptive, seemingly centered in the member who is most overtly dominating when in fact it may be the more quiet member whose withdrawal behaviors control the balance. Family counselor Terry Real demonstrated a case in which a verbally abuse wife would ceaselessly nag her husband about his failure to complete family chores (Stossel, 2004). The husband's pattern was to feebly say, "Yes, honey," to her demands, but never follow through. The children's self-esteem was adversely affected by the mother's tirades, and her behavior was apparently the source of the family's dysfunction. Yet, as Real pointed out, the recalcitrant husband held the cards in this system by encouraging his wife to nag him, turning her into the villain in the family. When directed by Real to either take care of his chores, or honestly say, "I can't do it now" to the wife, she became less frustrated, her nagging stopped, and the children collectively expressed a sigh of relief that the tension they suffered daily was dissipating.

Family counselors tend to see psychological symptoms like depression, anxiety, and eating disorders in terms of the roles they play within a family's power

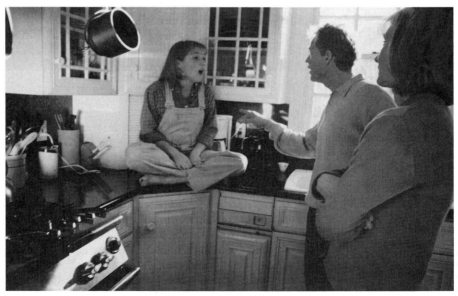

Counselors must help families to defuse their conflicts and build on their resources to develop more constructive communication patterns.

dynamics. For example, Madanes (1983) records the case of a depressed man whose symptoms were treated by resolving the hierarchical incongruity in his marriage. The husband had previously been dominant in the relationship, but as the wife developed outside interests and a career as a therapist, his own life and business began to fail. The husband's depression became a source of power in the marriage because the wife, as a professional helper, could do nothing to bring relief. The counselor's interventions focused on restoring a more balanced power hierarchy by reorganizing the way the couple dealt with each other. No longer useful as a form of one-upmanship, the depression vanished.

Balance of power between spouses can be viewed as a metaphor for other communications in the marriage. Consider a case in which the husband has all the power—in career, in decision making, in finances. The wife develops symptoms of depression. Husband tries to help but fails repeatedly. Husband becomes restricted in his own life by catering to wife. Wife indirectly controls husband and situation is reciprocal: Husband tells wife what to do about her life, then complains because she doesn't comply. Wife complains that husband is insensitive and can't or won't solve the problem. Both use power and helplessness, metaphors for submissiveness and rebellion.

Figure 10.1 describes another example of the power struggles within a family. The counselor initially plots the family organization, then identifies the problems of each member, and finally develops a series of interventions.

A child will often develop problems as a way to protect the parents from having to face their own difficulties. For example, the son in the family described here began to act out and became a common focus for the parents. In responding to the child's misbehavior, the parents were allowed to ignore their problem interaction pattern and the child felt powerful because he was keeping the family together. Although this intervention by the child kept the parents "together" in their interaction, it resulted in a serious family breakdown. As a counselor, you will often see families like this who present a "problem" child and view themselves as concerned parents who have no problems of their own. Counselors in a variety of settings observe this phenomenon, and it accounts for why even school counselors are now attempting more and more family counseling interventions (Davis & Lambie, 2005; Ho, 2001; Nelson, 2006; Vanderbleek, 2004).

SYMPTOMS AS SOLUTIONS

Family systems analysis provides a larger context within which to view the problems of the identified client. Rather than approaching treatment with the usual intention of promoting individual insight and then helping the client to make specific changes, the family counselor often looks at the behavior of the disruptive family member as helpful or constructive in some regard. The disruptive behavior continues because it is unconsciously supported and maintained by others within the family system.

Haley (1980) suggests that counselors, particularly when working with severely disturbed adolescents, view the child's disruptive behavior as stabilizing the family structure (such as in the case that began this chapter). The child's behavior protects the parents from each other, forcing them to find solace in sharing their frustrations

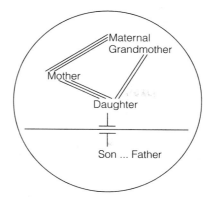

FAMILY STRUCTURE

Mother is overinvolved with grandmother and daughter.

Grandmother and daughter have a friendly alliance.

Father and son have a weak and peripheral affiliation.

Father and mother are minimally involved.

Father and son are both isolated from power in family.

Daughter and son are actively engaged in conflict.

The complete circle, above, represents a closed boundary separating family from influences of outside world.

FAMILY SYMPTOMOLOGY

Son is the identified client, who brought the family to counseling because of fighting at school and home.

Father is passive, withdrawn, uncommunicative, and depressed.

Mother is domineering, controlling, manipulative, and anxious.

Father and *mother* have marital problems; only son's acting out keeps them together.

Grandmother is lonely, isolated, and dependent on mother.

Daughter spends more time with *mother* and *grandmother* than with age mates; provokes her brother.

INITIAL THERAPEUTIC INTERVENTIONS

1. Solicit cooperation of mother, who is in control.
2. Build relationships with other family members and help them to tell their stories—and hear one another.
3. Rearrange coalitions with mother and father together against distracting influences of children and grandmother.
4. Invite father to take more power and control.
5. Strengthen bonds between mother and son, father and daughter, to equalize involvement.
6. Help grandmother to expand her social world. Help son to stop rescuing parents.
7. Open boundary isolating family from outside world.

FIGURE 10.1 | STRUCTURAL MAP OF FAMILY ORGANIZATION

over the inability to control the unruly behavior. All family members, therefore, must be seen together to clarify the power and hierarchy structures. The family counselor's role is to help the parents regain control over themselves and the adolescent.

Haley finds it helpful when working with disruptive children to assume the following: (1) The client's symptoms are serving a protective function; (2) the client has the capacity to assume responsibility for disruptive behavior (and is not a victim of external forces); (3) the power hierarchy of the family is confused, with the "little" people controlling the "bigger" people; (4) the real problem is the family communication pattern, not the young person; and (5) once power is restored to the parents and the child is no longer permitted self-indulgence and failure—once the confusions, inconsistencies, and conflicts in family communications are cleared up—then the child can act more normally and responsibly without destabilizing the other family members.

When the child's destructive acting-out behavior is diagnosed as the solution to another, more important problem within the family, then interventions can be directed toward helping the parents to resolve their conflicts. Once the child's "help" is no longer needed, the child can then revert to more appropriate behavior to deal with his or her own internal conflicts.

This particular conception of symptoms as solutions certainly doesn't apply to all situations. In fact, those applying a more constructionist approach would try not to make very many assumptions about families and their problems until the families' narratives are shared and understood. Some family therapies are more culturally and gender-sensitive in their approach, looking at issues of power, sexual politics, and collaboration in very different ways (Brown, 2004; Lyness, 2006; Robb, 2006).

INTERPRETING SYMPTOMS AS METAPHORS

Most communication has messages on two levels: *digital* and *analogical*. One part of communication is literal and content oriented, whereas another, deeper communication expresses messages of a more subtle kind. For example, when a woman says to her spouse at the dinner table, "You eat so fast I don't know how you can even taste or enjoy your food," she is, in fact, making a literal comment about her husband's table manners. But in addition to this digital statement, she may also be communicating metaphorically about another aspect of their relationship that is rushed without enjoyment: their sex life.

Now, the counselor has the choice of interpreting the disguised meaning of the communication or responding on a similar symbolic level. Haley (1973), in writing about Milton Erickson's preferred strategy, relates that "whatever the patient says in metaphoric form, Erickson responds in kind. By parables, by interpersonal action, and by directives, he works within the metaphor to bring about change. He seems to feel that the depth and swiftness of that change can be prevented if the person suffers a translation of the communication" (p. 28). The couple in this example may be requested to go out and have a slow, drawn-out, leisurely meal. This message and its subsequent action permit the partners to practice their foreplay in an indirect, minimally threatening situation.

| VOICE FROM THE FIELD

Training in family therapy really changes you on many levels. Sure it's cool to learn all the techniques you can use with clients. But far more than that, it sensitizes you to look more closely at all your relationships, especially with those you live with. When you're first learning how to do a genogram [a diagram of family relationships], you do one of your own family, and this is absolutely mind-blowing. The same is true when you learn to read family dynamics: You apply it all to your own family. At least I do.

At first it's scary. I mean all this dysfunctional stuff has always been going on that I've been oblivious to. Then after a while, this greater sensitivity helped me to be more understanding. The worst part, though, is that I can no longer get away with the games I used to play with my own parents since now I catch myself. It's just no fun any more.

Because people communicate on these different levels, the family counselor must learn to recognize the ways in which children and adults express different issues through their behavior. Presenting complaints or identified symptoms are thus often interpreted as something quite different from their surface messages. This theoretical construct is common to many individual therapeutic approaches, such as psychoanalytic and Gestalt counseling. The main difference may be that the strategic family counselor is less interested in explaining or interpreting the metaphor and instead prefers to operate on the same level as the family members.

DIAGNOSTIC QUESTIONS

One other unique contribution of the family systems perspective is the way it has encouraged practitioners to think diagnostically about client behavior. The narrative approach to counseling presented in Chapter 5, the solution-focused approach introduced in Chapter 6, and the systemic approach to diagnosis mentioned in Chapter 8 are all examples of different ways of asking questions. In some cases, the goal is to find out information not only about the symptomatic client's experience but also about how everyone in the family is affected and, in turn, affects the problem in their interactions. In other instances, especially in a narrative approach, the very act of asking questions is designed to promote changes in the ways that clients view their predicaments.

Operating strategically, the family counselor would be interested in sorting out the confusing connections among symptoms, metaphors, power hierarchies, and other relevant variables by asking some specific questions:

- What is the problem?
- When does the problem occur?
- Where does the problem occur?
- Where are various family members when the problem occurs?
- What is each member of the family doing when the problem occurs?
- What are the effects on each family member?
- What are the benefits to the client?
- Who in the family has had a similar problem?
- Where is the power (money, decisions, time)?
- Who is being protected?

The *genogram* is another useful tool for gathering information about family relationships and structures. It consists of a comprehensive map of all the members of a family over several generations, including their coalitions, conflicts, and connections. It thus provides a blueprint for the counselor in understanding the cross-generational themes that repeat themselves over time, as well as the current interpersonal conflicts that are evident in the structural map (Figure 10.1) presented earlier.

For example, using symbols standardized by McGoldrick and Gerson (1985) in their book on family assessment, Erlanger (1990) plotted a four-generation genogram of Lucy, a 75-year-old client (see Figure 10.2). A review of this chart reveals several issues that Lucy may wish to explore: her father's suicide, her son's alcoholism, her relationships with her aging husband and mother. All of this is clear before any efforts are made to include existing conflicts among family members.

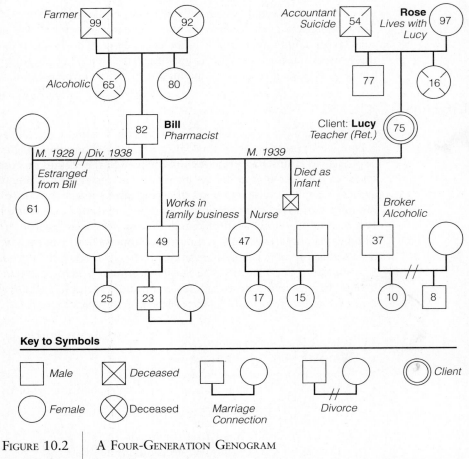

FIGURE 10.2 | A FOUR-GENERATION GENOGRAM

Source: Erlanger, M. A. (1990). Using the genogram with the older client. *Journal of Mental Health Counseling,* *12*(3), 321–331.

During the process of constructing a genogram, a number of issues will emerge, often in a nonthreatening way. You are simply taking a rather structured family history and learning as much as you can about patterns of relationships in the present and the past. Such background information will be critical to you later when you are attempting to unravel dysfunctional interactions that may have their origins in previous generations.

REFRAMING

Two types of diagnoses are useful in family counseling. The first variety includes applying those labels that help the counselor to grasp the processes and problems involved. We have already examined diagnosing client position, family hierarchy, communication style, and symptoms as solutions and metaphors in this context. But there is a second kind of diagnosis—the one communicated to the client. The counselor's initial task, therefore, is to define or reframe the present problem to the client or clients in such a way that it may be resolved.

Clients come into counseling sessions with preconceived notions of what is wrong with them and why:

- "My marriage is on the rocks because my wife wants to go back to school and start a career rather than taking care of the family."
- "My boy is having trouble in school because his teachers are too strict and don't appreciate his uniqueness."
- "I've never been able to hold a job because everyone in my family has always been lazy."

In the process of reframing, the counselor redefines the presenting complaint for the family, using both ingenuity and creativity to think on concrete and metaphorical levels. In the resulting working diagnosis, the counselor identifies issues that can, in fact, be responsive to change, so that the family will be more willing to work on them. There isn't much that can be done to help a client who is complaining about another person's behavior, unless, of course, the other person will come in for counseling and willingly change what the accuser dislikes. In initiating counseling for clients with the complaints quoted above, the most important task would be to reframe the client's perceived difficulties. The husband who wants compliance from his wife would be helped to view the problem more as a lack of communication: He hasn't conveyed his desires in such a way that his wife could understand (and accept) them. The problem of the boy having trouble in school would be reframed to say that, although he is clearly a talented comic, he is performing for the wrong audience. The person without a job would be helped to redefine his problem as a lack of skills and/or motivation rather than a lack of employable genes.

The value of reframing is exemplified in the case of a 35-year-old client who arrived for his session huffing and puffing, his face flushed, and his hand wrapped in a towel that was quickly turning red with blood. The flustered counselor, a tiny woman of 90 pounds, looked up at the 230-pound mechanic and responded, "Oh, I see you had some trouble. What happened?"

Still standing in the foyer, the man smiled with a glazed, stunned look and answered, "I locked my damn keys in the car and I got mad. And when I get mad I like to hit things. Anything. I can't help it. Boy, am I mad. Now, what's all this shit about you wanting to see me about my kid?"

The counselor went to her supervisor immediately following the session. She calmed down, at least enough to hear the more experienced clinician reframe the man's behavior: "What do you think about this guy? Blustering his way into a first session with his hand all bloody. This is funny. This is hysterical. This guy is no bully—this guy is a clown. Next time he comes in, treat him like a clown and see what happens. And, just in case you need me, I'll be close by."

During the next session the man responded with a burst of anger to the counselor's accurate confrontation about how he had been neglecting his son. He stamped the floor and rose with a menacing stare. The counselor, of course, was startled, but she regained her composure and looked at the humor in his behavior. She smiled, seemingly unaffected by his threatening behavior, thinking: "This guy really is funny."

The man anxiously demanded some explanation of the counselor's calm appearance. He was used to having people feel afraid of him. She told him compassionately how silly he really looked stamping around like a child; then, as an afterthought, she moved back a little and waited.

Yes, he agreed, he probably did look funny, but he does get what he wants by intimidating other people. He eventually admitted, though, that he hated himself for behaving so badly and appreciated the counselor seeing through the mask and allowing him to discuss his vulnerable feelings.

Although this was a risky strategy, it nevertheless demonstrated the power of reframing behavior, casting it in a different light. Not only is the client able to view his behavior as more manageable, but the counselor is also able to see the behavior in compassionate rather than threatening terms.

 ## VOICE FROM THE FIELD

Reframing is one of the strategies I most enjoy doing. I think it's because it gives me a chance to be creative—it's like I'm taking an experience my clients are distressed over and rewriting it as something not only not a problem, but even as something positive. In fact, it is a little like putting positive spin on things. I remember telling a husband and wife that her angry behavior towards him was the only way she knew how to get closer to him. She was hoping her anger would at least stir things up, maybe even start a fight—and the fight would at least create more intimacy than they were having now. The wife looked so pleased when I said this—suddenly, she no longer felt so guilty about her anger. And the husband—he

initially gave me this kind of puzzled "huh?" look. But when he asked his wife if my reframe was accurate, she nodded, and now he felt less upset with her anger!

Of course, you have to be careful not to create reframes that are too much of a stretch. I've done my fair share of reframes that sounded good, but really weren't true. I just wanted them to be true, and wanted the family to think more highly of themselves, with less guilt and blame. Sometimes it would work—the family believed the reframe, even though deep down I knew my reframe made no sense. And sometimes the family would all shake their heads—"Nah, we're not buying that one."

Another variation of reframing occurs in the narrative approach to family counseling. Called *externalizing*, the method is essentially the same; the counselor introduces another way of viewing the problem. Just as narrative therapy helps individual clients conceptualize their problems as outside them, family counselors enable family members see their symptoms as outside the family; in this way, everyone can work together as a team to defeat the problem (Monk, Winslade, Crocket, & Epston, 1997). This also prevents the family from blaming themselves or the identified client, because the enemy is now seen as being on the outside rather than the inside.

DIRECTIVES

The idea of deliberately telling clients what they should do goes against the grain of almost all counseling systems. Counselors are, after all, supposed to be neutral, objective, detached, and not prone to giving advice. A rationale for the violation of this golden rule is that such interventions are often successful. Furthermore, family counselors, by the very nature of their work, are more active, structuring, and directive than they would ever consider being when working with individual clients. Put all members of a family together in a room—particularly those who so are conflicted they had to ask for help—and the situation often turns chaotic. Unless the counselor is prepared to jump in and take the initiative, the family counseling session could make matters considerably worse.

A number of directive options are available to the family counselor. They may be designed to be either obeyed or disobeyed, depending on which is more likely to work. They can be simply and straightforwardly presented or explained in such a complicated and confusing way that the client will rebelliously do the opposite. The best directives are those that involve everyone in the family, are precisely described, provide sufficient motivation to encourage completion of the task, and are simple enough that they can be reasonably accomplished.

In using directives, the counselor seeks to initiate changes in the family structure by getting people to act differently. The goal is to realign the hierarchy of power along more desirable paths—for instance, with the parents in charge rather than the children or grandparents, or with both spouses on an equal footing. The process of initiating all directives usually involves (1) redefining the problem in a less threatening form and describing it in a way that allows resolution, (2) motivating and preparing the client to follow (or not follow) the directive, and (3) presenting the directive clearly, simply, and realistically, ensuring that all participants understand what they are to do or not do.

All directives (and for that matter all therapeutic interventions) are designed to help the counselor gain some control over the presenting symptoms and the family to attempt new solutions (Goldenberg & Goldenberg, 2008). The following tactical maneuvers are examples of those that require active counselor direction.

FORCING THE SPONTANEOUS

Many psychosomatic complaints, performance problems, and thought disturbances occur spontaneously, in spite of a client's attempts to control them. Trying too hard to fall asleep, reach orgasm, or stop a tic only makes things worse. Asking the client to cease behavior that is not within conscious control is not reasonable. Instead, the client can be directed to continue the behavior at will. A person who can't sleep may be told to stay up or to get up after 15 minutes and work on an important but nonstimulating task. The client is then able to make the first step toward resolution of the problem: If she or he can exhibit some control over the uncontrollable problem by exercising some choices around its occurrence, then the problem seems less ominous and not as wayward as the client originally believed. A paradoxical directive of this type allows the counselor to be successful, and the client perceives himself or herself as making progress. The client who complies with the suggestion is exhibiting control, and the client who doesn't abide by the directive to fail is then cured of the problem. This type of directive is safe for both the counselor and the client because it provides ample opportunity for positive outcome.

OPPOSITION THROUGH COMPLIANCE

In the physical world, when we attempt without success to solve a problem by a certain action, we will try something else—usually the opposite action. If we try to open a door by pushing it and it won't budge, we may try pulling it. If we attempt to loosen a screw by forcing it to the left and it doesn't move, we will try forcing it to the right. Yet when an attempted strategy doesn't work in emotional family struggles, with participants locked into no-win battles, a person will often try the same thing harder. If a wife fights for her independence in the marriage by repeatedly resisting her husband's orders and then discovers she is worse off, she will nevertheless struggle harder. If parents have attempted on numerous occasions to get their rebellious adolescent to comply with house rules and they have found that the youngster is only getting worse, the parents will demand even more compliant behavior.

This second category of directives takes the form of suggesting to those without power that the only way they will get any control is to back down. By deliberately taking a "weak position" and "giving in," they finally break the vicious, repetitive cycle. Thus, benevolent sabotage begins to defuse the conflict: "I'm sorry I burned your toast. I don't know what's getting into me." The powerless client is able to feel more dignity and control because she or he backs down by choice. The key to using compliant tactics effectively is to avoid sarcasm or overt game playing. The client must attempt a "one-down" instead of the "one-up" position that didn't work. Once the opposition ceases, the cycle is often broken, and the other family members no longer derive satisfaction from their positions. It's no fun to dominate if the other person won't fight back. And it's no fun to rebel if the others won't force compliance.

PRETENDING

A favorite ploy of Madanes in working with children is to direct the parents to encourage the symptom deliberately and to ask the child to pretend to have it. Much of the tension associated with the symptom is thereafter dissipated because everyone is "only pretending." Consider the case of a "28-year-old adolescent" who

■ | VOICE FROM THE FIELD

The thing you gotta be careful of with directive counseling is that these brilliant ideas usually come from behind a one-way mirror. What I mean is that when you see demonstration videos at workshops or read about cases in books, the presenters inevitably include these amazingly creative solutions to problems. Of course, they often came up with these interventions as part of a team. Sitting behind the one-way mirror is one or even more colleagues watching the session, talking among each other about all the possibilities, then calling on the phone into the session when they'd like to make a suggestion. It's a fabulous idea, naturally, one that changes the whole course of treatment.

When you read about this, or see it on a video, you think to yourself, "Wow, I gotta try that!" Then you get back to your own practice where you don't have the luxury of having the most brilliant minds in the city watching and contributing to your sessions, and the stuff you come up with on your own isn't nearly as sterling as what the master therapists invented.

Don't get me wrong. I think using directives and all are powerful strategies. It's just that it's damn hard to come up with them at the time. That's why you always need to be connected to a great supervisor to consult with.

was still so dependent on his father that he carried around a paging device so that his father could reach him at any time, usually to scream at him for some mistake he had made in the family business. The young man was constantly late, missed appointments, and botched orders, and each time his father would furiously bawl him out. Neither man much enjoyed the pattern, but each felt powerless to stop it.

The counselor directed the son to bungle something deliberately at least three times a day. He was to pretend to make mistakes so that his father could no longer determine when the young man was truly irresponsible and when he was only faking. The son improved after discovering that because he could control when he made mistakes, and pretend to do so, he could certainly refrain from such errors whenever he chose.

A way to involve other family members is to encourage them to criticize the person's "performance." Another pattern is thus broken, because instead of trying to deter the symptoms, they are now trying to help the person do them even better. With the introduction of directives to pretend, the metaphorical symptoms are no longer allowed to be part of reality. The problem diminishes because it is no longer taken seriously.

SLOWING DOWN

Whenever anyone tries too hard to do something, the task becomes more difficult. The directive to slow down is often most effective during initial interviews, when clients are apprehensive about being asked to do something they won't be able to do. If the presenting problem is resolved too quickly, before the clients have had the opportunity to make new adjustments or discover other ways of relating to one another, it is possible that the family structure will break down.

During the first session with a woman complaining of a marriage that is falling apart, the counselor specifically directs her to stop trying to fix things: "Leave things just the way they are for now. This way your husband, too, will have the chance to get involved in solving the problem. I know he's saying that he won't come in for counseling. That is certainly the case as long as you keep nagging him, but let's see how things change once you slow down. The marriage isn't comfortable anyway, so by backing off you can hardly make things worse."

The therapeutic circumstances are now programmed for success no matter what the outcome. The client immediately feels released from her sole responsibility for fixing the marriage. She can loosen up and take a deep breath. She also focuses on herself rather than trying to change her husband. And, if things don't improve immediately, the client will be more patient and willing to keep working.

It is not possible to review these various family therapy interventions without reflecting on the power they give the counselor. There are two issues involved here. First, the counselor is deliberately shaking up a family system, using the rationale that "stirring the pot" will at the very least engender some kind of shift in stuck family patterns. Although some family counseling theorists and researchers suggest that directives, pretending, and similar strategies do not adversely affect the client-counselor relationship (Betts & Remer, 1993; Gardner, Burr, & Wiedower, 2006), counselors need to be mindful that the impact of powerful interventions can be unpredictable.

Family counseling, as we have noted before, presumes that movement by one member inevitably starts a chain reaction that creates behavioral changes among the entire family. Family counselors need to be well trained and highly experienced in their ability to contain potentially adverse outcomes from their interventions. Virginia Satir has observed that systemic change inevitably initiates a period of chaos within the family, as it struggles to redefine boundaries, roles, and power hierarchies (Satir & Baldwin, 1984). The role of the counselor is to help the family manage the chaos stage successfully on their path to integrating changes into their daily functioning.

Second, counselors need to remain vigilant about not getting seduced by their own power. There can be a level of deceit and manipulation inherent in these interventions. For novice counselors, in particular, their use can be a heady experience. Good family counselors bring a spirit of humility to their work; boldness in counseling is a virtue only when tempered by counselors' self-monitoring of their personal issues regarding power and control.

COUPLES COUNSELING

See Companion DVD
Couples Counseling

Even if you never end up doing sessions with whole extended families present, you will inevitably do a significant amount of work with clients and their partners. This is especially true because problems in intimate relationships have been cited as the number one reason why people show up for counseling services (Johnson & Lebow, 2000). Since the advent of family counseling theory in the second half of the 20th century, couples counseling has generally been considered a specialized form of family counseling with the same conceptual frameworks and interventions. This view has been radically challenged by a virtual revolution in the field of couples counseling since the 1990s, spurred by the research work of such scientist-practitioners as John Gottman and Susan Johnson, who have forcefully argued that couples work is a distinct discipline, requiring its own models and intervention techniques. Current thinking about helping couples does incorporate family systems theory but is also looking at innovative approaches to working with couples; learning these new approaches requires a thorough study of 21st century scholarship and textbooks in this field.

Couples work can be among the most satisfying endeavors in the counseling profession. Most of us have had some personal experience with being a partner in a couple, and know firsthand the joys to be found in an intimate or romantic relationship, as well as the pain when relationships turn sour. The majority of couples come in for counseling when the relationship is on the edge of falling apart, when there is a yearning for regaining the intimacy experienced in the early phase of the relationship, but also because of the fear that the partnership has become unsalvageable. Despite their best attempts to save the relationship by themselves, it remains filled with fighting, emotional distance, unsatisfying sex, constant tension, and personal anguish. If there are children involved, the desperation of the couples can be even more intense, as the prospect of separating and its impact on their children looms increasingly as inevitable. Thus, when a couples counselor helps partners strengthen the bond between them, enhance the quality of intimacy in their relationship, and regain confidence that the partnership can last, the experience for the counselor can be immensely gratifying. Equally meaningful work is helping couples who have decided to dissolve the relationship to do so in a collaborative, respectful way, with each partner able to articulate the behaviors he or she contributed to the relationship's failure.

GOALS OF COUPLES COUNSELING

As with other forms of counseling, there is disagreement in this field in a number of areas, beginning with, "What is the goal of couples counseling?" Most state and national ethical codes require that counselors not violate client autonomy. Translated to the field of couples counseling, that means it is not your job to help the couple stay together; rather, your role is to help each partner take responsibility for his or her role in the relationship's difficulties, develop skills in communicating his or her emotional needs with honesty and directness, learn to fight fairly, and allow each person to become emotionally open and vulnerable with his or her partner—perhaps the essential requirement for intimacy. If you can help clients do all these things, you should feel good about your work regardless of whether the couple decides to stay together or not. You feel secure in the knowledge that even if they separate, they have learned valuable lessons from counseling that will help them succeed in their next relationship. This way of conceptualizing the role of the couples counselor ensures ethical practice, helps you maintain professional objectivity, and reduces the very real risk of feeling like a failure if the couple splits up, which is their decision, not yours. One way to hold a neutral stance regarding the outcome of the treatment is to remind yourself that you do not know what is ultimately best for the two people: Perhaps their own growth toward becoming more fulfilled and healthier human beings lies in pursuing separate paths.

However, some couples counseling theorists argue that maintaining this neutral stance toward the outcome of treatment is not only unrealistic for the counselor but detrimental to the therapy process itself (Doherty, 2009). One question they raise is this: Is it humanly possible for a couples counselor to help clients without being emotionally invested in the couple staying together? Our basic impulse, the motivating push that helps us do our best work, comes from our desire to see the relationship succeed. And if we don't care whether or not the couple stays together, is there not the risk we will somehow project our indifference onto the couple, undermining the couples' motivation to work on their relationship? A second argument comes from a religious perspective: Couples who were married in a religious ceremony have made a covenant with the God they worship. Regardless of the couples counselor's values regarding religion, some theorists believe the counselor has an obligation to help couples maintain a sacred agreement to remain together "for better or worse." Finally, there are some theorists who believe that all marriages can succeed—if both partners do the work necessary to repair the relationship.

DEALING WITH ANGER

Another key issue in the field of couples counseling is the counselor's role regarding couples who openly express anger toward each other. The traditional approach, still held by many counselors, is that anger is inevitably destructive to a relationship, and while angry fights will always occur from time to time, the counselor's role is to help couples find alternate ways of resolving differences. To that end, numerous interventions have been developed to reduce the criticism, name-calling, and various other hurtful behaviors couples routinely practice. These include rules for fair fighting and lessons in reporting anger as an alternative to expressing it.

Imagine a wife who is frustrated with her husband's failure to take out the garbage. This leads to angry commands such as, "You lazy good-for-nothing. You never take out the garbage. What's your problem!" The husband experiences this as nagging behaviors, which only serve to make him more recalcitrant.

Once the repetitive pattern is identified, the counselor teaches the wife how to express her anger in different ways, following three basic principles.

1. Report the underlying distress. Instead of saying, "*You never take out the garbage*," say, "*It upsets me…*"
2. Report the specific behavior that bothers you. "*It upsets me that you let the garbage pile up every night until the kitchen begins to smell.*"
3. Report the specific behavior you wish your partner to perform. "*It upsets me that you let the garbage pile up every night until the kitchen begins to smell. Please take it out at the end of the day before we go to bed.*"

Another anger-reducing technique is to teach couples "time-out" skills in which both partners realize they have power to end a fight by saying "We need a time-out to cool off; we can talk about this later." Crucial to these approaches to anger is that the couples counselor does not allow partners to fight during a session. The counselor takes firm control, stopping the couple when voices start to rise and partners throw out "zinger" statements or bring up past resentments not relevant to the topic being discussed. If necessary, the counselor will act like a preschool teacher with an unruly class, asking partners to stop their negative interaction, take a deep breath, and restart the discussion in a more civil tone. Additionally, the more couples practice these skills in a session, the better able they will be to use the same skills when

Voice from the Field

Growing up in my family, I had always believed that fighting and arguing was always a terrible thing. I heard my parents fighting and it was ugly, let me tell you. They would scream and slam doors and call one another names. When they finally got divorced, of course I was upset—but I was also relieved that we could have some peace in the house.

I avoided doing couples counseling for as long as I could. I didn't want to subject myself to couples being mean to one another, like my parents. The few times I saw couples together they would scream so loud that the walls would literally shake. One time a fistfight actually broke out in my office.

There was this one, older couple I saw for a while who seemed to always be fighting and screaming. They kept getting kicked out of their apartments because they were making so much noise and neighbors would complain. I tried my hardest to get them to stop yelling but nothing I tried seemed to work. It took me the longest time to realize that this was part of the interaction style. They were actually quite loving toward one another. They'd been married for over 20 years. I got a message from them a few years after I stopped seeing them. They were still fighting, but still doing fine. That was the one case that taught me that being passionate or volatile in a relationship didn't necessarily mean that it was doomed.

disagreements occur in their everyday life, enabling them to interrupt an imminent conflict before voices escalate and anger erupts.

While no theorist believes that angry fighting in front of children or rage-filled yelling are acceptable behaviors, many writers and researchers in this field are concluding that couples counseling should not be about stopping fights. Wile (1993) believes that fights are not only an inevitable part of relationships, but actually opportunities for the couple to strengthen their bond. After a fight, couples often talk honestly about how and why things got out of control and what role each of them contributed to the misunderstanding. The role of the couples counselor is to facilitate couples practicing this postfight processing in their couples session.

Gottman has conducted extensive empirical research on predicting couples who end up in divorce by analyzing their communication patterns. Several conclusions resulted from these long-term studies (Gottman, 1999; Gottman & Gottman, 2008):

- Anger itself was not a predictor of divorce; in fact, couples who expressed anger showed increases in marital satisfaction over time. Because partners get charged up with adrenaline when fights begin (especially men), learning "fair fighting" skills in couples counseling is impractical: In the heat of the moment, couples will express anger regardless of what they learned in a counseling session.
- If anger was not necessarily a bad thing for relationships, there were four kinds of negative interactions that were found to be destructive: criticism, stonewalling (when one partner turns away from the other or leaves the room in the middle of a disagreement), defensiveness, and contempt. It was the last two, in particular, that most powerfully predicted an unhappy marriage.
- While negative emotions were a normal part of marriage, relationships succeeded when the number of positive emotions expressed in interactions was higher than the number of negative ones. Simply put, anger is fine so long as people are nice to each other more often than they are angry.

- Successful couples were good at making up after fights. They had developed means to repair any damage that had been inflicted. Couples who tended to begin conversations with a "harsh start-up" (that is, a request or demand by one partner that is expressed in an angry or commanding tone of voice) were likely to have unhappy relationships.

THEORIES OF COUPLES COUNSELING

Couples counseling has been practiced as far back as the 1920s, and became established as a distinct profession in 1942 (Sperry, Carlson, & Peluso, 2006). As with individual counseling theories, numerous theoretical models have been developed, some adapted from individual theories (e.g., psychodynamic, cognitive-behavioral, humanistic, narrative, and solution-focused) and some stand-alone models rooted in the clinical experiences and/or research findings of particular counselors and theorists.

Couples counseling models can be categorized as "problem-solving" approaches (including behavioral strategies, communication skills training, and systemic interventions) and "acceptance" approaches (for example, Integrative Behavioral Couple Therapy, Emotionally Focused Couple Therapy, and Imago Relational Therapy). Problem-solving approaches focus on reducing the destructive interpersonal behaviors or on resolving specific dilemmas that couples describe as their presenting problem. Acceptance models focus on increasing intimacy and connection, solidifying relational bonds, and facilitating each partner's acceptance of the other partner's limitations and strengths. Acceptance models also tend to be highly integrative, fashioned from a synthesis of family systems thinking, psychoanalytic conceptualizations, and specific behavioral changes.

PROBLEM-SOLVING THEORIES

Behavioral theories emphasize teaching couples specific problem-solving skills, while giving couples homework assignments designed to increase the number of positive behaviors exchanged (Jacobson & Christensen, 1996; Dimidjian, Martell, & Christensen, 2008). For example, couples might be given the task of "catching your partner doing something nice"—recognizing and complimenting each other every day when someone demonstrates a caring behavior. Behavioral couples therapy had strong research support until the 1990s, when reevaluations of studies' findings showed only a 50% success rate and frequent relapses (Jacobson & Christensen, 1996).

Communication skills training is a staple of couples counseling interventions, utilized by many counselors regardless of their specific theoretical orientation. If you utilize this intervention, you would teach couples how to paraphrase, reflect, clarify, and empathize—and most important, listen without interruption or giving advice. (In other words, you teach them the same active listening skills counselors learn.) You would then assign couples the task of practicing active listening at home, recommending, for example, that couples choose a time during the week where each spends 20 minutes as either the speaker or the listener. The speaker talks about anything she or he wants, and the listener can do active listening but nothing else. The expectation is that with practice, couples will learn to hear each partner's feelings and respond empathically instead of defensively, thereby reducing the number of frustrating arguments.

Systemic models utilize similar constructs and interventions practiced in systemic family therapy. The counselor pays attention to the couples' interactional sequences, noting the "dance" of the relationship. If the husband repeatedly accuses the wife of chronically overspending on credit cards, the counselor might ask the husband how she reacts to his complaints. The husband might discover that she responds to his anger by getting depressed and going on shopping sprees to soothe her distress. Thus, a systems-oriented counselor might give the couple feedback on how the overspending problem is created by both wife and husband. One of the virtues of this approach is that neither partner feels blamed as the cause of the relationship difficulty, since both are equal contributors. If you are a systems-oriented counselor, your main intervention might be providing feedback and insights as to how each partner helps maintain the problematic behavior; however, you might also use more dramatic, hands-on strategies, directing the partners to change specific behaviors. For example, in the above example, you might direct the husband to stop complaining. He will probably react skeptically, thinking the overspending issues will only worsen. However, what actually happens is that she no longer needs to shop to alleviate her discomfort, reducing the behaviors that upset him and thus removing his need to complain. Now he feels better about her, and she feels better about him, and the counseling is deemed successful.

Acceptance models of couples counseling represent the major shift in thinking about the causes of couples dysfunction and the design of effective treatments. Rather than attempt to help partners resolve conflicts and reduce problematic behaviors, acceptance models emphasize helping each partner see each other realistically, appreciate the differences in their personalities, and increase their bids for more intimate connection—with the underlying assumption that a couple securely bonded will find their own solutions.

Gottman's *Gottman Method* approach requires that couples share and honor each other's personal dreams. Additionally, rather than force couples to stop their repetitive fights, Gottman asks couples to follow their arguments with a more intimate conversation about the fight itself (Gottman & Levenson, 2000; Gottman & Gottman, 2008). Gottman's treatment approaches are grounded in extensive research about the characteristics of successful and unsuccessful marriages. The popularity of his workshops throughout the country suggests that his model will find increasingly greater acceptance by counselors.

In the mid 1990s, Jacobson and Christensen, previously advocates of behavioral couples counseling, shifted gears and suggested an *acceptance and change* model, which they called *Integrative Behavioral Couples Therapy* (IBCT); counselors help their clients create a stronger relationship by accepting the personality traits each partner wants to change in the other as just "differences," rather than as problems. As couples increase their levels of intimacy, behavioral and communications-training strategies are incorporated into treatment in order to consolidate gains (Jacobson & Christensen, 1996; Dimidjian, Martell, & Christensen, 2008).

Emotionally Focused Couples Therapy (EFT) integrates attachment theory, systems theory, and client-centered empathy to help couples express their deepest fears about becoming close to each other (Johnson, 2004, 2008). Emotionally focused counselors identify the ways in which couples create negative cycles of interaction, and reframe hostile behaviors as a partner's protest that the relationship isn't closer. The counselor helps couples develop insights into their approach-distancing patterns, while using empathic listening to create a safe counseling environment where couples can articulate their fears of being rejected. Treatment ends when clients feel their relationship has become a secure base where each partner can confidently go for soothing and comfort. EFT has garnered strong empirical support and is becoming one of the most widely practiced couples counseling models (Simon, 2004).

Hendrix's *Imago Relationship Therapy* (IRT) builds on psychoanalytic concepts to explain how we choose mates who resemble our parents—with the unconscious hope that our partner will heal our childhood wounds. Relationship difficulties are caused, in part, by our disappointment in discovering that our partners cannot make up for old, family-of-origin wounds. If you are an IRT counselor,

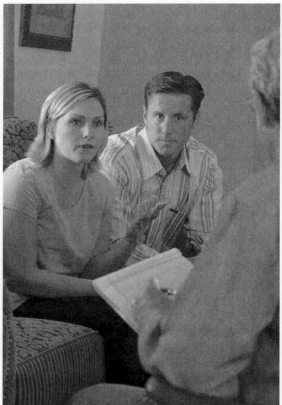

SW Productions/Photodisc/Getty Images.

Counselors must listen with equal attention to each family member's point of view, being careful never to take sides.

you help partners understand how they are projecting the negative traits of their parents onto their partners; the goal is to help each partner become conscious of his or her projections and see the other as the individual he or she really is (Hendrix, 1988, 2007).

Regardless of the theoretical orientation you use, there are some general principles most couples counselors would agree are critical:

1. *Establish clear goals and focus*. Because couples counseling tends to be a short-term process (three to six months), establishing clear goals and a focus for the treatment is critical. Moreover, the counselor and the couple need to be in sync about what the goals are, which may include improving communication, reducing fighting, resolving a specific conflict, enhancing their sex life, or dealing with infidelity. Sometimes couples have conflicting goals: One partner wants to make the relationship work and the other wants to leave. In this case, the counselor might focus on the common goal of helping both partners communicate their feelings clearly and expressing their underlying pain.

2. *Maintain balance*. Balance in couples counseling refers to two aspects of the process: The counselor avoids taking sides, and demonstrates an empathic appreciation for both partner's concerns and needs. Also, the counselor ensures that both partners have an equal opportunity to talk, interrupting one partner if necessary to give the other a chance to air his or her views. If the counselor determines that it would be helpful to see one of the clients in an individual session, the counselor will see both clients individually to maintain balance. When balance is lost, and one partner believes the counselor is taking sides with the other, the process inevitably fails. The challenge in maintaining balance is when privately you do take sides; Wile has observed that the art of couples counseling is being empathic toward the partner whom you secretly think is wrong (Wile, 1999).

3. *Do not allow verbal abuse in a session*. Regardless of your approach to anger and fights in sessions, you never allow people to intentionally hurt each other with abusive language.

4. *Assess for domestic violence*. It is essential for couples counselors to be educated in the signs of domestic violence and how to deal with it when they suspect abuse is taking place. Most theorists believe that partners should not be seen as a couple if spousal abuse is occurring; instead, the victim is referred for individual counseling and the abuser to a batterer's group.

5. *Stay calm* regardless of the intensity of the couple's arguing or covert tension. Remaining outside the drama the couple is engaged in can be the most difficult challenge for a couples counselor, especially beginners; however, the counselor's steady demeanor in the face of a couple's hostile interactions is a critical ingredient to the success of the process.

6. *Assessment of couples should be multidimensional regardless of theoretical orientation*. Couples counselors look at partners' family-of-origin beliefs about marital roles and expectations, circular systemic patterns, intrapsychic conflicts, and here-and-now communication processes.

7. *Be assertive when appropriate*. Couples counselors are not passive listeners; they are often more like film or theater directors, stopping clients from

| Voice from the Field

The best part of being a couples counselor is that you get to see what goes on at home right in front of you. It's almost like watching a scene in a film. When I counsel individuals, there's always that thought in the back of my mind, "Well, my client is complaining about how her boyfriend treats her, but I don't really know how he behaves—I'm just hearing her perspective." With couples, it's different, because you can actually see how they treat each other. So you can point out to them with confidence, "This is what I just saw happening—Sue, you got angry with Sam, and Sam, you shut down and moved to the side of the couch, and then Sue, you got frustrated and raised your voice. You must have been scared that Sam was pulling away from you again, like he does at home. And Sam, you seemed scared that you didn't know how to handle Sue's strong emotions, so you got as far away as you could." And then Sue and Sam say, "Yes! That's what we do all the time!" It's a great feeling when that happens.

I have to admit, I do struggle with couples who get angry. I grew up in a home where my parents were fighting all the time. They screamed at one another. They slammed doors. They threatened to leave each other. Of course, we were terrified our parents would break up.

What this means for me is that I have a hard time being in a room with people who are being mean and hurtful to one another. I know that sounds funny for someone in my line of work but I still have difficulty watching people yelling and screaming at one another. I have a low tolerance for that sort of thing and I don't put up with that behavior in my office. To a certain extent, this compromises my effectiveness because sometimes couples need to express themselves passionately. That part is fine with me, but not if it means raising your voice. So I enforce strict limits. I make people behave themselves when they are with me no matter what they might do when they are by themselves.

I know this means that I have to continue to work on my issues with anger in my own relationship. That's the other part I like about this kind of work; it forces me to work on my own marriage. My wife has noticed that I am gradually getting better handling her own anger. I'm convinced that the more I work on this in my home, the more effective I will be with couples. So it becomes a kind of upward spiral of growth for both me and my clients.

engaging in pointless arguments, choreographing their physical interactions so they face and talk to each other, and directing them in how to speak from the heart.

8. *Examine your own values regarding relationships*, your relationship behaviors, and your parents' relationship to ensure that you see your clients objectively and remain aligned with their goals, rather than with yours.

Working with partners or cohabitants brings up a number of other issues— violence, money issues, sexual dysfunctions, child rearing, lifestyle compatibility, role definitions, health, jealousy, fidelity, career, and leisure choices. Anything you would hope to do with one person in the room is infinitely more complex when you are managing the interactions between two people who may already be locked into resentments and heated battles. This presents a series of new clinical challenges as well as ethical conflicts.

ETHICAL ISSUES IN COUPLES AND FAMILY COUNSELING

If you have gotten the impression that marital and family counseling are powerful treatment methods that can often promote "cures" in a matter of weeks, that is indeed true. It is because these modalities are so potent, however, that they bring with them a number of moral dilemmas for the practitioner. Another critical issue is the matter of secrets; what do you do when one member of a family or couple calls you on the phone and reveals something that he or she does not want other family members to know? Some counselors hold a "no secrets" policy, believing that all secrets are toxic to family relationships and must be brought out into the open, even if the counselor must be the one to do so. Others argue that a "no secrets" rule discourages a client with an important secret from disclosing it to the counselor; these advocates of an "I will hold your secret" policy take the position that hearing secrets from an individual member at least affords the counselor an opportunity to encourage the client to come forward to the family. Then, there is the "split the difference" view, in which counselors explain to family members that the counselor will only reveal secrets that are germane to the family's growth. Thus, if a spouse reveals in an individual session an affair conducted decades earlier, the counselor will hold the secret; but the counselor will disclose a more recent infidelity. Which policy would you hold? All are ethical, but none are ethically simple.

A later chapter will focus on ethical and legal issues as they relate to the practice of counseling, but we nevertheless wish to mention briefly some of the conflicts you will face in your work as a marital and family counselor. In addition to the secrets issue, Southern, Smith, and Oliver (2005) list two other particularly complex moral and ethical dilemmas:

1. Family counselors typically "join" with the family system, thereby increasing the chances of being invited to family rituals and celebrations. Is it ethical to attend?
2. Family counselors conceptualize the whole family as the client, and the psychological issues of one member are a symptom of the entire family's dysfunction. However, in order for the counselor or client to collect reimbursement from a health insurance organization, one member must be identified as a patient and given a DSM diagnosis. What is the ethical course of action?

There are other ethical issues as well for marriage and family counselors; some may already have occurred to you:

- Is it ethical to be deceitful and manipulative (using paradoxical techniques, for example) if it is for the client's own good?
- If your primary function is to treat family problems, what about the individual goals of each member, which may conflict with those of the others?
- Because family conflicts frequently involve value issues related to fidelity, sexuality, promiscuity, divorce, child rearing, and life priorities, how can you possibly keep your own values in check regarding how you believe people should behave?
- Because family counselors are often highly directive and dramatic in their interventions geared toward breaking up dysfunctional patterns, aren't there greater risks for doing harm?

Last, but by no means least, is the area of family violence and the special ethical problems it raises. The abuse of children, spouses, and the elderly creates

problems not only for the victims and perpetrators but also for the helping professionals caught in the middle who are trying to stabilize explosive situations (Green
& Hansen, 1989; Huber, 1994; Sommers-Flanagan & Sommers-Flanagan, 2007).
Counselors have to sort through a number of conflicting loyalties: (1) to state laws
that mandate the reporting of abuse, (2) to the family member(s) who are the perpetrators and are requesting help, and (3) to the victims (or potential victims) of
the dangerous behaviors. While ethical counselors agree that the needs of the victim come first, the process of dealing with all three "stakeholders" can take an
emotional toll on the clinician.

Both the American Association for Marriage and Family Therapy (AAMFT)
and the International Association of Marriage and Family Counselors (IAMFC)
have developed ethical codes for this specialty. In addition to the universal ethical
issues that all counselors face (confidentiality, conflicted loyalties, social responsibility, competence), these codes will help guide you to sort out dilemmas as they
emerge, often in consultation with your supervisor.

SEX COUNSELING

Sex counseling can be a subspecialty of couples counseling or a profession of its
own, although the confluence of two forces may diminish the number of counselors
who specialize only in sex therapy. On the one hand, the advent of drugs like
Viagra® have medicalized sexual issues like erectile dysfunction, so that clients seeking help for sexual problems are increasingly likely to go to their physicians rather
than counselors. At the same time, the field of couples counseling is recognizing that
sexual issues are often inextricably linked to intimacy difficulties, as well as to societal pressures on couples to experience unrealistic levels of sexual engagement and satisfaction. Thus, when clients come to a couples counselor with sexual concerns (and
many come to couples counseling for this reason), the counselor is likely to initially
conceptualize the problem in terms of intimacy issues, rather than as a sexual dysfunction problem.

Having said this, it is still important that counselors are familiar with behavioral interventions designed to increase sexual satisfaction; these interventions, dating back to the pioneering work of William Masters and Virginia Johnson in the
1960s, can be highly effective when integrated into a couples counseling treatment
plan that also addresses intimacy and communication issues.

Joanning and Keoughan (2005) suggest that couples counselors follow a specific
decision-making process when conceptualizing the best way to approach sexual problems. First, determine the nature of the sexual problem. If it is primarily a relational
issue, proceed with one of the couples counseling models described above, followed
by sexually oriented behavioral interventions. If it appears to be isolated from intimacy issues, proceed right to behavioral interventions combined with sex education.
If the sexual problem appears to be organically caused, refer to a physician, but with
the proviso that the couple return to couples counseling if medical treatment does
not completely resolve the couple's distress.

VOICE FROM THE FIELD

Learning the techniques of sex counseling and education is the easy part. I mean, it's not brain surgery or anything. There are these structured programs that teach you about the techniques and all. The hard part, though, is confronting your own attitudes and values and beliefs related to sex that might get in the way of your work with people. That's why the training almost always includes experiential-type groups where you look at your own sexual issues and get used to talking about sex in an open, honest way.

One standard way that they often start the training is that they put the words penis and vagina on the board and have everyone in the room yell out all the names they can think of for those body parts. It's

hysterical. People start out saying the standard ones but then they end up blurting out their own pet names for their private parts. While everyone is laughing, they don't realize that what the exercise is supposed to do is desensitize you to sexual terms so that you can talk about them to couples without shame.

If couples you're working with sense that you feel the least discomfort talking about sex—I mean any aspect of it—they won't deal with their stuff. They are looking to you for guidance and the best way to offer it is to be really calm and matter-of-fact about the subject.

SENSATE FOCUS

If there is one behavioral intervention for sexual difficulties that all counselors should be familiar with, it is *sensate focus*, a sequence of exercises designed to enhance each partner's awareness of his or her body while eliminating the performance anxiety frequently associated with sexual difficulties. After the counselor has assessed for and addressed intimacy issues, the counselor will next introduce the sensate focus sequence in the treatment, essentially a prescribed series of progressive exercises that the couple will do at home. Initially, all pressure is removed by specifically prohibiting the couple from any further attempts at intercourse. They are absolutely forbidden to try, thereby removing the threat of failure. The sensate focus exercises involve sensitively and non-demandingly giving and receiving nongenital pleasure through touching. Very gradually, the couple add to their repertoire by engaging in any number of sensual experiences the couple finds interesting and pleasurable. For example, the couple may begin with mutual back rubs for one week, followed by non-genital touching and mutual pleasure in other areas of the body. Only when the couple feel comfortable conducting these sensual experiences does the counselor recommend moving toward sexual activity. This sequence might start with light genital stimulation without orgasm, followed by genital touching to orgasm, intercourse without orgasm (or erection), and, finally, intercourse to orgasm. Throughout the exercise sequence, the counselor encourages the couple to move at their own pace, reminding them that pleasurable sex does not depend on either intercourse or orgasm.

If the couple feel blocked at any point in the sequence, the counselor assesses for psychological issues that may need to be unearthed and resolved; these can include stern "sex is dirty" messages learned in childhood, sexual abuse, rape, or other traumas that one or both partners associate with sexuality. If we know anything about human sexuality, it is that it is a highly complex biological and psychological phenomenon, fraught with emotional and social issues. Regardless of the cause of sexual distress, the main points all counselors want to communicate to their clients are that patience with each other is essential; that partners need to respect each other's differences with regard to their sexual needs and desires; and that every couple defines their own vision of optimal sexual activity in the relationship.

SUMMARY

In this chapter you have learned about the basic theory and techniques of marital, family, and sex counseling. Most counselors are faced with many clients who experience adjustment problems in these areas. Professionals who work with children and adolescents in particular need knowledge and expertise in family counseling. The major focus of these techniques is to clarify the system of relationships occurring in marital and family interactions and to identify opportunities to interrupt dysfunctional patterns. In working with family systems, counselors attempt to help clients restructure relationships toward developmentally healthy goals and to reduce the impact of destructive systems of relationships. Counselors must skillfully blend specific marital, family, and sex techniques within the framework of individual and group counseling skills.

SELF-GUIDED EXPLORATIONS

1. What are some experiences from your family of origin that have influenced you to become a counselor?

2. Using the following notations, create a genogram or structural map of your family relationships. Clearly highlight the coalitions, boundaries, conflicts, and patterns of communication.

☐ Male family member	- - - - Weak relationship
◯ Female family member	═══ Dependent relationship
◎☐ You	⋀⋁⋀⋁ Conflicted relationship
═══ Strong relationship	

3. The concept of *reframing* is central to the practice of family counseling. In this process, you attempt to recast the way a problem is viewed so that it is easier to resolve. For example, a mother keeps pestering her son about doing chores that he consistently avoids. The more she nags him, the more obstinate the boy becomes. Once the counselor reframes the mother's behavior as a way of showing love and caring, the boy stops feeling so resentful toward the mother's intrusions. Think of a problem or conflict in your life that could be reframed in more constructive terms.

4. Couples counselors need to have a definition of a healthy relationship.
   (a) Reflect on what a healthy relationship means to you. What ingredients constitute the basis for a fulfilling intimate partnership?
   (b) Reflect on your own or your parents' relationship. What are its strengths and weaknesses?

5. Record and transcribe 10 minutes of your relationship or your parents' or another couple's. Count how many statements could be considered criticism, defensiveness, stonewalling, or contempt.

6. Everyone agrees that strong families, marriages, and partnerships are characterized by love. Yet, love is an extremely subjective term and one that is hardly ever used by family and couple counseling theorists. Clients say they want more love in their relationships but often are vague if you ask them what exactly do they want. What is your definition of love?

7. What are some sexual issues that a couple might present that would be uncomfortable for you to deal with? Imagine that a client walked in presenting that very issue. How would you help this person?

FOR HOMEWORK

1. Arrange to interview several "normal" families. Explore their family dynamics, coalitions, cross-generational issues, decision-making style, and other factors that you have learned are important in healthy family functioning. Be sure to look at strengths of the family and individual members, as well as any problem areas.
2. The literature that concerns the subject of training family and couples counselors is in general agreement that the two best films illustrating family systems are *Ordinary People* and *When a Man Loves a Woman*. View one of these films, and ask yourself the following questions:

(a) What is the family's homeostasis? In other words, what is the role of each family member when he or she is behaving in his or her typical patterns, as depicted in the first 20 minutes of the movie?
(b) Which character in the family is challenging homeostasis by changing her or his typical behavior in the system?
(c) When one person changes, everyone else is forced to change also, or the family will come apart. How do the other family members in these films react when one of the characters changes?

SUGGESTED READINGS

Becvar, D. S., & Becvar, R. J. (2008). *Family therapy: A systemic integration* (7th ed.). Boston: Allyn & Bacon.

Blume, T. W. (2006). *Becoming a family counselor: A bridge to family therapy theory and practice*. New York: John Wiley & Sons.

Carter, B., & McGoldrick, M. (2005). *The expanded family life cycle* (3rd ed.). Boston: Allyn & Bacon.

Gehart, D. R., & Tuttle, A. R. (2003). *Theory-based treatment planning for marriage and family therapists*. Pacific Grove, CA: Brooks/Cole.

Gladding, S. T. (2006). *Family therapy: History, theory, and practice* (4th ed.). Upper Saddle River, NJ: Prentice Hall.

Goldenberg, I., & Goldenberg, H. (2008). *Family therapy: An overview* (7th ed.). Belmont, CA: Brooks/Cole.

Hertlien, K. M., Weeks, G. R., & Gambescia, N. (2008). *Systemic sex therapy*. New York: Routledge.

Johnson, S. M. (2004). *The practice of emotionally focused couple therapy: Creating connection*. New York: Brunner/Routledge.

Long, L. L., Bryant, J. A., & Thomas, V. R. (2005). *Sexuality counseling: An integrative approach*. Upper Saddle River, NJ: Prentice Hall.

Long, L. L., & Young, M. E. (2007). *Counseling and therapy for couples* (2nd ed.). Belmont, CA: Brooks/Cole.

McCarthy, B., & McCarthy, E. (2003). *Rekindling desire*. New York: Brunner/Routledge.

Nichols, M. P., & Schwartz, R. C. (2007). *Essentials of family therapy* (3rd ed.). Boston: Allyn & Bacon.

Sperry, L., Carlson, J., & Peluso, P. R. (2006). *Couples therapy: Integrating theory and technique*. Denver, CO: Love.

CHAPTER 11 | CAREER COUNSELING

KEY CONCEPTS

Vocational choice

Work functions

Meaningful work

Occupational Information Network

Employability skills

Life coaching

Career identities

Holland personality types

Postmodern career counseling

Social learning theory

Career education

Computer-assisted guidance system

Historically, career development has been the principal domain of counselors. It is through the process and techniques of vocational guidance that the counseling profession was first introduced and implemented in numerous settings. In recent years, however, there has been a gradual yet perceptible shift in emphasis from vocational issues to more personal and emotional concerns (Andersen & Vandehey, 2006). Career decisions are also looked at in a much broader developmental, relational context (Phillips, Christopher-Sisk, & Gravino, 2001; Schultheiss, 2003), and with a more culturally responsive focus (Flores & Heppner, 2002; Niles & Harris-Bowlsbey, 2009).

This means that when someone comes in to deal with some career-related issue, you will also likely end up exploring family, cultural, gender, and related issues that are part of the bigger picture of their lives.

You would only have to consider the complexities of your own career transition right now (yes, you are in the throes of a major life transition) in order to appreciate what must be done in order to work through this developmental stage to a satisfactory conclusion. You are studying to be a counselor and, as such, there are many side effects, ripple effects, and consequences as a result of this choice. Certain financial resources are sacrificed to pursue this dream, monies that could be spent elsewhere. Your family and friends are also included as part of this journey, whether they wish to be or not. As you learn and grow and make changes in the ways you think and behave, the effects have far-reaching impact on all your other relationships. It would thus be impossible to talk to you only about your ultimate career aspirations without delving into your relationships, your family, your financial situation, your personal values, and what gives your life meaning. That is one reason why career counseling cannot take place without considering the personal, familial, and cultural context for a person's choices and lifestyle (Jackson & Scharman, 2002).

CAREER DEVELOPMENT: A CASE EXAMPLE

The nature of how systemic, cultural, and gender factors influence career decisions are illustrated in the life of one of us (David) who briefly describes his personal story. You will see how some of the choices he made were inextricably woven with personal issues, involving his past growing-up experiences and his present significant relationships.

> I grew up in a small town where my parents were deeply involved in the civic life of our community, conveying to their children the value of service and "giving back." Consistent with the Jewish culture of first and second generation immigrants from Eastern Europe, they also strongly encouraged me—pushed would be a better word— to get the best education possible, and to set my sights very high. Whatever I did, I should be the best at what I do. Needless to say, I worked hard in school to get accepted to a good college, and once there, found I loved the experience. There was something about the academic life that I just felt at home with.
>
> At some point in college, I needed to think seriously about a career choice. I was torn between two choices: becoming a professor of English literature, which would have enabled me to continue to stay in college, more or less permanently. My second interest was in becoming a journalist for a small town newspaper, a vocation that would reflect the values my parents had instilled in me. I sought advice from professionals in both fields, and the two men I talked to both expressed how these careers led to nothing but low salaries and unhappy lives. I just accepted their counsel and gave up these dreams—only years later did I realize that both were particularly unhappy men whose personal pain was unrelated to their vocation.
>
> I happened to be a movie-lover, a passion also learned from my family experiences; every time a classic old film was on television, the whole family would get together and my father would rhapsodize over what made these films so great. One day, reading a news story about a famous director, I had a thought—I love movies—why not become a filmmaker? Even maybe a Hollywood director? I floated the idea to my parents, and

Time Out for Reflection

Note how already in David's story there are strong influences from his culture, gender, and parental values that "pushed" him to pursue particular paths. It is also significant that David consulted two mentors, both influential men in his life, who dissuaded him from following his own passionate interests.

they were delighted well beyond what I had expected; my father in particular was in heaven. It was as though I was going to fulfill some dream of his own.

After college, I got a masters degree in film, and embarked on a career path that I hoped would eventually land me in Hollywood. In my 20s and early 30s, I achieved some success as first an educational filmmaker, and then working for a company that produced movies for television. Meanwhile, I worked on my own screenplays, hoping one would launch me into "the big time." But there was one problem: I was miserable. I didn't know exactly why. Though I had glimmers that maybe I was pursuing goals that didn't fit me well, I didn't want to take a good look at them. Instead, I worked harder and harder in my film career, simultaneously developing a host of physical ailments—stomach pains, headaches, insomnia—you name a stress-related symptom and I had it. My wife insisted I see a counselor; I agreed, with the idea of finding a specialist in career counseling who could help me either enjoy the field I was in, or direct me to a different vocation.

Fortunately for me, the counselor appreciated the relationship of career to personal issues; with her help, I saw how I was trying to fulfill my parents' need to have a son who could reach beyond the small town limits of their lives and fulfill hopes and dreams they had given up. I was denying the part of me that loved university life. At the same time, I wasn't utilizing some of the best values I had learned from my family—values about making a life focused on helping people. Lest you think I had these realizations in a couple of weeks, let me be clear—the process of really looking at myself entailed quite a bit of struggle and tears before I finally felt ready to let go of this whole movie career fantasy. But once I did, my symptoms disappeared virtually overnight. A burden lifted. And after several sessions devoted to reviewing career options with my counselor, I knew what I wanted to do—become a counselor myself. My only hesitation was that counseling seemed like something women do, not men, while filmmaking was very much a masculine endeavor. One more issue to discuss with my counselor! By the following fall, I was clear in my choice, and enrolled in a graduate program in counseling.

But the story doesn't wrap up neatly here. A career change in what was now my late 30s inevitably shook up the status quo of my life. I needed my wife to support me financially and emotionally, and though she tried hard to do both, she also felt resentment at the burden I was placing on her. I tried to relieve the guilt I felt for not contributing financially to the family by writing scripts in between classes and studying; ironically, the scripts were well-received, film industry job offers started to arrive, and I ultimately found myself working a day job as a screenwriter while taking counseling classes at night. I was making money again, but neglecting my marriage. What saved us from splitting up were the skills I was learning as a counselor—my ability to empathically listen to my wife's feelings of resentment and loss, while taking responsibility for my part in contributing to them.

Eventually, I completed a doctoral program, but now again faced what would seem to be a tough choice: it would be impossible to do an internship and maintain

■ | TIME OUT FOR REFLECTION

You will recognize other themes that have emerged in David's narrative. Since pleasing his parents, especially his father, was so important, he found himself internalizing career aspirations that were not his own. It was not until almost 40 that he discovered how unhappy he was working in a job that provided status, but little in the way of satisfaction. No matter how miserable he might have been, he was still reluctant to seek help until such time that his body rebelled and his wife pressured him to take action. Again there are systemic factors at work that brought David to this point.

a screenwriting career at the same time. Something had to be given up. You know what? It was an easy choice. I knew from my work with my counselor what I really wanted to do with my life. I enthusiastically started and completed the internship, worked for several years as a counselor, and then applied for a university teaching position in counselor education. That's where I am today, happily, and expect to continue until retirement—although, I've learned that when it comes to careers, nothing is ever definite.

As you can see, there are numerous factors involved in David's career development, including his family's values, cultural values, lifestyle issues, exploration of career options in young adulthood, the positive and negative role models he encountered, issues of personal growth and psychological separation from family, midlife career change implications, gender role issues, marital issues, and, throughout, the need for honest self-reflection. The complexity of David's story, the shifts in career direction and the complicated family and personal issues that involved every chapter in his journey, is not unique. Indeed, in the 21st century, such complexity has become the norm. Keep this in mind as you study this field because, traditionally at least, many of the theories of vocational choice have tended to be rather limited and microcosmic in their view of human experience. They also have reflected a period of North American culture in which a person training for a stable life career was the norm, manufacturing and industry were primary employers, and discrimination against women and minorities was accepted. A number of changes have taken place as both scholars and practitioners are making efforts to adapt traditional theories and develop new ones that are much more reflective of diverse cultural populations and gender differences for both men and women (Flores & Heppner, 2002; Sharf, 2006; Zunker, 2006).

In spite of the changes taking place in the field, there is still a myth among many counselors that "real" counseling is personal/emotional and that vocational/career counseling is somehow a second-class cousin that requires fewer skills and is more "routine." This attitude is not only false but dangerous. As you will see in this chapter, much of your self-esteem and many of your needs are met by career activities. To achieve a modicum of personal fulfillment, you must participate in effective life/career planning. Individuals who experience vocational chaos (such as unemployment, underemployment, and job dissatisfaction) report high stress, relationship difficulties, and low self-esteem. It is likely that you have experienced these conditions as well at some point in your life, if not this very minute. You can therefore relate to the feelings of uncertainty, anxiety, and fear often associated with these changes.

VOICE FROM THE FIELD

I think if they ever really told us what the impact of going back to school would be on our families, friends, stress levels, and economic situations, many of us never would have continued. At first, it didn't seem to be such a big deal. I'll just take a counseling class or two. It's only a few nights a week. No big deal.

But it's not just the time commitment that is so disruptive—or even the extra financial burden. When you get into this field, you not only learn things, but you also change your basic values and attitudes. So much of what we do is about learning

and growth. It's all very exciting, too. The problem, though, is that sometimes people get left behind.

I come home from school all excited about the things I'm learning. I'm working hard to be more open, to express myself more often. But if my friends and family are still stuck in the same old routines, then it can drive a wedge in our relationships. Even worse, I've heard from lots of classmates how their families are really threatened by them going back to school. I can really see that, too. Any career change like this creates a whole lot more problems, just as it solves others.

THE FUNCTIONS OF WORK

"Rich man, poor man, beggar man, thief. Doctor, lawyer, Indian chief." From our first day at school, we became eligible for that eternal question from well-meaning relatives—that question that still plagues (and will always nag) us: "What do you want to be when you grow up?" As if we had to grow up to be something—or as if we wanted to be something we are not—or as if we had to grow up. But even Peter Pan lost that fight.

Work is supposedly what we have prepared, educated, and trained ourselves to do. Long ago we shed our existence as hunter-gatherers whose only job was to find enough to eat. Now we are specialized. Everyone, and I mean *everyone*, is engaged in some purposeful, productive activity. Some receive financial remuneration for their efforts—they sell their time and talent. Others work for internal rewards or receive other forms of compensation by way of a cooperative division of labor. But labor we all do. Even the children are working—mastering new skills, taking in new knowledge. They may sometimes work in places called playgrounds, but we are not for a moment deceived that these little people are not laboring away at their age-related developmental tasks. They are working their bodies, testing their minds, and learning about cooperation, competition, and a million other things they will later find useful after they "grow up" and work in a "real" job.

Work is more than a source of income. For most people, vocation is very much tied into their sense of identity, self-image, and self-worth. Jobs are a measure of status, a major object of devotion of one's time and energy. They are a testing ground for skills and information that have been accumulated over a lifetime. They are the source of many friendships.

People who are satisfied in their work are those who are often most content with their lives. Lonely, depressed, anxious, problem-ridden people—those who seek a counselor's help—are often those who are not content with their life's work, whether that role is one of homemaker, student, or corporate executive. Career frustration, job stress, and discontent with one's decisions and current vocational development are thus major preoccupations for many people and therefore a significant part of a counselor's work.

If you think back to a time when you were not engaged in meaningful work, when you felt unappreciated or understimulated, when you were frustrated or bored on the job, you are well aware of how this dissatisfaction affects every other aspect of your life. You are also probably aware of how bleak and hopeless the future can sometimes seem, how alone you feel in your struggles, and how confused you can be about which direction to take. If only there had been a counselor available to help you sort out your desires and goals, offer support and encouragement, and structure plans to make needed changes, it might have made a difference.

ROLES OF COUNSELING

If work is what you have to do and play is what you want to do, then a major goal of counseling is to teach people never to work a day in their lives. Some people are able to adopt an attitude that helps them to enjoy their jobs, to have fun, and to feel fulfilled. When the alarm clock rings, they jump out of bed, eager to begin their day. Yet others, working in an exactly equivalent position, feel only dread, boredom, and disgust with what they do for a living. Take the case of the Pickens brothers described by Terkel (1972) in his book, *Working*. Both boys have paper routes. They both get up at the same time and basically do the same things. Yet note how the difference in their attitudes about their jobs affects their perceptions. One boy plays; the other works.

CLIFF: It's fun throwing papers. Sometimes you get it on the roof. But I never did that. You throw the paper off your bicycle and it lands someplace in the bushes. It'll hit part of the wall and it'll go booooongg! That's pretty fun, because I like to see it go booooongg!

TERRY: I don't see where people get all this bull about the kid who's gonna be President and being a newsboy made a President out of him. It taught him how to handle his money and this bull. You know what it did? It taught him how to hate the people in his route. And the printers. And dogs. (Terkel, 1972, p. 161)

These different attitudes about the same exact job are indicative of the choices people make in how they treat their work. Some people are immensely satisfied; some are burned out. Counselors spend a lot of their time helping people, whether children or adults, to think and feel differently about what they are doing. Attitude is all-important in any activity, and certainly in one that can become as routine as going to work. The ultimate goal of almost every person, and therefore every counselor who is giving assistance, is to wake up with energy and excitement, with enthusiasm and anticipation for the day's events that lie ahead.

Counselors help people with career indecision on a number of fronts. Developmental problems such as career immaturity are resolved by exploring the client's interests and career alternatives and applying decision-making strategies. Situational problems such as job stress are worked on within the context of a supportive, problem-solving relationship to develop alternative responses. And chronic problems such as psychological dysfunctions are resolved in longer-term counseling to initiate more extensive personality changes. In each case, counselors strive to develop more positive attitudes, as well as to accomplish the following objectives.

VOICE FROM THE FIELD

I am a career counselor at a university career center. I like to joke that the reason I got hired is because I've had nearly 20 different jobs in just as many years, but only one real career. Having struggled with career issues myself, I can completely relate to someone who is lost and searching. Often, our careers are attached to our self-esteem and vice versa. Individuals are sometimes at their lowest during periods of unemployment or when they are lacking career fulfillment. Being able to explore with someone what they would like to be engaged in, and providing them the tools to achieve their goals, is satisfying. As a career counselor I receive lots of thank yous and I know immediately if I have helped someone. There is nothing more gratifying than to hear back from a student saying that

they implemented a strategy that I suggested and "they got the job."

On the flip side, sometimes I encounter students who are not willing to take the steps necessary to improve their situation. Many times, I will provide several different approaches which will help them only to find that they will have excuses why each one won't work. When I encounter someone who has a defeatist attitude, it is obvious that there are other personal and/or environmental issues involved which are holding this person back from reaching their goals. At these times, I try to be empathetic and hope that they will overcome their limitations (perhaps with personal therapy) and learn to move beyond them.

FACILITATING SELF-AWARENESS

The first step is to help clients discover what they really want and need—to become aware of what they value most. Many people who require career development assistance aren't exactly sure what is most important to them, or if they do know, they certainly haven't matched their priorities with their current work.

Clients may be asked, for example, to rank-order the following work values according to personal preference:

- long vacations
- opportunities for advancement
- big money
- security
- variety of tasks
- friendly coworkers
- creative opportunities
- physically active
- flexible hours
- lots of responsibility
- status
- independence
- minimum of pressure
- benevolent boss
- power
- chance to help people

This type of self-exploration, whether related to values clarification or other forms of increased self-awareness, helps people to continue the process of deciding what would be the most meaningful work and what options are realistic given their skills, abilities, interests, and opportunities.

BECOMING FAMILIAR WITH THE WORLD OF WORK

Whatever structure is used—a Career Day, guest speaker, reading and research, online computer dialogue, experimentation, on-site visit to a workplace, or even the use of stories with embedded work values—the stated task is to help people become more aware not only of themselves but also of career options that are possible (Andersen & Vandehey, 2006; Heitzman, Schmidt, & Hurley, 1986). A person might ask herself, "Given the parameters of a profession that allows me to work with people, use my verbal fluency, and structure my own time, what jobs are likely candidates?" or, "Which careers would involve being outside, using my creative energies, and moving around a lot?"

The *Occupational Information Network (O*Net)*, the online service developed for the U.S. Department of Labor, lists 949 job titles. Occupations can be searched using six different descriptors (worker characteristics, worker requirements, experience requirements, occupation-specific information, workforce characteristics, and occupational requirements). High growth professions can be accessed separately, with a full array of data regarding growth projections. Every job in the database can be examined in great detail, helping the searcher eventually narrow down the choices to realistic possibilities.

Because of the sheer numbers of available jobs and the complexity of matching aptitudes, interests, values, and required educational level to accurate career information, the use of computer career information systems has become widespread. These systems allow users to access job information based on education, values, interests, and other user variables, greatly simplifying the task of becoming familiar with the world of work. Although these career information systems are useful, they cannot replace a trained counselor who can assist the client in understanding, interpreting, and applying the information.

TEACHING DECISION-MAKING SKILLS

Because career development is an ongoing life process, it is hardly functional to focus only on finding a first job for a client. More and more often, people are making radical changes in what they do for work, sometimes enjoying two, three, four, or even more distinctly different careers during their lifetimes. People make decisions to try different careers for a number of reasons—early retirement, boredom, desire for growth, new interests, or in the case of women and minorities who have been closed out of certain sectors, new opportunities. In particular, many individuals at midlife are faced with the need to make career decisions; some do so for personal growth, whereas many others face forced career change because of structural factors in the workplace (Perosa & Perosa, 1987; Sullivan, 1999). Many companies have been taken over, with duplicate positions being eliminated. Budgetary issues have forced other firms into a reduction in workforce; some companies have eliminated entire departments in an attempt to sharpen their focus and reduce overhead; and some have simply gone out of business. In each of these cases, many high-performing individuals find themselves needing to make often unanticipated career decisions.

People must learn to make quality decisions about when and how they should initiate career changes. As we get older, more established, and more secure, taking new risks becomes increasingly difficult, especially because career decision making affects family dynamics.

The counselor can help by teaching people how to make intelligent decisions. The process often involves learning to collect and assess useful information, generating alternative courses of action and predicting their probable consequences, narrowing the field to a plan of action, taking risks, and dealing with the aftershock of change. The counselor is the one who helps organize this process.

TEACHING EMPLOYABILITY SKILLS

In challenging economic times, with limited job opportunities and increased competition in the marketplace, it is even more important to teach clients skills for adapting to a fluid and flexible work environment. Clients are helped to develop personal marketing strategies to sell themselves and their potential during interviews. They are also encouraged to work on overcoming inertia, resisting procrastination, relieving job-related stress, building an interpersonal support system, and avoiding feelings of frustration and failure.

In other words, the goal of all career-counseling efforts ought to be to provide skills for making and implementing decisions throughout the lifetime. How these decisions ought to be made and, in fact, how people even develop vocationally are topics of considerable debate. The key feature, regardless of the approach, is to help prepare clients not only to deal with the most impending career choice, but also to generalize this new knowledge and skills for the purposes of working through future issues in any domain.

LIFE COACHING

Nowadays, some counselors are taking on a far more creative and flexible role in order to facilitate career development throughout the life span. The specialty of "life coaching" differs from traditional counseling in a number of ways:

Counseling	Coaching
Past and present oriented	Future oriented
Identifies problems	Identifies skill deficits
Therapeutic role	Consultant role
Focus on thoughts and feelings	Focus on goals and dreams
Builds on strengths	Builds on weaknesses
Licensed professionals	Unlicensed and unregulated

Rather than having clients come to the office to talk about their career-related concerns, a life coach would most likely visit the person in the workplace or home.

For me life coaching is mentoring, passing on lessons I was fortunate enough to learn to those ready for them. I start by asking clients to define what success will look like for our work together. Next they identify their passions—"what they love to do." Next we clarify what is nonnegotiable in their professional endeavors. With this foundation we create job templates. Finally is the most important part—an action plan—what they are going to do Monday morning. I've learned if you don't have a definitive career path in mind, you can't figure it out in your head. It will evolve through the serendipity of interacting with people who either have jobs you want or know of people who do. As the Buddhists say, what's important is the journey, not the destination. Self-empowerment is the final ingredient. This is the part I enjoy the most—reflecting back the obvious talents and gifts my clients have and asking them to write down success stories to remind themselves of what they've forgotten.

The coach functions less like a therapist and much more like a personal trainer, consultant, and mentor. Very specific goals are identified. Action plans are set in motion. But rather than waiting on the sidelines for the weekly report, the coach follows up progress via the telephone, Internet, and personal visits. Although a relatively new field, it is gaining increasing legitimacy as a counseling specialty; it has a governing professional association, the International Association of Coaching (IAC); an ethical code; and the active support of Martin Seligman, one of the country's preeminent psychologists and former president of the American Psychological Association (International Association of Coaching, 2009; Wright, 2008).

THEORIES OF CAREER DEVELOPMENT

Here is just what you didn't need at this point—*more* theories. You've been introduced already to general theories of counseling, theories of development and learning, theories of group counseling and family counseling, theories of assessment and treatment. Now come more theories of career development. Before you are exposed to new names, new concepts, and new theories, remember that all of this is just designed to provide you the tools you need to help people navigate the complex, turbulent waters of work. Don't overconcern yourself with memorizing names and terms at this point; focus instead on the very interesting ways that have been devised to explain how and why people end up doing the kinds of work they do.

Just as there are a number of theories that attempt to explain learning processes, personality styles, cognitive development, abnormal behavior, social functioning, and models of motivation and change, so too are there varied approaches to vocational development that counselors are required to familiarize themselves with.

Pertinent questions may come immediately to mind:

- How do people make career choices?
- Which variables are most influential in making career decisions? What parts do genetics, the environment, and cognitive and emotional responses play in career development?
- What makes some people happy and others so miserable in their work?

- How does work fit within the larger context of life satisfaction?
- What roles ought counseling to play in the shaping of career development?

Clearly these questions need answering—if not for our own peace of mind, then to better enable us to help clients select fulfilling occupations and learn the skills for remaining satisfied and productive. As we review each of the major theories of career development, try to approach the subject with the same critical eye you applied to glean useful concepts from other counseling models. Look for concepts that make sense and help explain this complex process of development. Note the value and applicability of these ideas to your own career choices and confusions.

THEODORE CAPLOW'S THEORY

The first and certainly the simplest theory we will attend to is one based on the notion that career choices are random events, accidents, or errors resulting from being at the right/wrong place at the right/wrong time. The sociologist Caplow (1954) believed that birth order and the accidents of inheritance (parentage, race, nationality, gender, and background) strongly influence your chosen occupation.

When people are asked how they ended up in their current profession, their responses are often muddled. Answers such as these are not uncommon:

- "I don't remember. I always wanted to be an electrician. My dad is one. And his father was too."
- "My cousin got me this job, and it seemed kind of easy to stay with it."
- "I didn't really intend to go into psychology, but there were no girls in business administration. So, at orientation, I walked out the door and psychology happened to be across the hall."
- "I didn't have much choice. In our town there were only two options for a girl—waitressing and working in the mill."
- "I was just walking down the street when I saw this sign that said, 'Help Wanted.'"

Many of our life's decisions are affected by quirks of fate and the "roll of the dice." If we were to subscribe to a theory of random movement, however, there wouldn't be much point in having counselors to provide guidance and encourage self-responsibility.

DONALD SUPER'S THEORY

For Super (1957), a person's self-concept is all-important in determining vocational development, a process that he viewed as ongoing and orderly through successive stages. An occupation is the individual expression of one's interests and abilities at a particular time. As a person's preferences and skills evolve, so does his or her career, reflecting the changing self-concept.

Super introduced his theory in a series of 10 propositions (1953) about the nature of developing career identities:

1. People differ in their abilities, interests, and personalities.
2. They are qualified, by virtue of these circumstances, for a number of occupations.

3. Each of these occupations requires a characteristic pattern of abilities, interests, and personality traits, with tolerances wide enough to allow both variety of occupations for each individual and variety of individuals in each occupation.

4. Vocational preferences, competencies, situations, and self-concepts change with time and experience, making choice and adjustment a continuous process.

5. This process may be summed up in a series of life stages, characterized as those of growth, exploration, establishment, maintenance, and decline.

6. The nature of the career pattern (that is, the occupational level attained and the sequence, frequency, and duration of trial and stable jobs) is detected by the individual's parental socioeconomic level, mental ability, and personality characteristics, as well as by the opportunities to which he or she is exposed.

7. Development through the life stages can be guided partly by facilitating the process of maturation of abilities and interests and partly by aiding in reality testing and in the development of the self-concept.

8. The process of vocational development is essentially that of developing and implementing a self-concept; it is a compromise process in which the self-concept is a product of the interaction of inherited aptitudes, neural and endocrine makeup, opportunity to play various roles, and evaluation of the extent to which the results of role-playing meet with approval of superiors and peers.

9. The process of compromise between individual and social factors, and between self-concept and reality, is one of role-playing, whether the role is played in fantasy, in the counseling interview, or in real-life activities such as school classes, clubs, part-time work, and entry jobs.

10. Work satisfaction and life satisfaction depend on the extent to which the individual finds adequate outlets for abilities, interests, personality traits, and values; they also depend on establishment in a work situation and a satisfying way of life.

Super recognized that people differ in their personalities and unique strengths and therefore choose occupations that will permit them to use their competencies. The pattern of development begins during adolescence with the *exploratory stage*, in which a person uses fantasy, play, and role experimentation to help clarify the emerging self-concept, and moves tentatively onward in the early 20s to a first job. The *establishment stage*, through experimenting and trying out various options, helps the person to discover an occupation well suited to satisfy personal needs. The self-concept adjusts to fit the stabilized career choice. Stability may or may not last into the *maintenance stage*. During the 1950s, when Super was writing, there were far more opportunities and less mobility and economic pressure, and it was more the norm to continue evolving in a single career. In today's times of high unemployment, greater flexibility, and changing situations, the maintenance phase may involve a return to earlier developmental tasks in the search for personal and professional satisfaction. The *decline stage* is characterized, naturally, by dealing with reduced energy and trying to maintain one's position until retirement. Later in his career, Super (1990) saw counselors as aiding an individual's progressive development across the whole life span, helping to facilitate the maturation of ability, improving the self-concept, encouraging reality testing, expanding interest, and negotiating a compromise between fantasy and reality and between the various roles that are played throughout life.

JOHN HOLLAND'S THEORY

Whereas Super focused on self-concept, Holland (1973) believes that career choices are expressions of the total personality. Satisfaction thus depends on the compatibility of a person's work situation and personality style.

Holland rested his theory on four major assumptions:

1. Individuals can be categorized into six different personality types—realistic, investigative, artistic, social, enterprising, or conventional—depending on interests, preferences, and skills.
2. Environment can also be classified into the same six types and tends to be dominated by compatible personalities.
3. People search for environments in which their personality type can be comfortably expressed; artistic people search for artistic environments, whereas social people look for social environments. They wish to exercise their skills and abilities, express their attitudes and values, and participate in agreeable problems and roles.
4. The behavior of an individual is determined by the interaction between personality type and environmental characteristics. If personality type and work environment are known, the outcomes of vocational choice, achievement, and job changes can be predicted.

The six different personality types that Holland described predispose people to do well in certain careers that capitalize on their strengths. Certainly these personality types do not describe everyone, but they do provide a structure for understanding why some people do better than others in particular jobs. The following is a more detailed description of each type.

1. *Realistic.* This person is logical, objective, and forthright. Preference is given to dimensions such as physical prowess, aggression, and domination. A realistic type prefers activities in which to manipulate objects, tools, machines, and other tangible things. This person is likely to be emotionally stable but less sociable and inclined to select technical, agricultural, or trade occupations. He or she is practical and tends to have underdeveloped verbal and social skills but highly developed motor skills. The realistic person chooses careers such as laborer, farmer, carpenter, engineer, or machine operator. The realistic environment allows realistic people to perform preferred activities and be rewarded for technical abilities.
2. *Investigative.* By relying on intelligence and cognitive skills, this personality type is a problem solver. Socially aloof and introverted, the investigative individual prefers intellectual tasks that require academic proficiencies. He or she also tends to be analytical, critical, intellectual, methodical, precise, rational, and reserved. This person exhibits traits of creativity, independence, and self-confidence but is often not realistic or practical. Career choices for this type include scientist, scholar, research worker, and theoretician.

I know that many students don't much like their careers class. I probably never learned to hate it because I started doing it before I had ever had a vocational theory course. I came into it as a "career" by accident, learned about it by modeling other counselors and by doing it, and liked it because I was never subjected to being bored by it by a tired university professor who'd rather be teaching something else. I mean, wouldn't everyone rather teach anything but voc? I figured out on my own what was important in vocational counseling, and later had that validated by many of the theories when I finally began to read them. Also, by learning about it "from the trenches" I saw what was actually done in the real world, not what books said was done. In my experience, more than any other type of counseling, there is a big gap between what is done in career counseling and what books say is done.

3. *Artistic.* This is a sensitive, impulsive, creative, emotional, independent, and nonconforming individual who values cultural activities and aesthetic qualities. This person may develop competencies in art, drama, music, writing, and language and avoid structured situations. Not surprisingly, a creative type chooses careers such as actor, writer, musician, and artist.

4. *Social.* This person is highly skilled at dealing with other people. She or he is usually accepting, responsible, cheerful, nurturing, and caring. If you have noticed a similarity between this type and yourself or your classmates, it is because this category is most often descriptive of those who choose helping professions. Take note, however, because this type often evades intellectual or physical tasks, preferring to use strengths in interpersonal manipulations.

5. *Enterprising.* This person uses highly refined verbal skills for leadership and sales professions such as marketing, business, and politics. He or she is enthusiastic, energetic, dominating, persuasive, extroverted, and aggressive. Much concern is devoted to attaining status, power, and leadership roles. Some examples of enterprising vocations are business executives, salespeople, politicians, and promotional workers.

6. *Conventional.* This type of person prefers activities that are routine, structured, and practical. A conventional type is self-controlled, orderly, inhibited, and efficient. Examples of conventional vocations include bankers, bookkeepers, office workers, and clerks.

To a large extent, Holland believes that there is a real relationship between personality and educational/vocational decision making. He further believes that interest inventories are really personality measures. Members of a vocational group have similar personalities, and each vocation tends to attract and retain people with similar personalities.

Because people in a vocational group have similar personalities, they respond to situations in like ways and therefore tend to create characteristic environments. Vocational satisfaction, stability, and achievement depend on the congruence between an individual's personality and the environment in which he or she works (Holland, 1996).

Robert Hoppock's Theory

Hoppock (1976) stressed the function of the job in satisfying personal needs, but his theory has attained wide popularity also because of his efforts to integrate ideas from a number of other theories. Vocational development begins with the first awareness that a job can help meet one's needs and continues as the person is better able to anticipate how potentially satisfying a particular career could be as compared with others. Once a person becomes aware of other jobs that could satisfy personal needs, then occupational choices are subject to change. The degree of job satisfaction can be determined by assessing the difference between what a person wants from a job (emotionally, financially, and so forth) and what she or he actually has attained.

Hoppock describes his composite theory in 10 basic postulates:

1. Everyone has needs: basic physical needs and higher-order psychological needs such as self-esteem, respect, and self-actualization. People vary in the pattern of their need structures, and the individual reaction to needs influences occupational choice.

2. People tend to gravitate toward occupations that serve their perceived needs. A person who has a strong need for power and status will be influenced to seek occupations that have them. Few people are controlled by a single need; most have a variety of needs that act in concert to influence occupational choice.

3. Individuals do not necessarily have to have a clear intellectual awareness of their needs for those needs to affect occupational choices. Individuals with self-understanding and insight may understand the forces that influence them, and others may simply experience pleasure or satisfaction in certain occupational areas.

4. Life experiences help to develop a pattern of individual occupational preference and, as such, suggest a developmental perspective on vocational choice. Contact with occupations occurs both experientially and vicariously, supporting the need for both work or occupational experiences and occupational information, especially during the years of formative development.

5. Given the great diversity of occupational choices, the individual must develop effective decision-making skills based on solid self-awareness and a rich informational base. A trial-and-error process of occupational experimentation is usually not appropriate. The number of occupations and the extensive training many of them require preclude that approach.

6. Self-understanding is the basis on which occupational choice rests; thus it is a primary goal for career counseling.

7. Understanding the self is only half of the occupational choice process; one must also have accurate and thorough information about available occupations. A person cannot choose a career without the knowledge that it exists. Likewise, accurate information dispels stereotypes and myths about the activities involved in various types of work.

8. When a person's needs are met by a job, then he or she experiences job satisfaction. Money is not the only need satisfied by a job; other higher-order needs are just as crucial to satisfaction as basic security needs. For a worker to perform effectively and with the motivation to deliver quality, the ratio must

be positive. Industrial and assembly workers are often good examples of this principle: Although they may be well paid, many do not have higher-order needs satisfied; as a result, their performance on the job is low, the quality is erratic, and absenteeism is a problem.

9. Individuals can delay need satisfaction if they perceive their job as having the potential to satisfy their needs in the future. Opportunities for advancement and career mobility are, therefore, important if a firm wishes to maximize satisfaction.

10. If the balance between needs and satisfaction is unfavorable, then a worker will change jobs if another position appears to offer the potential to meet needs more fully.

In using Hoppock's theory of occupational choice, the counselor's role is to: (1) stimulate the client's self-awareness of interests and needs, including the clarification of values; (2) promote insight into that which gives life personal meaning; (3) provide accurate and complete occupational information; and (4) help match the client's perceived strengths and weaknesses with occupations likely to provide maximum need satisfaction. Hoppock's theory has a number of implications for counselors:

- The counselor should always remember that the needs of the client may differ from the needs of the counselor.
- The counselor should operate within the framework of the client's needs.
- The counselor should provide every possible opportunity for the client to identify and to express his or her own needs.
- The counselor should be alert in noticing and remembering the needs that the client reveals.
- The counselor should help the client gather information about occupations that may meet his or her needs.
- The counselor should help the client to anticipate how well any contemplated occupation will meet the client's needs.
- The counselor should stay with the client through the process of placement in order to provide the further counseling that will be needed if the desired job is not available.
- The counselor should follow up with the client some months after placement in order to see how well the job is meeting the needs that the client thought it would meet.

ANNE ROE'S THEORY

On the basis of her intensive investigations of scientists' early childhoods, Roe (1957) created a theory that emphasizes need satisfaction in career choices. Persons from child-centered, rejecting, or accepting homes are predisposed to compensate for (or duplicate) in their jobs experiences that they missed (or enjoyed) in their childhood homes.

Roe suggested that the emotional climate of the home is one of three types: (1) emotional concentration on the child, (2) avoidance of the child, or (3) acceptance of the child. Emotional concentration on the child has two extremes: overprotecting

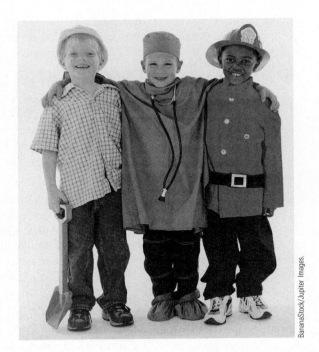

BananaStock/Jupiter Images.

According to Anne Roe's theory of career development, early childhood fantasies form a strong motive for later employment choices.

and overdemanding. Overprotecting parents limit exploration by the child and encourage dependency. Overdemanding parents set very high standards for the child and rigidly enforce conformity.

The avoidance type is divided into those ranging from rejecting to neglecting. A rejecting parent resents the child, expresses a cold and indifferent attitude, and works to keep the child from intruding into his or her life. A neglecting parent is less hostile toward the child but provides no affection or attention and only the bare minimum of physical care.

An accepting pattern is divided into casual acceptance and loving acceptance. Casually accepting parents are affectionate and loving but in a mild way and only if they are not otherwise occupied. They tend to be easygoing. Lovingly accepting parents provide much warmth, affection, praise, and attention. They encourage the child and help in an appropriate way.

These six subdivisions produce, according to Roe, two types of vocational behavior. The categories of loving, overprotective, and overdemanding tend to produce a major vocational orientation toward persons. The remaining categories—casual, neglecting, and rejecting—produce a major vocational orientation away from persons. The theory has generated considerable research, which has overall failed to bear it out. This may be in part because of misunderstandings and misinterpretations about what Roe intended (Brown, Lum, & Voyle, 1997). In any case, any theory that is more than 40 years old is going to have some problems being

■ | VOICE FROM THE FIELD

Why do I like vocational counseling? It's challenging. It appeals to the detective or investigator in me, sorting through data and theories to try to help someone get clarity about decisions they want to make. It's personal counseling, in the most personal sense. What's more personal than the work one invests one's life in? If work isn't going well, it impacts the person's life, not just their work. If it is going well, the same is true.

Probably on a personal level, it appeals to me because the goal is relatively concrete—clarifying, deciding, narrowing choices. I also like functioning in the role of an expert. A vocational counselor needs to be a bit of a frustrated research librarian because he or she needs to know a lot of information about the world of work. I like that, too.

applied to contemporary life without adaptations. Nevertheless, Roe is still responsible for calling attention to the ways that jobs fulfill needs that were not met in early childhood.

JOHN KRUMBOLTZ'S THEORY

Krumboltz (1978) developed a social learning theory that attempts to synthesize the factors that influence career decision making. First, Krumboltz acknowledges the impact of genetic endowment—how race, gender, cultural and physical characteristics, native intelligence, and abilities limit some choices and expand others. Not everyone can choose to be a professional basketball player, brain surgeon, or ballet dancer, regardless of motivation or interest. Second, environmental factors play a part in career development. The economic climate, occupational opportunities available, labor laws, union rules, technological developments, family resources, educational systems, and other variables outside the individual's control influence occupational decision making. Third, previous learning experiences (in behavioristic terminology, *conditioned stimuli* and *reinforcers*) shape the person's attitudes and interests toward various professions. Some children are reinforced by their parents for reading, others for their physical or mechanical skills.

A final factor to be considered, according to Krumboltz, is a person's "task approach skills," which are his or her performance standards, work habits, unique perceptions, and abilities to alter problem-solving strategies flexibly according to the demands of the situation.

Krumboltz summarizes the responsibilities of a counselor in the career development process as helping people to: learn a logical sequence of career decision-making skills; arrange a series of exploration experiences that will provide needed information; and make informed choices about the consequences of what has been learned.

Subsequent development of this theory has led to several other practical applications that can be used in counseling (Mitchell & Krumboltz, 1987; Zunker, 2006):

1. Career decisions should be based not only on present interests and abilities but also on others that can be developed.

2. Structured learning experiences can be customized for clients so that they can expand the range of their choices and opportunities.
3. Efforts should be undertaken to prepare people for a changing world in which new skills and abilities will need to be developed.
4. Career counseling should be integrated into all counseling efforts rather than just restricted to occupational choices.
5. Cognitive restructuring methods should be employed to help people to think differently about their choices and situations.

LINDA GOTTFREDSON'S THEORY

Gottfredson (2002) proposed a theory that differentiates itself from previous developmental models in three significant ways: (1) She perceives the decision-making process beginning as early as age 3, and in general emphasizes childhood and adolescence as key phases in exploring and choosing career options; (2) although she was not the first to stress the importance of matching a career to one's self-concept, she has looked at the role of the social self-concept—how one sees one's self in terms of gender and social class; (3) she believes that decision making is not so much a matter of finding what occupation best fits one's self-concept, but rather a process of rejecting possibilities, a winnowing away of unacceptable alternatives that ultimately concludes with a career choice in adolescence or in young adulthood.

Gottfredson termed the narrowing of interests children experience as *circumscription*, which begins in preschool and continues through the middle and high school years. The way in which children cognitively process their career thinking is linked to four stages of childhood development, each stage reflecting levels of growing cognitive complexity:

Stage 1: Orientation to Size and Power (ages 3–5). In the first stage, children are learning through observation about play and adult occupational activities. They see the world in dichotomous terms, big (adults) versus little (children); they note as well that big people, the ones who have jobs, are also the ones who hold power in children's terms. Preschool children are already beginning to think about careers, as they give up the fantasy goals of early childhood ("I want to be a princess when I grow up") in exchange for the occupations adults actually perform.

Stage 2: Orientation to Sex Roles (ages 6–8). In this stage, children begin the process of sex-role stereotyping and reject career options that appear incompatible with their own gender. Peer influences begin to exert pressure if a child begins to express interest in a career that is not considered "appropriate" for the situational/cultural context. A second-grade boy, for example, who talked about wanting to be a nurse (his mother was a nurse) was teased by classmates until he changed his preference to one that was considered more "manly."

Stage 3: Orientation to Social Valuation (ages 9–13). As children's cognitive processing becomes increasingly abstract, they are also becoming sensitive to issues of prestige and social class, and which occupations are associated with status among adults. The process of elimination continues, as early adolescents reject careers that are too low in prestige but also try to think in job terms consistent with the social class to which they belong. In the earlier example of the second-grade boy who said he wanted to be a nurse, the boy experimented with disclosing a number of other preferences—a "plane mechanic," an inventor of video games, a house builder. Even at his early age, he learned that he received the most approval from adults and peers when he said he wanted to be a doctor for children. Children in middle school and junior high school tend to express interest in career possibilities that not only match their interests, but also are infused with perceived status.

Stage 4: Orientation to the Internal, Unique Self (age 14 and older). At this stage, the decision-making process shifts from narrowing down choices to reflecting on which occupations match one's emerging sense of identity, abilities, interests, and values. Nevertheless, choosing careers that are gender congruent and adequately prestigious continues to be important. Circumscription is now replaced by *compromise*, as adolescents and adults find a balance between careers that fit their self-concepts and careers that are realistically accessible to them (e.g., enough jobs are available in that profession).

Understandably, Gottfredson's suggestions for career guidance begin with establishing elementary school programs that help children explore a full range of career possibilities while restraining them from engaging in the limiting process of circumscription. Throughout the school years, teachers and counselors need to discourage sex-role stereotyping of career options and facilitate more open and flexible attitudes regarding the fit between gender and vocations. Gottfredson's major concern is that children and adolescents will unnecessarily restrict their career options; a primary role of counselors is to ensure that individuals have not foreclosed on certain career possibilities because of lack of information or rigid thinking.

While research related to Gottfredson's theory has been limited, she is credited with filling important gaps in the career literature (Niles & Harris-Bowlsbey, 2009). In particular, the notions that the career decision making begins in the preschool years and that sex-role stereotyping is a significant factor in career choice are issues that may have continuing relevance for career-oriented program development and for career counselors in the exploratory processes they facilitate with their clients.

POSTMODERN THEORIES

Postmodern theories in general look at how we give meaning to both our inner worlds (thoughts, feelings, values, etc.) and to external reality: The *constructivists* emphasize how our minds make sense of reality, while the *constructionists* are interested in how meanings are created through the interactions of individuals (in particular via language) in the various social contexts (e.g., our culture, our families, our communities) in which we live. *Narrative* theorists focus on how we give meaning to our actions by creating stories—essentially plots of our lives in which we are the central characters. All three of these postmodern approaches share the premise that meanings are fluid—our subjective interpretations, meanings derived from social discourse, and meanings embedded in our personal narratives can all change. In contrast to the positivist paradigm that presumes the existence of an objective, measurable, and fixed reality, postmodernists argue that humans create their own reality and, by definition, can create different realities throughout their lifetimes (Brott, 2001).

Rather than try to match our specific skills with a particular vocation, a post-modern career counselor would want to explore with us the meanings we give to various careers, as well as how we define our own interests. A counselor may have a client whose father, a Latino immigrant, was an engineer in a city's public works system; the career of a civil servant was talked about as a secure hedge against the insecurities of life. The dominant social discourse placed high value on a union job that offers lifetime employment in exchange for a limited salary. Another client, growing up in a privileged home where high expectations of financial success were placed upon her, might have learned to devalue working in the public sector. In both cases, the counselor would want not only to explore how the client learned to ascribe meanings to different careers, but also to facilitate the client's discovery of what the client really wants, which may be consistent or in conflict with the dominant discourses of his or her childhood.

As a way of exploring "what one wants," the constructionist career theorists Campbell and Ungar (2004) recommend that clients focus on four tasks:

1. *Explore dominant story lines and preferred futures.* The dominant story line is the one we grew up with in our primary social environments, including home, school, and culture. Calling our career goal a "preferred future" emphasizes both the uncertainty inherent to life as well as an openness to inventive ways of experiencing the essences of our goals, even if we do not achieve our original career choice. They cite the example of a school board executive who wanted to become a veterinarian, imagining the latter career to be a more satisfying life. With the help of the counselor, the executive discovered that the essence she was seeking was to be of more tangible help to others, a goal she could achieve in a variety of ways, including in her current post. Envisioning her preferred future left open several paths to occupational satisfaction.

2. *Develop flexible goals that reflect positive uncertainty.* There is never one way to achieve a life goal, or, as narrative counselors would put it, write the next chapter in your own story. Clients need to be optimistic about finding career satisfaction while remaining grounded in the reality that they may require detours to get there.

3. *Explore creative ways of integrating seemingly multiple and conflicting discourses.* Within the various social contexts of our lives, we inevitably hear conflicting messages and themes about who we are and the nature of various occupations. Moreover, dominant social discourses may conflict with our personal life goals (e.g., our parents might want us to get an MBA and we want to become counselors). Clients to need sort out these various messages, and collaborate with the counselor in developing a storyline that makes sense to them.

4. *Develop a contingency plan of the alternative paths available for reaching their preferred futures.* Knowing that clients will most likely need to take a variety of paths to reach their preferred futures, counselors can help them explore backup plans for how to deal with the obstacles they encounter as they pursue their vocational hopes.

Within the postmodern camp, there are a variety of schools, all with different as well as overlapping emphases. Common to all of these ways of thinking is a belief that humans are agents of their own life and responsible for converting intention into action (Chen, 2006); that the meanings we ascribe to vocations cannot be understood outside the various social contexts in which we live; and that the role of career counselors is to facilitate not only clients' understanding of the source of their views regarding various occupations, but also clients' understanding of the value they give to their own skills and dreams.

CAREER EDUCATION

Direct counseling service is only one way that counselors provide help to people; as with other specialty areas, practitioners are also called on to function in the roles of consultants and teachers. Career education, career development, and vocational assistance are lifelong processes that often require supportive services at various developmental levels. It is an ongoing process that has crucial significance in elementary, secondary, and postsecondary schools. In addition to professionals who work in school, college, and university settings, rehabilitation counselors are also involved in career education programs, most of which have several components:

1. *Every learning experience has career implications.* Career education must be accepted as an institutional responsibility rather than a function of the counseling and guidance staff.
2. *Skill training is necessary for entry into an occupation.* Educational experiences should have a work-related skills component attached to them. Counselors should be ready to work with clients and other professionals to structure appropriate skill-related activities.
3. *Cognitive and experiential ways must be provided in order for students to understand work-oriented values.* The counselor must help the student to gain self-understanding, knowledge of alternatives, awareness of values, and decision-making skills in both cognitive and experiential ways.
4. *Opportunities must be provided for observing work environments.* Individuals must have the opportunity to develop experiences and knowledge about the world of work. Counselors can coordinate with students, employers, and educational institutions to create these opportunities.
5. *The interrelationships among home, family, community, and societal values should be identified.* The impact of these values on career decisions and preferences needs to be clarified.

Each of these general components requires the assistance of counselors who provide information as needed, consult with other personnel, and structure activities and experiences designed to facilitate career awareness, self-understanding, and occupational information.

ABILITIES

Individuals must have an understanding of their abilities in order to identify potential areas for job exploration and career development. In order to participate fully in the career development process, people must recognize both the need to develop basic academic skills and the need to maximize potential abilities. In an era of rapidly changing technology and job obsolescence, the task of identifying abilities will extend well into the adult years. Most adults will confront periods of unemployment in their lives, and practically everyone will experience work adjustment problems at some time or another. A thorough understanding of abilities, including needs for remediation, will be helpful to both students and adults as they participate in the career development process.

INTERESTS

A knowledge of interests (and the personality tendencies they suggest) will be helpful to individuals as they attempt to match aptitudes with available occupations. Interests are often the key to occupational satisfaction; people whose interests are not represented in their occupational choice can suffer much unrest and dissatisfaction. It is also important for the counselor to emphasize that abilities and interests are not always neatly related and that interest alone is not a sufficient condition for job satisfaction in positions requiring abilities that the client lacks.

VALUES

Values are an important factor affecting career development. Occupations that reflect values similar to those held by clients can lead to greater job satisfaction, especially with regard to motivation and job performance. The ill-defined or poorly defined values of many clients can interfere with effective decision making. Counselors must help clients to clarify their values and relate them to abilities and interests. Clients who are aware of the relationship among values, interests, and aptitudes can be described as vocationally mature and more likely than others to experience job satisfaction and career advancement.

CAREER DECISION MAKING

See Companion DVD
A Career Center

In some ways, career development—and certainly career choices—can be viewed as a decision-making process. Clients who are unable to integrate knowledge about the self with occupational information will make sporadic progress in career choice. Helping clients to develop refined decision-making skills is an essential dimension of occupational assistance.

Some clients will come to career counseling aware of the skills involved in decision making. For others, knowledge may be absent or fragmentary, requiring the counselor to assess the client's level of decision-making skills and provide appropriate information. Most decision-making models contain several specific steps:

1. *Defining the problem.* The counselor helps clients explore various aspects of a stated vocational issue. Specific counseling skills are used to elicit information, establish priorities, and crystallize salient points. It is essential that sufficient time be spent on this step because it will set the tone for future progress. Problem identification may need to be done at several stages in the process.
2. *Finding and using information.* Once the vocationally related problem is identified, the counselor assists the client in gathering useful information.

Sources might include testing; occupational, vocational, and educational information; and a computer-assisted job search. The counselor must also help the client to use the information in an appropriate manner by interpreting tests, clarifying misunderstandings, and generating conclusions.

3. *Creating alternatives.* In this step, the counselor and client combine forces to identify as many alternatives as possible. Those that are clearly inappropriate are excluded, and the remaining alternatives are examined in the light of information on aptitudes, interests, values, and availability.

4. *Developing plans.* In this stage, plans that may be either tentative or firm, depending on the client's needs, are developed. The planning stage should be detailed and sequenced and should have contingencies built into it. This is a crucial step in decision making because it translates the information into action-oriented steps.

5. *Implementing plans.* Implementing and following through on plans are primarily the responsibilities of the client, although the counselor should be available for consultation and support. Sometimes clients experience difficulty at this stage, and the counselor should intervene to determine whether there are flaws in the plan or whether personal counseling is needed.

6. *Evaluating plans.* Evaluation helps the client to determine the effectiveness of the decision-making process and to feed results into a new problem formulation. Counselors should emphasize to clients that they are ultimately implementing a process as much as a specific decision. Vocational decision making is a lifelong undertaking that requires continual refinement and development.

Counselors must be familiar with the decision-making process both generally and specifically as it is applied to career decision making so they can identify particular problems in a client's decision-making style. Career counseling, however, must focus not only on decision-making skills but also on techniques to correct the embedded or underlying difficulties in making decisions. For example, a family systems approach may be appropriate for individuals whose pattern of enmeshment interferes with career decision making; for others who exhibit irrational beliefs and attitudes, cognitive restructuring may be indicated. Career counselors must be flexible and insightful as they diagnose the multiple variables affecting career decision making and be versatile in designing treatment approaches for specific problems.

The process of career education and vocational choice is highly complex. Counselors can help clients to perform this crucial lifework in a systematic and objective fashion, providing information and assistance at critical points. The ultimate goal of career education is to assist individuals in optimizing their resources and in making vocational choices that are likely to lead to job satisfaction and career development.

TRENDS AND ISSUES IN CAREER COUNSELING

The world of work is rapidly changing and evolving, requiring major adjustments on the part of the labor force and vocational counselors. For example, there is little doubt that the fundamental nature of our society has changed from an industrial base to an information base. Whereas once upon a time our economy was driven by the manufacture of tangible goods, other countries (China and India, for example) are becoming the world's new industrial powers—while the marketplace in the United States and other Western nations is increasingly dominated by service-oriented jobs. Outsourcing of thousands of jobs to foreign countries, free-trade agreements between industrialized and developing nations, the explosion of the Internet and other means of worldwide instantaneous communication—all are part of the globalization phenomenon that is changing irrevocably the vocational options available to us. Amid these dramatic shifts in our economic structure, two classes of workers are emerging: (1) skilled and specialized service, professional, and technical workers who form an elite and highly employable class, and (2) an underclass of workers without employable skills (Brown, 2007). These forces are likely to create technical problems and labor shortages in addition to the human problems created by dislocations. Vocational counselors must be ready to respond to all of these issues, particularly those involving retraining and the use of technologically dense systems.

Changes in the Workplace

The ways we function in our jobs change almost every year. If we look only at ways we communicate the written word, we can appreciate how quickly we are forced to adapt. For decades, business documents were typed by secretaries, who were in great demand if they had rapid typing skills. When computers and word processing software replaced typewriters in the 1980s, that demand shifted from typing abilities to mastery of word processing and spreadsheets. In the 1990s, fax machines replaced the mail as the quickest vehicle for document delivery, which in turn were replaced by email, but you still had to be at your computer to send and read them. In the 21st century, texting and smartphones like the BlackBerry and the iPhone changed all that, enabling us to write to one another as we walk across campus, down corridors, and along sidewalks. As we write this very chapter, corporations are in a desperate competition to develop new technologies for transmitting the written word.

Similarly, as the pace of change accelerates, many workers are likely to experience unemployment and job elimination because they were unable to adapt quickly enough. Career guidance professionals will have major responsibility for helping workers who become occupationally obsolete to cope with the stress of transition and dislocation and to develop marketable skills through retraining and retooling.

As women increasingly enter the workplace, counselors must be aware of issues pertaining to sexual harassment, salary inequities, dual-career families, and the need for child care. Estimates of sexual harassment, for example, have found it to be widespread (11,000 incidents were reported in 2005 alone), resulting in damage at both the individual and the institutional levels (U.S. Equal Employment Opportunity Commission, 2006). Career counselors must develop educational programs for women to assist them in responding to these and many other issues as they gain equality and opportunity in the workplace.

Additionally, career counselors must recognize that the majority of the new workers entering the labor market will be women and immigrants. These groups are overrepresented in areas experiencing the least amount of growth and are less prepared educationally for the fastest-growing segments of the labor market. This change illustrates the challenges for career counselors who must develop programs to improve the educational and employability levels of these new job seekers. Innovative procedures must be developed in response to the career development needs of women, minorities, and immigrants.

WORK AND LEISURE

As productivity increases through the application of technology to work, efficiency is likely to increase, meaning that people will be able to work fewer hours (even if they are not yet choosing to do so). In fact, productive work may become a relatively scarce resource. To compensate for decreased demands of work, individuals must develop the skills and abilities to use leisure in a manner that will be personally fulfilling.

Work and leisure must be seen not as antithetical but as psychologically related aspects of a career. Career counselors must recognize the importance of leisure as they help clients to engage in life/career planning that will include creative and fulfilling ways in which to use their time. Leisure can be used effectively once the misperception of leisure as nonproductive is eliminated. Some of the productive uses of leisure might include alternative ways of seeking fulfillment, techniques for managing discretionary time, and resources for reducing stress and maximizing consciousness. Leisure, then, must be seen by the vocational counselor as a companion concern to work.

CAREER COUNSELING IN HARD TIMES

During the latter part of the first decade of this century, a devastating economic crisis reverberated across the globe, bringing about massive job losses, the eradication of people's savings and investments, and a climate of prolonged financial anxiety in both developed and developing countries. Although severe, this crisis was not the first time Americans experienced such a downturn: a painful recession occurred in the early 1990s, an even more severe one swept the United States in the early 1980s, and the Great Depression of the 1930s persisted for over a decade. We can reasonably predict that at various points in your career, there will be other downturns, and your counseling skills—whether as a career specialist or mental health practitioner—will be sorely needed.

Much of what we know about how individuals and families are affected by economic hard times comes from a longitudinal study of Iowa farmers who lost their fields and jobs in the 1980s farm crisis (DeAngelis, 2009). Conger and his colleagues (Conger, Conger, Elder, & Lorenz, 1992) videotaped and surveyed struggling families and identified a painful downward spiral: Falling incomes led to stressed-out parents, whose relationship became strained, thereby transmitting their stress to their children. The parents' emotional reactions to their economic plight (e.g., depression and anxiety) also adversely affected their parenting abilities. As the children suffered, their school performance declined, ultimately leading to less rewarding jobs when they entered the work force as young adults. These findings have since been replicated in a number of other studies, involving different populations (Conger & Donellan, 2007; Scaramella, Neppl, Ontai, & Conger, 2008).

Shallcross (2009) informally surveyed professional counselors during the most recent economic crisis, listening to their reports about their clients who still had their jobs. The theme that emerged was these individuals were experiencing a damaged work-life balance: clients were putting in longer hours and scared of being perceived as dispensable. Moreover, the email-based interconnectivity of our wired age meant they never felt they could risk detaching from their jobs and focusing on other areas of life.

Clearly, if ever there is a time when a counselor's services are needed, it is during economic hard times. Career counseling skills remain valuable, as laid-off clients learn to use their forced down-time to explore alternate career goals, perhaps discovering new and more satisfying interests. Counselors can also teach clients new job-seeking skills, while being mindful of the fact that job opportunities are realistically limited.

Here are some more suggestions of how counselors can be helpful in hard times (Christensen, 2009; Rollins, 2009):

- Teach relaxation techniques to reduce the stress of being out of work or looking for jobs in a scarce market.
- Explore with clients where their meaning and identity come from, helping them to differentiate the meaning that comes from career versus from family or other important life pursuits.
- Attend to their marital/partnership and family relationships, which are frequently stressed during difficult economic periods.
- Help them develop effective coping strategies and monitor the potential for self-destructive coping (e.g., substance abuse).
- Facilitate the expression of grief, as they come to terms with the reality of career loss.
- Above all, instill hope. Remind clients that a crisis by definition comes to an end, and out of crisis new opportunities, for both career pursuits and personal growth, can emerge.

THE IMPACT OF TECHNOLOGY

Computers and the Internet have already affected career and vocational counseling more than any other specialty within the counseling and guidance field. Increasingly, academic institutions are utilizing computer-assisted guidance systems (aka CAGS), which are capable of providing every service traditionally offered by career counselors, including the dissemination of information, vocational testing, computer-generated interpretation of tests, databases for searching for job information and opportunities, and advice on vocational planning, résumé writing, and interviews (Brown, 2007; Niles & Harris-Bowlsbey, 2009). Some of the most widely used CAGS are the Career Information System (CIS), Guidance Information System (GIS), DISCOVER, and CHOICES.

CAGS do require the involvement of a human counselor for assisting clients in using these systems effectively, and they are expensive, so only organizations like universities can afford them. More so than CAGS, it is the Internet that raises the question of what will be the role of career counselors in the future (and whether there will be a role). All the things CAGS do can be found somewhere on the Internet, if one learns to search for them. Sites (e.g., monster.com) initially developed as online databases of employment opportunities now enable any computer user to take vocational assessment tests online and receive helpful advice on a variety of matters related to finding a job. Traditional vocational tests like the Myers-Briggs, Strong Interest Inventory, and Kuder Occupational Interest Inventory can be taken on the Web, usually for a small fee. Even the U.S. government has gotten into the act, with the creation of O*NET, an immense database of occupational titles that also allows users to "crosswalk" (link from one database to another).

Nevertheless, career counselors need not change vocations and start seeking career advice themselves. There are many things that neither CAGS nor the Internet can do, but real human beings can do very well:

- Only human career counselors can provide a supportive environment for individuals struggling with a career decision. The key word here is "struggle": It is important to remember that the decision-making process can be an emotionally difficult one—for some, leading to intense distress—and only a trained counselor can provide the calming presence and empathy required for reducing a person's anxiety.

- Difficulties with choosing a career are often rooted in underlying emotional issues, which only a counselor can detect. Paying attention to a client's nonverbal behavior, for example, can provide clues that signal to the attentive career counselor that other issues besides vocational ones need to be explored. In some cases, the counselor will make the decision to refer the client for therapeutic counseling.

- Effective career decisions cannot be made without looking at the contextual factors in a person's life—for example, how a specific choice is likely to impact one's role in the family or how other family members will be affected. Counselors can help clients explore their career goals as part of a more comprehensive portrait of both their immediate life situation and their overall life dreams.

- While computers can administer and even interpret tests, only a career counselor can help a client explore the meaning of test results; it is the exploration process as much as it is the test results that facilitates a discovery of satisfying career possibilities.

- A career counselor can guarantee confidentiality regarding the data clients report when taking inventories or completing other instruments; the Internet, on the other hand, is not a secure environment.

- Finally, only humans can pat you on the back and say, "Don't worry. It's going to be OK. We'll work together to find something that fits for you and then develop an action plan so you can land that job."

It is still crucial, however, that counselors are highly skilled in the use of computers and other technologies, which will only become more sophisticated and effective as tools that can assist counselors in their work. The National Career Development Association (NCDA), a division of the American Counseling Association, established knowledge competencies in 1997 that still remain relevant:

1. Counselors need to have knowledge of the various computer-based guidance and information systems as well as the services available on the Internet.

2. Counselors need to know the standards by which such systems and services are evaluated (by organizations like the NCDA).
3. Counselors must be able to ensure that computer-assisted guidance is conducted ethically.
4. Counselors need to discern which clients are likely to profit from computer-assisted guidance.
5. Counselors must be able to evaluate and select computer guidance systems that meet local needs (NCDA, 1997).

SUMMARY

In this chapter we have examined the value and diversity of career counseling. Almost every client you ever see, for whatever presenting complaint is brought into session, will have career issues that are directly or indirectly related to the initial concerns. So much of life's meaning and a person's sense of worth is related to career satisfaction. Even if you never specialize in this aspect of counseling you will still regularly assist clients with the ongoing choices they make about what they do for work, and how they process these experiences.

The importance of career counseling will only increase with the impact of technology on our society. The counselor's role in a high-tech society is to help individuals assimilate the effects of change, thereby allowing them to develop to their fullest potential.

SELF-GUIDED EXPLORATIONS

1. List some of the most helpful things that people have said to you in your life regarding work and careers.
2. What are some of the things people have said to you about work and careers that have not been very helpful?
3. The circumstance in which you presently find yourself—taking a counseling class—is the result of a number of forces and factors that have affected you in particular ways. Describe as many influences as you can identify that have shaped your conscious and unconscious choice to be where you are now.
4. Counselors often use guided visualizations to help people identify their goals. Here's a simple one you can do to connect with your personal career fantasy. Sit in a quiet, dark space, with minimal distractions. Close your eyes and focus on your breathing for about two minutes. Just notice whatever physical sensations you

experience as you inhale and exhale. Next, imagine you are walking down a hallway, with a door at the end. Imagine yourself opening the door, and on the other side of the door, you can see yourself engaged in a work activity in the place where that kind of work would occur (e.g., a counseling office). Most important, this person—you—is feeling wonderful as she or he is engaged in this task. The feeling could be joy, peace, excitement, fascination, contentment—any positive feeling that comes up for you in your visualization.

What did you see yourself doing? Was it what you expected? Or something different? Even if this image of yourself is not how you ordinarily imagine your future, there might be information in your visualization that will give you some fresh insights.

5. Rank-order the factors that would be most important to you in a job.

_____ Variety of tasks

_____ Supportive coworkers

_____ Subsidies for further education

_____ Good salary and benefits

_____ Opportunities for creativity

_____ Job security

_____ Minimum of pressure

_____ Excellent supervision

_____ Promotional opportunities

_____ Lots of responsibility

_____ Attractive office

_____ Freedom of movement

How have these rankings helped you decide what you will focus on when you look for a job after graduation?

FOR HOMEWORK

Talk to several different people of various ages and socioeconomic backgrounds to find out what it is about their work that they find most and least satisfying. List the principal factors that you discovered are most significant.

PBS has broadcast excellent biographies of American presidents in their series *American Experience*, and all are available on DVD. View any one of these. Two especially compelling ones are *FDR: An American Experience* and *Harry Truman: An American Experience*. Notice the complexity of Franklin Delano Roosevelt's or Harry Truman's career path. What forces—social, cultural, and psychological—shaped their career choices and circuitous paths to the presidency?

SUGGESTED READINGS

Anderson, P., & Vandehey, M. (2006). *Career counseling and development in a global economy*. Boston: Lahaska Press.

Brown, D. (2007). *Career information, career counseling, and career development* (9th ed.). Boston: Allyn & Bacon.

Capuzzi, D., & Stauffer, M. (2006). *Career counseling*. Boston: Allyn & Bacon.

Colozzi, E. (2009). *Creating careers with confidence*. Upper Saddle River, NJ: Prentice Hall.

Gibson, R. L., & Mitchell, M. H. (2006). *Introduction to career counseling for the 21st century*. Upper Saddle River, NJ: Pearson Prentice Hall.

McMahon, M. (2006). *Career counseling: Constructivist approaches*. New York: Routledge.

Niles, S. G., & Harris-Bowlsbey, J. (2009). *Career development interventions in the 21st century* (3rd ed.). Upper Saddle River, NJ: Pearson Merrill/Prentice Hall.

Shahnasarian, M. (2005). *Decision time* (3rd ed.). Alexandria, VA: American Counseling Association.

Sharf, R. S. (2006). *Applying career development theory to counseling* (4th ed.). Belmont, CA: Brooks/Cole.

Terkel, S. (1979). *Working*. New York: Avon.

Zunker, V. G. (2006). *Career counseling: A holistic approach* (7th ed.). Belmont, CA: Brooks/Cole.

CHAPTER 12

ADDICTIONS COUNSELING AND PSYCHOPHARMACOLOGY

KEY CONCEPTS

Addiction

Drug culture

Prevention programs

Medical model

12-step programs

Therapeutic model

Cybersex

SSRIs

Benzodiazepines

PROFESSOR: So, in our last discussion, we talked about where you could work with your counseling degree, and at the end, you were feeling a little confused. Getting clearer now?

STUDENT: I think so. I'm beginning to see myself actually doing counseling. So I hope you're not going to ask me another one of your elliptical questions.

PROFESSOR: Ah, you know me well. So here it is. What do the substances people get addicted to, and the drugs psychiatrists prescribe, have in common?

STUDENT: Hold on! You're not telling me that the drugs that people take to destroy their lives are no different than antidepressants! I strongly disagree with that.

PROFESSOR: And well you should. Pharmacological drugs can save lives. No question about that. But try to answer my question.

STUDENT: Well, I'll go with the obvious first. You can get addicted to both?

PROFESSOR: Not a bad answer, but not quite accurate. For example, some people get addicted to alcohol, but most don't. Some of the psychopharmacological agents, antianxiety medicines in particular, are highly addictive, but lots of others are not.

STUDENT: How about this one: All of these drugs get "pushed"—drug dealers push street drugs, corporations sell you alcohol and cigarettes, and pharmaceutical companies push their pills with advertising.

PROFESSOR: There's a lot of truth there. But we also need to be careful to distinguish between illegal activities and businesses' need to market effectively their legal products. Let me ask you a question by posing a question.

STUDENT: Uh, oh. Here you go again. I knew this would happen.

PROFESSOR: All of these substances, legal and illegal, helpful and destructive, answer the same question millions of people ask themselves every day. What we need to know is, what is that question?

STUDENT: I'm really confused now.

PROFESSOR: The question is: How can I change the way I feel? So many people can't get through a day without feeling stress or depression; so many struggle with their emotions day in and day out, and are desperate to fix their pain. Maybe it's the times we live in. Maybe its genes and biology. Maybe a little of both. We just don't want to feel what we feel. And we reach for something—sometimes anything—as a solution. Unfortunately, the answer for too many of us is ingesting highly addictive substances that have terrible side effects and consequences. For others, legitimate medicines prescribed by psychiatrists or family doctors are the hoped-for answer. It's the question that remains the same.

THE PERVASIVE CONDITION OF ADDICTION

Almost everyone has some kind of addiction—if not to drugs or alcohol, then to gambling, cigarettes, risky behavior, exercise, television, computer games, the Internet, adult videos, work, shopping, and so on. The key issue here is not just whether you are addicted but if that attachment interferes with the satisfaction and productivity of life.

There is probably no presenting complaint that will be brought to you as a counselor that is more common than some form of addiction—and quite likely none that you will find more frustrating to treat. The incidence of addiction to drugs and alcohol is staggering, estimated to cost the nation billions of dollars alone in economic loss, not to mention the debilitating effects on physical, social, and family life (Doweiko, 2009). One out of five Americans has five or more drinks per day, and over 23,000 die in a year from alcohol-induced illness (U.S. Department of Health and Human Services, 2008). The use of the violence-inducing drug methamphetamine, which can be manufactured from cold medicine plus chemicals you can buy at any hardware store, has quadrupled since 1992; child welfare workers throughout the country are increasingly placing children in foster homes because of the meth use of their parents (National Association of Counties, 2005).

When you add to substance abuse problems the many other addictions common to contemporary life (computers, video games, excessive exercise, eating disorders, workaholism, etc.), you can appreciate the magnitude of the problem. Increasingly, for example, more and more people are becoming hooked on the Internet, with Americans spending over 12 billion dollars a year on Internet pornography alone (Young, 2008). As with any other addiction—from excess television viewing to abusive levels of daily exercise—these problems are often chronic, intractable, and even life-threatening.

SYMPTOMS OF ADDICTION

An addiction is defined as a persistent, chronic, and intense focus on a single behavior pattern that feels (or is) out of control. Whether in the case of a drug or an activity, there are a number of symptoms in evidence (DSM-IV-TR, 2000; Stevens & Smith, 2008):

1. Persistent and frequent thinking about the activity throughout the day
2. Significant interference with enjoying other important aspects of life
3. Inability to control, cut back, or stop the behavior, even after becoming aware of debilitating effects
4. Restlessness or irritability when attempts are made to cut back the behavior
5. Feelings of anxiety or agitation if behavior is stopped for a period of time
6. Use of the addiction to escape or avoid other responsibilities
7. Dishonesty or exaggerations when reporting the incidence of behavior, minimizing the problem to self and others
8. Engaging in high-risk behavior that jeopardizes emotional or physical safety
9. Intense mood swings associated with the activity, ranging from euphoria to shame, guilt, and depression

It is no wonder that addiction counseling is one of the fastest-growing specialties in the field, spawning its own professional associations (International Association for Addictions and Offender Counselors, National Association of Alcoholism and Drug Abuse Counselors), its own certification bodies, and journals. In addition, self-help groups proliferate around the world to provide needed support systems—not only the familiar Alcoholics Anonymous, but also hundreds of other groups devoted to one addiction or another. Finally, as our prisons become overcrowded with people whose only crime is drug possession, states may increasingly turn to substance abuse programs as a less expensive alternative to housing drug offenders in jails. Voters in Arizona, California, Hawaii, and Washington, D.C. have all passed initiatives mandating that first- and second-time nonviolent drug possession offenders can receive treatment instead of incarceration; this trend may lead to increasing job opportunities for counselors skilled in working with addictions (Drug Policy Alliance, 2003).

Among the various addictions that you will encounter as a counselor, surely treating alcohol and drug abuse will be among the most challenging. This will be the case not only because of the physically addictive properties of mind-altering substances but also because our culture is so steeped in drug-related behavior. In fact, three of the most common substance addictions in our society actually have their own institutions devoted to supporting the behavior: coffee houses, bars, and cigarette breaks.

VOICE FROM THE FIELD

There's nothing my counselor could have done to help me when I was using. [Laughs.] There's nothing anyone could have done. And a whole bunch of people tried, I gotta tell you. [Laughs again, but he's not smiling.] I was in detox I don't know how many times. I was in and out of I don't know how many places. I saw more people like you than you could imagine. They all did their best, I know. Shit, I felt sorry for 'em all. That's why I played their games and all. I knew what they wanted—what they wanted me to tell 'em. So that's what I did.

So what did it take? Hey, good question. I guess that's why I want to be a counselor now to figure it out. I don't think anyone really knows. I think with me it was just that I hit bottom. Nothing left to lose. I had no money left to score. Couldn't risk gettin' caught again stealing stuff. My friends were sick of me, my good friends anyway; I always had buddies I could get high with. Who knows? Maybe some of the counselors did help me. Kind of a delayed reaction. [Laughs.] I do know, though, that when I got ready to get clean, that was it! I've never looked back since.

DRUG USE AND DRUG ABUSE

Everyone without a drug habit, raise your hand. Now, let those who are smugly confident that they hold nothing in common with your basic drug addict (and so are holding their hands quite high) consider the following:

1. A drug can be any substance ingested into the body that produces an altered state of consciousness or change in body chemistry.
2. Andrew Weil (1972, 1998), a noted pharmacologist, and Michael Winkelman (2001), an expert in shamanic counseling, have theorized that all humans have an innate drive to alter their consciousness. From spinning in circles as children to eating spicy foods as adults, the goal is to experience sensory overload. For some people, it is stimulants like coffee, amphetamines, or even chocolate that light their fire; others prefer to medicate themselves with "downers" like alcohol or Xanax.
3. Drug use not only is common among human beings but also is found among other creatures. When animals in Africa are subjected to crowding, poaching, and other stressful conditions, they resort to intoxicants. Elephants will munch fermented fruit. Grasshoppers will literally get high (given their jumping prowess) after eating marijuana. Peruvian llamas are fond of cocoa leaves. Rats, when given choices between plain water and alcohol, prefer the booze, especially at bedtime.
4. The difference between drug use and drug abuse is a matter of degree (see Figure 12.1). Once a need for drugs has been established, in order to maintain

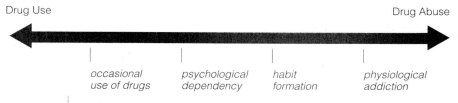

FIGURE 12.1 | CONTINUUM OF DRUG BEHAVIOR

VOICE FROM THE FIELD

I was working with a client determined to go "cold turkey." And she had good reason to be serious about this; years of alcohol and cocaine abuse had damaged several internal organs. Her physicians had made it plain—stop or die. Wanting to stop and being able to stop are not the same; as strong as her fear of death was her fear of what life without drugs would feel like. This woman had underlying chronic anxiety, depression, and ADHD, and her drug use had pretty effectively masked these symptoms. Plus, her evening buzz was the one thing in life that she looked forward to, and helped her get through her dreary day job.

I devised a multifaceted treatment plan that would make her day something to look forward to without the help of booze and coke. I did vocational counseling, exploring with her jobs that she might actually enjoy. She learned meditation to relax and the effects of walking in nature to soothe her over-stimulated system. Time at the gym gave her an endorphin rush, and some pride in her newly buff body. But the most helpful intervention turned out not to be any of these traditional interventions. Listening to her complaint about losing the ritual of the after-work drink, I suggested we invent a nonalcoholic, not-too-sweet cocktail that would allow her to maintain her nightly ritual. It was some weird mix of sparkling water with various flavorings, and she loved it. And I learned to appreciate how important the ritual of drinking was to the person who had been sipping alcohol at the end of the workday since she was 18.

effective functioning, addiction and physiological dependence prevail. The most widely used (and probably abused) drugs are those that happen to be legal. Coffee, cigarettes, chocolate, and cola beverages all contain sufficient quantities of amphetamines to create full-fledged addictions.

5. Almost every person alive has some oral addiction, and the world is filled with regional choices. Whereas alcohol has permeated every known culture (except that of the Eskimo, who live in a climate too cold to grow anything), more exotic drugs are found in every region. Cocaine originated in the Andes of Peru and Bolivia, coffee and hashish in southern Arabia, peyote in Mexico, opium in India and Mesopotamia, and, of course, tea in China.

It may now be evident that most people ingest drugs in some form, whether as food additive, beverage, medication, or intoxicant. Although the biological mechanism underlying drug use is not clearly established, one theory suggests that drugs have psychomotor stimulant properties that activate positive reinforcement mechanisms within the brain. This results in pleasurable sensations that are more powerful than those occurring naturally (Kalivas, 2003).

There are many factors that determine whether a person can safely and responsibly use drugs (such as an occasional cup of coffee or glass of beer) or will abuse addictive substances (heroin, for example) or become psychologically dependent (as is common with marijuana). Counselors are often required to work with these various forms of drug use and to make a determination with the client as to which behaviors are self-destructive and out of control.

The subject of drug use and abuse merits its own chapter in an introductory counseling textbook for a number of reasons. First, most people, and especially clients who tend to be externally controlled, regularly use drugs in some form. Often alcohol, marijuana, coffee, tobacco, or excessive food is a troubled person's effort at self-medication for distressing symptoms. The externally oriented addict denies responsibility for problems, blames others for experienced misery, and feels that, because someone else has created the emotional pain, an externally available substance will fix things. The unfortunate part is that such a person is perfectly correct. Drugs do provide immediate relief. They dull pain and are great distracters. While using drugs at moderately abusive levels (whatever that means), people can still function through their day in a purple but painless haze. (See Table 12.1, which illustrates reasons for drug use and abuse.)

Many people engage in mood-altering behavior to create a sense of euphoria or well-being or to block out unpleasant events. Counselors must recognize that drug taking is a behavior and follows patterns that can be understood and modified to the same extent as any other. The behavior will persist if it minimizes discomfort or maximizes pleasure and satisfaction. Nothing will decrease the hold of drugs unless there is an adequate substitute for the feelings drugs provide. Counselors need to assess and observe a client's behavior to determine whether the client is displaying symptoms of abuse and reliance on mood-altering substances. A final reason for studying drug counseling is that our knowledge of what causes addiction and what treatments are effective is continually expanding. Indeed, for both researchers and drug counselors, the field has stirred up widely divergent views. Some argue that no treatments have been proven to work, while others cite studies demonstrating the efficacy of one or more interventions. Traditional therapeutic interventions have been tried with varying success, as well as have highly dramatic and creative interventions. The adherents of the 12-step approach assert that addiction is a spiritual disease and only participation in AA and similar groups make change possible (Vaillant, 2005). Other experts will tell you that 12-step programs have never been proven to work (Stevens & Smith, 2008).

TABLE 12.1 | REASONS FOR DRUG USE AND DRUG ABUSE

Why People Use Drugs	Why People Abuse Drugs
Euphoria	Biochemical predisposition
Availability	Physical addiction
Cultural exposure	Maintenance of intoxication
Pain suppressant	External control
Boredom	Habituation
Rebellion	Social reinforcement
Entertainment and curiosity	Poor self-image
Enhancement of reality	Addictive personality
Peer pressure	Escape
Stress reduction	Impulsivity
Social lubricant	Instant gratification
Self-medication	Few perceived options

■ | Voice from the Field

I've never understood how people in our field can have such disdain for addicts. Sometimes, you hear them made fun of and all. You see, there's basically two kinds of drug counselors: those who are recovering addicts themselves but who don't have much formal training, and people like me who have a degree but no direct experience as an addict. Sometimes, it feels like war in that each group thinks they have more credibility. Obviously, though, both points of view are valid. But I don't think you need to have been a drug addict and lost everything in your life in order to know what it feels like to be out of control. I think almost everyone knows that feeling. I think all of us, at one time or another, have had a problem with impulse control or whatever.

I'm pretty disciplined about a lot of things in my life. I eat right and exercise regularly. I never got into the drug scene and I don't drink very often. But still, I don't know what I'd do without my lattes and all. You can laugh, but I'm serious. I just don't think I could give up coffee for anything. Maybe that doesn't sound like a big deal, but it does give me an idea of how hard it would be to quit. And I use this to understand clients better. That's why I don't judge them so much.

There are those who see addicted clients as difficult, resistant individuals, typically in denial of their problem—which results in a situation that requires counselors to remain constantly on the lookout for manipulation and trickery (Craig, 2004). Another school believes that patient, compassionate, person-centered interventions are the only kind that have a chance of truly helping (Blume, 2005). Thus, drug counseling is a specialty rife with controversy, which makes it incumbent that counselors stay current with the research as well as make their own choices as to how to conceptualize both clients and their treatment.

OUR DRUG CULTURE

People are constantly encouraged to purchase drugs to feel better and to buy products that help with weight loss. The implicit—if not explicit—message is that comfort and ease are of maximum importance. There is little glorification of the hard work or discipline involved in maintaining a healthy body. Advertising has clearly had some impact on drug use in our society. Ads on television and in other media promise to make you feel happier, younger, sexier, more attractive, and less tense. They persuade people to buy over-the-counter drugs as a means of relief from suffering and to create a desirable personal image. Advertisements clearly imply not only that the use of these drugs will create wonderful results but also that the drugs are harmless.

Although legislators try to keep current in providing protection for the consumer, our society continues to approve and even encourage use of substances such as caffeine, alcohol, and tobacco. Although the latter is becoming less than fashionable these days in North America, its use is increasing in other parts of the world. The acceptance of alcohol as an appropriate drug by all citizens over a certain arbitrary age encourages the development of a milieu in which drug use is considered normal.

Almost all drugs are available to adolescents, not only on the street but also on the school grounds. It is not uncommon to find younger teens sniffing glue and older ones digesting prescription stimulants and highly-addictive painkillers during school hours (National Institute on Drug Abuse, 2009). Marijuana use is so prevalent among adolescents that it is often considered normal by school officials. There is also frequent use of methamphetamine ("meth" and "crystal meth"), especially in the Southwest, Northwest, and upper Midwest, although nationwide its use appears to be slightly declining (Prah, 2005).

Depending on the setting in which you practice, and the specific population that you work with, you must educate yourself about the various substance abuse problems that will be most common. This will alert you to watch for physical signs (fatigue, sleep disturbances, confusion); emotional symptoms like mood fluctuations, unprovoked hostility, and uncooperativeness; interpersonal signs such as hanging out with deviant groups; and those symptoms related to impaired work or school performance (Windle, 2001).

EFFECTS OF DRUG ABUSE

There are many negative physical effects that result from drug abuse. These symptoms are in addition to the relationship casualties that usually occur as the abuser alienates friends, family members, and coworkers.

1. Death has to be at the top of the list. Reports of drug overdoses occur in the newspapers so routinely that they are no longer news. Suicide is certainly a distinct possibility for a person in an altered state of consciousness, and it is not unknown for people to die from convulsions while withdrawing from barbiturates.
2. Through neglect, disinterest, and distraction, the diet of a drug abuser often suffers. Many drugs tend to stifle the appetite; other drugs (narcotics, alcohol) lead the user toward malnourishment.
3. Disturbances of sleep are common results of introducing artificial stimulants or depressants into the bloodstream. Certainly anyone who has had a few cups of coffee before bedtime or who has fallen asleep while still feeling the effects of alcohol knows that the quality of sleep is impaired. The loss or disruption of sleep presents added dangers for the drug abuser, whose perceptions and reactions are already less than optimal.
4. Many other physical symptoms can develop as a result of long-term drug use. Naturally, after foreign substances are ingested, the body reacts. Some problems are the result of the ways in which the drugs are introduced into the body. For example, nasal damage results from repeated snorting of cocaine, lung damage has been reported in marijuana smokers, and skin disorders occur in those who inject heroin. A variety of musculoskeletal, respiratory, gastrointestinal, and central nervous system disorders are also possible— even likely—after long-term drug or alcohol abuse. In addition, almost every system of the body is affected: Neurons are destroyed, neurotransmitters are sidetracked, genetic material is altered, and disease is more likely.

ADOLESCENT DRUG USE

Many counselors interpret the drug abuser's behavior within the context of family dynamics. The family is sometimes stabilized in its distraction by and attention toward the abuser's behavior. The family has its scapegoat. And the abuser has feelings of control, at least over making others feel powerless. Everyone continues helplessly along, unable to break the destructive patterns that bind the family members together.

The significance of such early use of drugs relates to the development of crucial social and personal skills in adolescence. This is a difficult time, and drugs are an available way to ease pain and discomfort. Unfortunately, they also increase anti-social behavior, block completion of normal developmental tasks, and sometimes lead to the development of a deviant lifestyle. Frequent drug abusers often appear as withdrawn, alienated, and generally unhappy.

The frequency and intensity of adolescent drug use are of concern to the counselor. Early identification, treatment, and support are crucial to reducing the negative effects of drug and alcohol use in the next generation. Adolescent drug users present a troubled profile to counselors. They are unable to invest in or derive pleasure from personal relationships, work, or school or to direct energy to future goals.

Working with adolescents on drug abuse and alcohol use is sensitive and complex, requiring counselors to provide a nonjudgmental, supportive environment while simultaneously attending to the client's resistance. Treatment approaches can be outpatient, inpatient, and residential, although inpatient treatment appears to be the least often utilized. Outpatient treatments tend to involve 12-step programs, cognitive-behavioral interventions, and family therapy, which can reduce levels of denial, shame, resentment, guilt, anger, and insecurity (Burrow-Sanchez, 2006). In some cases, adolescents are placed in long-term residential programs or "therapeutic communities," where they can be monitored 24 hours a day; and in addition to receiving individual and group counseling, they can develop support networks among their peers, which can play a role in the treatment (McNeece & DiNitto, 2005).

PREVENTION

Although treatment of substance abuse receives considerable attention, it is through prevention efforts that counselors can have the best potential to affect alcohol and substance abuse problems. Prevention programs are especially important in schools because substance abuse often begins with school-age experimentation. Early and frequent prevention activities can provide the needed knowledge and skills for children to learn alternatives to substance use and abuse. Because students find counselors to be creditable resources, there is an opportunity for counselors to broaden and expand their involvement with primary prevention in the school.

In designing prevention programs, counselors need to determine whether the program is *primary, secondary*, or *tertiary*. Primary prevention programs are designed for adolescents with little or no experience with substances, secondary prevention targets beginning users, and tertiary programs work with the experienced, highly abusing, or dependent teen (McNeece & DiNitto, 2005). Prevention programs can focus on alcohol and drug education, social resistance, and social skills training. Focus should be directed toward understanding the reasons why people use drugs, especially variables like self-confidence, self-control, and impulsivity. Prevention programs designed to help build skills can be an important aspect of what counselors do.

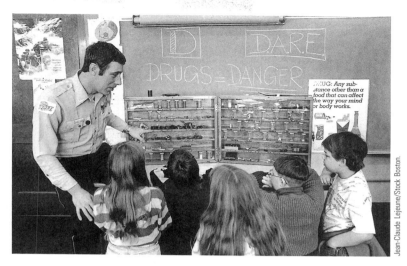

The best way to deal with substance abuse problems is a prevention program that equips children with the necessary attitudes and skills that will immunize them against future addictions.

Effective prevention programs have the following characteristics:

- They go beyond simple information sharing and publicity about substance abuse.
- They include parent and family involvement.
- They are long-term commitments, not Band-Aid approaches.
- They are integrated into a holistic concept of healthful living.
- They are closely connected with positive school climates.

Involvement with prevention activities provides the counselor with multiple opportunities to influence the substance abuse problem at the earliest stage before it becomes a negative factor interfering in the lives of adolescents and adults.

THE FUTURE IS NOW: NEW ISSUES IN COUNSELING

INTERNET ADDICTION

Earlier in this chapter, we defined addiction as a pattern of behaviors that could be applied not only to substance use but to activities as well; increasingly, researchers are labeling a variety of activities or behaviors as potentially addictive, including gambling, overeating, sex, and shopping (Griffiths, 2001; Kottler, Montgomery, & Shepard, 2004). Many of the DSM-IV-TR's criteria for substance dependence can also be applied to behaviors, and the DSM establishes a precedent for the existence of behavioral addictions by including pathological gambling as a mental disorder (DSM-IV-TR, 2000). In the 21st century, one of these self-destructive behavioral patterns that counselors are likely to encounter is Internet addiction.

For many of us, surfing the Internet has become as much a part of our daily lives as turning on a TV or listening to music; computers with Internet access are in our homes, dorms, offices, schools, hotels, cafes, and libraries. The latter two locations make it possible for even the most economically disadvantaged to get on the Web. When the Internet was first developed in the late 20th century as a government and academic tool for exchanging knowledge, did its founders ever imagine the day when people would suffer from Internet addiction? Yet, that is exactly what appears to be happening, and counselors are increasingly reporting seeing cases of Internet addiction in their offices (Mitchell, Becker-Blease, & Finkelhor, 2005). Internet addiction can impair lives, destroy relationships, and tear apart families in the same way that substance abuse can; you are likely to face many clients in your practice whose lives are being negatively impacted by their need to surf.

For most of us, the Internet remains simply a source of entertainment and information; addicts, on the other hand, may spend 40–80 hours a week on the net, with sessions lasting up to 20 hours. They may also surf well into the evening and early morning hours, resulting in fatigue-related school and job problems. Particularly at risk are college students, who may have unlimited, free Internet access in their dorms as well as large blocks of time in which to surf (Young, 2004).

According to Young (2004, 2008), the diagnostic criteria for Internet addiction are similar to those for substance abuse. Counselors would assess by asking the following questions:

1. Are you preoccupied with thoughts about going online?
2. Are you spending increasing amounts of time online?
3. Have you unsuccessfully tried to cut back your hours online? If you do cut back, do you feel moody, depressed, or irritable?
4. Is your Internet use jeopardizing your relationships, schoolwork, or job performance?
5. Are you lying to others about how much time you spend on the net?
6. Do you go online as a way to escape other problems?"

While there are several forms of Internet abuse (e.g., online gaming addictions, compulsive Internet shopping), arguably the most serious problem in terms of affecting mental health is cybersex—addiction to seeking, perusing, and possibly masturbating to online pornographic imagery. Cybersex can cause emotional distress (guilt and/or anxiety) and seriously impair intimate relationships, whether the user's engagement in pornographic surfing and viewing is excessive or minimal (Mitchell, Becker-Blease, & Finkelhor, 2005; Philaretou, Mahfouz, & Allen, 2005; Young, 2008).

What makes cybersex so compelling? According to Carnes, Delmonico, and Griffin (2001), there are six components that cause any kind of media to lure our attention; all forms of media contain one or several of these, but only Internet pornography contains all six. It is Intoxicating—users get a feeling of euphoria; Integral—Internet access is so integrated into our lives, it is impossible to avoid; Inexpensive—most people can afford monthly service charges, or have free access; Interactive—we can use a mouse to go to the next screen or respond to other Web site commands; Imposing—the amount of pornographic sites and images appears virtually unlimited; and Isolating—we can view pornography in private, without having to visit the adult section of a DVD store or bookstore. Another theory is that cybersex becomes a compulsive quest for a sexual image that is a perfect match for the viewer's internal fantasy visualization of love. When the match is found, the gratification is so fleeting and disappointing that the cybersex addict embarks on the search once again (Philaretou, Mahfouz, & Allen, 2005).

Delmonico (2002) developed a treatment protocol for cybersex addiction that would seem to make sense for any kind of Internet overuse.

- Counselors need to help users reduce access to their computers. For example, you can suggest they move the computer to a spot where others can see them watching.
- Counselors must help their clients recognize they have a problem, and make the cybersex addiction a central focus of their treatment.
- Counselors can explore with them to find out if the Internet is being used to self-medicate for depression or anxiety. If so, addressing these issues, as well as providing a psychiatric referral for possible medication, would be appropriate. Similarly, issues like grief and loss, shame and guilt, or childhood traumas may underlie the addiction and may need to be explored.
- Counselors should bring in the family so they can be part of the recovery and support effort.
- Counselors can help clients explore their sexuality and find other means of expressing it and seeking gratification.

Some kind of spiritual faith—a client's connection to an organized religion or a belief in a higher power—can be of help in the same way that 12-step programs frequently are helpful as an adjunctive element of substance abuse treatment. Throughout the process, counselors need to make sure they create a collaborative relationship with the cybersex addict; it is essential that counselors reflect upon any negative judgments they may have regarding sexual addictions, as well as examine their own behaviors and temptations when it comes to Internet surfing.

PRINCIPLES FOR COUNSELING THE CHEMICALLY DEPENDENT

MEDICAL MODEL

Historically, alcoholism was considered a moral problem, by both the medical field and society in general. In some ways, it still is. Have you ever passed a drunk panhandler in the street, and walked briskly passed him, making no eye contact as he begged for money? We have all done this, and chances are we made a snap negative judgment about this person's character. In the medical field, however, the moral model changed dramatically in the 1950s and 60s because of the work of E. M. Jellinek (1952, 1960), a physician who argued that alcoholism should be viewed as a disease, similar to diabetes or cancer. More recently, two lines of research have lent some support to biological models: (a) Gene studies have indicated that some individuals may be born with a propensity for becoming alcoholic. Schuckit (2000) has argued that 40% to 60% of an individual's risk for alcoholism may be the result of genetic inheritance, and more recent research has found biochemical markers in the human body that predict a genetic predisposition (Peterson, 2005). (b) Research in brain chemistry has suggested that substance abusers may have lower levels of neurotransmitter dopamine receptor sites than the normal population, and may therefore have an innate propensity for experiencing pleasure from

VOICE FROM THE FIELD

I'm consistently struck by how self-critical—that's being too mild—how self-hating so many of my substance abuse clients are. It's painful and terribly sad to listen to them describe themselves as failures as parents and partners, disappointments to their own parents, and hopelessly defective as human beings. I can see how externalizing their drug addiction, seeing it as biological illness rather than one more piece of evidence of being weak and flawed, offers a little relief.

Yet, I can't help thinking of this one client, a man in his 40s, who consistently needed me to validate his belief that his abuse was a medical problem, not a psychological one. I gave him the validation he sought, but it was a trap; every time I said, "Yes, you have an illness and we can treat it," he heard it as, "I don't have to deal with the damage I've done to my family and friends. I couldn't help it." It's a very tricky dilemma for me as a counselor; on the one hand, I don't want to confirm his worst view of himself, and on the other, I don't want to collude with responsibility-avoidance. I can see this will be a struggle for me so long as I work with this population.

certain addictive substances (Doweiko, 2009). Neither of these research avenues suggests that biology is the sole cause of substance abuse, but rather a predisposition that may be exacerbated by family conflicts, peer pressures, or other life stressors.

These new views of alcohol and substance abuse have had a profound impact on treatment implications. In the medical model favored by many hospital, mental health, and clinic settings, the abuser is helped through a detoxification program that may include forced abstinence, intensive psychotherapy, family support groups, social skills training, and possibly medications to help with withdrawal symptoms. Acamprosate, Antabuse, and naltrexone, as well as some antidepressants (Prozac, for example), are prescribed drugs that may help some alcoholics stay sober and prevent relapses (Anton et al., 2006; Herbeck, Hser, & Teruya, 2008). They are, however, effective only if the person agrees to take the preventive drugs on a regular basis and can live with the side effects. As such, their usefulness is limited. Medications are more likely to be helpful depending on how long the person has been drinking excessively and whether therapy or counseling are used as supportive adjuncts (Swift, 1999). In the medical model, treatment can take place on an inpatient and outpatient basis. However, the preponderance of research evidence points to such outpatient approaches as cognitive behavioral therapy and the person-centered motivational interviewing model as more effective than inpatient treatment and deliverable to the client at a fraction of the personal and monetary cost (Miller, Zweben, & Johnson, 2005). Because the medical model approach absolves the client of responsibility for his or her condition, the counselor works intensively on issues related to self-control and compliance to the prescribed program. Efforts are also directed toward helping clients understand the full implications of recovering from a chronic "disease" or genetic predisposition. You may read this and have an instinctive negative reaction to the idea of "absolving the client of responsibility." But if you put yourself in the shoes of these clients, you can imagine how much better you would feel about yourself as a person if you thought your addiction was caused by genetics or brain chemistry instead of your being a bad person. Proponents of the medical model would argue that removing addicts' shame and guilt for their problem makes it more likely they will seek and make good use of treatment. For the counselor, conceptualizing addiction as a disease can make it easier to maintain a nonjudgmental stance toward clients, a core condition for successful outcome with this population just as it is with any other kind of person in counseling.

AA/NA Model

The Alcoholics Anonymous/Narcotics Anonymous (AA/NA) model has become such a widely used component of addiction treatment that it is essential that counselors understand what it is all about and are familiar with 12-step language. Arguably, a professional treatment plan for a substance abuser should contain referral to a 12-step group, despite the fact that this model is both controversial and lacks strong empirical support. While AA began in the 1930s specifically to help alcoholics, the 12-step model has grown to the point that today there are specific groups for almost every kind of addiction, including narcotics, overeating, and gambling.

This model is somewhat compatible with the medical approach in that the abuser is labeled as helplessly addicted forever unless complete withdrawal is initiated. Unlike the medical model, however, advocates of AA and similar programs view substance abuse as a spiritual problem, characterized by an addict's false pride, self-absorption, sense of entitlement, and, most prominently, determination to deny the very fact of addiction. Consequently, a core emphasis of 12-step programs is the addict's acceptance of a "higher power," a belief critical to addressing the addict's spiritual void. Because addicts tend to maintain the narcissistic attitude that they are the center of the universe (similar to how a child sees the world), accepting the existence of a higher power requires letting go of this belief (Doweiko, 2009). Such acceptance is also a humbling experience, and advocates of the model believe that humility is necessary for spiritual recovery. Belief in a higher power, however, is only the first step in recovery; 12-step models insist that addicts make major changes in their attitudes and behaviors toward others. Despite the model's view that addicts are helpless against their disease, taking personal responsibility for one's recovery remains a central focus.

Twelve-step programs are similar to therapy groups; participants speak from the heart about their struggles with addiction and receive support from group members. Anonymity is crucial in facilitating participants' feelings of safety when making painful confessions. Each member is assigned a "sponsor," a group member who is available 24 hours a day for support and guidance. Recovery requires addicts to complete all 12 steps, and relapse necessitates going back to the beginning. Addicts are never actually cured, but remain "in recovery" their entire lives. Use of any mind-altering substance, including physician-prescribed medications, is considered a return to addiction. You will hear clients say things like, "I'm 9 years in recovery" or "5 years sober"— statements that reflect their appreciation that sobriety is a life-long struggle. Clients may tell you they are "working the program" (going through the steps) or simply are "in program" (participating in a 12-step group).

Working with abusers requires familiarity with the 12 steps, given the likelihood that your client will be either a current or past participant in a group. Stevens and Smith (2008) have divided the steps into five components. First (steps one through three), addicts must accept their helplessness against the disease of addiction, appeal

VOICE FROM THE FIELD

It's a funny thing, this whole substance abuse counseling business. You've got to be very careful what you do, and how you do it. I'm not talking about with clients but within the community. A lot of what we do in counseling is in direct opposition to what they do in NA or AA. Here we're trying to teach people they can take control of their self-destructive patterns, and AA groups often teach them to turn over the control to a Higher Power. They can't help the way they are and so should turn themselves over to God. For some people, this is an outstanding plan. They take like ducks to water with the 12-step program. But other people just drop out, and they get really confused with the messages they get in counseling versus those they get at AA.

to a higher power for help with recovery, and honestly acknowledge their personal limitations. Second (steps four through seven), addicts must undergo rigorous self-examination, making a personal inventory of all the ways they have harmed partners, family, friends, and coworkers. Addicts also must begin to own the feelings that they had used substances to suppress and self-medicate. The third component (steps eight and nine) is that addicts actually make amends to those they have hurt, thereby restoring damaged relationships and relieving shame and guilt that may underlie the addiction. Fourth, addicts must regularly attend group meetings. Some AA members will attend weekly; others attend almost every day. When traveling, they go to meetings in that city. Finally, addicts need daily affirmations to assist in their lifelong process of recovery. They are encouraged to memorize phrases like "One day at a time" or "Let go and let God" (Stevens & Smith, 2008).

Two criticisms of the 12-step model are most salient. One is the rigidity of the model: its insistence that (a) it is the only effective path to recovery; (b) addicts must abstain from all substances for the rest of their lives; (c) addicts must accept the higher-power concept. Second, 12-step programs' emphasis on external control may conflict with the values of therapeutic counseling. Participants may learn to substitute one form of dependency for another: Whereas they may no longer abuse drugs or alcohol, they nevertheless must go to meetings in order to maintain the cure; indeed, research suggests that 12-step programs are only effective when participants attend meetings at least weekly and remain committed to long-term participation (Fiorentine & Hillhouse, 2003; Johnson, Finney, & Moos, 2006). It is for this reason that individual counseling can be even more helpful in conjunction with AA and NA programs, giving focus to issues of autonomy, independence, and self-control.

Counselors need to be familiar with local AA/NA resources and to make referrals in a manner likely to result in client attendance at a meeting. It is also extremely important that the work you do in counseling complements rather than opposes the 12-step programs. Riordan and Walsh (1994) suggest several guidelines for making referrals to AA:

1. *Whom to refer.* Most clients, except those with significant pathology, are appropriate referrals.
2. *Making the referral.* An AA referral should be based on a complete assessment and a recognition that outpatient treatment is indicated. Support should be offered so the client does not feel rejected.

3. *Timing the referral.* A referral should be made as soon as practically possible. Often a referral at a point of reduced denial is useful; for example, following a binge or other adverse consequence.

4. *Be aware of labeling.* Many clients are offended by the label of alcoholic. Consider neutral ways to refer to the problem without glossing over real issues. Also consider that while abstinence is often preferred (and a requirement of AA/NA), some clients can manage with controlled use.

5. *Personalize the referral.* It is helpful to have materials available and give written instructions on how to get to the meeting; the client might even make the first contact from the counselor's office. Establish a follow-up session after the initial referral to process the experience.

6. *Prepare the client.* Help the client to understand what to expect and explain the difference between a religious and spiritual program. Emphasize the anonymity of the meeting. Encourage the client not to make a decision about involvement in the first one or two meetings. Be aware of the variety of meetings, times, and locations. Each meeting has a distinctly different "culture" and composition. Warn clients that they may need to visit a half-dozen or more different meetings to find one that feels right.

7. *Attend meetings.* It is useful for counselors to attend "open" meetings to get a more complete understanding of the AA experience.

Occasionally, some clients will not be well suited for AA because they don't care for the religious emphasis or are unwilling to engage in complete abstinence. Fortunately, alternative programs are available. In the case of those who want the benefits of a more secular support group, a number of other groups exist such as Secular Organization for Sobriety (SOS) and Self Management and Recovery Training (SMART). For those who are interested in reducing their drinking but not stopping altogether, they may find assistance at Moderation Management or DrinkWise.

THERAPEUTIC MODEL

See Companion DVD
Motivational
Interviewing

In the therapeutic model, the various approaches to counseling are applied to the specific problems of substance abuse or addiction. The two approaches that have earned widespread recognition are *motivational interviewing* (Miller & Rollnick, 2002) and *relapse prevention* (Marlatt, 1985). Motivational interviewing's increasing popularity in the addictions field may stem from its being a brief treatment model (two to four sessions), which makes it appealing to insurance companies and HMOs seeking to minimize health care costs (Heather, 2005). However, another factor may be its humanistic, non-adversarial, person-centered approach, putting it in sharp contrast to the aggressively confrontational strategies employed by many in the substance abuse treatment world (Madison, Loignon, & Lane, 2009). Counselors who prefer a therapeutic style inspired by Carl Rogers, with its emphasis on empathy and collaboration, may be drawn to this model. Motivational interviewing also presumes that many alcoholics can successfully reduce their consumption to moderate levels, a stance squarely in opposition to the AA model, which demands total abstinence. Clients who are loathe to give up the social pleasures of the occasional drink may be more likely to participate with this approach. Finally, there is a considerable body of research demonstrating its efficacy (Carroll et al., 2006; Hettema, Steele, & Miller, 2005).

Motivational interviewing presumes that the substance abuser will only change when motivated to do so. Abusers remain addicted out of choice; they prefer the benefits of substance abuse to sobriety. At the same time, many abusers also have dreams and goals in life, which they can never achieve so long as they continue their substance use. Thus, abusers experience an inner conflict or ambivalence about their drug use, a discrepancy between their addiction and their deeper hopes for themselves. The role of the counselor is to assist them in resolving this conflict by helping abusers recognize these hopes and goals, and appreciate how their addiction holds them back.

The model emphasizes that the counselor cannot push or confront clients into giving up their addiction; only clients can take responsibility for change in their lives, and they cannot do so until they are ready to change, wanting to accomplish their goals more than they want their alcohol or drugs. From this perspective, addicts who minimize their substance abuse are not "in denial," but more likely have not reached the desire-to-change stage, and no amount of counselor confrontation will make them get there. Indeed, advocates of this model believe that confrontation is counterproductive, increasing clients' resistance to change by promoting defensiveness and lack of self-confidence. Instead, motivational interviewing counselors remain gently empathic toward whatever feelings, values, or goals clients describe; as with any client-centered approach, the counselor maintains a stance of nonjudgmental acceptance, including acceptance of clients' unwillingness to give up their addiction. Lack of readiness to stop using drugs and alcohol is validated as understandable and normal. Thus, the goal is to create in the counseling relationship the conditions where clients can examine the consequences of their behaviors and, on their own, arrive at the decision that it is time to give up their addictive lifestyle (Britt, Blampied, & Hudson, 2003; Lewis & Osborn, 2004; Sommers-Flanagan & Sommers-Flanagan, 2009).

The motivational interviewing approach has a natural theoretical link with the process of change model developed by Prochaska, DiClemente, and Norcross (1992; Prochaska & Norcross, 2010). The two models are often cited together in the literature on motivational interviewing, although for any counselor, the process of change model is useful in understanding how change actually occurs. These authors suggest there are five stages to change, and clients must pass through all five in order to alter behaviors.

1. *Precontemplation.* Individuals in this stage do not recognize themselves as having a problem, and only come for counseling because they are pressured by a spouse or employer, or mandated by a judge.
2. *Contemplation.* In this stage, substance abusers recognize they have a problem and are beginning to weigh the pros and cons of their addictive behaviors. They are not ready to change, but are giving the idea serious consideration.
3. *Preparation.* Individuals in this stage intend to take action and change their behaviors, but still haven't committed to taking the major steps necessary.

4. *Action.* The "action" stage reflects overt behavioral changes, with successful alteration of their addictive behaviors. They feel like they are actually doing something about their problem.

5. *Maintenance.* In this stage, substance abusers have been abstinent for more than six months and are trying to avoid relapsing, which for some will be a lifelong process.

From a person-centered perspective, you can see the value of using this approach to conceptualize the client's readiness to change. The counselor's role would be to understand and validate the client exactly where he or she is along this continuum, gently nudging but never pressuring the client to move to the next level.

RELAPSE PREVENTION

The underlying premise to the relapse prevention model is that it is normal for substance abusers to return to some of their old patterns following treatment. The initial setback is termed a "lapse," and when the setback evolves into a complete return to substance abuse, the individual is said to have "relapsed." Research does suggest that most substance abusers will experience a lapse, and many do relapse (Polivy & Herman, 2002). Unlike the AA model, where relapse is seen as failure, relapse prevention advocates reframe relapses as opportunities to learn more effective coping strategies.

Marlatt, who first developed the model in the 1980s, noted that recovered abusers who experienced a lapse would get caught up in a vicious cycle: Their "failure" led to self-blame for using again and a perception that they could not control their desire for mood-altering substances. Together, these negative attitudes increased the likelihood that the individuals would use alcohol or drugs to relieve their distress, thus resulting in a full relapse. To minimize the risk of a return to the old self-destructive patterns, Marlatt and his colleagues developed a cognitive-behavioral therapy using a variety of interventions designed to help individuals avoid this downward spiral (Marlatt & Gordon, 1985). Drug and alcohol counselors utilizing this model would take the following steps:

- Assess the high-risk situations the client is likely to encounter that would facilitate a lapse. These include negative emotions, interpersonal conflict, and social pressures (e.g., certain friends, drug dealers, favorite bars, parties where alcohol or drugs are used).
- Challenge the client's expectations that using the substance will be a positive experience.
- Educate the client about the nature of lapses and relapses, to remove some of the shame associated with lapses and reduce the likelihood of using substances to relieve the shame.
- If the client has experienced a lapse, assess whether he or she sees it as a personal failure and, if so, help normalize it and minimize feelings of decreased self-efficacy.
- Design a program of cognitive behavioral interventions aimed at helping the client cope effectively with high-risk situations.

- Encourage the client to make significant lifestyle changes that include relaxation techniques.
- Teach the client to replace negative addictions with positive ones like aerobics at a gym or regular running (Stevens & Smith, 2008; Witkiewitz & Marlatt, 2004).

As with any cognitive-behavioral therapy, the treatment is short term, and requires that the counselor work collaboratively with a client who is ready to make changes. Occasionally, clients will need booster sessions to help solidify their coping strategies. Research does support the efficacy of this model, particularly with alcoholics. While clients do tend to experience lapses, their new coping skills decrease the probability of a full relapse into previous substance use patterns (Witkiewitz & Marlatt, 2004).

The apparent efficacy of both client-centered and cognitive-behavioral approaches, theories that you will most likely study at some point in your counseling program, means that even as a novice counselor, you may have a sufficient knowledge base to provide real help to clients dealing with substance abuse issues. In addition to these two theories, other theoretical models presented in Chapters 5 and 6 could conceivably be applied to substance abuse programs. For example, some counselors might delve into repressed conflicts underlying the drug symptoms, or perhaps concentrate on issues related to self-control. Regardless of the therapeutic model, however, there are some general rules that will help counselors in working with alcohol/drug abusers in particular or addictions in general:

1. Recovery from addictions is unlikely without some support system as an adjunct to counseling.
2. Group counseling modalities are often helpful in providing support, positive modeling, motivation, intimacy, and constructive confrontation for substance abusers.
3. Family counseling strategies help the counselor to recruit more power and support, to collect more information about the problem, and to resolve conflicts that are sabotaging recovery. The concept of family can also be expanded to include a wider network of friends, associates, and concerned others who wish to be involved. Among some indigenous groups, there is a wide network of extended kin, related by blood and affiliation, who are all involved in providing family support (the New Zealand Maori, for example, call this *whanau*; the Hawaiian *ohana* is similar in concept).
4. The counselor should explore the motivation for using alcohol by examining the availability of nonchemical incentives.
5. Alcohol and drug abuse is often a form of self-medication in which the client attempts to cope with debilitating depression or anxiety. Attempts should be made to identify and treat the underlying pain that is being anesthetized.
6. Time can be spent productively helping clients to grieve the time they've wasted, even the childhood they've lost. Help addicts resolve their feelings of shame and anger, leave the past behind, and move forward.
7. Physical exercise programs that involve daily structured commitments are often helpful in creating more positive addictions. Activities such as biking, running, swimming, and aerobics have been found to reduce tension, increase productivity, improve confidence, and provide an alternative to drugs.

VOICE FROM THE FIELD

I was pretty discouraged when I first began my job in a treatment center. From reading the research on drug addictions, I saw that 98% of teens who go through treatment fail. Yet the place where I worked claimed to have a 75% to 80% success rate. But that's only as they leave the center. When they do follow-up three months later, they find that most of them relapse.

Still, there are several things you can do to increase the chances that counseling will be helpful. I learned the hard way. First, you have to be honest with them and you have to talk to them at their level; if you sound any way like a counselor, they will shut you out.

You have to stand up for them. They interpret loyalty as caring. For instance, when a lampshade was broken, the program director refused to let up on them until he found out who did it. I stood up for the kids and he backed down. That really made a difference in my relationship with them.

Treatment is all about setting limits. Strength gets their attention. Then, you have to follow through on what you said you were going to do. The limits should be balanced with showing that you care for them—really care. If they don't think they matter to you, you don't have a chance to help them.

8. Work extra hard in developing trust with the client, so that confrontations can be made without provoking client resistance and defensiveness. Watch for manipulation, deceit, and lying, which are not uncommon among those who are used to saying anything in order to relieve physical or psychological cravings. When these behaviors do occur, be careful to avoid judgment or becoming adversarial toward your client.

9. Rules and limits are often needed to structure acceptable and inappropriate behavior within the sessions. For example, the counselor may refuse to work with the client unless she or he can agree to maintain sobriety for at least eight hours prior to any session.

10. Because drug and alcohol abuse is often associated with low self-esteem, considerable work should be spent helping the client to improve confidence and self-worth.

11. Work on identity issues, because addicts often use "totalizing descriptions" of their own essence: I am an addict. A narrative counseling approach would locate the problem—the addiction—outside the individual ("The addiction is seducing you") but would also make certain that the clients did not confuse their behavior with who they are as human beings.

12. Varieties of adventure and constructive risk taking other than the drug-induced kind should be substituted. As the person finds more fulfillment in a career, course of study, hobby, intimate relationship, social network, travel experience, or any other passionate project, the need to use drugs for excitement or boredom decreases.

13. If the client cannot or will not practice complete abstinence, offer a compromise program of moderation. A number of self-help organizations such as Moderation Management and DrinkWise are having limited success with people who would otherwise drop out of treatment altogether.

14. Make sure to consider the factors and consequences of addiction as they affect a client's financial status, career, relationships, and stress levels.

15. Consider gender and cultural differences as a context for the addiction or substance abuse. Alcohol abuse, for instance, may have different meaning for

some women who have histories of sexual or physical abuse (Van der Walde, Urgenson, Weltz, & Hanna, 2002).

16. Regardless of the treatment model employed, systematic follow-up of cases is critical, ideally for up to two years after sessions have ended.

Regardless of the specific program that the counselor adopts for those clients who are struggling with the temptations of drug and alcohol use, this specialty has become a big part of the mandate of professional helpers. The demand for qualified experts in this field will only continue to grow at the pace with which children, adolescents, and adults abuse chemical substances.

PSYCHOPHARMACOLOGY FOR COUNSELORS

"I've just been so depressed lately," a new client says to you by way of introduction. "I just don't have any energy lately. I'm tired all the time. And I've just lost all hope."

You have already reviewed the intake forms and note several significant factors about this case. First of all, the client has already seen a number of medical specialists to rule out any physical problems such as a neurological disorder or endocrine imbalance. Secondly, he has been in therapy previously for depression, without satisfactory improvement. Thirdly, you note there has been a history of depression in the family: His mother was depressed, as was one of his siblings. While all of these factors don't definitively point to an organically based depression that might respond to antidepressant medication, you do start thinking that an evaluation for meds might be indicated.

After securing permission, and getting a signed release, you call the client's primary care physician who admits she had thought of the same thing, but before she tried antidepressant medication she first wanted to see if this patient responded to therapy alone. You applaud this conservative approach, especially realizing how rare it is that a physician would not routinely prescribe drugs for someone who reported depression.

"So," the doctor says to you, "what would *you* recommend that we do with him?"

As a counselor, you have hardly had medical training, nor have you spent extensive time studying psychopharmacology, much less biochemistry and drug interactions. Yet you are being asked to recommend a medication for a client and you are not sure how to respond to the question.

Of course it is beyond the scope of counseling practice to prescribe medications, but your skills as a competent professional should be informed by knowledge about basic psychopharmacology. There are times when doctors (especially general practitioners) will ask you what you'd recommend. But far more commonly, you must know when medication for depression, anxiety, and other disorders might be indicated and refer the client for tests and evaluation. Furthermore, you must also be aware of the influences, side effects, and experiences of various drugs when your clients have been taking them.

In this section, we briefly introduce you to psychopharmacology for counselors. We recognize that, like most of the chapters and subjects in this text, you will likely take a whole course or workshop on this topic. This overview is intended to provide you with a general background that will help reduce the complexity of this field when you devote further study to it in the future.

The use of mood-altering drugs, known as psychotropic medications, has become so widespread in our culture that you can be assured you will be seeing clients taking medication, or a combination of medications. So many people are taking drugs for depression, for example, that antidepressants are among the top-selling drugs in the United States (Herper & Karno, 2006). You may also be in the position of deciding whether to refer a client for possible medication. As counselors, regardless of our personal views on whether using medication is a "quick fix" that enables clients to avoid the hard work of exploring their issues, or a necessary adjunct to counseling, it is our duty to have adequate familiarity with the field of psychopharmacology.

There are several reasons why familiarizing yourself with psychopharmacology is not only desirable but also mandatory for you as an ethical professional (King & Anderson, 2004). First, ethical codes insist that you stay up-to-date on scientific knowledge related to clinical practice. Second is the issue of informed consent: Ethical practice means you need to describe to your clients not only how you practice but also the alternative treatment options available to them; psychotropic medications are one such alternative. Finally, there is the concept of standard of care, defined as the "knowledge, skill, and judgment [each counselor must have] common to other members of their profession" (Corey, Corey, & Callanan, 2007, p. 193). What this means is that if you fail to discuss psychopharmacological options with your clients, or neglect to consider a medication referral for a client whose problem might respond to drug treatment, you are probably practicing below the minimum standard of care in our current world.

Imagine that a depressed client does not respond to all of your best efforts (yes, it does happen!), and the depression makes him unable to keep his job. A year later, his family doctor suggests an antidepressant, which relieves him of depression. Now, the client turns around and sues you for malpractice, claiming your incompetence deprived him of a year's wages and caused emotional suffering. If you had failed to discuss medication possibilities with the client, and never referred him for a psychiatric evaluation, you might well lose the case (King & Anderson, 2004).

Counselors play a major role in collaborating with medical professionals to ensure that clients get the best possible care. For many clients, actual time spent with a psychiatrist for medication purposes consists of a one-hour initial evaluation, and 15-minute follow-ups—at best once per month, and in many cases once every six months. Those 15-minute sessions can go something like this:

DOCTOR: "I see you're taking Lexapro and Wellbutrin. How are you feeling?"

PATIENT: "Pretty good. I'm not getting as depressed as I used to. But I still have a hard time getting up in the morning. And my sex life still isn't what it used to be."

DOCTOR: "OK. I'm going to increase your Wellbutrin dosage to 300 mg, and give you a prescription for something that should help with your sex drive. Let's reschedule for two months from now and see how you're doing."

Of course, not all psychiatric consults are this brief and superficial, but the main point is that it will often be up to you to monitor carefully how clients are experiencing and responding to medications prescribed by their doctors.

VOICE FROM THE FIELD

There is this one psychiatrist I know who is a real jerk. He's got the interpersonal skills of a toad but he is a brilliant chemist. He is also very, very cautious in what he prescribes. More than half the time that I refer clients to him because I think they might respond to medication, he sends them right back and says, "No way, you gotta do the work with this one. I'm not letting you off the hook." I've worked with other psychiatrists who automatically dole out drugs to every client I refer to them; it's like I'm the one who is prescribing, which makes me very uncomfortable.

One other advantage of sending my clients to this one psychiatrist I just mentioned, who is somewhat less than warm and engaging, is that they come back to me so much more grateful and appreciative for what I do for them. That's just an added benefit.

Moreover, in many cases, the client will not be working with a psychiatrist (aka psychopharmacologist), an expert in psychotropic drugs, but rather with an internist or family physician who prescribes medication without a focused expertise in how these medications work. Cost-containment measures by insurance companies and HMOs have meant that primary care physicians, rather than specialists in psychopharmacology, increasingly do the work of prescribing psychotropic drugs. This trend is increasingly true for children and adolescents who are most frequently put on medications by pediatricians (Brown & Sammons, 2002).

You can begin to see why you will play such an important role in the client's medication treatment. Indeed, a good part of your counseling is likely to involve discussions around medications. Many clients will need to talk about their complex feelings about being on drugs—in particular, the shame they may feel about needing a medication and their fears about possibly unpleasant side effects or long-term harm. In order to perform these tasks effectively, you will need to be competent in the following areas:

1. Determining whether a referral to a psychiatrist is needed. For example, you may assess that your client's depression is not being sufficiently alleviated by counseling, and an antidepressant would be of help.
2. Staying current with research on counseling treatment alternatives to medication.
3. Referring clients to psychiatrists in your area whom you trust and who prescribe medications only when they are absolutely needed and indicated.
4. Conducting a professional conversation with the psychiatrist or primary care physician about your client's situation—using precise language, keeping the discussion brief, and not revealing more confidential information than what is necessary for the physician to know.
5. Knowing the difference between normal and abnormal side effects for the most commonly used drugs.
6. Encouraging your client to take the medication as prescribed (called "compliance") and being aware of the negative effects clients are likely to experience when they digress from the prescribed regimen.
7. Helping your clients manage the withdrawal stage when they discontinue medications. (For many people, discontinuation is a difficult process, involving a temporary return to the previous symptoms and additional unpleasant withdrawal effects.)

To gain the necessary competence in these areas, you will need to take a course in psychopharmacology (at a university or as a continuing education course) and read at least one good psychopharmacology text; some recommended readings are included at the end of this chapter. You will want to have this text available to you wherever you conduct counseling, and every several years purchase the most up-to-date version.

PSYCHOPHARMACOLOGICAL TREATMENT FOR EMOTIONAL DISORDERS

Although you will have the opportunity to study the neurophysiology of drug effects, as well as psychopharmacology, later in your training, we will review some of the major emotional disorders you are likely to encounter and how medications are often used to treat them. As counselors, we have a general bias in favor of addressing life's problems with skills, relationships, and psychological solutions. However, despite our belief that drugs are *way* overprescribed, we still think it is important for you to understand the range of options available. As often as not, you may help your clients make informed decisions about going off medications that are no longer necessary (if they ever were).

In the sections that follow, we don't expect you to memorize, or even learn, the names of the various drugs and what they are for. Rather, we simply wish to introduce you to the various challenges you will encounter and how medications have sometimes been found useful in helping to manage the symptoms.

MEDICATIONS FOR DEPRESSION

The most commonly prescribed medications for both major and moderate depression are the class of drugs known as *Selective Serotonin Reuptake Inhibitors* (SSRIs); common brands are Prozac (generic name, fluoxetine), Paxil (paroxetine), Zoloft (sertraline), Celexa (citalopram), and Lexapro (escitalopram). Knowing generic names is important because research studies only discuss drugs with this terminology. Other popularly prescribed medications, known as atypical antidepressants, include Wellbutrin (bupropion), Effexor (venlafaxine), and Cymbalta (duloxetine). Some clients may be taking an earlier class of antidepressants, called *trycyclics*, mostly out of favor with contemporary physicians and given only to clients for whom the SSRIs are ineffective.

The SSRI class of drugs operates by increasing the transmission of the neurotransmitter serotonin across neuronal synapses (the spaces between neurons). Serotonin influences mood regulation (primarily inducing a calming effect), sleep and arousal, and regulation of physical pain (Sinacola & Peters-Strickland, 2006). This is (hopefully) experienced by the individual as a reduction in depression (Greenfield, 2000; Julien, 2008).

The problem with any drug, especially those that operate on the central nervous system, is that there are inevitable side effects. Some are merely annoying (dry mouth, tiredness, constipation) and some feel catastrophic (weight gain, insomnia, lack of sexual drive). Some clients report an unpleasant flattening out of their emotional lives; although definitely feeling less depressed, they perceive that their positive emotions lose intensity as well (Julien, 2008).

VOICE FROM THE FIELD

It is not that the drugs didn't work for me, because they did. I tried everything first and was very reluctant to use any kind of medications. I don't even like to take aspirin if I can help it. So you can say I was resistant. Okay, I was adamant that I didn't want to take anything. But the depression got so bad, and I felt so out of control, that my therapist convinced me to give it a try.

Now I just feel kind of numb. The part I really don't like is that I can't cry anymore, even if I want to. It feels like I'm emotionally constipated or something. I'm sure as far as my friends and family are concerned, I must seem much better to them. But inside I feel weird, like it isn't me anymore.

Although SSRIs are intended to be calming, some clients experience agitation, anxiety, and a feeling described as "jumping out of my skin." These side effects tend to occur in the first few days of taking the drug, and often subside after the client's system adjusts. Commonly, prescribing physicians will reassure their worried patient that these unpleasant sensations will pass, and their patient—your client—gamely tries to wait it out. No one, however, should have to endure truly uncomfortable sensations; intense side effects are often a sign that a specific drug is not a good fit for that person's particular brain chemistry. If clients complain to you about side effects, encourage them to contact their physician and address any feelings they may have about "bothering" their doctor. Sexual side effects, on the other hand, are an unfortunate reality of taking these medications, and not a sign of a biochemical mismatch; however, some physicians will prescribe Viagra™ or similar drugs to counteract the SSRI's negative effects.

Counselors also need to know that antidepressant medications need to remain at fairly constant levels in the blood in order to remain effective. If clients tell you they have stopped taking the drug for any reason, you need to explore their reasons for discontinuing. It is important to explain the importance of sticking to the prescribed regimen, and to encourage discussing any desire to stop with their physician. Finally, counselors should be aware of the "poop-out" effect, the euphemism many psychiatrists use for the phenomenon of an antidepressant ceasing to be effective. Sometimes, the prescribing physician will raise the dosage, but drugs can stop working even at the maximum dose, at which point the physician may switch to another medication, until that drug "poops out" as well. This experience can be frustrating and frightening for the depressed client, who dreads the day when no medication will be helpful; it will be your job to support clients through this experience, while staying abreast of new counseling approaches that might be helpful alternatives to medications.

MEDICATIONS FOR BIPOLAR DISORDERS

For decades, the most popular drug for bipolar disorders has been lithium, a naturally occurring salt that reduces both depression and mania for individuals with this condition. Despite its widespread use since the 1970s, what makes it work remains unclear. On the other hand, its side effects are very well known, including gastrointestinal distress, weight gain, skin rashes, increased urination, and difficulties with memory and concentration. It is no wonder, then, that clients prescribed

| VOICE FROM THE FIELD

It frankly scares me how unprepared some of my clients are for the withdrawal effects of taking antidepressants. A woman I was working with had told her physician she was going through a hard time, and the doctor promptly gave her a bag of drug company samples of Paxil. Well, the drugs seemed to help, and after a year of taking them, she called the doctor, who said it was fine to stop. Three weeks later this poor woman was way more depressed than she had ever been, and could barely get out of bed to come to see me. We tried to figure out what was going on in her life that was causing this relapse. Fights with her husband? Feeling like she wasn't a good enough mother?

Worries about her aging Dad? Nothing seemed to explain the deep, dark hole she was in. Finally, we agreed she should see a well-known psychiatrist in our community with a specialty in antidepressant medications.

The psychiatrist knew right away what was going on—my client was experiencing a rebound depression from getting off SSRIs too quickly. What a relief for my client to know she wasn't going crazy. And what a relief for me, too, because I didn't know what to do and was getting pretty scared. And what about all those other people taking these drugs who don't have the luxury or the money to see the best psychiatrist in town?

lithium often stop taking it against their doctor's orders. Some clients will discontinue it not just because of the side effects, but because it is working too well to reduce mania, which at times can be a pleasurable experience, not unlike taking a street drug to get high. Counselors play a critical role in psychopharmacological management of bipolar disorders by monitoring for a return of manic or depressive symptoms, which may indicate noncompliance. The consequences of getting off of lithium can be severe: reckless, destructive behaviors if the client becomes manic again, and potential suicidal tendencies if depression reoccurs. Counselors need to educate clients as to the risks of discontinuation and remain sensitive and compassionate toward the suffering engendered by lithium's side effects.

Drug companies continue to develop alternatives to lithium, including Depakote (valproic acid), Tegretol (carbamazepine), and Lamictal (lamotrigine), and research studies have supported their efficacy (Adams, et al., 2009). All of these drugs have their own side effects, including sedation, rashes, and stomach distress, but tend to be easier to tolerate than lithium. Some psychopharmacologists address bipolar disorders by combining a variety of drugs, including antidepressant and antianxiety medications.

Most important for counselors is an appreciation of the fact that bipolar disorder is a biologically based condition that requires medication. With ordinary depression, medication is an option, but counseling may be preferable; the same cannot be said for bipolar illness. Any signs of mania in a client are an automatic red flag for psychiatric evaluation.

MEDICATIONS FOR ANXIETY

The most frequently prescribed antianxiety drugs are a class of medications called benzodiazepines; common brand names are Klonopin (clonazepam), Ativan (lorazepam), and Xanax (alprazolam). All of these drugs have similar effects, calming both the mind and the muscles, and eliminating such anxiety symptoms as racing thoughts, obsessive thinking, insomnia, feelings of panic, and heart palpitations. Differences among the various brands involve how sedating they are (the more sedating ones tend to be prescribed for insomnia) and their half-life—how long it takes for the drugs to be metabolized and eliminated from the body. Some clients will be prescribed SSRIs for anxiety, in particular Paxil and Zoloft, both of which also have calming properties.

The primary side effect of the benzodiazepine family is oversedation, which is why it is commonly prescribed for sleep disorders. In the elderly, these drugs can also cause cognitive impairments and loss of balance. The most serious drawback to this class of medications is that they are highly addictive when taken for long periods of time and/or taken in high doses. As with any addictive drug, clients can experience increasing levels of tolerance, requiring higher doses to maintain the same level of effectiveness. Moreover, withdrawal can be very difficult (even more so than withdrawing from heroin!). Consequently, most physicians will give patients no more than a two-week supply, with instructions to take them "as needed" instead of on a regular basis. When clients have been taking high doses or using the drug over a sustained period, the tapering-off process must be very slow, and rebound anxiety is common.

The best approach for a counselor is to refer clients for possible benzodiazepine medication when they are experiencing intense, life-interfering anxiety, triggered by a specific, short-term situation. For example, a client who has just purchased a house, and is so overwhelmed by anxiety after completing the deal that he or she cannot function at work, may be a candidate for these drugs. Clients with a history of ongoing substance abuse generally should not be referred for this

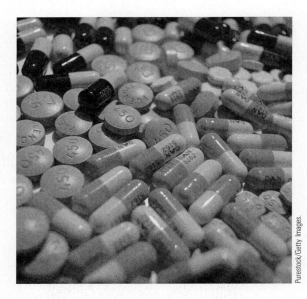

Psychotropic medications have become ubiquitous in our culture.

VOICE FROM THE FIELD

I will never forget a young woman with a new job as a secretary at an accounting firm. She was concerned that her male supervisor was making sexual overtures to her, including sending her inappropriate e-mails. She was quite distressed, and I did a good job of calming her anxiety and exploring options with her. We role-played how she might confront him, and explored her legal options if the confrontation failed. When she revealed her childhood sexual abuse, I was even more empathic, appreciating how this current violation was stirring up painful memories. I was pretty proud of the way I was handling this.

And then, while reviewing her chart, I noticed she was taking an antipsychotic, meaning it was quite possible everything she was telling me was a delusion. Or was it? I honestly didn't know. But I did know that I could not proceed with focusing on the surface problem without being assured that she was not experiencing paranoid delusions. In the next session, I casually asked her how many offensive e-mails this man had sent her during the past week (for some reason, it never occurred to me to ask her this before). When she told me a thousand, I knew I was in a whole new ball game, and, in fact, I was not the appropriate health professional to help her.

kind of antianxiety medication. You will learn many other methods for reducing stress and anxiety in your clients, including cognitive restructuring, hypnosis, relaxation training, meditation, mindfulness, exercise, and others, but there may be times when medications do help during times of transition; and anxiety impairs functioning.

MEDICATIONS FOR PSYCHOTIC DISORDERS

Although counselors typically are not the prime health care providers for people with psychotic disorders like schizophrenia, you may work with clients on antipsychotic medication. For example, you may be providing adjunctive supportive counseling to a mentally ill client, or conducting family therapy where one member has a psychotic disorder. Moreover, physicians sometimes prescribe low dosages of antipsychotic medications, along with SSRIs, to treat depression. Thus, familiarity with this class of medications is essential.

In the 21st century, the first line of treatment has become Risperdal (risperidone) and Zyprexa (olanzapine); you may also have clients taking Seroquel (quetiapine) or Clozaril (clozapine). Though all of these medications have fewer side effects than the previous generation of antipsychotics, they can still cause such symptoms as sedation and weight gain (Sinacola & Peters-Strickland, 2006).

As with any medication, awareness of these side effects is essential; for example, what may appear to be a psychologically rooted depression may actually be caused by the drugs. However, the most important role of the counselor is to help clients stick to their medication regimen despite their desire to quit when the symptoms abate. Counselors can also teach clients and their families about the need for compliance and the near certainty that the symptoms of the illness will return once medication stops. This means helping clients and families cope with the challenges of side effects and exploring ways of motivating clients to stick to their treatment plan.

PSYCHOPHARMACOLOGY AND CHILDREN

The issue of whether to encourage clients to consider medications becomes even more challenging when counseling children and adolescents. Many parents will understandably want to know if taking a medication for depression or attention-deficit/hyperactivity disorders (ADHD) constitutes a health risk to their child. They may have heard horror stories about the effects of these drugs, yet are equally disturbed by their child's symptoms. As a counselor, you need to be current with what the research says about both a medication's risks and efficacy, helping parents separate frightening anecdotes reported in the news from the actual data about how these drugs impact children's lives. The medical field sometimes refers to this kind of decision making as a risk/benefit issue; you must discuss with parents whether benefits of psychotropic medications outweigh the potential health risks of taking these powerful drugs. You also need to encourage the parents to discuss the risk/benefit issue with the prescribing physician.

One of the most controversial fears among the public has been that anti-depressants cause young people to kill themselves. Actually, it is very difficult to prove that a medication *caused* a depressed child's or teen's suicide, since depression alone could very likely have been the reason. Another possibility is that in some cases, a child may have abruptly discontinued taking a medication and experienced a severe withdrawal-caused depression, which led to suicide (Julien, 2008).

The Food and Drug Administration does have real concerns about the potential for antidepressants to cause suicidality in adolescents, and in 2003, it issued a "black box" warning label on all antidepressants, which declares that these medications may raise the risk of suicide in children and adolescents (Raz, 2006). According to one research study, in the year following the addition of this label, suicide rates among teens rose 14%, presumably because the warning discouraged physicians from prescribing the antidepressants which might have reduced suicidal attempts (Gibbons et al., 2007). Similar conclusions have been reached in other studies demonstrating that antidepressants decreased suicide rates among both teens and adults (Olfson, Shaffer, Marcus, & Greenberg, 2003). Ultimately, it will likely take many years before there is general agreement within the medical community regarding the safety of these drugs for children.

Regardless of the inconclusiveness of research on medication safety, counselors can take certain steps to ensure that children and adolescents minimize the risks of taking medication.

- Decide if the child's symptoms constitute a threat to the child's health; for example, depression with suicidal thoughts, self-mutilation (i.e., cutting), and eating disorders might all warrant medication. In these cases, a referral to a psychiatrist/psychopharmacologist specializing in childhood disorders is appropriate. The counselor should also be aware of counseling approaches for these conditions that could serve as potential alternatives to medications or in combination with drugs.
- Discuss with the parents both the benefits and the risks of medications. Consistent with ethical counseling practice, review with them options besides medication.

- If the parents choose to pursue medication treatment, obtain the necessary releases and discuss the medication plan with the physician.
- Familiarize yourself with the drugs prescribed.
- Assist parents in having meaningful discussions with their child's physician. Support the parents' right to ask questions, and help them devise a list of concerns they want to address.
- Because you will be in a better position to observe the child's reactions than the physician, monitor for signs of increased depression and suicidal ideation, agitation, and any behavioral changes that give you concern.
- Stay current with ongoing research in this area. For example, it is conceivable that there will be new evidence that these medications are riskier than previously thought.

COUNSELOR SELF-REFLECTION

All counselors need to reflect upon and get clarity about their own values regarding the use of psychotropic medications. Although counselors never make the actual decision to put a client on medication, we do make the choice about whether or not to refer clients to a physician for a medication evaluation. Moreover, clients often ask us to share our views about medications, and we need to be clear about our values before responding. Sorting out these values has been made especially complicated by the bombardment of media messages both we and our clients receive regarding the pros and cons of medications. On the one hand, we see the constant barrage of television commercials promoting medications for depression, anxiety, social phobias, and insomnia. On the other hand, news media regularly feature stories about the dangerous side effects of these medications, including suicide and homicide. The issue is especially complicated when we work with children. Counselors also need to be aware of the potential for recommending drugs out of frustration with the slow pace of counseling, or from feelings of inadequacy and of having failed our clients. Conversely, counselors sometimes avoid discussing medication for fear that clients will leave counseling once the medication relieves their symptoms.

For many counselors, the question comes down to: What intensity of clients' suffering indicates to the counselor that medication referral is warranted? Certainly, there are situations when it is imperative to refer to a physician, such as when a client is severely depressed, feelings of anxiety are overwhelming and unrelieved by talk therapy and behavioral exercises, or the client has a neurobiologically based condition like bipolar disorder or schizophrenia. However, in many other cases, the decision to refer is not clear-cut.

Jack is a 75-year-old man whose wife of 50 years died one year ago. Jack's grief has been extremely painful; he misses her terribly, cannot find pleasure from any of the things that used to interest him, and spends most of his days blankly watching television. Jack comes in for counseling, and you correctly assess him as suffering from a grief-related depression. You assess for suicide, and Jack makes it clear he has no desire to die, just to get over the pain of his loss. Do you refer him for medication? Some counselors might say no: Grief is a normal and necessary

VOICE FROM THE FIELD

I've always been very antidrug. I'm suspicious of big pharmaceutical companies, and believe they play down the side effects. I don't like all the advertising convincing people they should be taking pills they don't really need. As a counselor, I'm a strong believer that talking things through and getting to the bottom of issues is a much better approach than putting potent chemicals in your body. At least, that's how I used to feel. Then, some of my clients decided to try medications on their own, especially the SSRI antidepressants. I was amazed at the difference it made. Not for everybody, but an awful lot of clients who had been struggling with depression for most of their lives were now feeling pretty good for the first time. I'd like to think it was all the hard work of counseling that made the difference, but frankly, I'm not sure. I still think counseling is the best treatment for most psychological problems, but more and more I'm supporting my clients' decisions to try medications.

response to profound loss, and the best course of action is to help Jack in his mourning process by encouraging him to talk about his feelings and memories of his wife. Another counselor might take a different point of view: There is no need for Jack to suffer. He may not have that many years ahead of him—why shouldn't he be able to enjoy them to the fullest?

What choice would you make as Jack's counselor? Both paths are clinically legitimate, but reflect different philosophies about human life: One sees some kinds of suffering as an important experience in life; another sees all suffering as unnecessary pain. As you can see, something as simple as a medication referral can have profound implications for the client, and is strongly influenced by the counselor's value system.

SUMMARY

Addictions present some special challenges for the counselor for a variety of reasons: (1) The effects of the drugs are intrinsically rewarding and resistant to extinction; (2) there may be pressure from peers to continue the abuse; (3) abusers tend toward irresponsibility, and may try to manipulate the counselor or act uncooperatively; (4) abusers are ambivalent in their motivation because the drugs do work—in spite of side effects—to temporarily reduce symptoms of boredom, anxiety, or depression.

Because of these and other factors contributing to an addict's situation, the counselor should develop a multifaceted treatment program to combat resistance on physiological, psychological, family, and cultural levels. Motivational interviewing, relapse prevention, 12-step programs, therapeutic communities, and group and family counseling have all been used with some success. However, even with the best resources available, prognoses for chronic drug and alcohol abusers are guarded.

In this chapter, you have also learned the fundamentals of psychopharmacology; as drug treatments become increasingly acceptable to clients, parents, and the counseling profession as a legitimate primary or adjunctive treatment, it has become ethically incumbent upon counselors to have a reasonable level of knowledge regarding the use and side effects of these medications. Moreover, counselors are often in a better position than physicians to discuss and monitor medication use with clients. The decision of when to refer for medication can be a complex one; the counselor's personal values, the client's values, research findings, and rigorous assessment of the client's psychological needs all come into play.

SELF-GUIDED EXPLORATIONS

1. Relive a time in your life when you "self-medicated" yourself for some sort of stress. This could have included the use of substances (alcohol, illicit or prescription drugs, coffee, cigarettes, etc.) or some other activity designed to provide escape (sleep, isolation, exercise, food, etc.). Describe the positive and negative impacts that experience had on your life. How did you decide to stop or cut down?

2. Describe a close friend or relative whose life was significantly changed as a result of drug/alcohol abuse. What impact did this behavior have on you and others who were close to him or her? What finally made a difference in helping him or her to stop?

3. Two different positions argue that: (1) addiction is a genetic predetermination and disease that we can do little about—except to abstain from all temptations; (2) addiction is a choice based on our refusal to accept responsibility for our behavior. Create a dialogue between two proponents of these positions, each trying to convince the other of the respective accuracy of his or her position. Which position are you most sympathetic to? Defend your position by coming up with some evidence.

4. Recall a time when you were depressed or anxious and wishing there was a way to escape your emotional pain. How miserable would you have to feel before you wanted to try psychopharmacological answers? Would you ever reach this point, and if not, why not?

FOR HOMEWORK

1. Attend several different open meetings of Alcoholics Anonymous, Narcotics Anonymous, or some other self-help support group devoted to addictions. Consider ways that this research will help you to integrate your own counseling efforts with the work being done in these groups.

2. Visit a physician's office and count the number of drug company advertisements you see. Look for them in waiting room magazines, on wall calendars, pens, coffee mugs, etc. Describe the psychological impact you experience from your observations.

3. View one or more of the following films about drug abuse: *Clean and Sober, Rush, Leaving Las Vegas, When a Man Loves a Woman,* or *Permanent Midnight.* Observe the ways in which the main characters use self-denial and manipulative behaviors in order to maintain their addictions. At what point in their stories did they have an opportunity to turn away from drugs, but continued? In your view, what was the reason they didn't stop even though they were paying a high price for their drug use?

SUGGESTED READINGS

Blume, A. W. (2005). *Treating drug problems.* New York: John Wiley & Sons.

Craig, R. J. (2004). *Counseling the alcohol and drug dependent client: A practical approach.* Boston: Allyn & Bacon.

Doweiko, H. E. (2009). *Concepts of chemical dependency* (7th ed.). Belmont, CA: Brooks/Cole.

Harrison, T. C., & Fisher, G. L. (2009). *Substance abuse: Information for school counselors, social workers, therapists, and counselors* (4th ed.). Boston: Allyn & Bacon.

Hedges, D., & Burchfield, C. (2006). *Mind, brain, and drug: An introduction to psychopharmacology.* Boston: Allyn & Bacon.

Juhnke, G., & Hagedom, W. B. (2006). *Counseling addicted families: An integrated assessment and treatment model.* New York: Routledge.

Julien, R. M. (2008). *A primer of drug action* (11th ed.). New York: Worth.

McNeece, C. A., & DiNitto, D. M. (2005). *Chemical dependency: A systems approach* (3rd ed.). Boston: Allyn & Bacon.

Peele, S. (1998). *The meaning of addiction: An unconventional view*. San Francisco: Jossey-Bass.

Preston, J. D., O'Neal, J. H., & Talaga, M. C. (2008). *Handbook of clinical psychopharmacology for therapists* (5th ed.). Oakland, CA: New Harbinger.

Sinacola, R. S., & Peters-Strickland, T. S. (2006). *Basic psychopharmacology for counselors and psychotherapists*. Boston: Allyn & Bacon.

Stevens, P., & Smith, R. L. (2008). *Substance abuse counseling: Theory and practice* (4th ed.). Upper Saddle River, NJ: Pearson Merrill/Prentice Hall.

Thombs, D. L. (2006). *Introduction to addictive behavior* (3rd ed.). New York: Guilford.

Van Wormer, K., & Davis, D. R. (2008). *Addiction treatment: A strengths perspective* (2nd ed.). Pacific Grove, CA: Brooks/Cole.

Weil, A. (1998). *From chocolate to morphine*. Boston: Houghton Mifflin.

Counseling Diverse Clients

CHAPTER 13

KEY CONCEPTS

Multiple cultural identities

Dominant cultural identity

Multiculturalism

Cultural sensitivity

Personal biases

Prejudices

Cultural identity development

Social justice

Marginalization

Gender roles

Body image

Boy Code

Cultural immersion

Aging

Sexual orientation

Differently abled

Religion versus spirituality

Working with diverse populations requires the skills needed for all counseling, plus knowledge about and sensitivity to the needs of particular groups. The same counseling skills are used with women as with men, just adapted differently; the same theories of change apply to the physically handicapped as to the athlete but with certain modifications. Depression or anxiety may not feel qualitatively different to a Latino, African-American, or white person but may be expressed quite differently. Group dynamics operate in similar ways in groups of children, middle-aged adults, and older adults, but with significant differences. Gay men and lesbian women feel loneliness, frustration, or anger just as do heterosexuals. The delinquent, disabled, or drug-addicted clients all respond to empathy, confrontation, and other therapeutic strategies, depending on the counselor's finesse and sensitivity.

Yet in spite of these similarities, every client you will ever see requires you to adapt what you do—and how you do it—to a unique cultural context. Each person's ethnicity, religious and spiritual orientation, gender, sexual orientation, life stage, and primary cultural identities will challenge you to be sensitive and flexible in the ways that you work. To complicate matters further, often the differences you will see within particular identified groups will be so diverse that generalizations are next to useless. Nevertheless, your job is to (1) examine and explore your own cultural identity, (2) educate yourself as completely as you can about the cultural context for each client's experience, (3) learn about the effects of oppression on minority and disadvantaged groups, (4) acknowledge and confront your biases and prejudices with regard to particular groups, and (5) adapt all your counseling knowledge and skills in such a way that you can help diverse clientele. This is a tall order, indeed, but one that is absolutely necessary in order for you to function effectively and ethically.

MULTIPLE CONCEPTIONS OF CULTURE

Traditionally, chapters, books, and discussions about multiculturalism referred to a person's ethnicity or race. Yet "culture" involves a set of multiple identities for most individuals (Robinson, 2007; Slattery, 2004). Each person is not only strongly influenced by his or her ethnic/racial background but also the culture of his or her gender, religion, socioeconomic class, geographical location, first language, sexual orientation, political affiliation, profession, and similar identities. In fact, to some clients you will see, their choice of social group (Alcoholics Anonymous, Shriners, gang affiliation) or leisure activity (coin collector, softball player, snowboarder), or even factors related to their appearance (tattoos, clothing), may be the most defining characteristic of their cultural identity. Table 13.1 provides examples of cultural groups as they are defined by their norms, rituals, characteristics, traditions, and shared beliefs.

A client walks in the door and speaks with a particular accent, or has a particular skin color, or exhibits features of some identifiable group. You may immediately assume that being African American, Native American, Latino, or Vietnamese is the person's dominant cultural identity (and so make further assumptions about the best way to structure the sessions) but you may be sorely mistaken. It is extremely important that you approach this whole subject of multiculturalism with a truly open mind and heart so you are best positioned to truly learn about any given client's experiences and multiple cultural identities.

TABLE 13.1 | SOME EXAMPLES OF CULTURAL GROUPS

Race (African American, Native American, Chinese)
Country of origin (Mexico, Cuba, Chile)
Language (Gaelic, Spanish)
Political affiliation (Republican, Communist, Green Party)
Gender
Sexual orientation
Living situation (widowed, divorced with children)
Club (sorority, Harley Davidson)
Hobby (gun collecting, fantasy baseball, cooking)
Physical characteristics (blonde, tattoos, obese)
Physically challenged (hearing impaired, dwarfism, wheelchair bound)
Afflicted (HIV, multiple sclerosis)
Profession (athlete, police, counselor)
Religion (Mormon, Jewish, Southern Baptist)
Church/temple affiliation
Age (baby boomer, Gen-X, newly retired)
Alumni (Harvard, Marines, Peace Corps)
Geography (New Yorker, Southern Californian, Texan)
Victimization (Holocaust survivor, incest survivor)

Initial sessions may very well be devoted to asking questions such as the following:

- What would be helpful for me to know about you in terms of your cultural background?
- What are some of the groups with which you most closely identify?
- What is it that I need to know in order to understand where you come from and what is most important to you?

Your challenge is to learn as much as you can about the unique cultural background, history, and traditions of each client you see. This is not an additional burden on your job but rather a privilege of the profession that comes with the territory. Every client who walks in affords you the opportunity to learn about a variety of cultural identities that previously may have been beyond your experience. A skydiver comes in complaining of chronic anxiety. A Haitian immigrant is depressed because she misses her family back home. An Orthodox rabbi has just been diagnosed with inoperable cancer. On the way to helping them work on their issues you become an expert in their lifestyles. You learn all about their worlds, their languages, their beliefs and values. And all throughout this process you become more knowledgeable and wise.

VOICE FROM THE FIELD

I think it's the atmosphere of political correctness that makes it difficult to talk about the real issues in this field. I mean, we are all required to undergo cultural sensitivity training or whatever. Every journal is filled with articles on the subject. But I wonder how much really changes.

For lots of white counselors like me, we've just learned to pretend we aren't as racist as we really are. We pretend that we're all liberal, enlightened souls, but that's a load of bull. I'm not saying things aren't better than they were, but the truth is that the people I help the most are just like me. They look like me. They believe in the same things. The real challenge is to help the ones most not like me. That's really hard because I'm not working in areas in which I feel most comfortable and familiar.

BEING CULTURALLY SENSITIVE

See Companion DVD
Cultural Sensitivity

In one sense, the idea of multiculturalism runs contrary to some of the themes from the American idea of the great melting pot. Many people adamantly hold to the belief that people are essentially similar and any emphasis placed on the differences between "us" and "them" borders on discrimination. One major injustice inherent in that belief is the notion that if we are all the same, then what works for me obviously must also work for you. A counselor who operates from this belief system will undoubtedly play out the dynamics of domination and hegemony that the minority client has learned to distrust or abhor. This subtle bias in action looks harmless enough, but it may have dire consequences. Consider the interaction between a white, male school counselor and his Japanese-American client:

COUNSELOR: I heard about the death of your brother. I'm really concerned about our last few sessions because it seems that I've been doing most of the talking. I can imagine that you are feeling really sad right now, but you seem so disconnected. How can I help you explore your feelings? You know it's okay to cry in my office.

CLIENT: [Looking down at the floor]: I don't know.

The counselor obviously holds to the notion of Western values that successful intervention requires the client to have a cathartic emotional process. However, for the Japanese-American client, the expression of intense emotion and the exploration of his problem outside the family unit run contrary to his cultural values. Understanding clients from their unique cultural perspective has been the impetus that has driven the multicultural movement. Moreover, the definition of culture has evolved to describe more than racial and ethnic barriers to now include social class, gender, age, sexual orientation, and physical capabilities.

Make no mistake, multiculturalism is one of the most powerful and enduring movements in the profession in the past two decades. No longer is it acceptable to have only one course on multicultural issues; the subject is ideally infused into *all* courses and textbooks because it is considered so critical to understanding each client's world and planning for respectful, appropriate interventions.

Pedersen (2001) described multiculturalism as the "fourth" force in counseling, complementing the traditional three forces of psychodynamic, behavioral, and humanistic as explanations for human behavior. The multicultural perspective emphasizes the

■ | VOICE FROM THE FIELD

I'll be honest. For a long time, I resisted the whole idea of multiculturalism. It wasn't a political thing—I just felt I had struggled so much to learn counseling skills and theories, and now, the idea that I had to adjust them for different clients seemed too overwhelming. I guess I wanted to master the basics first. It was hard enough getting those right! And frankly, some of my professors implicitly supported my resistance. I remember one who would say, "Empathy is empathy, nonjudgmental acceptance is nonjudgmental acceptance, and genuineness is genuineness—that's what makes counseling work and that's all you have to know, no matter who is the client."

Well, I can tell you from experience, it's not all you have to know. I learned to do all of those things pretty well, and still, clients whose skin color was different from mine would quit after a couple of sessions. Obviously, I was doing something wrong. So I had to get over my laziness, start going over my multicultural textbooks again, and think about what would make clients from different cultural backgrounds comfortable. Yes, it was extra work, and yes, it paid off. And, you know what? It didn't turn out that I had to abandon the core conditions of good counseling. I just had to be conscious of the cultural rules my clients brought with them into the process. And appreciate that I was operating with Euro-American values, and it was arrogant for me to think those were the only ones that mattered.

value of diversity and the recognition that all people—and therefore all counseling relationships—are shaped and influenced by cultural patterns of thinking and acting. Therefore, the daunting task of working with a diverse population of clients is a complex endeavor. The counselor needs to have an awareness of the client's cultural worldview, while concurrently relating to the client as a unique individual. Furthermore, effective counselors approach this relationship with an understanding of the counterproductive personal and cultural barriers that they may also present.

Clients are both alike and different. It is only through a connected humanness that counselors can positively assist clients. The need to blend a clear understanding and respect for myriad cultural patterns with a recognition of the universal human qualities that connect individuals is a core requisite for counseling diverse clients.

Culturally sensitive counselors have been identified as having several qualities (Arredondo, 1999; Baruth & Manning, 2007; Lum, 2007; Robinson, 2007):

1. They embrace the concept of cultural pluralism and are extremely committed to learning all they can about racial/ethnic groups different from their own.
2. They are aware of how their own ethnicity and cultural backgrounds influence their practice.
3. They realize the extent to which they are not only enriched but also limited by their own ethnic and cultural heritage, a circumstance that can be remedied only through greater openness to new experiences.
4. They have developed a perspective in which each person is seen as a unique individual with values that have been influenced by the cultural context of the environment in which he or she was raised.
5. They are extremely flexible and eclectic in the ways they work with people, depending on where the client comes from and what he or she needs. Furthermore, this flexibility is manifested not only in the kinds of alliances that are

I can't tell you how often I've gotten myself in trouble by assuming that a client is a particular way based on what I think is the person's cultural background. I see someone who is black and I would think, okay, this is someone who has likely experienced oppression and discrimination because of his skin color. Then I find out he is also gay, and that cultural identity is far more important to him than being black. Then, there was another time in which I was working with a corporate executive who was also black and I again assumed that this must be important to him. Yet every time I tried to bring up racial stuff in sessions, he kept saying that this wasn't a big thing to him where he worked; it was his corporate culture that most strongly identified himself. At first, I didn't believe him; I couldn't believe him because my own race is so important to me. But over time, I've learned to be very careful to watch and listen and learn from clients rather than to assume that they hold particular values because of the way they look or speak.

created and the interventions that are chosen but also in the ways they live their lives.

6. They recognize the influence of cultural background on a client's concepts of *power, growth, time, solution,* and other terms that are part of the counseling vernacular.

7. They are relatively free of prejudices and biases that tend to stereotype people and free of the ignorant or patronizing attitudes that tend to alienate them.

8. They are aware of and sensitive to the client's worldview and work to clarify it and understand it in assessment, diagnosis, and treatment selection.

When you put all this together, what you've got is a template for relating more effectively and sensitively to all your clients. As a society, we have reached a point where these qualities are not only part of a culturally skilled and competent counselor, but anyone who seeks to help others. Table 13.2 summarizes 10 points to keep in mind when working with your clients.

TABLE 13.2 | DOING A CULTURALLY SENSITIVE INTERVIEW

1. Help the client to tell his or her story.
2. Monitor any assumptions you may have about this person that might be based on your first impressions or past experiences with others who may appear similar.
3. Use open-ended questions and probes to elicit information related to multiple cultural identities.
4. Flesh out the context and background using reflective listening skills.
5. Ask the client to teach you what you need to know and understand in order to be helpful.
6. Communicate your intense interest and convey what you've heard and understood.
7. Make sure that your communication style is sensitive, respectful, and appropriate to the particular values of your client.
8. Match your language and behaviors to those of your client.
9. Watch your biases and internal judgments as they arise during the conversation.
10. Deal with issues of marginalization, power, and oppression (if indicated and appropriate).

There are some clients I see who I think I should pay rather than the other way around. Their stories are so, so interesting. Their life experiences just blow me away—the things they have seen and done. There was this one guy who, when he was a teenager, was recruited to fight in Palestine. He kept this to himself his whole life. Didn't even tell his wife and children. Yet it was such a formative part of his life. I ended up learning a whole lot about that part of the world during that time period in history. I not only heard this client's stories but I ended up reading books so I could better understand his world. I've had other clients who are prostitutes, or stockbrokers, or actors, or litigators, and with each one of them, I end up learning so much about their inner worlds. Oh, the books I could write on what I've learned.

INFLUENCE OF BIASES

Are you biased? Of course you are! Think about it. How do you define happiness? How would you describe a psychologically healthy person? Your answers to most questions about human behavior, religion, philosophy, or health are rooted in your worldview. Is it your job to convince the indigenous client that his depression is not caused by demonic spirits but rather by his irrational belief system? Do you think that if you confronted the client about his ideas he would come back for a second session?

Even if you don't believe people who are different from you are substandard, such individuals may very well have sufficient injustice in their lives to sense such feelings from you—feelings that maybe even you are not aware of. So, although your desire to treat all people as equals is laudable, you may still unconsciously and unintentionally be harboring a number of biases and prejudices that can easily be picked up on by others who have trained themselves to be more than a little cautious—especially about people who look like you.

Members of diverse populations know they have some unique issues, and a counselor who fails to acknowledge them will likely be perceived as ineffective. Furthermore, biases and prejudices move in both directions. Picture yourself as a white male counselor in professional practice. You've analyzed your biases and beliefs. You are especially aware that as a member of the majority culture, your beliefs reflect the ideas of those in power and have not exactly been sympathetic to those who have experienced oppression.

Imagine, for example, that thus far in your efforts to establish a practice you have only three clients and the bills are piling up. Your 4:00 P.M. appointment shows up and you are excited about this new referral, an African-American 40-year-old lesbian. You run through your list of dos and don'ts as a multiculturally sensitive counselor before you invite her in and open the session with a warm greeting. She immediately sits down and wonders how this straight, uppity white boy can possibly understand her world, let alone help her! You have about 10 minutes (if you're lucky) to prove yourself.

Biases, stereotypes, and prejudices are indicative of the often instinctive and automatic cognitive processes that we use to understand the world (Fiske, 2005;

VOICE FROM THE FIELD

I work with teenagers who are getting in trouble in school—they're too aggressive, too sullen—the diagnosis would be Oppositional-Defiant Disorder. Their teachers complain to the parents, who then bring their kids to me, wanting me to fix them. Most of these kids grew up in pretty tough neighborhoods, the kind you want to avoid at night unless you have to live there.

When I listen to their stories, my heart breaks for them, and I throw diagnostic jargon out the window. Wouldn't you be angry and sullen if you grew up listening to drive-by shootings as you tried to fall asleep? Seeing your mother wired on meth carted away to jail?

Or never having a real home—getting tossed from foster home to foster home? Forget psychological "issues"; I'm thinking, what happens to a child's nervous system when she or he grows up never being able to feel safe?

How do I handle this? You know, all I do is listen, and admire the amazing resilience these kids have for just surviving, for coming to school every day and trying to stick it out the best they can. I make the hours we share a safe refuge from the storms that have dominated their lives. I try not to appear shocked by some of their horror stories. And I let them know I am humbled by their courage.

Hayes, 1996). In essence, we seek to categorize others in an attempt to understand ourselves. By observing what we are not, we can define who we are. Problems with biases and prejudices arise when we are intolerant about people's differences. When we adamantly adhere to the notion that our way is the "right" way—whereas others are wrong, corrupt, or naïve—we exhibit a rigidity that can only be destructive to our relationships with those unlike us.

In one sense, biases and prejudices are the most natural thing in the world. Throughout history, human beings have been notoriously intolerant of others who are not of their "tribe," and have killed one another with abandon. Just consider all the ethnic and cultural wars that have taken place: Assyrians versus Babylonians, Romans versus Carthaginians, Moors versus Spaniards, Boers versus English, Iroquois versus Algonquins, Paiutes versus Utes, Croats versus Serbs, Turks versus Armenians, Japanese versus Koreans, Peruvians versus Ecuadorians, Hutu versus Tutsi, Khmer Rouge versus Cambodians, Irish Catholics versus Protestants, Union versus Confederacy, Bloods versus Crips, Arabs versus Jews, Romans versus Christians, Montagues versus Capulets, Hatfields versus McCoys.

Historians have estimated that since the Holocaust, there have been as many as 50 documented cases of genocide in which one group or another has tried to do its best to wipe out others of a different religion or skin color or geographical region (Stone, 2004). It would seem that there is even a human tendency to expend our energy doing everything we can to protect resources on behalf of others who are members of our "tribe" and who therefore share our gene pool—and to do everything we can to prevent others "not like us" from enjoying the benefits of limited resources (Wright, 1994).

So, it's senseless to deny that you have biases toward one group of people or another. Notice whom you gravitate toward at a party and whom you naturally move away from. Such attraction/repulsion may not be based on skin color or physical features, but often you will find yourself preferring to be around others who share your basic values, socioeconomic class, or even professional affiliation.

VOICE FROM THE FIELD

I'm sick of do-gooders who think they are being helpful but don't have a clue about what is going on with the people they are trying to help. There were some architects who got together to volunteer their time to design economic public housing for the inner city. They built these low-slung, modern-looking buildings not at all like the usual concrete towers that are in most cities. They had courtyards. They were decorated in bright colors. Very attractive. The problem was that nobody would live in them. They were built according to the aesthetic tastes of the architects, many of whom were minority people but from a very different socioeconomic class. Their worldviews never considered that the so-called public spaces, the courtyards, allowed gangs to patrol freely. And the walls of the buildings might have been quite nice to look at, but they were too thin to stop bullets from penetrating. They never stopped to consider what the people really wanted who were going to be living in the housing project.

Any one person or group of people who differs from societal norms almost inevitably faces covert and overt forms of discrimination. Differences can be as obvious as physical characteristics or more subtle, such as education level, religious affiliation, or marital status. Discrimination can be as obvious as preventing African Americans or women from voting or owning property. Covert discrimination occurs more subtly but is just as harmful. An individual may not get a job because of sexual orientation, ethnicity, or gender. A child may not be picked to answer a question in school because he belongs to a lower class or is black. There are countless ways in which people from diverse populations are quietly and discreetly discriminated against.

Some biases and prejudices result from the awareness that "bad" things can happen to all of us; the discomfort we experience at seeing a disabled or mentally ill person is often related to our own fears. Rigidity of thinking, fear of the unknown, avoidance of risks, and many other self-defeating behaviors likewise contribute to an individual's inflexibility.

There is also a danger that counselors who work with large numbers of people will class them in groups rather than seeing them as individuals: "I was seeing this Jewish housewife yesterday..." or "What do you do to get around the resistance in Asian families..." or "I've got this deaf guy on my schedule..." But that's our point. Their generalizations are likely to breed misconceptions.

How would you describe the following people: a Latina, a high-school dropout, an African-American teen, a truck driver, a priest? When you think of these people, what images do you see in your head? What experiences have you had with people who carry these labels? If a member of a culture different than your own were to walk into your office, you might make a snap judgment about that person. This is not only a natural phenomenon but a useful one as well. Our survival, at least in the past, was based on making instantaneous and accurate judgments about who was safe and who was dangerous. We carry within us this legacy in which we are constantly making assessments and predictions about people based on our prior experiences with others who *appear* similar.

The problem, of course, comes when—in light of new, more complete information—you don't alter your initial judgments; you retain your prejudices and refuse to see individuals as who they really are rather than as members of a group.

VOICE FROM THE FIELD

I used to think I had personally never experienced discrimination. My grandparents were immigrants, and struggled in America, but my father was a successful businessman, and even though I was a minority in my school, I grew up with every advantage. Sure, I was called some names on playgrounds from time to time, but my parents would just tell me those people were just ignorant, and I would forget about it.

Then, one day my teenage son was given the assignment to interview me about my experiences with discrimination. He started asking me a bunch of questions about what it was like as a kid. At first, I said I wasn't going to be of much help. But I went along with it, and as I started to recall those moments when cruel things were said, I could feel the tightness in my throat—the counselor in me immediately recognized the feeling as a sign of tears I'd buried for a long time. And then as we talked, he asked me about the places I've lived in my life, and this realization hit me—I've lived in four states, and in every one, I've chosen without thinking to live in communities where people looked like me and shared my core values. Because, I guess, those were the places where I felt safe. And here I was thinking that I had never been affected by my cultural heritage!

It is not uncommon for people to believe that although they are prejudiced against a certain group of people, they never let that belief interfere with their work. It is unlikely that anyone who has strong biases or prejudices is completely able to conceal those feelings from others. In counseling, for example, diagnostic biases abound (Baruth & Manning, 2007), leading, for example, to consistent misdiagnoses with minority groups (Aklin & Turner, 2006). For example, African Americans and Hispanics tend to be over diagnosed with schizophrenia and under-diagnosed with mood disorders (Rosenthal & Berven, 1999; Whaley & Geller, 2007). Diagnosticians are also often seen to have a bias against lower-class patients. A diagnosis of severe psychosis is more likely to be bestowed on a lower-class patient than on a middle-class patient, given similar manifestations of pathological symptoms.

Counselors, regardless of their sex, rated female clients with unusual career goals as being more in need of counseling than those with conforming career goals (Sinacore-Guinn, 1995). This finding raises an important issue: Bias is not necessarily directed toward someone who is different from us—the opposite sex, in this case—but can also be directed toward people who are like us. The societal expectations, norms, and socialization processes operate systematically to define appropriate roles for women, African Americans, senior citizens, and disabled persons. Prejudices and biases can be and are formed against any conceivably definable group of people: WASPs, veterans, Ku Klux Klansmen, gays and lesbians, hunters, blue-collar workers, executives, middle-class suburban housewives, and BMW owners are all groups of people for whom certain stereotypes have been established in our society. There are, of course, many more.

IDENTITY ISSUES

How would you describe your own cultural identity? Are you a woman, a man, Latino, white, African American, gay, Southerner, or Methodist? Or are you a gay Hispanic man, an African-American woman? If you are white, what does that mean to you? Are your European roots especially important to you? What would a counselor need to know and understand about your cultural identity in order to be helpful to you?

Or would you describe your cultural identity as something completely different? Think back to how you developed your sense of yourself and your culture. Does the definition of your culture differ from how others would see you? In fact, we would dare to guess that your cultural identity could be comprised of many cultures. Researchers have argued that multiculturalism can be delineated into mutually independent categories and that a cultural identity is much more complex than association with a single group (Schmidt, 2006). To further complicate the issue, there has been much discussion about the applicability of the male Eurocentric treatment models to members of diverse populations (Slattery, 2004). Gilligan (1982), Jordan (2003), and Comstock (2005) have argued eloquently that women's identity must be considered from a relational rather than an autonomous viewpoint. What, then, is the process for identity development of a disabled Hispanic girl?

Developing a positive identity is a universal human challenge often compounded by membership in a minority group or groups. Pervasive numbers of "isms" (ageism, sexism, racism) in society can act as barriers to positive identity development. Many individuals feel alienated and different when they do not live up to expectations because of cultural differences. In order to help clients build a positive sense of personal identity, counselors must be aware of alternative models for identity that are culturally broad and inclusive.

Facilitating identity development is a critical issue for counselors working with diverse clients. The presence of a clear and directed identity is essential for fostering growth and development. Counselors must be aware of the limitations for many clients of traditional developmental theory and be able to work with alternative patterns if they fit more appropriately.

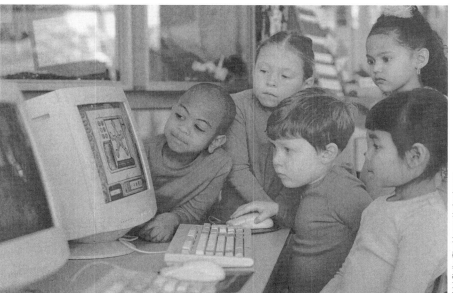

Ariel Skelley/Blend Images/Jupiter Images.

Children from various cultural groups may develop their primary identities through different influences, including their neighborhoods, families, schools, clubs, friends, and media.

VOICE FROM THE FIELD

Is there such a thing as a "positive bias"? Because I've got one. You see, there's a particular kind of client that I actually prefer... someone I instinctively look forward to working with. It's always the same: a person who is well educated and articulate, someone in touch with feelings. Probably a woman, since she's more likely to talk about feelings. I like clients who are a bit feisty, who stir things up, who challenge me, but who, when it comes right down to it, are women of action. There's nothing worse than someone who talks and talks but never changes anything.

Who don't I like to work with? Well, in my experience, older men can be a pain in the butt. They just didn't grow up during a time when counseling was acceptable. They don't know how to be good clients. They want me to tell them what to do.

Because God is important to me, I have a hard time working with anyone who doesn't feel the same way. It's not that I can't help that person, it's just that my feelings come through. I know it.

CONFRONTING YOUR BIASES

The idea we are about to introduce is provocative and may spark some defensiveness: It is our belief that *everyone* is a racist; and *everyone* has biases and prejudices toward others. What we mean is that you prefer to hang out with folks who are "like me" and avoid people who are "not like me." These are people who are part of your "tribe," your identified peer group. This may not be based on skin color, or religious preference, but it is certainly based on shared interests, values, and preferences. Just consider the immediate impressions you might have, and prejudgments you might make, about someone described to you as: "Republican," or "a rodeo cowboy," or "a Seventh-Day Adventist," or a "transsexual." It is difficult, if not impossible, to avoid forming some initial expectation. Furthermore, such impressions are in many ways highly functional.

Confronting your prejudices and biases is an important component of your counselor training (Ivey, D'Andrea, Ivey, & Simek-Morgan, 2007; Pope & Vasquez, 2007; Schmidt, 2006). You can do great damage to clients who may already be feeling somewhat vulnerable and insecure. If they sense and feel your critical judgments of them (and these are very hard to hide), it may further erode their already fragile self-esteem.

COUNSELORS AS ADVOCATES FOR SOCIAL JUSTICE

Let's say you have devoted yourself to becoming a culturally sensitive counselor. You've educated yourself on cultural traditions, you respect worldviews different from your own, you are careful to adjust your counseling interventions so as not to offend your client's values, and you are highly cognizant of how your clients from marginalized backgrounds have suffered from discriminatory practices. As a result, your clients feel understood, more self-aware, and, because of your help, empowered to pursue their goals.

But the reality is that many of your clients from minority cultures will leave your office still facing barriers to achieving those goals. They go out into the real world, only to discover once again that the social and political obstacles remain;

there is the job they may not get because of their accent; the bullying their children can be subjected to on school playgrounds; the cop that pulls them over for no legitimate reason. They come back to your office discouraged, maybe even depressed. Is it enough for you to once again listen compassionately and use your counseling skills to reduce depressive symptoms? Or is some other intervention required, one that may even extend beyond the walls of your counseling office?

Proponents of social justice counseling argue that the role of the counselor includes not only empowering your clients on a psychological level, but also actively confronting the social injustices and inequalities that impact your client's well-being (Crethar, Rivera, & Nash, 2008; Kottler & Marriner, 2009). The notion that counselors have responsibilities to address systemic inequities has been closely intertwined with multiculturalism since its beginning. Some have argued that social justice is the core of the multicultural competence movement (Arredondo & Perez, 2003). The meaning of social justice, as it relates to the counseling profession, varies among different authors and is difficult to precisely define, but one thing is clear: to be a counselor means to be an active advocate for those clients whose individual aspirations and access to economic resources have been restricted by the dominant culture (Pieterse et al., 2009). This means advocating on behalf of the oppressed and marginalized, whether in your community or on a global scale.

While the need for counselors to intervene on behalf of marginalized clients has been generally endorsed, there exists a diversity of opinions on how counselors can put advocacy into practice. Roysicar (2009), for example, calls for counselors to become active in politics or volunteer their time to community organizations aimed at redressing social inequities. Other authors suggest counselors combine self-reflection regarding one's biases, knowledge of the various ways in which social injustice impacts the lives of marginalized cultures, and collaborative involvements with schools, mental health, and community organizations (Constantine, Hage, Kindaichi, & Bryant, 2007). Advocacy competencies that provide a framework for how counselors can make a difference (Lewis, Arnold, House, & Toporek, 2002) include:

1. *Client/Student Empowerment.* Counselors help clients and students recognize their strengths and learn how to advocate for themselves.
2. *Client/Student Advocacy.* Counselors work with community agencies, community leaders, and school authorities to provide resources and support for clients.
3. *Community Collaboration.* Counselors can use their listening skills to facilitate collaboration among community groups. For example, a counselor helping a child being bullied because of his minority status might bring together school and local leaders, help them identify their common goals, and lead a discussion on how to prevent bullying (Lopez & Paylo, 2009).
4. *Systems Advocacy.* This competency recognizes that institutions can be resistant to change and suggests counselors use their training in addressing client's resistance in therapy to address systemic resistance at a school or community level. This might include empathizing with local leaders' concerns and guiding them towards an action plan that would initiate change at a systemic level.
5. *Public Information.* Counselors can use their communication skills to disseminate information through media outlets about the negative impact of social injustice on human development.

6. *Social/Political Advocacy.* Counselors need to recognize the larger social problems that require political action to address. They can then identify community leaders and legislators who can impact the political system; communicate to them the need for social change; and actively support them in their change-making efforts.

Some have pointed out that implementing all of these guidelines can lead to counselor burn-out, and clinicians would be wise to collaborate with organizations that are willing to carry much of the burden (Ratts & Hutchings, 2009). What is important is that counselors appreciate that clients' mental health difficulties can be rooted at both the micro-level (emotional conflicts, irrational beliefs, ineffective coping strategies) and the macro-level (social and political forces that impinge on clients' well-being). True helping sometimes requires that we conceptualize client problems at both levels, and martial our energy, skills, and courage to facilitate change not only in our clients' internal worlds but in the external, real world we all share.

As daunting as this responsibility might appear at first, it is remarkably easy to begin your own social justice commitment. It just takes one small step to make a difference in your community or among any oppressed group, and your efforts may start while you are still a student. There are many inspiring stories of individuals who, with little or no training, felt inspired to begin small, modest programs that blossomed into global enterprises helping thousands of people who would otherwise have never received help. (Examples of such inspiring stories can be found in several sources (Kottler & Marriner, 2009; Mortenson & Relin, 2007; Wood, 2007).)

As one example, Jeffrey has been working with groups of counseling and health students to support lower caste girls in remote regions of Nepal who would otherwise be at-risk to be sold into slavery because their families are too poor to feed them. Initially the project began by offering one scholarship to an academically gifted girl who could no longer afford to attend school (it costs only $100 to support a child for a year). The project (www.ghimirefoundation.org) has now grown to support more than a hundred girls in eight villages around the country, all the result of students and counselors working collaboratively to intervene with some of the most neglected children in the world.

You don't have to go to Nepal in order to begin your own social justice project; it just takes a little bit of imagination and the commitment to follow through within any community that needs help.

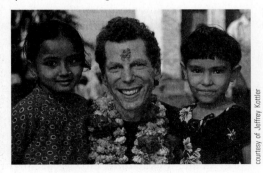

Jeffrey in Nepal.

COUNSELING WOMEN

About three-quarters of the clients you will see are going to be women. This is not because females are inclined to have more problems than men but because they are often designated as the "identified clients" in their families, the ones who seek help on behalf of others. Furthermore, the whole enterprise of counseling is much more congruent with the values of women: Clients are expected to be self-disclosing, to share feelings openly, to be vulnerable, and to admit to weaknesses. These are tasks not often associated with male socialization.

Though women are not definable as a minority group, they have been subjected to similar marginalization, discrimination, and prejudice that minorities have experienced. This is true not only from the perspective that most counseling theories were invented by white males and reflect their values and biases, but also that most positions of power and influence have been controlled by men as well. Although this trend is changing (it is now rare for a man to be elected president of the American Counseling Association, one professional group whose members are primarily female), inequalities still exist in many sectors.

With a few notable exceptions (Melanie Klein, Anna Freud), men created most of the foundational theories of this field, some showing biases regarding the roles women should play. Certainly Freud's portrayal of the "weaker sex" as dependent, hysterical, and inferior established a precedent. Most of the theories that followed continued to reinforce conventional stereotypes of women as sex objects who need counseling for their boredom.

Women are more likely than men to be diagnosed with major depression, and when they are depressed, they stay depressed longer. The books of Sylvia Plath, Virginia Woolf, Doris Lessing, Alice Walker, and other writers document the depressive episodes all too familiar to women who feel powerless, ignored, abused, and neglected in their lives. Eriksen and Kress (2008) noted that women are more likely than men to be diagnosed as suffering from dependent and histrionic personality disorders. Research evidence has found a sex bias in the diagnosis of borderline personality disorder, which is characterized by emotional volatility (Boggs et al., 2005). Horsfall (2001) observed that the criteria for these and other disorders in which women predominate are caricatures of traditional female roles—that is, diagnoses that describe women who are overconforming in their efforts to satisfy gender stereotypes. Thus, favorite labels include such terms as *hysterical*, *passive-dependent*, and *anorexic*, which all describe the symptoms of a woman trying too hard to be subordinate, emotional, dependent, and skinny. Counselors need to be aware of the danger of creating additional problems for female clients by labeling overconforming behavior as pathological.

Then there is the whole concept of body image. Women strive to fulfill some ideal concept of how they should look and in the process often develop distorted images of their body and poor self-concepts. Eating disorders are a particularly dramatic example of the attempts of women to live up to the ideal standards of body image created by Western culture (Behar, 2006). Almost all models are tall and thin. While striving for this narrow conception that beauty is slimness, some women lose control of their original goal to become thinner and eventually their ability to accurately assess their own body shape, so that no amount of weight

VOICE FROM THE FIELD

I like working with men, and there's a good reason for it. As a male counselor, I have a pretty good idea of the way men think, especially to avoid feelings, because I've spent a lot of time tuned in to my own thoughts doing the same thing. So I can say to a guy, "OK, here's what I'm guessing is going through your head right now. You tell me if I'm wrong. It's something like this …"—and I get it right more times than not. It's a satisfying feeling. And it facilitates trust, so as the work progresses, I can start approaching real feelings without the client getting resistant.

My biggest problem is with teenagers, regardless of sex. Honestly, it's not because they can be sullen and uncooperative, but because of what it brings up in me. Too many uncomfortable memories of my own adolescence. There's some stuff I don't think I'll ever get over, and I'd just as soon spare myself reliving some pretty painful times.

loss satisfies the desire to experience themselves as thin. One prevalent consequence is anorexia nervosa, or drastic weight loss to the point of starvation. This disorder has been associated with the degree to which women conform not only to society's image of beauty but also to its definition of feminine behavior; thus, women who silence their own needs and refrain from expressing anger may be more likely to experience disturbed eating patterns and become preoccupied with their body shape (Piran & Cormier, 2005). Adolescent girls are particularly vulnerable to this eating disorder, which is reinforced when parents, teachers, and sports coaches encourage them to lose weight (Behar, 2006). Bulimia, or compulsive food gorging, is another way women ruin their bodies through abusive eating habits, often the consequence of rejection and a poor self-concept. Eating disorders have proven to be highly challenging to treat effectively; cognitive behavioral, psychodynamic, family systems, and group modalities have all been adapted to cure anorexia and bulimia, yet full recovery remains elusive for about half the women with eating disturbances (Kalodner & Delucia-Waack, 2003).

Serious questions are often raised about the validity of counseling interventions with women on the grounds that the personality theories from which they derive are authored by men and focused primarily on male concerns. Concepts such as "penis envy" and "Oedipus complex" and stereotypical portrayals of women as emotional and nurturing make it more difficult for them to attain the autonomy and independence so prized by most psychological theories.

Two counseling models have been designed to specifically address both women's internal dynamics and the psychological consequences of living in a still-male-dominated society. Feminist counseling stresses enhancing women's empowerment, and facilitating exploration of the impact of patriarchal social structures on their lives. For example, counselors working from a feminist perspective would note a client's tendency to suppress anger in favor of the more socially acceptable feminine responses like sadness or forgiveness; her angry feelings would be normalized and validated, and, together, counselor and client might discuss how socialization forces taught her to dismiss her authentic feelings. Interventions like assertiveness training, self-defense classes, and psychoeducation about handling finances might also be used to help clients practice newly discovered feelings of empowerment in real-world situations (Sharf, 2008).

■ | VOICE FROM THE FIELD

I was leading this group mostly composed of women, when one member was discussing her frustrations related to her husband's nonresponsive behavior. I interrupted her several times, essentially saying to her that rather than complaining and blaming, what was she going to do about it? Okay, I admit it: As a man I was identifying with the husband a lot.

The group member ignored me and kept on with her story. I looked around the group and saw a number of female heads nodding in agreement, or perhaps they were just indicating that they were with her. I sure wasn't, because I interrupted her again, this time to ask her where things were going because I was noticing myself (and the other men) becoming bored with the monologue.

She looked me straight in the eyes and said to me: "What is it with you guys—is it so hard for you just to listen to me? I don't want you to fix me. I don't want you to push me or interrupt me. I don't ever feel that men hear what I am saying." Wow! That sure got my attention. Forever after, I have been considering the multitude of ways that men and women do speak different languages.

The second approach that is gaining increasing acceptance in the counseling field is relational-cultural therapy (RCT), first developed by Judith Jordan and her colleagues at the Stone Center in Wellesley, Massachusetts. As we discussed in Chapter 5, RCT theory presumes that women's emotional distress is associated with disconnections, from both vital interpersonal relationships (e.g., family-of-origin figures and past and current intimate partners) and aspects of their own emotional lives. In contrast to traditional models where psychological health was associated with individuation, RCT counselors believe that relationships are an essential component of people's existence, and that women's natural growth is toward connection and mutuality rather than autonomy and self-reliance. Counselors using this model emphasize an empathic counseling relationship, in which counselors explore women's past history of painful disconnections and reflect their yearnings for more fulfilling relationships. Well-timed self-disclosures by counselors regarding the emotional impact clients are having on them serve to enhance clients' feelings of empowerment within a relational context. Finally, clients are helped to strengthen their relational resilience, so they can tolerate the disappointments and temporary disconnections that are inevitable in intimate relationships (Jordan, 2003).

Women are often more frequent victims of poverty and domestic violence. We have witnessed this not only in North American culture but in most countries around the world. Women who live in impoverished conditions are unable to gain access to such support systems as child care, health care, and counseling, so they are more likely to develop serious problems before they receive help. Although women are frequent victims of domestic violence, they are reluctant to reveal their experiences or seek help, in part because victims fear they will be judged and criticized for participating in an abusive relationship (Fugate, Landis, Riordan, Naureckas, & Engel, 2005). Women who survive an abusive relationship often experience grief, depression, and a sense of guilt and shame. The family is not a safeguard against violence for women because violent incidents directed toward women often involve family members.

VOICE FROM THE FIELD

I do a lot of couples counseling, and the single most frequent complaint I hear from husbands is that their wives are too "emotional." Of course, you can guess what their wives' reactions are—tears or anger, as though they are falling right into the trap. And there is a part of me that wishes some of these women could turn it down a notch. Just saying these words indicates that I'm the one who's fallen into the trap—the trap our society has created that labels emotionality as pathological.

One of the current theories on the evolutionary purposes of emotion is that it is an adaptive signaling system, meaning it's the brain's way of cueing people there might be danger present, so that they will check their surroundings and determine if a real threat exists.

If it does, they can take some sort of action to protect themselves and their families. From this perspective, "emotional" women actually have highly sensitive danger-alert mechanisms. A million years ago, in cave-people times, they'd be the survivors and the rest of us less emotional types would be eaten alive. Somehow, though, the meaning of emotion has changed over the years, and as men eventually dominated social structures, emotions became something negative. Now I reframe "emotionality" as a gift, sort of like being extra intelligent or unusually compassionate.

It's such a relief for the women I work with to hear their emotions framed this way; their whole lives, people have accused them of being too "sensitive," until their own emotional life became shameful to them.

Current lifestyle issues such as juggling roles, coping with poverty, and responding to violence—combined with developing an identity and positive self-concept in the shadow of theories that discount many aspects of the female experience—demonstrate the importance of acquiring and using knowledge and insight in the counseling of women. In particular, female counselors must be careful not to assume that being female correlates with understanding the problems and concerns of all women.

COUNSELING MEN

While men notoriously underutilize counseling services, you will see male clients, although they may not be happy about needing your help. Men usually come to counseling because they are in a crisis state and, frequently, because someone else has pushed them into it. A wife demands her husband get counseling as an ultimatum in their marriage; a judge orders a man who has hit his partner to get anger management counseling; an employer orders a man whose job performance has deteriorated to deal with his alcoholism. Other men come to counseling when their depression or anxiety have become unbearable, and hiding their pain from themselves and others is no longer possible. Men in midlife may be experiencing an existential crisis, terrified of their looming mortality and struggling to redefine themselves. Some men, at any age, may need help sorting out their sexual orientation (Englar-Carlson & Shepard, 2003; Rabinowitz & Shepard, 2002).

Regardless of the reason for a man's getting psychological help, counselors need to be sensitive to the particular issues men face arising out of their socialization experiences. Keep in mind that many men learned throughout their childhood to avoid any experience that might feel "feminine" to them, and, as noted in the previous section, the counseling experience is a feminine one by definition; it requires the self-disclosure of vulnerable feelings, the admission of needing help from others, and openness to forming an intimate relationship with a counselor. Making the counseling experience a safe and inviting one for the male client requires skill and sensitivity, including the recognition that some traditional counseling interventions such as feeling-eliciting probes may be inappropriate, at best creating therapeutic impasses and at worst inciting your client to exit counseling prematurely.

Effective male counseling begins with an awareness of the internal conflicts many men face arising out of their socialization experiences. Most men learned in childhood and adolescence the traditional male gender role. Four components of this role have been identified: A man must be "The Sturdy Oak," which means never showing weakness; he must "Give 'Em Hell," demonstrating aggressiveness and bravado; he needs to be "The Big Wheel," achieving status and power; and, above all, he must demonstrate "No Sissy Stuff," never displaying qualities associated with women, such as dependence, warmth, and empathy (David & Brannon, 1976). Men learn these rules in the locker rooms and playgrounds from their peers, and at home from their parents or other family members when they are told "Big boys don't cry" or similar messages. Pollack (1998) referred to the rules boys internalize as "The Boy Code," and the rules are enforced by shame—every boy can recall an experience of humiliation when showing vulnerable feelings in front of peers and family.

Living according to this code is virtually impossible; every man experiences hurt, self-doubt, and the need for support from others. Every man needs to share painful feelings, and be soothed by the comforting words of an understanding friend or family member. Thus, many men frequently experience a gender role strain or conflict, torn between their authentic needs and yearnings, and their fear of being unmanly. Boys and men differ in how rigidly they conform to the traditional rules of masculinity; some are more comfortable with expressing feelings and vulnerability than others. But it is unlikely that any boy grows into manhood without knowing the rules and experiencing some gender role conflict (Robertson & Shepard, 2008; Shepard, 2004).

These socialization pressures may play a role in men's emotional struggles as well. Trying to live up to the traditional male role has been associated with depression and overall psychological distress (Hayes & Mahalik, 2000; Liu & Iwamoto, 2006; Shepard, 2005), and also may contribute to substance abuse (Blazina & Watkins, 1996); because men learn not to seek emotional support when they are feeling sad or depressed, they may self-medicate with alcohol or other addictive drugs. The fact that men are taught not to cry or show negative feelings also means they lose the opportunity for family members to recognize their pain and come to their aid. Some men get so little practice expressing tender feelings that they struggle using the language of feelings; as a result, their intimate partners find them emotionally unavailable or inadequate for providing words of support. This leads to stresses in relationships.

One particularly insidious consequence of male socialization that counselors need to be aware of is masked or hidden depression (Cochran & Rabinowitz, 2003). Because displays of weaknesses are considered unmasculine, some men who are experiencing depression may externalize their distress rather than display sadness, tears, and other mood symptoms that are the typical signs of depression. Instead, depression manifests as irritability, substance abuse, anger, withdrawal from others, and even domestic violence; thus, you may see a male client referred because of difficulties with abuse or anger, but if the underlying depression is not addressed, the behavioral problems are likely to persist. Depression is a particularly dangerous mood disorder for men because men tend to be effective in their suicide attempts, using guns or other quick-acting lethal means rather than making the "cry for help" suicide gestures that women tend to use (e.g., taking pills, or cuts to the wrist) and that may allow time for someone to come to their rescue.

In the last several years, researchers in the field of male counseling have begun developing models designed to make counseling more effective for boys and adult male clients (Englar-Carlson & Shepard, 2005; Kiselica, 2003; Kiselica, Englar-Carlson, & Horne, 2008; Rabinowitz & Cochran, 2002). As with any client, developing a working alliance is the first and perhaps most important step, and involves the following:

1. The physical environment should be male friendly; if you are practicing in an agency or private office, make sure there are male-oriented magazines in the waiting room. Check the counseling office you are using to see if it has too many feminine touches; something as innocuous as flower prints on the wall can confirm his fears that counseling is a female-oriented experience. For adolescent boys, conducting sessions on a basketball court or walking in a park may be helpful; boys tend to talk more freely when engaged in other activities.
2. Engage in small talk and appropriate self-disclosure; talking about the parking situation, the building you are in, and other superficial subjects may put the male client at ease.
3. Respect your client's comfort level with regard to self-disclosure. Do not confront a man's reluctance to express feelings or reveal shameful matters until you feel confident that the male client feels safe in the counseling relationship. Part of a good assessment is to note his initial use of feeling-oriented language; if the man uses words like "sad" and "fearful" early on, he may have no problem with feeling-oriented empathy and questions. On the other hand, if he tends to say "I think" instead of "I feel," and avoids feeling-language, it may take more time before he is ready to engage in the discourse typical of counseling. That's why your basic "How does that make you feel?" question can create discomfort; the language of feeling not only violates socialized role norms, but may be a challenge for him to use competently.
4. If a male client is ambivalent about being in counseling, whether in individual, couples, or family contexts, discuss his ambivalence with him. Explore his fears about what counseling entails, and normalize his uneasiness as understandable given his expectations that counseling reflects female values, not traditional male ones.

As with any client, men benefit the most from counseling when their strengths are reflected as well as their problem areas, and the strengths associated with masculinity—appropriate self-reliance, decision making in crises, self-sacrifice, codes of loyalty and honor, to name a few—all should be affirmed. Finally, men's capacity for forming intimate relationships, for learning to express feelings, and for allowing themselves to experience healthy dependence on others should never be short-changed or dismissed as being deficient due to the biological differences between men and women. Men have the same deep yearnings for closeness and connection that women do, and the counseling relationship can be the ideal laboratory for helping men learn how to meet these essential human needs.

■ | VOICE FROM THE FIELD

I think the most important lesson I've learned from working with men is that they do not have to "feel" in order to be feeling something. What I mean is, if you interpret minimal displays of emotion as avoiding feelings, and work extra hard to help him have a cathartic experience, the client is more likely to freeze up than show strong emotions. For example, I worked with a man struggling over a difficult divorce. You'd think he'd be in a lot of pain, and he was, but he was determined not to show it in front of me. Why? Because he was already humiliated by his wife's leaving him for someone else, and to now cry over it in the presence of a counselor would have been doubly humiliating. He was desperately trying to hold on to his pride, which was very shaky at the moment, and I would have done him no service by undermining the pride he had left.

I want to be clear on this point: I'm not suggesting I believe he should keep his feelings inside. That won't help him at all. But my talking about how painful it must be for him, and how I could imagine what he must be going through, allowed him to simply say, "Yes. That's what it's like for me." For this client, that was expressing emotion. At the same time, I said to him, "I really admire your courage in keeping yourself together through all of this. I also want you to know that it's OK for me if you don't." He gave me just the tiniest nod in reply, but enough to let me know he understood. He had permission to let go, but also he was in control, and for a male client, maintaining some control in the face of overwhelming pain is just as important as releasing his inner burden.

COUNSELING ETHNIC MINORITIES

The United States is a nation of diverse cultural groups, a few of which control most of the power and resources. A number of traditionally disadvantaged minority groups—notably Latinos, African Americans, Native Americans, and Asian Americans—have been underrepresented not only in positions of prominence but also as counseling clients. There is probably no issue in the field considered more important right now than attention to the ways in which counselors can better serve minority groups in their educational, vocational, and personal pursuits.

Although lip service is often given to this "politically correct" professional issue in counseling education, it seems that often the changes initiated are cosmetic rather than substantial. Perhaps a chapter is included in a book such as this one. You take a class and go to a few workshops to increase your multicultural sensitivity. The public celebrates Martin Luther King Day or Cinco de Mayo. Employers sponsor workshops in cultural sensitivity. We recognize Black History Month. Certainly this is better than nothing, but it's not nearly enough.

Researchers ascribe much of the failure and ineffectiveness of mental health programs to the lack of recognition given to the needs of minority groups. In reviews of the literature pertaining to treatment of minority populations, researchers came to several conclusions (Robinson, 2007; Schwartz & Feisthamel, 2009):

1. Minority clients are diagnosed as having more severe disturbances and pathological conditions than white persons—a finding that is not surprising considering that most tests of mental illness are culturally biased and most diagnosticians are not members of minority groups.
2. Minority clients will tend to use mental health services only in cases of emergency or severe psychopathology, again skewing the perceptions of clinicians, who may be used to working with normal or neurotic whites but

VOICE FROM THE FIELD

I travel a lot. I try to spend as much time as I can visiting places I've never been before. I used to travel abroad to do this when I was younger, but lately, I've learned that there is so much to see within driving distance. I say that I am visiting places but I'm really far more interested in meeting people, especially those from different cultures. I don't care much for museums or tourist spots; I am drawn to places where people hang out. In fact, lately when I travel I arrange for home-stays rather than antiseptic, homogenous motels. I give up a little privacy, sure, but I learn so much about people living with them for a few days or a week.

My counseling training has served me well during my travels. I have become so skilled at asking the kinds of questions that get people to open up. I listen carefully. I communicate to the people that I meet that I am so interested in their lives, and especially their stories. I think more than anything else I do—workshops I've attended, classes I've taken, supervision—these travels have taught me to be more open and understanding of my clients' experiences.

---

very disturbed minorities. It is a cultural norm, for instance, among South American populations to handle most psychological problems through the resources of the family and church, relying on counselors or therapists only in extreme cases.

3. Minority clients more often drop out of treatment prematurely, usually within the first few sessions. Whether this tendency is a function of poor motivation or due to a difference in how they are treated is not clear.

4. In inpatient settings, evidence does indicate that African-American clients are treated differently than whites, more often receiving stronger medication, seclusion, restraints, and other punitive "therapies"—and less often receiving recreational or occupational therapy.

5. Minority group attitudes toward psychological disturbances are markedly different from those of whites, more often stressing the roles of organic factors. Latinos, for example, may have more faith in the power of prayer than in counseling for healing what they believe are inherited illnesses. The expectations of some minority clients may not, therefore, be conducive to success, because so often the faith and hope that are so important are not operating at high levels.

6. Many people feel more comfortable and prefer working with others whom they perceive as similar (particularly with regard to race or ethnic background). Yet there are relatively few trained minority counselors who are available to serve this need.

7. With minority clients, and particularly with those of the lower class, counselors must adapt their strategies and interventions to cultural differences. Eye contact and attention patterns can be interpreted variously as resistance, passivity, or aggression, depending on the client's culture.

8. Counseling can be viewed as a form of social control, because its goals are most often to help deviants better adjust to the cultural norms of the majority. For the minority client this sort of adjustment presents special problems, because more conflict can result from the clash between subcultural values and those of the majority.

VOICE FROM THE FIELD

When I was an intern, I was given the most "difficult" client in the agency, an African-American man in his early 30s who had seen three previous interns, making them think twice about their new careers because of his powerful outbursts of rage. He would yell in sessions, and I mean, really yell. He'd yell about the bosses who were treating him unfairly, he'd yell about his father who had abused him as a child, and worst of all, he'd yell at me, this white guy who presumed to want to understand him. I would gingerly try to say something empathic, and I'd get back, "You can't possibly understand me! Where do you come off thinking you can! Where do you get the arrogance to think you could ever possibly know what I've been through!"

You bet I was scared, too. Not that he would hurt me. Just that I would wilt under the ferocity of his anger. The worst thing I could have done would have been to confront his insistence on seeing himself as a victim. He would just have exploded some more, even if it were true. Instead, I was honest with him. "I don't think I could ever understand what you've been through. I'm a white guy who has gotten every break. But I do want to try to understand. Can you help me?" He gave me this odd, puzzled look, as though saying, "Who is this weird white guy?" But he softened a bit, and began to tell me his life story. I won't give you the details, but I will tell you that I wept. And felt his anger was totally understandable. And I told him that. Did his outbursts go away? If only our jobs were that simple! But they slowed down in frequency, and we gradually became very close, until, of all my clients, he was the one I missed the most when I completed my internship.

Recognizing your cultural biases is only the first of several steps to ensuring effective treatment of minority clients. Counselors must also be highly motivated to educate themselves about other cultural groups. Counselors, especially European Americans, need to be prepared to self-disclose to clients their emotional reactions to clients' stories of oppression and racism; such disclosures may strengthen the counseling relationship and encourage minority clients to elaborate on their experiences of discrimination and victimization (Burkard, Knox, & Groen, 2006). Finally, counselors must develop the cross-cultural intervention skills to work with each client as an individual. By endlessly focusing on the differences among various ethnic groups, counselors can fall into the trap of neglecting the uniqueness of each member of the group. A person's ethnic identity is only one of several contextual variables that can help counselors understand and work with clients. Similarly, understanding the cultural heritage of clients is a necessary but insufficient condition for attaining true empathic contact.

A serious need exists not only for increased awareness of racial and ethnic minority groups but also for educational programs that can prepare counselors to work with these groups (Abreu, Chung, & Atkinson, 2000; Baruth & Manning, 2007; Kress, Eriksen, Rayle, & Ford, 2005). Promoting multicultural development basically involves three stages: awareness, knowledge, and skills (Pedersen & Carey, 2003). Thus, as students of counseling, you must continue to develop awareness of your own attitudes, acquire knowledge about different cultures, and develop skills for interacting with persons from various backgrounds. These steps are equally important for all students and practicing counselors, regardless of race or ethnic origin. Belonging to the same race or culture as your client does not mean that you know or understand all the experiences of other members of that group.

| VOICE FROM THE FIELD

I remember one time I was doing a group that included some Native American participants. I thought I was being so sensitive to their needs and I went to extraordinary lengths to accommodate them as best I could and make them feel welcome.

Then one day I noticed that one of the Native students was absent. She didn't come back the next time either. But I figured it would be intrusive or insensitive of me to push things. Still, I was a bit bewildered by her behavior, just dropping out like that without the courtesy of a phone call. Honestly, I was angry.

I later learned that there had been a death in her family and according to her traditions, she was required to drop out of all normal activities so she could devote herself to a year of mourning. When I asked the other Native participants why she didn't have the courtesy to tell me what had happened, they told me that it wasn't her place to tell me, but my place to ask.

In addition to the need for awareness and understanding, counselors must also develop specific skills for working effectively with clients of different backgrounds (Baruth & Manning, 2007). Although the literature on this topic is becoming extensive, there is unfortunately little consensus about the actual behavioral criteria that represent expertise in multicultural counseling. At least a set of multicultural competencies considered desirable if not mandatory for any competent practitioner is beginning to evolve (Arredondo & Perez, 2006; Ponterotto, Alexander, & Grieger, 1995).

Becoming a competent multicultural practitioner is especially difficult because there are so many diverse populations, each with its own characteristics. Even the grouping of "Latino" or "Asian" is misleading because there are so many differences in subgroups. A Japanese, Vietnamese, Filipino, or Chinese person—or a Mexican, Brazilian, Salvadoran, or Cuban person—might be greatly offended by some assumptions that they are all similar in their cultures. As a student you may consider designing a step-by-step approach that involves first learning about the customs of each and every cultural group that might be represented in your practice. Better yet, arrange immersion experiences in which you "join" the culture on an experiential level. The goal, for each and every one of your clients, is to become an expert on their worlds. Each new client represents an opportunity for you to learn as much as you can about a new culture—including its customs, values, and worldview.

Again we want to stress that this is not an additional burden and responsibility of your work—it is a privilege and one of the most satisfying parts of the job. Counselors are not the highest-paid professionals around, nor do they receive the same kinds of perks as other professionals, but they do enjoy the tremendous benefit of learning so much about different people and their experiences. Some would say that this is the best part of the job.

COUNSELING THE AGED

When most of you will be at your peak of professional productivity, a disproportionate part of the North American population will be considered elderly citizens. There is little doubt that the single specialty within the helping professions that is most likely to flourish, if not explode, will be counseling older adults. The number of people over 65 has increased sevenfold: from 1 in 30 Americans in 1900 to an expected 1 in 5 Americans by 2020. Life expectancies will continue to lengthen, stretching normal life spans well into the 80s and perhaps 90s. Age 65 will be considered a part of the productive rather than the retirement years. Older citizens will dominate the consumer markets and they will control a significant part of industry, families, and lifestyle. And with these changing roles, opportunities, and expectations will come new problems of adaptation—and important responsibilities for counselors to aid the aged in this adjustment and in the resolution of age-related conflicts (Maples & Abney, 2006).

Although there are more similarities than differences in counseling old and young people, the assessment process is more complex with the mature client and specialized competencies are necessary. Not only are there more life experiences to take into account, but the diagnosis may be affected by underlying medical or physiological problems.

These special diagnostic problems are more than compensated for by the tremendous satisfaction that geriatric counselors experience in their work. In a sense, you get to hang out with the wise elders of society and learn from their life experiences. Certainly, there are also many challenges—such as the possibility of stirring up all kinds of countertransference feelings.

Some models of aging view older people as helpless, disabled, and burdensome to society. There are special facilities where the aged may be cleaned, clothed, and fed until they die. Institutional environments of this type are often viewed as depressing places where people wander about, forgetting who or where they are. The more agile can play cards, turn the channels on the television, or even shuffle along for walks outside the home.

Alternative conceptions of aging view older persons as senior adults with a wealth of valuable experiences and skills accumulated over a lifetime. Elders used to be considered the wise men and women of the community to whom the young would come for advice and assistance; now they are the elderly—the shuffleboard and Depends generation. Old age is a time of physical changes—hair thinning and turning white, skin losing its moisture and smoothness, the body actually shrinking in size, muscles becoming flabby and losing their strength. Joints become progressively stiff, bones are fragile, the heart is less efficient, and the arteries that circulate blood work like a slow train. Digestion is slowed, reaction times are diminished, and lungs work at less than peak efficiency and bring less energy-providing oxygen. All the senses lose their precision, and the older person, receiving less information from vision, hearing, taste, touch, and smell, is thus more isolated, irritable, and moody.

Yet the effects of these symptoms of physical deterioration are often slight and the stereotype of the elderly person as being slow moving and fragile, with dulled and distorted perceptions, is hardly accurate. From observing a number of biochemical and physiological changes in the elderly, researchers have concluded that slowed intellectual, perceptual, and mental behavior, particularly in those who are free of debilitating diseases, need not necessarily restrict functioning levels in major life areas. That does not mean, however, that you shouldn't make adjustments in the ways you work with this population. In fact, it would probably be advisable to alter assessment techniques, the length of sessions, and even the sorts of methods you employ. Still, the aged retain the capacity for self-awareness and insight. They respond to reinforcement. They may be a bit more cautious in their mental and

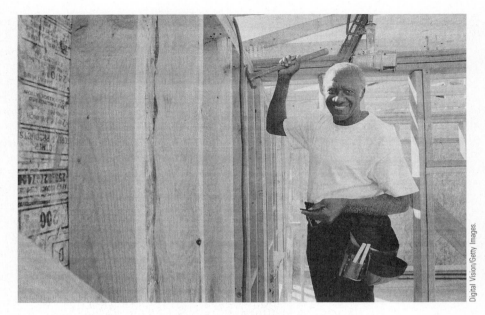

Digital Vision/Getty Images.

A nonretired senior working at the height of his professional life. For some active and productive people, youth is more a state of mind than chronological age.

physical movements, but they still think, feel, and act—and wish to do so more effectively.

Traditionally, at least at the time that Erik Erikson was formulating his theory of psychosocial development, later maturity was a time for a resolution of the crisis of despair and for introspective integration of one's life. The elderly were supposed to be giving meaning to their life's work and preparing themselves to accept the inevitability of death. At age 81, himself engaged in this final life stage, Erikson revised many of his thoughts about old age to place much more emphasis on the creative, productive elements supposedly restricted to earlier stages (Hall, 1983). Through their roles in grandparenting, volunteer work, and involvement in intimate relationships, older people can retain the playfulness, joy, and wonder that were so much a part of childhood.

B. F. Skinner, another influential thinker of the 20th century, also wrote about his own struggle to maintain his desired levels of effectiveness and to avoid growing old as a thinker even though his body stubbornly persisted in its progressive decline. "Old age is like fatigue, except that its effects cannot be corrected by relaxing or taking a vacation" (Skinner, 1983, p. 241).

The older adult must learn to accept his or her incapacities and to find alternative ways to accomplish the same goals and to meet the same needs. Death, certain and inevitable, is a difficult issue for the older person as it looms ahead, closer and closer. Some people become crippled by their fears; others welcome their final deliverance. Yet when old persons are given the opportunity to talk through their fears, most are able to resolve the developmental task, accept what they cannot change, and go on about the business of living fully in what time remains. When

VOICE FROM THE FIELD

Part of my job involves visiting some senior citizens' homes, and I'm telling you I had to throw everything I learned out the window. I see the residents in groups, trying to get them to talk about their struggles. Gee, most of them are just so lonely, or at least it looked that way. Later I learned that loneliness is more a problem for younger people, actually.

Anyway, I'd get the group going and it was like a circus. They'd all interrupt one another. This one guy would start rambling all over, which seemed to be okay since nobody was listening anyway. At first, I felt so useless 'cause I couldn't use all the skills I'd been trained in. Once I let go of those expectations, though, I found that I really could help them by just listening to their stories and helping them to do that for one another. Most of these folks didn't want to change; really, they didn't need to. But they did feel a very strong desire to be heard.

discomfort arises in confronting the topic of death—with relatives, friends, nurses, doctors, or counselors—it is important to distinguish who exactly is uncomfortable, the older adult or the counselor.

Dying is the last developmental task for everyone. Whether it comes unexpectedly, with or without pain, during sleep or sex, death is patiently waiting. Woody Allen (1976) freely admits, "It's not that I'm afraid to die. I just don't want to be there when it happens" (p. 106). In our technological age, where dying can be a prolonged process measured in the slow beeps of monitors and the drips of an IV, counselors can, at the least, help make the experience easier.

Throughout history the aged have always served the important function of passing on wisdom from one generation to the next. Whether in the role of teacher, guru, shaman, or grandparent, the elders have taught their accumulated knowledge, experience, and skills to youth so that they too might survive life's tests. The aged are responsible, through storytelling and the sharing of life experiences, for maintaining family and ethnic traditions. It is through listening to accounts of their own mistakes, failures, and weaknesses that, they hope, their protégés will learn to avoid similar traps.

When it comes to counseling the aging population, there are a number of specific interventions that have been demonstrated in research to be effective for elderly individuals suffering from emotional distress. Myers and Harper (2004) summarized these interventions as follows:

1. Treatment plans need to be modified, including increasing the length of sessions and length of overall treatment.
2. Counselors need to appreciate the complexity of the issues the elderly are dealing with; simple DSM diagnoses may not be sufficient for categorizing their distress, given the real-life issues of loss and change that are part of everyday life for this population.
3. Anxiety is quite common for the elderly, and counselors need to be alert for symptoms reflecting this form of distress. Research suggests that the elderly are highly responsive to treatment for anxiety disorders.
4. Treatment plans that include life-review interventions are especially helpful for depression.

5. Counselors can be helpful by normalizing concerns like depression, insomnia, and anxiety, given their prevalence for this population.
6. Finally, elderly people who have completed counseling often benefit from long-term support groups that can prevent relapse.

Publications about adult development and aging are plentiful; as counseling students, you will be able to read and learn much about the issues involved in counseling the elderly. Even if this is not an area of special interest, you will find it necessary to acquire some background knowledge and skills because the number of older people who will be needing and seeking services will continue to grow. Aging is a natural part of the developmental cycle; that should not be ignored when you work with this special population.

COUNSELING LESBIANS AND GAY MEN

For most of our nation's history, negative social attitudes and a pattern of stigmatization institutionalized in laws and the mental health system have kept lesbian, gay, and bisexual (LGB) people an invisible or hidden minority (Dworkin & Gutierrez, 1989; Fassinger, 1991). And while LGB persons may be more open about their sexuality in some of our large cities, the risk of condemnation and discrimination is still powerful in many if not most communities—so much so that it is virtually impossible to know how many Americans have a lesbian or gay sexual orientation (Baruth & Manning, 2007). The mental health profession has traditionally not treated this population with more acceptance than society in general has; homosexuality was viewed by psychiatry as a mental illness until 1973, and it wasn't until the publication of DSM-III-R (1987) that all references to homosexuality were declassified. Thus, the counseling and development needs of gay men and lesbians have not historically been addressed, and even today, most counseling students do not feel their training program has prepared them to work with gay and lesbian clients. (Burkhard, Pruitt, Medler, & Stark-Booth, 2009).

There are many issues unique to this population of which you will need to be aware (Barret & Logan, 2002; Murphy, Rawlings, & Howe, 2002).

IDENTITY DEVELOPMENT Gay and lesbian clients may often struggle with varying degrees of acceptance of, and satisfaction with, their sexual orientation. While several models have been proposed that describe a series of developmental stages, most stages include moving from a point of confusion to comparison with others, acceptance, tolerance, then pride and synthesis (Schmidt, 2006).

COMING OUT There are some different issues presented in counseling for those who have publicly disclosed their sexual identity versus those who keep that part of their lives private. Some clients may request support in their efforts to deal with others' reactions to their lifestyle.

OCCUPATIONAL/CAREER ISSUES Discrimination in the work arena is a reality for many gay, lesbian, and bisexual people, and counselors must be sensitive to the special

VOICE FROM THE FIELD

Homosexuality always went against my basic beliefs and my religious training. I just thought it was wrong. On a personal level, I had even stronger reactions. Then I discovered that one of my clients, whom I already had a very close relationship with, admitted to being lesbian. I tried not to show the shock on my face—or the revulsion. But the strange thing is that I already cared so much for this woman that learning her sexual preferences didn't seem to matter much to me. She was such a good and honorable person.

I learned so much about her history and way of life. Eventually, I'm proud to admit, I even overcame my own biases against people who live alternative lifestyles. I still feel uneasy about the whole thing, but maybe that's because of my own issues related to my own sexuality. What's amazing to me is that, previously, I could never have imagined myself working effectively with this population. Now I quite enjoy the challenge of delving into areas in which I have had little experience.

life/career planning issues that arise. Counselors must be aware of occupations or professions that are more tolerant of sexual orientation, be sensitive to the dual career issues of lesbian and gay couples, and be knowledgeable about the special resources available to gays.

RACIAL, ETHNIC, AND REGIONAL ISSUES   Gay men and lesbians have historically experienced discrimination and violence as a result of living in a homophobic and heterosexual society. When social class and racial issues are added, gay individuals may experience double- or triple-minority status with increasing attendant discrimination. Geography and regional differences also affect the gay subculture and may affect the available resources and networking opportunities for gay people. Counselors must be knowledgeable about these issues and be prepared to offer support and encouragement to gay clients experiencing multiple layers of discrimination.

ISOLATION   An openly gay lifestyle in a heterosexist society can result in a feeling of isolation and a fear of discrimination and rejection. Counselors must recognize the dangers of an isolated lifestyle and encourage gay people to develop a full and wide pattern of interaction with both gay and nongay individuals.

EMOTIONAL DISTRESS   Individuals may experience high levels of distress directly related to their orientation. Experiences of discrimination and prejudice as well as feelings of exclusion from mainstream society have been linked with depression and suicidal tendencies, substance abuse, anxiety, and other psychological concerns (Zakalik & Wei, 2006).

COUPLE ISSUES   Gay and lesbian individuals need to affirm the validity of their lifestyles and their commitment to their primary partner. In addition to the special issues that confront gay/lesbian couples, there are the typical types of conflicts and stresses inherent in all intimate relationships. Counselors must be cognizant of the special challenges and strengths of the gay/lesbian couple as well as the more traditional problems of all couples.

Voice from the Field

I'm an openly gay man, but it took a long time to get there. I was still refusing to accept myself when I began my internship. I had one huge fear—I'd be assigned a gay client who would see through me, and say something. I have no idea where this fantasy came from. After all, clients talk about themselves, not confront their counselors about their sexual orientations. Probably, some part of me was hoping I'd get challenged, so I would have to deal with it. Of course, eventually I did get assigned a gay man, a guy in his early 30s who was struggling with issues with his partner. I tried to listen as though everything was normal, but I simply couldn't be present. The hardest thing I ever had to do in my life, professional or personal, was talk about this with my supervisor, because there would be no way of getting around the truth. But I knew that if I was going to be the counselor I wanted to be, I had to deal with this. I was positively shaking in supervision that day, but the great thing about this field is how accepting people are, and that's how my supervisor was with me. She made it so much easier.

As for my client, he never brought my sexuality up. I don't think he gave me much thought at all, frankly; he was way too wrapped up in his own anxieties. So he'll never know how important he was to my life.

HIV   The role of the counselor in working with AIDS issues has two major focal areas: (1) providing services to HIV-positive individuals and (2) providing education to non-HIV-positive individuals regarding practices designed to prevent AIDS.

This role of health educator is a new and complex one for counselors, yet it is essential because HIV is a largely preventable disease. Counselors must be prepared to discuss sexual practices frankly and to provide information to assist in prevention efforts. AIDS education programs must increase awareness of the risks associated with the disease, promote an understanding of the principles of "safe sex," and encourage the necessary behavioral controls to confront denial and increase the probability of implementing AIDS prevention behaviors.

Antigay Violence   Hate crimes against gays and lesbians have been prevalent throughout history. They range from verbal insults and slurs to acts of violence, including murder. This reality exacts a toll on the gay person's self-esteem and can lead to depression and feelings of hopelessness, shame, and guilt. Counselors must provide support to the victims of antigay abuse and work with them to counteract the negative effects on their self-esteem. Counselors can also help their clients to direct their feelings into positive, activist channels to counter antigay violence.

Perhaps the most challenging aspect of working with gay and lesbian as well as transgender and bisexual clients is confronting your own biases and prejudices related to these populations (gay and lesbian counselors may have to address their own biases and prejudices toward straight people). This means addressing your own internalized homophobia, as well as any beliefs or personal convictions that may trigger for you a degree of discomfort when talking about this subject (Murphy, Rawlings, & Howe, 2002; Plummer, 1999; Schmidt, 2006). You may even hold rather strong ideas about moral issues related to one's sexual orientation. Just as with every other group that is mentioned in this chapter, you can do great harm to people if your personal biases leak into sessions and clients sense your criticism and disdain (Campos & Goldfried, 2001).

VOICE FROM THE FIELD

When you're working with HIV clients, you have to lose your squeamishness. If a guy recently had sex, for example, you have to ask him very direct questions. Did he use a rubber? Did he protect himself?

With another family I'm seeing how the kids are dealing with their mom's AIDS. She's close to death. As I reflect on my session with them, I see how nervous and unsure I was with them. The simple fact is that I'm afraid to talk about death with them. Death is the enemy. I want to feel differently, but deep down inside there is mostly fear that surrounds a nugget of wonder. It's a small nugget, maybe, but that whisper drives me to search further.

COUNSELING CLIENTS WHO ARE PHYSICALLY CHALLENGED

Clients who are physically challenged, or disabled, generally become involved in counseling through rehabilitation services provided to assess the needs of the client and establish a program of physical and emotional restoration. Career exploration and the establishment of training goals are a major focus of rehabilitation efforts, helping individuals to prepare for alternative forms of meaningful work (Corrigan, Jones, & McWhirter, 2001). Counselors need to recognize, however, that these individuals may have emotional problems not necessarily related to their abilities or disabilities.

People with disabilities are often able to participate fully in life as a result of social, political, and technological developments. Today we are challenged to think of disabled or handicapped people as "differently abled" as a way to remove the stigma associated with such conditions. In one sense, we are all "temporarily abled" persons in that the conditions in one's life are variable and likely to change over time. Such a perspective can be discouraging in that it emphasizes lack of control over our individual fate, or it can be reassuring in that it assumes that we can adapt to whatever happens.

When Erik Weihenmayer became the first blind mountaineer to scale Mount Everest, he was attacked by the elite climbing community as being a danger to others. He was considered too handicapped by his lack of sight to assess weather conditions or take care of himself. Responding to one of his critics—Ed Viesturs, one of the premier Everest experts—Erik responded:

> He hadn't seen the 16 years I'd been climbing, learning rope management, crevasse rescue, and avalanche safety; he surely hadn't seen the days spent on big walls when my teammates hung from anchors placed by the blind guy. Or the years I spent becoming independent, learning to build snow walls, cook meals on gas stoves, and set up tents in whiteouts. Viesturs hadn't seen any part of my life except that I was blind. (Weihenmayer, 2001, p. 55)

That is one of the major problems that physically challenged people face: They are not seen for who they are, or what they can do. They are their handicaps—the blind guy, the dwarf, the lady with no hands, the boy in the wheelchair, the albino. This is really no different from the way that so many of us are labeled or reduced to a single label based on our physical or racial features.

Counselors need to be knowledgeable about and sensitive to the issues faced by clients who are disabled in many various ways. This includes familiarity with the unique cultures of each group that may include language, customs, norms, and rituals just as for any other group we have studied. For example, the deaf community has a complex set of language and cultural dimensions as rich and complex as any ethnic group (Filer & Filer, 2000). Counselors also need to feel comfortable talking about the disability itself, and the role it plays in the client's identity. Open discussion of a person's disability can be emotionally troubling for counselors, leading either to the avoidance of questions and reflections regarding the disability, or, conversely, to an overemphasis on the role it plays in the person's life (Smart & Smart, 2006). Here again, the solution is continual self-reflection on the part of the counselor with regard to his or her own feelings about, stereotyping of, and biases toward the disabled.

In addition, family members of disabled individuals may experience guilt, anger, resentment, and insecurity because they do not know how to handle problems related to the disability. These symptoms may be manifested by siblings as well as by spouses and parents. Because the disabled family member requires extra assistance and attention, other family members may not be comfortable asking to have their needs met. The counselor can help the family develop ways to manage time, money, and emotional resources so that everyone can receive appropriate attention and support.

Disabled children, in particular, can provide especially difficult challenges for the parents and the other children (Morison, Bromfield, & Cameron, 2003). Seligman (1983) points out that, because disabled children need excessive caretaking, other family members must bear the responsibility and burden, often neglecting themselves and one another in the process. But it is certainly not always the case that the presence of a disabled child adversely affects the family. Often the experience encourages brothers and sisters to develop a sensitivity and caring that they will maintain their whole lives. Counselors must realize, however, that the "identified client"—the disabled child—may not be the only one with problems.

This reminder is but a specific application of the principle that holds true for most presenting problems that occur in a family: When one person develops symptoms, they inevitably disrupt the daily lives of everyone else. Particularly when the disabled individual is making a poor psychological adjustment, the added strain and stress place the other children at risk for developing problems. In addition to feeling guilt and resentment, they may also act out as a way to win attention according to family norms that emphasize being taken care of. For all these reasons, it is often advisable to work with the disabled in the context of their families.

THE FUTURE IS NOW: NEW ISSUES IN COUNSELING

COUNSELING CLIENTS WITH STRONG RELIGIOUS/SPIRITUAL VALUES

In a Gallup poll, 72% of Americans reported that they strongly believe in God, and an additional 14% are pretty sure God exists; only 3% reported clearly atheistic beliefs (Newport, 2006). We are a very religious country, arguably more so than any other developed Western nation, and yet it is only within the last decade that authors in our field have suggested spirituality could play a role in counseling, and that knowledge of religious and spiritual values should be part of a counselor's multicultural training (Briggs & Rayle, 2005).

Religion and spirituality are rooted in many of the cultural and ethnic heritages of Americans, and are a significant part of many people's identity, worldview, and values; multicultural competence requires us to be sensitive to our client's religious/ spiritual heritages, current beliefs, and the role these beliefs play in their coping strategies for handling both major stressful events and the daily challenges of life. For most Americans (and therefore, many, if not most, of our clients), religion and spirituality are interwoven throughout the life span, beginning with the rituals that may have accompanied our birth; the moral teachings of our youth; both the positive and negative associations with religion and religious institutions internalized in our childhood and adolescence; our connections to our immediate and extended family members, among whom there may be a variety of religious views; the rituals that marked key milestones of our development (e.g., confirmations, Bar/Bat Mitzvahs); our weddings; the births of our children; our struggles with partners when religious values conflict; and the ways in which we deal with issues of death and dying with regard to not only family members but to our own leaving of this world. Moreover, the fact that values, rituals, and the role of religious institutions within community life differ among ethnic groups (e.g., Native Americans, African Americans, Hispanics, Asian Americans) adds further emphasis to the need for counselors to bring knowledge and sensitivity to the religious/spiritual life of clients.

As a new field of inquiry in the profession, you might expect debate and controversy, and with this particular subject, the debate begins with the definition of religion and spirituality. The focal point of agreement appears to be that they are overlapping but distinguishable concepts. Spirituality can be defined as a yearning for experience beyond the boundaries of self and for being connected in some way to the vast and unexplainable universe (Baruth & Manning, 2007). It may also be a search for wholeness, and purpose and meaning in one's life (Hage, Hopson, Siegal, Payton, & DeFanti, 2006). Religions are characterized by their specific beliefs and practices, requirements for membership, and social organizations (Miller & Thoresen, 2003). From this perspective, one can be spiritual without a religious affiliation, but could also integrate spirituality into religious life, seeking meaning and transcendence through participation in organized religion and its various rituals and liturgies.

There are some very good reasons why knowledge of the role of religion and spirituality in counseling is just now being addressed by the counseling profession, and why the integration of religion into the counseling profession still sparks debate and controversy.

1. Disagreements over religion and counseling historically began at the birth of our profession; Freud, though connected to his Jewish heritage, was primarily atheistic in his beliefs, and, consistent with his psychoanalytic principles, believed religion was a transference of feelings for one's father extended to the concept of a supreme father. On the other hand, his protégé and colleague, Carl Jung, the son of a pastor, believed deeply that people need to engage in religious experience in order to maintain psychological balance in their lives (Rychlak, 1981).

2. The amount of blood shed over the centuries in the name of religion is horrific, and appears to be continuing unabated; it is sometimes difficult to separate out the value of religion in people's lives from the destructive energy unleashed historically by religious institutions and currently by religious zealots.

3. The goals of counseling, with its emphasis on tolerating the ambiguities and uncertainties of life, determining one's own beliefs and values, self-actualization, and personal responsibility, may conflict with religious views that emphasize values derived from both religious dogma and the surrender to a higher power for direction and meaning in life.

4. The majority of counselors, though affiliated with a religious denomination, do not themselves participate in organized religion (Walker, Gorsuch, & Tan, 2004).

5. Mental health professionals tend to prefer constructs that can be translated into observable phenomena that can be measured and tested; religion and spirituality are vague concepts that are a challenge to researchers' need to operationalize constructs.

While the role of religion in politics has focused media attention on the religious life of many Americans, it is also the scientific study of the relationship of religion and spirituality to mental health that has brought religion and spirituality to the attention of the counseling profession. Studies have shown, for example, that regular church/service attendance is correlated with positive emotions, optimism, caring behaviors, social support during times of crisis, a sense of purpose and meaning, and even lower mortality rates (Powell, Shahabi, & Thoresen, 2003). A review of the research by Russell and Yarhouse (2006) found associations between religious commitment and reduced rates of suicide, substance abuse, and depression as well as higher rates of psychological well-being.

For counselors, the central concern is how one can best be sensitive to the religious/spiritual beliefs and heritages of clients, and at the same time maintain a healthy boundary between one's own beliefs in this arena and those of the client. Several authors have addressed this and similar issues, which can be summarized in the form of the following recommendations for effective practice (Briggs & Rayle, 2005; Hage, 2006; Schmidt, 2006; Slattery, 2004; Walker et al., 2004):

1. Reflect on your own religious and spiritual values, including your biases toward a specific religion or to the idea of religion in general. Briggs and Rayle (2005) suggest students ask themselves the following questions: (a) What are your views concerning religion and spirituality? (b) How do you believe these views will affect your counseling role? (c) How will you be able to empathize with clients who have differing spiritual values than your own? (d) How will you keep your own spiritual values/beliefs from inappropriately influencing the counseling relationship? (Briggs & Rayle, 2005, p. 50)

2. Assess for clients' spiritual and religious functioning, and recognize when their values are relevant to the presenting issue. As part of this task, it is important to appreciate what is normative within a religious culture, so that you do not pathologize what may be an accepted belief within that tradition.

◼ | VOICE FROM THE FIELD

The client was a 42-year-old Orthodox Jew, a mother of five, struggling with a crisis of faith. Politically liberal, and open about her views, she found herself being shunned by the congregants of her synagogue, who were on the opposite side of the political spectrum. It wasn't a matter of simply changing her place of worship; she lived in a Boston neighborhood dominated by Orthodox Jews. The members of her synagogue were her neighbors, the parents of her children's friends, and her employers. How is it possible, she wondered aloud in our sessions, that people who worship God in the same way I do would treat me this way? What was the point of religion if believers had no compassion for someone who disagreed?

Let me say right off the bat—I knew nothing about Orthodox Judaism. But I do have some pretty strong negative feelings about rigid believers in anything—religion, politics, you name it. I could feel my own anger toward her neighbors, and I could sense my desire to nudge her toward leaving her spiritual community. Fortunately, I had been well trained by my teachers that I was experiencing countertransference and could harm my client if I didn't deal with it. I needed consultation, and not just from my supervisor, but also from an expert in Judaism who could help me appreciate the issues she was dealing with.

I learned an amazing amount, especially about how Jewish rituals and prayers were interwoven into every aspect of her daily life—prayers in the morning, rituals around eating and preparing meals, prayers in the afternoon, prayers and rituals at the end of the day. I recognized that a change in her spiritual and religious life could rock the foundation of her very existence. I would have to help her be very patient with her spiritual crisis, affirming her right to go back and forth with her choice, and never, never push her in a particular direction, even inadvertently. So I just reflected, reflected, and reflected some more, staying with her wherever she was through months of her agonizing self-examination. Eventually, she found a way to separate her private spirituality from the behaviors of her neighbors and chose to continue her adherence to Orthodox Judaism. Her politics remained the same, and if she was shunned—well, that was God's way of testing her faith. My respect for her is enormous and I'm grateful for what she taught me, not just about her religion, but also about the emotional costs of examining your religious values.

3. Familiarize yourself with the different belief systems and the role of religion among the various cultural groups you work with. This endeavor is no different from learning any other facts about different cultural worldviews and beliefs.

4. Join with clients in using their spiritual language, without abandoning or imposing your own beliefs. You can demonstrate your commitment to entering your client's subjective worldview, without sharing and implicitly pushing your own values. When your beliefs are different from the client's, be open about it (briefly!) and maintain a stance of curiosity about his or hers.

5. When clinically appropriate, recommend interventions like prayer or meditation that have been demonstrated in research as helpful and are also consistent with the client's own practices. At the same time, use spiritual and religious interventions very cautiously, and retain firm boundaries about your role as a counselor; you do not have to engage in religious rituals, pardon sins, or give blessings (Hage, 2006).

6. Make it safe for clients to talk about their religious and spiritual beliefs; as you might expect, that means remaining empathic, nonjudgmental, and staying alert for any subtle signs you might express that could discourage clients from sharing their views. You also need to make it safe for clients to reject their

faith, if they so choose; clients who have suffered a traumatic loss (e.g., death of a child) may question their religious teachings, resulting in either abandoning them or reaching a new perspective on them. Your role is to facilitate them in this process, without an agenda for an outcome, even if it conflicts with your own religious values.

7. Remember that religious and spiritual beliefs are only a part of a person's worldview and value system, and explore with clients the overall role their values play in their lives and their sources of meaning and purpose.

SUMMARY

In one sense, every client you see represents a special population with unique problems and challenges. Nevertheless, some client groups in particular have suffered more than their fair share as a result of discrimination and prejudices. Furthermore, several of the diverse populations discussed in this chapter have tended to underutilize counseling services. That is one reason why the role of being a counselor includes not only prevention and treatment, but also advocacy. Your job is not only to help your individual clients but also to help the world become a more equitable place for people of all backgrounds and experiences.

The complexity of the problems and special considerations for each group is evidenced by the amount of literature detailing the characteristics and methods of treatment. The challenges facing you as a counselor include learning about each of the diverse populations, developing the specialized skills needed for counseling diverse individuals and families, and understanding your own biases and how they affect your thoughts and behavior with clients.

SELF-GUIDED EXPLORATIONS

1. Describe the cultural, ethnic, religious, gender, and racial influences that have helped to shape your identity. If you were going to work with a counselor, what would you want him or her to know and understand about your cultural background?

2. Your perception of reality is influenced a great deal by how you have been indoctrinated throughout your life by family members, teachers, books, media, and most of all, your cultural identity. List as many of these "social constructions" as you can think of that have shaped who you are and what you most value.

3. Pretend that you wake up tomorrow morning a different race and color than before you went to sleep. After the initial shock wears off and you begin the normal business of resuming your life, what will be most difficult for you to adjust to?

4. In what ways do you feel limited by your gender? What would be different in your life if you were a member of the opposite sex?

5. Describe a time in your life when you felt oppressed by someone. Now imagine going to someone for help who resembles others who have abused you.

FOR HOMEWORK

ASSIGNMENT 1:

One way to broaden your cultural perspective is through watching certain movies with strong multicultural themes. Examples might include any of the following films: *West Side Story, Birdcage, Joy Luck Club, Philadelphia, White Man's Burden, Once We Were Warriors, Hoop*

Dreams, Priscilla: Queen of the Desert, Fools Rush In, Six Degrees of Separation, Secrets and Lies, Dangerous Minds, Mi Familia, Black Robe, Songcatcher, American History X, My Left Foot, Hurricane, My Big Fat Greek Wedding, Crash.

Get together with several classmates, friends, or family members and watch a few of these movies (or others you can think of) together. Talk to one another afterward about what the films stirred up for you. Speak to one another—not as film critics, but as reactors to the cultural themes highlighted.

Assignment 2:

Explore a culture that you know little about, one that represents a group you may see represented in a future counseling job. Study this culture from several different viewpoints through reading, interviews, observations, and *immersion* experiences. It is crucial that you enter this culture through *direct contact* with as many facets as you have the time and inclination for.

Write in your journal describing what you learned about the culture, and what you learned about yourself during the process. Connect these insights to other themes from class and your text.

Assignment 3:

Read some novels with strong multicultural themes. For instance, in Barbara Kingsolver's book,

Poisonwood Bible, or in Michael Dorris's book, *A Yellow Raft in Blue Water,* there are prevalent themes dealing with developing a cultural identity.

Assignment 4:

Take a transformative trip in which you immerse yourself in a different culture. You need not go far from home, just somewhere that presents opportunities for you to experiment with different parts of who you are. Ideally, the most potent environments for personal change are those that:

1. Insulate you from usual influences so you are free to experiment with alternative ways of being.
2. Foster some sort of emotional activation in which you are strongly aroused by what you are experiencing.
3. Force you to face some of your fears as well as new challenges.
4. Get you out of your normal routines and comfort zone so that you feel lost and have to find your way.
5. Provide "teachable" moments that are memorable and impactful.
6. Force you to solve problems or overcome obstacles in new ways.
7. Structure opportunities to reflect on the meaning of the experience.
8. Allow you to transfer what you learned to other aspects of your life.

Suggested Readings

Anderson, S. K., & Middleton, V. A. (2005). *Explorations in privilege, oppression and diversity.* Belmont, CA: Brooks/Cole.

Barret, B., & Logan, C. (2002). *Counseling gay men and lesbians: A practice primer.* Pacific Grove, CA: Brooks/Cole.

Baruth, L., & Manning, M. L. (2007). *Multicultural counseling and psychotherapy: A lifespan development* (3rd ed.). Upper Saddle River, NJ: Prentice Hall.

Bieschke, K. J., Perez, R. M., & DeBord, K. A. (2007). *Handbook of counseling and psychotherapy with lesbian, gay, bisexual, and transgender clients* (2nd ed.). Washington, D.C.: American Psychological Association.

Dorris, M. (1998). *A yellow raft in blue water.* New York: Warner.

Ellis, C. E., & Carlson, J. (2008). *Cross cultural awareness and social justice in counseling.* New York: Routledge.

Englar-Carlson, M., & Stevens, M. A. (2006). *In the room with men: A casebook of therapeutic change.* Washington, D.C.: American Psychological Association.

Hogan, M. (2007). *Four skills of cultural diversity competence—A process for understanding and practice* (3rd ed.). Belmont, CA: Brooks/Cole.

Ivey, A. E., D'Andrea, M., Ivey, M. B., & Simek-Morgan, L. (2007). *Counseling and psychotherapy: A multicultural perspective* (6th ed.). Boston: Allyn & Bacon.

Jordan, J. V., Kaplan, A. G., Miller, J. B., Stiver, I. P., & Surrey, J. L. (1991). *Women's growth in connection: Writings from the Stone Center.* New York: Guilford.

Kingsolver, B. (1999). *The poisonwood bible.* New York: Harper.

Kottler, J. A., & Marriner, M. (2009). *Changing people's lives while transforming your own: Paths to social justice and global human rights.* New York: Wiley.

Lee, C. C. (2006). *Multicultural issues in counseling: New approaches to diversity* (3rd ed.). Alexandria, VA: American Counseling Association.

Lum, D. (2007). *Culturally competent practice: A framework for understanding diverse groups and justice issues.* Belmont, CA: Brooks/Cole.

McAuliffe, G., & Associates (2008). *Culturally alert counseling: A comprehensive introduction.* Thousand Oaks, CA: Sage.

Morgan, O. J. (2007). *Counseling and spirituality: Views from the profession.* Boston: Lahaska Press.

Rabin, C. (2005). *Understanding gender and culture in the helping process: Practitioner's narratives from global perspectives.* Belmont, CA: Brooks/Cole.

Robinson, T. L. (2005). *The convergence of race, ethnicity, and gender: Multiple identities in counseling* (2nd ed.). Upper Saddle River, NJ: Prentice Hall.

PROFESSIONAL PRACTICE

PART 4

ETHICAL AND LEGAL ISSUES

CHAPTER 14

KEY CONCEPTS

Confidentiality

Public welfare

Ethical codes

Divided loyalties

Multiple relationships

Sexual misconduct

Clinical misjudgments

Professional negligence

Informed consent

Privileged communication

Tarasoff decision

Duty to warn

Mandated reporting

Managed care dilemmas

Standard of care

Scope of practice

Counselor impairment

Ethical decision making

Civil, criminal, and mental health law

CLIENT RIGHTS

You have been working with a young client for three months. He was at first wary, reticent, and cautious. It has taken patience and careful use of your trust- and relationship-building skills to break through the resistance.

Finally he is beginning to talk and share something of his life with you in the counseling sessions. Yet each time you begin to make progress, he draws back into his shell with a defensive remark: "You shrink types are all the same. You get your kicks out of prying into other people's lives." You repeatedly reassure him, reminding him of the sanctity and privacy of your office and the confidentiality of your relationship. He has tested your integrity a number of times and has attempted to probe your attitudes and values. You have responded by keeping the focus on him. You have thus spent a disproportionate amount of counseling time reaffirming your trustworthiness.

Finally your persistence and patience pay off. After much hesitation and several false starts, he slowly discloses his secret, meanwhile closely monitoring your reactions to him. He is satisfied as to your neutrality and acceptance of him (which you are consciously controlling) and so continues to describe his problem. This 16-year-old boy has quite a successful career selling various drugs to other kids in the junior and senior high school. He has no intention of quitting. In fact, he loves the work. He explains that finally he has power, respect, and friends. He likes the excitement and the risks. He enjoys having his "clients" dependent on him. And he can't complain about the money. No, he certainly has no intention of quitting this lucrative "career." There is one thing about which he is adamant: He does not want you to tell his parents. You inquire as to his reasons, and suddenly his voice becomes soft, hesitant—he reveals to you that his father has beaten him repeatedly. He warns you that if anything is said, his father is likely to retaliate with another beating. In a plaintive voice, he asks you for reassurance: "You were serious when you said everything you say in here is privileged communication, and nothing disclosed will ever leave this room. Right? You did really mean it, didn't you?" You have but a moment to respond, to decide on one of several possible courses of action:

1. Because the most sacred principle of counseling is to protect the confidentiality of the client, as well as to act in his best interests, you have no choice but to honor your commitments. It is, after all, not your purpose to tell people how to live their lives or to judge them. Also, the laws of your state and the ethical code for counselors are quite clear: Criminal activity disclosed by a client, unless a specific person or group is threatened with bodily harm, remains confidential.

2. On the other hand, his parents have a right to information that would protect the health and welfare of their child; does that rule apply here? Plus, your own values tell you that his parents should be informed of this; if it were your son, you would want to know if he were involved in illegal activity.

3. But if you do tell his parents, your client will no longer trust you, and it's doubtful he'll reveal anything else of importance to you; in fact, there's a good chance he'll just quit counseling, giving you no chance to help him change his behaviors.

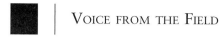

VOICE FROM THE FIELD

I'm required to attend a continuing education class in ethical and legal issues every two years in order to maintain my counseling license. And every two years I dread going. These experts, often lawyers, blast you for four to six hours on all the ways you can screw up, and end up being sued by clients or losing your license. If I heeded their advice, I'd see every client as a potential litigant, and would be too afraid to try any new or interesting intervention for fear I'd be accused of practicing unprofessionally. I'd be worried so much, there'd be no joy left in counseling.

But I do appreciate what these teachers are trying to do: They want me to be absolutely up-to-date on the latest ethical and legal rules, and it is true that they seem to keep on changing. And they really are interested in risk management—helping me minimize the risk of unethical behavior, before I do something that could get me in trouble. They've got a point, and their scare tactics work; I now keep great records of every session after I found out that it was illegal not to have thorough records! The trick is, finding a balance between managing risk and keeping my focus on doing the best counseling I can.

4. Also, if you do say anything, are you putting the boy at risk of being beaten by his father? Ethical codes permit you to withhold information from parents if it puts the client in danger; yet, all your instincts tell you that the "beating" story was fiction, made up to deter you from talking to his parents. The problem is, you just can't be 100% sure.

5. If the boy was beaten in the past, do you have to file a child abuse report with the local child protection authorities? That could precipitate a whole sequence of events, including an investigation of the father and potentially the removal of the boy from his home. Yes, the laws require you to file a report when you hear evidence of abuse. But do you really want to go down that road at this point?

6. Now you're back to thinking that maybe you should do nothing. The counseling relationship ought to continue as it has been developing. It is to be hoped that he will alter his behavior as he gains insight into his self-destructive acts and learns more socially acceptable ways of earning money and social approval.

You can appreciate why making ethical decisions is one of the most challenging aspects of our field, and how every decision involves therapeutic goals, state laws, institutional policies, and even personal feelings toward the particular client. The most difficult aspect of making ethical decisions such as this is that there are rarely single, perfect solutions.

PROFESSIONAL CODES

Professional codes of ethics are published by a number of organizations that work with counselors, such as the American Counseling Association, Association for Specialists in Group Work, American Association for Marriage and Family Therapy, American Psychological Association, National Academy of Certified Clinical Mental Health Counselors, National Association of Social Workers, and American Association for Sex Educators, Counselors, and Therapists. These guidelines, however, are often difficult to apply to individual cases, are sometimes contradictory,

VOICE FROM THE FIELD

Sometimes I'm not sure who my client is. It's supposed to be the children who are part of my caseload, but then the teachers in my school think I should be more accountable to them; they get mad if they think I'm taking the side of a child against them. My principal thinks that I work for her. If I don't please her with what I'm doing, she can make life very difficult for me. Then the parents of my kids feel that they are the ones I should be responding to. So, what do I do when I'm pulled in all these different directions? Everyone has their own agendas.

and are challenging for the professional organization to enforce. Furthermore, the field is so fragmented in its various licensures, certifications, and governing bodies that practitioners are often left to sort out the confusion for themselves. To make matters still more confusing, you must not only reconcile various ethical principles but also deal with the often conflicting cultures of the mental health system versus the law. For these reasons, ethical rules cannot just be memorized; rather, ethical behavior must be learned and decision-making skills developed to be internally consistent and yet compatible with acceptable societal and professional standards.

Ethics can be particularly frustrating to discuss in relation to the counseling profession. The nature of the field—its young history, conflicting theoretical base, and emphasis on the ambiguous and abstract content of the human mind—makes it difficult to define sanctioned professional behavior, much less enforce such professional standards. Practicing counselors sometimes have conflicting opinions about what constitutes acceptable standards of behavior. Each practitioner uses different labels and terms to describe the processes and has different goals and techniques. Depending on the state or country in which the counselors reside, the institutions in which they work, their training, type of degree, and client needs, they can differ widely in what may be described as "ethical conduct." You would get no such impression from studying the ethical codes of the profession, wherein each point is neatly organized, numbered, coded, and set down in dignified, precise language. Many experienced practitioners have spent their whole careers attempting to set forth these standards of acceptable conduct.

There is a distinction between the ethical decision making of the beginner and that of the experienced practitioner. Whereas the seasoned expert has logged years of therapeutic hours, the beginning counselor is starting out in a haze of confusion. It is difficult enough to track client statements, analyze underlying meanings, plan intervention strategies, and respond effectively without having additionally to contemplate open-ended moral issues and ethical conflicts. It is for this reason that we urge you to read and study your professional ethical codes and follow them to the letter. It is only with vast experience and intensive study that a scholar or practitioner can expect to improvise individual moral decisions based on solid empirical and philosophical grounds. And even those with such wisdom may believe, or publicly announce, something different from what they actually do within the privacy of their offices. The problem is further compounded by the often conflicting demands from a number of sources.

DIVIDED LOYALTIES

Who exactly does a counselor work for? Counselors learn in school that it is the clients. As professional helpers, counselors are to be their advocates, to hold their trust and confidence and protect their rights. However, sometimes loyalties are divided between two or more constituents. If the client is a child, counselors may be answerable to the parents for their actions, often a source of conflict when the parties disagree about the best course of action. If counselors were to comply with parental wishes and keep them informed of their work, inevitably they would lose the trust of the child. If they are uncooperative with the parents, the parents may sabotage the child's efforts or remove the child from counseling. To complicate matters further, counselors must answer to their school, agency, or institution for their actions. Counselors are also subject to the personal preferences of supervisors and the norms of the colleagues with whom they work. Then state and federal laws regulate behavior, sometimes against the welfare of clients and the best interests of institutions. As has been previously mentioned, professional codes of various organizations also regulate behavior. And through them all come the urgent whispers of your own inner voice.

Within each individual are many competing loyalties. The fact that ultimately you answer to yourself for your actions—not to a judge, the government, or your boss—would seem to simplify the matter. Yet it is further confounded by your responsibility to various parts of your own history (for instance, a client you once failed, on whose account you promised yourself to act differently thereafter) or to the shapers of your values and formulators of your conscience (parents, grandparents, mentors, teachers, and friends).

AREAS OF ETHICAL DIFFICULTY

Ethics could quite legitimately be discussed under the topic of "fear." The subject is not usually given much thought until the prospect arises that something could go wrong. Ethics is the analysis of good versus bad choices, moral versus immoral motives, helpful versus harmful action. The ethical implications of a problem are considered the last step of therapeutic decision making. Ethical consequences of behavior are usually examined only after a narrowly avoided mishap or the threat of a problem. Ethical discussions are often postmortem autopsies, analyses of what should have been done or what will be done next time.

It is more useful to consider ethical issues, their implications, and possible resolutions before they occur, during a time when personal and professional needs and beliefs can be rationally thought out and decisions made about behavior. Predicting and identifying the conflicts that are likely to develop in the practice of counseling allow examination of implications, exploration of personal values, and an opportunity to evaluate several preferred responses. This preparation can demystify the process and diminish much of the fear and apprehension that will arise during a crisis.

Right now, what is the ethical conflict *you* fear most? What situation might occur within a session that would create for you a moral nightmare of confusion and frustration? To help stimulate self-exploration, here is a review of some of the

VOICE FROM THE FIELD

I have to tell you, I was shocked when my supervisor told me not to file a child abuse report after my 12-year-old female client told me her father touched her where he had no right to. Basically, the supervisor was encouraging me to break the law. Believe me, that was a risk I didn't want to take. But he was adamant; the agency should make every effort to keep families together unless the evidence of abuse is absolutely clear and the girl is in serious danger. Over and over he'd say the same thing in our meetings—once the county child protective services shows up at her house to do an investigation, your client will never trust you again. You'll probably never see her again. So how would you be helping anyone?

I see his point. It makes perfect sense. Except for one thing. It's the law that I report. It's not just a clinical decision. My future is on the line. So I'm going to err on the side of obeying the law and hope that whatever happens, I can work it through with my client and keep her trust. Oh, there's one more thing. What if she is being abused? I'm not taking any chances with that, either.

major ethical dilemmas in our field, as well as common problems that frequently present themselves in the first year of practice.

MULTIPLE RELATIONSHIPS

One consequence of the ambiguities inherent to ethical decision making is that authors, ethicists, moral philosophers, and leading clinicians in our field engage in ongoing dialogues about what constitute ethical breaches. These dialogues may lead to changes in ethical thinking within the entire profession, and ultimately may manifest as revisions in the official ethical codes that govern one or more professional associations. Such a process is currently occurring around the issue of *multiple relationships*, defined as a helper participating in a nonprofessional role with a client or with someone close to the client (Welfel, 2006). Also known as *dual relationships* (recent literature tends to use the "multiple" designation, so we will adhere to this trend), these professional/nonprofessional interactions may include the following:

- When a business relationship also exists between the counselor and client
- When the counselor serves multiple roles in the client's life as a supervisor, colleague, or instructor
- When there is nonerotic physical contact (hugs, stroking) that may be misinterpreted
- When bartering for a fee takes place
- When clients are seen outside the office
- When the counselor becomes friends with a client
- When there is romantic or sexual interaction between counselor and client

A related concept in the ethical literature is the notion of *boundaries*, the rules and borders that govern the professional relationship—for example, the counselor's office, the focus in counselor-client conversations on the client's issues, and the exchange of payment for services. Any time counselors depart from the commonly accepted practices in terms of the counselor-client relationship, they are committing a *boundary crossing*; when a boundary crossing is harmful to a client, it constitutes a *boundary violation*. Boundaries serve to provide structure for the counseling process, a safe environment for the client, and sufficient emotional distance between counselor and client that treatment will work (Welfel, 2006).

Historically, all multiple relationships have been considered unethical boundary violations because of the harm they can do to a client (Cottone & Tarvydas, 2007). Generations of counselors have been advised that they must make every effort to avoid stepping outside the confines of the professional role, lest they damage a client, or leave themselves vulnerable to accusations of malpractice or client exploitation. At the same time, many in the field recognized that multiple relationships and boundary crossings were not by definition unethical; the problem was only when such relationships endangered the client's well-being. For example, organizations like the American Psychological Association state in their ethical code that multiple relationships should be avoided only if they are exploitative of the client or impair the counselor's objectivity and judgment (American Psychological Association, 2002). In short, the issues of multiple relationships and boundary crossings have continually remained a challenge for counselors when trying to determine the border between ethical and unethical behaviors.

At the heart of the ethical concern around multiple relationships is the power differential between counselors and clients; it can be difficult for clients to resist a counselor's invitation to engage in a nonprofessional relationship, whether clearly exploitative (e.g., a sexual relationship) or seemingly benign (e.g., allowing a client to pay for a session by doing some home repairs for the counselor). Clients who may feel inwardly troubled by such offers may be reluctant to say no, submitting to the counselor's wishes because he or she is an authority figure. You can imagine how clinically harmful this would be for clients whose reasons for seeking counseling may be their unassertiveness or previous victimization. Similarly, clients who have experienced traumatic abandonment in their past may agree to a nonprofessional relationship out of fear of another abandonment by someone who is supposed to care about them.

Take for example the issue of hugging a client. We routinely attend continuing education workshops by counseling ethics experts who advise the audience never to hug. You may be saying to yourself as you read this, "But why should an innocent hug be unethical?" Your own counselor may even have hugged you after a session, and you may have experienced the gesture as natural and comforting; indeed, hugging can be accepted practice in some orientations. But there is a counterargument: A client who was sexually abused by a parent may misinterpret your hug as a sexual overture, regardless of your gender. A client whom you have hugged after particularly painful sessions may come to expect it every week, and experience rejection and abandonment feelings if you don't offer it. For the counselor, a hug may represent a countertransference moment where it is the counselor who actually needs the hug, perhaps to be soothed by the client after a tense session, or because the counselor feels guilty that she or he didn't do enough to rescue the client from painful feelings. The ethics of hugging are still debated within the profession, but it is important to appreciate the legitimacy of arguments that hugs and similarly "innocent" gestures can be harmful to clients. It's the strength of these kinds of arguments, as well as those on the opposing side (e.g., the argument that hugging a client can be a helpful act of compassion and reassurance), that makes sorting out your own ethical choices both a complicated and essential task.

Moleski and Kiselica (2005) reviewed the more moderate positions on multiple relationships and boundary crossings, and identified at least three ways in which they may be not only ethically acceptable, but potentially beneficial to the counseling relationship: (1) Counselors in small towns and rural areas need to be able to see clients with whom they may have social contact outside of sessions; it is pragmatically impossible to avoid such dual relationships; (2) culturally sensitive counseling requires counselors to attend rituals (e.g., weddings) and accept gifts from clients where such gestures are indicators of respect and gratitude; (3) with some clients (e.g., adolescent boys), sessions may be more effective if held in restaurants, gyms, and playgrounds, where clients are often more comfortable discussing vulnerable emotions.

We need look no further than the most recent version of the American Counseling Association's Code of Ethics (American Counseling Association, 2005) for evidence that this line of thinking is impacting the rules on ethical behavior. When the ACA revised the code, it added a paragraph describing "potentially beneficial interactions," which may include attending formal ceremonies, purchasing services provided by a client, and mutual membership in community organizations.

How, then, do counselors, beginning and experienced, make good choices when the potential for boundary crossings develops? Corey, Corey, and Callanan (2007) and Herlihy and Corey (2006) offer some suggestions for the perplexed:

1. Always consider the question, "Whose needs are being met?" If it is the counselor's, then the boundary crossing is unethical.
2. Remember that the rules regarding multiple relationships are premised on the ethical principle that counselors *must first do no harm*. The counselor's responsibility is to rigorously examine his or her motives before crossing a boundary, and determine whether it may place the client at risk.
3. Discuss any potential multiple relationship with a client before engaging in it, including a review of the risks and benefits, and then secure the client's consent.
4. Seek supervision or consultation when contemplating entering a multiple relationship, or when a problematic one exists.
5. Always document any multiple relationships and boundary crossings in your case notes.

Another route to ethical decision making regarding multiple relationships and boundary crossings has been proposed by Austen, Bergum, Nutgens, and Peternelj-Taylor (2006), who argue that the word "boundary" is itself a problematic metaphor, and that there are other ways to think about these issues that may be more helpful. They suggest two alternative metaphors: As counselors, we build "bridges" to our clients, and our role is to reflect on how we can build a strong and safe bridge that allows us to enter the world of the person on the other side. The authors suggest that using a bridge metaphor emphasizes, rather than limits, the paths to connection between ourselves and our clients. A second metaphor is the counseling relationship as a "territory," a space in which both counselor and client travel. Clients enter this new territory in a vulnerable state, uncertain of the rules and parameters guiding a safe passage. Counselors practice ethically by continually reflecting on the moral implications of traveling in this territory along with the client; the metaphor helps remind us of the need to be vigilant regarding the rights and safety of the clients who share the territory with us.

SEXUAL IMPROPRIETIES

Do you fear being seduced by a client?

F. Scott Fitzgerald's *Tender Is the Night*, a classic in American literature, popularized the theme of the inevitable magnetism between a vulnerable, idolizing young client and her omnipotent therapist, each attracted to the other during the intimacy of a therapeutic encounter. Only within the last few years have many clients had the courage to publicize their experiences of seduction with former and current helping professionals, experiences that constitute the most damaging form of multiple relationships helpers can engage in. Before you act indignant and rush to swear that it could never happen to you, first consider the dynamics that operate in many counseling situations: (1) The client feels helpless, vulnerable, and confused; (2) the client has few satisfying relationships in his or her life; (3) the client feels undying gratitude to the counselor who has provided crucial help at a desperate time; (4) the client has disclosed the most intimate details of her or his life; (5) the counselor is worshiped by the client as a professional who at once appears so omnipotent, warm, affectionate, and understanding; and (6) the counselor's attraction is magnified by the inequality in power and control of the relationship. Add to this potent mix the variables of countertransference, involvement, respect, and affection that the counselor will come to feel for some clients, and you have a potentially explosive situation. That may be why as many as 12% of counselors have engaged in sexual misconduct with their clients (Celenza, 2005).

This explanation is not meant to excuse or pardon unprofessional conduct that is a dangerous, abusive, and exploitive breach of trust, but rather to encourage a healthy amount of legitimate apprehension about such situations. It is not altogether impossible for a counselor to find that a grateful hug has turned unexpectedly amorous. Often, in such intense situations, emotions don't respond to a half-prepared conscience. A counselor must be constantly aware of the detrimental results that are likely to follow sexually intimate entanglements with clients. The negative consequences will often cancel the previous therapeutic effects and send the client into a tailspin of mistrust of professionals who use their power to their own advantage. It may be helpful to rehearse and role-play sexual encounters, including responses that can be made to romantic or sexual overtures from clients. For example: "I have a confession to make. The only reason I keep coming to counseling is that I am so attracted to you. You have helped me so much. I owe it all to you. You are so different from other people I have known. How do you feel about me?" What is your response?

- "Ah. Our time is about up. Maybe we can continue next time."
- "How would it be helpful to know my feelings?"
- "You're feeling attracted to me because I've been helpful to and supportive of you, and you're hoping that I am attracted to you."

VOICE FROM THE FIELD

I remember the first time a new client told me about her previous counselor's unethical behaviors. The client was in her late 30s and immediately likeable—not the kind of person you expect would want to deceive you. She told me she had invited her boyfriend to sit in on a couple of sessions with her and her counselor, and she could sense immediately that her counselor had a crush on him. "Well," my new client spit out with disgust, "the next thing you know, that woman told me she had decided to work with my boyfriend, and she would refer me to another counselor—you. And two weeks later, my boyfriend broke up with me!" My heart went out to her, and I

was really shocked, especially since I knew the counselor had a sterling reputation. She was even someone I sent clients to.

The more I got to know my client, the more I began to doubt her story. It was just that she told me a bunch of things that didn't add up. And she made it clear she did not want me to talk about any of this with her ex-counselor.

The sad thing is, I can't refer to this counselor anymore. I just don't trust her enough. And I don't trust my client, either. Whatever actually happened, everybody loses.

- "It is not appropriate for you to think about me personally. We have a professional relationship, and it is necessary that we keep our relationship nonpersonal in order to work together effectively."
- "Since your personal feelings seem to be getting in the way of our professional relationship, perhaps we should discuss the possibility of your working with another counselor."
- "Your place or mine?"

No matter how you look at the situation, with levity or seriousness, this incident may test the resolve of the most experienced counselor. As with all other ethical behaviors, it is insufficient merely to memorize a moral commandment: "Thou shalt not be sexually involved with thy client." You must thoroughly and genuinely believe it as a guiding principle—an internal, personal belief that certain behaviors are crucial to maintaining professional standards. The fear of being caught is not enough to prevent a problem. The counselor must understand the responsibilities, moral obligations, and consequences that come with the territory.

Time after time, research has demonstrated that sexual/romantic entanglements between client and counselor are almost always harmful, no matter what the circumstances or how they are justified (Pope & Vasquez, 2007; Somer & Nachman, 2005; Sommers-Flanagan & Sommers-Flanagan, 2007). This is true even if the personal relationship begins after the professional one has been formally terminated—because there are always lingering dependency and attachment issues. Most licensure laws prohibit romantic relationships between counselors/therapists for a period of two years after treatment has ceased. And there must still be clear indications that such a relationship will not be harmful.

CLINICAL MISJUDGMENTS AND FAILURES

Are you fearful of making a terrible mistake that might hurt a client and unsure about whether you would take responsibility for the consequences? Making

Everyone has their "worst moment as a new counselor" story, and here's mine. I'm a male counselor and I know exactly the kind of woman I fall for—what she looks like, sounds like, acts like. And, of course, one day, she walks into my office. I knew I was in trouble. I could feel myself turning on my most compassionate counselor's voice, leaning a bit closer to her in my chair, saying things that I thought were particularly wise and meant to impress her, not help her. And when she said, "I'm amazed at how well you understand me. I'm really looking forward to our next session," I literally glowed inside. A few weeks later, after a session with her ended and she left, I felt this pain in my chest, which I recognized immediately as heartache.

At this point, I was ready to put an end to my career right then and there. I went to talk to my supervisor about it, my face red with shame. I could barely get the words out to describe what was going on, and cringed in anticipation of his scolding. The moment was just excruciating.

He smiled. "Welcome to the life of a counselor." (And here I began to breathe again.) "Seriously, though, I'm not worried that you're going to have sex with this person. So relax. But now we have to deal with this, or you will soon find yourself in a cozy, warm, and very comfortable relationship with this client. You'll be so afraid of her not liking you that there's zero chance you'll help her really look at herself."

mistakes is inevitable in counseling. Some of the time we are working without a clear, detailed map of the desired direction for the counseling process. Clients often don't know themselves what is troubling them, and they frequently mask their true feelings as a defense. Sometimes the deception is even deliberate, part of an elaborate game-playing scheme intended to test the counselor's ability to see through the cover-up.

The counselor's judgment is further subject to error by the relatively low reliability and validity inherent in counseling techniques. Practitioners disagree as often as they agree on the diagnosis of a client; even when they do agree on the diagnosis, they may still choose different treatment plans. Consecutive consultations with different therapeutic helpers might well yield quite different diagnostic assessments. Suppose a client presents symptoms of irritability, listlessness, low energy, failed performance at work, lack of sex drive, and loss of appetite; these symptoms may be diagnosed in a number of ways, ranging from anorexia nervosa to depression to an acute stress reaction. Errors are possible not only in the conclusions drawn about a case but also in the way chosen for working with the client.

The issue in this discussion is not whether mistakes and misjudgments will occur (many of which will hurt clients), but what can be done about them. What is gained by apologizing to the victim? For example: "I'm awfully sorry. But, ah, remember when I said that it would be best to confront? Well, ah, I've thought about it and think that might not be the best alternative." What would be the likelihood of keeping a job if you rigorously reported every mistake to the supervisor? "Boss, I messed up again. This time, when I should have been supportive, I started confronting. I'm afraid the client won't be coming back." The important part of such ethical conflicts is, first, learning from mistakes to prevent repeating the same errors and, second, minimizing or reversing any negative effects on the client, possibly by seeking counsel from a peer or supervisor or perhaps by admitting to the client the problem and solutions.

It is easy to hide transgressions. No one else will ever know what goes on within the privacy of the office. Clients usually don't challenge a process so mysterious that almost anything can be viewed as potentially therapeutic from at least one theoretical point of view. It becomes all the more essential, then, to develop and internally monitor professional behavior from an ethical perspective. The individual counselor's awareness of and commitment to ethical principles will, in the final analysis, determine the ethical content of interviews.

In processing and working through misjudgments and failures in counseling, several things should be considered (Dillon, 2003; Kottler & Carlson, 2003; Kottler & Hazler, 1997; Duncan, Miller, & Hubble, 2007):

1. Failures are inevitable and unavoidable.
2. Counselors often avoid and deny their mistakes and misjudgments by calling clients resistant, pretending that they have everything under control, and blaming factors outside of their control.
3. Failures are often caused by variables related to the client (unrealistic expectations, toxic personality, poor motivation), counselor (rigidity, arrogance, poor skill execution), therapeutic process (transference, pace, inadequate alliance), and extraneous variables (lack of support, enmeshed family).
4. Mistakes and misjudgments can be worked through by considering the client's secondary gains from remaining stuck, the counselor's personal issues, what has been overlooked, which interventions have been most and least helpful, and what outside resources can be tapped.
5. Discussing mistakes with the client offers a chance for the counselor to discover where the treatment has veered away from the client's goals and then to make the necessary adjustments.
6. Failures can provide wonderful opportunities for both counselor's and client's learning and growth, if processed constructively.

An important distinction should be made between mistakes and small failures and professional negligence or malpractice that represents a serious failure of competent practice and puts clients at risk. A mistake that rises to the level of negligence is one in which the counselor did not meet *the standard of care*, defined as an adequate quality of professional treatment that would be expected of other competent counselors (Welfel, 2006). Moreover, to be negligent, you must have actually harmed the client in a way that can be legally established. Don't get us wrong; some counselors do commit acts of negligence, and you should do everything possible to practice within the standard of care. However, do not confuse the mistakes and failures that are an everyday part of our profession—and virtually inevitable during your novice years—with malpractice and negligent counseling.

Deception and Informed Consent

Would you ever deliberately lie to or deceive a client, even if it were for his or her own good?

Counselors stand for truth, honesty, sincerity, and genuineness. But influence is also an important counseling skill. Is it justifiable to manipulate a client into experimenting with a new behavior? Is it ethical to disguise a trap waiting for the unsuspecting client? Is it even appropriate to water down the truth with clients? Although students may respond with a resounding chorus of "NO," most experienced counselors will reluctantly admit that therapeutic deception may be necessary when it is intended for the benefit of the client.

When a client straightforwardly asks a direct question (for instance, a low IQ client asks, "Do you think I'm intelligent?"), we are confronted with the inevitable choice of whether or not to tell the truth. The client might not yet be ready for the truth or, alternatively, might respond poorly to protective lies. The counselor must make a choice representative of his or her ethical standards and live with the consequences of the choice. While you are making your own decisions as to your preferred response, consider the following case.

The client is a young woman, inhibited, rigid, fearful, and shy. She is petrified of anything remotely spontaneous, because the outcome is not 100% predictable. She is also terrified of anything that might require her verbal performance, for failure (which she very loosely defines) would certainly crush her already fragile ego.

The counselor quickly (and probably accurately) decides that the vicious cycle of self-defeating beliefs ("I can't do it because I'm _____") can be broken only by encouraging her, just once, to try acting differently from the way she has in the past. If she would pretend, even within the safety of the session, to be somewhat playful and spontaneous, she could not continue to use the excuse "I can't do it," because she would have revealed an exception to her self-defeating behavior.

Role-playing would obviously be the technique of choice for encouraging the client's creativity and spontaneity, but she is vehement in her refusal to try it. The counselor agrees to back off, and discussion continues in other directions until an opportunity arises. The client, in talking about her mother's endless complaining and cackling, starts to change her voice in imitation of her mother, thus initiating spontaneous role-playing. The counselor need only change roles and start imitating the client, knowing that it will provoke her continued performance as her mother. After having previously promised not to pressure her into role-playing, the counselor now has an easy chance to trick her into trying it, obviously for her own therapeutic growth. Is the counselor ethically justified in proceeding—when he has said he would not—because the outcomes are so potentially desirable?

In this case the counselor chose to stop the action, disclose aloud the temptation to be manipulative, and then deal with the reactions. The client felt so grateful for the maintenance of trust that she was then able to experiment slowly, not at the same dramatic level as would have been possible in the incident of spontaneous role-playing, but well enough to make progress. For every example in which honesty produces the best results, there are also cases in which other, less direct actions might also be defensible.

The principle of *informed consent* is based on the notion that clients have a right to freely enter counseling, without any form of coercion or manipulation. They have a right to be provided with clear, accurate, and comprehensible information on such things as the limits of confidentiality, fee policies, limitations and dangers of treatment approaches, alternative treatment models, access to records, counselor qualifications and training, and the right to refuse treatment. By describing to clients, in writing, the relevant information they need to know before commencing counseling, the clinician ensures clients are making a fully informed

VOICE FROM THE FIELD

I'm a big believer in dotting every "i" and crossing every "t" when it comes to being ethical. So my informed consent forms are very thorough. I give my clients plenty of time before the first session so they can read them, and the first thing we talk about is whether they understood what they signed. And I make sure that my informed consent forms make it clear in writing that counseling is often an uncomfortable process, and clients may need to feel some emotional distress as part of resolving their issues.

You would have thought that clients would ask me questions about this, or maybe even decide counseling isn't for them. But the funny thing is, no one has ever brought it up. I'm not sure why—whether they are so anxious before their first session that they really don't read the forms carefully, or whether people have come to accept the fact that pain is part of growth. In either case, I know I've done the right thing in letting people know in advance there are risks to engaging in this kind of work.

choice when they consent to proceed (Welfel, 2006). Informed consent also does not stop once the counseling begins; if counselors make adjustments in a treatment plan, or change the theoretical model being utilized, clients need to know, and terminate if they so desire. Like the issue of multiple relationships, the notion of informed consent is in a state of flux, with an increasing emphasis on fully apprising clients of exactly what they should anticipate from the counseling experience. Pomerantz and Handelsman (2004) suggest that counselors add to their informed consent office forms such facts as the name and nature of the theoretical orientation they use, how it compares with other forms of treatment, what percentage of their clients improve and what is the evidence for the success rate, how government regulations will influence confidentiality policies, and how much information they will disclose to a managed care company. This range of information is significantly more comprehensive and detailed than what was expected of counselors 10 to 15 years ago, and reflects the growing trend in the field to treat clients as consumers of a service.

CONFIDENTIALITY AND PRIVILEGED COMMUNICATION

Are you worried that you may inadvertently or deliberately violate your client's confidence?

Struggles with maintaining confidentiality are among the most common ethical dilemmas that counselors face. Not a week will go by when you won't be tested in some way—parents wanting to know what their child said to you, another professional calling you for information about a previous case, a current client you are seeing who has AIDS and is sexually active, another client who threatens suicide and may carry out that threat, or even a colleague or a spouse who casually asks you about a client you are seeing. Yet as challenging as these dilemmas seem to you, you can make things easier for yourself by thoughtfully preparing responses to the situations that trouble you the most.

In a situation such as the one presented at the beginning of this chapter, a counselor may struggle with whether or not to break a previous promise because the client is committing a crime. Ethical dilemmas do arise because of a conflict between what is best for the client and what is best for other people. In a landmark court case, now referred to as the Tarasoff decision, a counselor failed to warn a murder victim of potential danger from his client and was held responsible and ordered to pay damages to the victim's parents. Although the judgment was eventually overturned, the case has brought much attention to the limitations of confidentiality. Counselors in most states are now required to do several things if they have direct knowledge of possible harm to an identifiable victim. They must make reasonable efforts to warn the victim and they must notify appropriate authorities.

In addition to counselors' ethical obligations to uphold a promise of confidentiality, they may have an ethical and legal responsibility to breach the vow (1) when the client is a danger to himself or herself or others, (2) when the counselor is so ordered by the court, (3) when it is in the best interests of a child, elder, or dependent (i.e., unable to care for herself or himself) who is a victim of abuse, and (4) when case consultation or supervision is needed. Unfortunately, the courts do not offer to counselors the same protection they do to others whose communications are privileged, such as lawyers, physicians, clergy, and spouses. That is one reason why at the beginning of every counseling relationship you are required to inform your clients about the limits of confidentiality. It is also one reason why we are often forced to make painful decisions about times when our previous vow to maintain secrecy with clients should be overruled by an even more pressing moral imperative to protect human life.

Inadvertent slips that reveal confidential information are quite another matter. There is no justifiable excuse. That is not to say that we are not constantly tempted to share information with friends, spouses, or colleagues. But we must endure the isolation of not being able to talk about our work in any revealing detail because clients deserve to have their information protected by professional, ethical behavior.

You should also understand that while confidentiality is an ethical issue that concerns keeping the content of communications private, privileged communication is a concept that refers to the legal arena. There are certain exceptions to privilege that you should also know about, meaning certain instances when the client waives or surrenders his or her right to privacy. This can occur in situations such as worker compensation cases, child custody evaluations, sanity hearings, and other legal proceedings. It may also be the case if you are sued for malpractice or if the client is a minor and you believe that his or her rights must be safeguarded.

RECENT TRENDS

Because ethical and value issues in counseling are reflective of contemporary culture, the standards for professional practice continue to evolve. Some of the most common violations of ethical behavior as well as those dilemmas that are likely to be most salient in the future are continually evaluated by counseling ethicists, and ethical codes and laws are regularly revised. The following situations are ones that you should be especially vigilant about monitoring closely.

DUTY TO WARN   You will be asked to assess the potential dangerousness of your clients, to determine whether they have the potential to harm themselves or others. This potential can include the threat of physical violence, or it could conceivably

VOICE FROM THE FIELD

The client was a young man in his late 20s, who came to me because he couldn't make up his mind whether to marry his girlfriend. I helped him deal with his fears of commitment, and he decided to marry her. The next thing I know, I've been invited to the wedding. Well, I have a policy about this. I first discuss with the client what it might actually be like for him when I show up. Will my presence make him uncomfortable? How will he introduce me? And if he still wants me to come, I will—I'd be honored, in fact, to share this wonderful event with him. But he should know in advance, I will show up for a few minutes and then leave—because even if he doesn't realize it, I know how emotionally complicated it will be for him to have his counselor at his wedding. I would never take the chance of making him feel self-conscious at such a precious moment in his life. I'll just be that strange person sitting in the back of the church, who ducked out right after the "I dos."

apply to the dilemma of working with a client who is HIV infected. If you believe there is imminent danger, you will be required to take action, which could involve warning potential victims, initiating commitment proceedings, or even calling the police. All of those choices, of course, violate your vow of confidentiality, so your assessments must be accurate.

General guidelines recommend the following (Cottone & Tarvydas, 2007; Isaacs, 1997): (1) Take a detailed history, assessing potential dangerousness of a client; (2) document very carefully any progress made in counseling; (3) consult with supervisors for additional input; (4) if necessary and indicated, obtain client's cooperation in warning the potential victim(s); (5) contact authorities if in your professional judgment the client poses a threat to self or others. In addition, it is useful to prepare ahead of time for such challenging cases that, hopefully, you will never have to deal with. This includes having appropriate referrals ready, having informed consent forms that specify the conditions under which confidentiality may be breached, keeping abreast of the laws and policies that govern your practice, and consulting with more experienced colleagues (Standard & Hazler, 1995).

The duty-to-warn rules are often subject to legislative actions and court decisions; that is, regardless of your association's ethical codes, judges and lawmakers in your state may either expand or narrow the conditions under which the counselor is required to break confidentiality. This is particularly true in the area of HIV-related reporting issues, where regulations regarding when it is acceptable to warn the partner of an infected client can vary from state to state or among the different associations' ethical codes. Welfel (2006) cautions counselors not to respond to their emotional or intuitive feelings regarding breaking confidentiality to prevent HIV-spread; any decision needs to made extremely carefully, keeping the welfare of the client in mind.

REPORTING CHILD ABUSE The law is clear: If you suspect that emotional or physical harm is being inflicted on a child, you must report it to the authorities within 24 hours. The ethical dilemma, however, is, what to do if you believe obeying this law may be harmful to your client. When you report child abuse to your community's child protective services agency, you may be initiating a sequence of events that can traumatize the child. Investigators may show up unexpectedly at the child's home; one or both parents may be arrested; the child may eventually be removed from the home and placed in foster care. Yet in spite of the possible negative consequences that may result from reporting suspected child abuse inaccurately, we advise you to follow your state's laws when it comes to abuse if there is any reasonable evidence of it. It is not your job to assess whether the accusations are true or not, but merely to allow authorities the opportunity to investigate the case. By failing to report suspected abuse, not only do you put yourself at risk for violation of law, but you also may negligently allow children to be harmed.

TECHNOLOGY USAGE As more and more client information is stored on computers in schools and agencies, it is becoming increasingly difficult to restrict unauthorized access and guarantee the confidentiality of records. Although computers are making life much easier for counselors as a way to store records, access files, process paperwork, and look up needed information, they are also lacking in safeguards to protect clients' rights to privacy. A number of ethical and professional hazards have been raised, including compromised confidentiality and the validity of information received. Internet communications are hardly secure and almost any self-respecting hacker could gain access to the record system to retrieve desired information.

As more and more counselors are engaging in counseling services via the Internet, telephone, and videophone, additional ethical and legal concerns are being raised (Koocher, 2007; Shaw & Shaw, 2006). In most cases, liability insurance may not cover such professional activity. Additionally, usually you must be licensed in the state in which the client is a resident. Finally, however much more convenient and accessible such services might be, you must be aware of the limits of such a professional activity—one that gives only limited visual cues and restricts you to receiving information that cannot be assessed with face-to-face interactions.

In 1996, Congress passed the *Health Insurance Portability and Accountability Act* (HIPAA), which defined new rules of confidentiality, informed consent, and record keeping applicable to any practitioner or agency that transmits client information electronically. Given our culture's increasing use of computer technology for all text and data communication, it is likely that either the agency you work for or your own practice will need to comply with HIPAA regulations. HIPAA was designed to encourage electronic transactions while simultaneously adding safeguards to protect the confidentiality of health care users (Corey et al., 2007). While giving clients enhanced rights to view their health care records, HIPAA also clarifies the distinction between official client reports and psychotherapy notes (your informal thoughts and analyses regarding clients).

RELATIONSHIPS WITH FORMER CLIENTS Although ethical codes are quite clear about the inappropriateness of becoming romantically involved with a client, or even conducting a friendship with a client at the same time he or she is in treatment (dual relationship), there is a recent trend to also restrict relationships with former clients. This issue is complicated by confusion as to when counseling actually ends: Is it after the last scheduled session? Or is it when the client stops thinking of you as a professional (which could take a lifetime)?

It is also important to keep in mind that it is not acceptable to end a therapeutic relationship expressly for the purposes of beginning a personal one. This is especially important because it is so difficult to determine when a therapeutic relationship is really over—not just with regard to the termination of scheduled sessions, but also with regard to the client's fantasies about the relationship.

All professional association ethical codes prohibit sexual relationships for at least two years after termination, and the American Counseling Association goes one step further in banning both sexual and romantic interactions for five years. However, other sorts of personal relationships, including friendships, are less clear. The situation is compounded by life in rural areas and small towns where it is much more difficult to compartmentalize relationships.

MANAGED CARE   "When I first went into private practice it was my dream to have a full caseload. Now I have more clients than I can possibly see but I am making far less money than when I was working for a salary. I feel like an assembly line, turning out stamped products as fast as I can."

As this practitioner complains, insurance carriers, preferred provider organizations, employee assistance programs, health maintenance organizations, and government-administered health programs have to some degree changed the profession into a business. With slashed budgets, even community agencies are being forced to participate in these programs.

All of a sudden, what is best for clients is no longer the only concern; now counselors must consider the realities of what third parties mandate in terms of counseling plans and even length of treatment. Nowhere is this ethical dilemma more prominent than when it comes time to fill in a diagnosis on the appropriate forms.

Assume, for example, that a client presents symptoms that resemble what is known as a personality disorder. In the interests of accuracy, if you should enter a diagnosis of "borderline or narcissistic personality disorder," two things are likely to occur: (1) Your client will not likely have treatment approved because these intractable conditions are not supposed to be amenable to counseling, and (2) your client will be stigmatized for life with a label in the file that can be accessed by any number of sources in the future. This client is also feeling depressed about his condition, so perhaps you might legitimately call the problem "adjustment disorder with depressed mood." Sure, it is a bit of a stretch—but aren't you doing this to protect the client's rights?

Ethical dilemmas such as this one are becoming increasingly a part of the ways counselors function. Managed care organizations are forcing them to amend the ways they are used to working. In some cases this is a good thing, because counselors are now required more and more to demonstrate their effectiveness and to operate more efficiently. Yet sacred therapeutic relationships are now intruded on by administrators and review boards, who are telling counselors what they may do and how long they may do it. If they don't follow their instructions, the organization may decide to cut off all support entirely.

CONFRONTING COUNSELOR IMPAIRMENT   In spite of best intentions and training, almost all clinicians experience some type of impairment or dysfunction in their lives. These lapses of conduct occur because of drug addictions, life transitions, traumas, poor training, pathological personalities, burnout, or, stated more directly: "holes" in one's conscience.

VOICE FROM THE FIELD

I know a lot of counselors hate managed care and HMOs. I've even heard them talked about at conferences as "the enemy." I can appreciate their feelings—after all, having a faceless organization telling you how many sessions your clients need can sometimes be a serious interference with our goal of providing the best possible care. But I think there really is another point of view to consider. Let's be honest—a lot of counselors will drag therapy on for as long as they can, so the money keeps coming in. And some clients are there for personal growth, which is terrific, but should their employers have to pay for that? I tell my clients that if you are using your managed care insurance to pay for counseling, the goal is to get you back to working as productively as possible; that's why your company is paying for your health care. Once we reach that point, the counseling can stop. And if you want to continue our work to look at deeper issues, I'll support that 100%, but you will have to pay for it out of pocket.

Even as a beginner you have an obligation not only to uphold ethical conduct but also to help other professionals who might be experiencing degrees of impairment. Although initially compassion and empathy should be employed to help an impaired counselor get needed help, at times you may be forced to take more proactive steps that include reporting the ethical breach to licensing boards and professional organizations or even protecting clients who might be in jeopardy.

RESOLVING ETHICAL CONFLICTS   Most ethical codes specify that if you become aware of a colleague who is engaging in unethical or unprofessional conduct you must take appropriate steps to intervene and protect the safety of others who may be harmed by this behavior. That guideline seems relatively clear but is, in fact, quite difficult to execute effectively.

Let's say you find out from a client that a former counselor did some things in session that were strange at best, and highly unprofessional at the very least. Do you report this behavior to the local licensing board and the practitioner's professional ethics board? The first step is usually to informally resolve the suspected violation by contacting the colleague and communicating your concerns. But in order to do so, you would first need the permission of your client to breach confidentiality (and often clients do not want to do that). Once you have attempted this informal resolution, then you may report the violation directly to the proper authorities. They will then investigate the case and make a determination about whether some sort of action need be taken.

MAKING ETHICAL DECISIONS

See Companion DVD
Making Ethical
Decisions

You will be confronted on a regular basis with the necessity of making ethical decisions. When an ethical issue emerges, you will have to make a virtually instantaneous decision; little opportunity will exist for careful analysis and thoughtful reflection. Thus, the first recommendation in making ethical decisions is to anticipate. It is essential to develop a reasonably clear ethical style based on analysis and reflection that will guide decision making, and to develop a capacity for making sound moral decisions that are compatible with the consensual standards created by the profession and consistent with your own professional identity, sense of personal virtue, and cultural factors (Cottone & Tarvydas, 2007; Remley & Herlihy, 2010).

One of the reasons that practitioners are often broadsided by difficult ethical dilemmas is because they fall into one of several traps (Steinman, Richardson, & McEnroe, 1998):

1. *The common sense trap.* This naïve orientation is based on the idea that if you merely study the ethical codes you will be well prepared to handle anything that comes up. In truth, while the codes provide guidance, most difficulties arise because of personal interpretations of rules and laws that are not necessarily based on consensual standards.

2. *The values trap.* Some counselors confuse ethical standards with their own values and religious and moral convictions. Under the myth that they are being ethical, they attempt to impose their own strong beliefs on their clients, without respect or sensitivity to their clients' unique cultural values.

3. *The circumstantiality trap.* "You have to understand the situation before you judge whether I was right or wrong." Ah, the old excuse that the reason you ran the red light is that you were.... There is always some good excuse. Making sound ethical decisions is certainly based on contextual circumstances, but never to the point where a client's rights or safety are compromised.

Keeping these traps in mind, the ethical decision-making process involves a number of sequential steps that would be most helpful for you to study (Corey, Corey, & Callanan, 2007; Grosso, 2009; Welfel, 2006).

1. *Recognize that there is an ethical conflict.* In order to make a decision about something you must first be aware that a decision needs to made. Studying ethical issues helps sensitize you to those situations that qualify as a legitimate dilemma in need of some resolution.

2. *Describe the problem.* After recognizing that an ethical decision needs to be made, it is useful to specify the parameters of the issue, figure out what is at stake, consider what harm can result to whom, and anticipate consequences. Gathering and organizing this information will give you some sense of the time parameters involved before a decision must be made and action taken.

3. *Identify appropriate ethical standards involved.* Consult the ethical codes for guidance. If there is clear and definitive instruction, act accordingly. If the ethical guidelines are ambiguous or unclear, consult with peers and supervisors. If the particular ethical standards fit the situation but the mandated actions seem "wrong," get further supervision and reflect on whether any ethical traps apply.

4. *Review professional literature.* Another source of information, if not wisdom, that you will wish to check out is the scholarship that has been undertaken in relation to your ethical conflict. It is highly likely that many others before you have struggled with similar issues and have chosen to research various alternatives and their consequences.

5. *Reflect on personal morals and values.* Is your ethical decision in the best interests of your clients, or is it to meet your own needs? Often breaches of

There's just so little time to think about things when a situation comes up. You're taken by surprise a lot, just not expecting to face some ethical issue. Or at least that's true with me. I've read the codes through and through. I've gone to mandatory refresher courses required for keeping my license. I've read books and articles on the subject. Sure, I talk to people about it all the time. Really, I think that's what counselors talk about the most—beside complaining, I mean. But still, I get caught by surprise. You're just kind of in a comfortable position, listening, nodding your head, thinking hard about stuff, then before you know it, there it is: Your client just confessed something, or just told you something, and bells start going off in your head. Like you know you're supposed to do something, but for the life of me, I can't figure out what that should be. I think to myself, "Damn—why me again?"

I usually try to stall for time because I don't do well under pressure like that. I want to buy some time. Then as soon as the client leaves I talk to as many people as I can to find out what I should do or how I should handle the situation. Sometimes that even makes things worse, because everyone has a different answer. But eventually I'm able to sort things out and respond decisively the next time the client comes in.

ethical conduct—and poor decisions—are made when counselors fail to recognize the extent to which they are attempting to meet their own needs in the guise of helping others.

6. *Deliberate and decide.* Frame a preliminary course of action. Document the process you followed. Consult with peers and supervisors for feedback. Consider the consequences of your actions and alternative plans if things do not proceed as anticipated.

7. *Take action.* This is where you follow through on the informed, intentional decision that you have made through careful research and planning.

8. *Reflect.* Ethical dilemmas are opportunities for systematic growth and moral development. Review the situation as it developed. Consider other ways you could have responded. Identify what you learned from the situation and what you resolve to do differently in the future. If indicated, "publish" the results by informing others (verbally or in writing) what they might learn from your experience.

In addition to the introspective analysis that leads a person to select a defensible moral choice, the decision-making process should also take into account the guidelines established by professional organizations and the legal system. Most of these sources mandate the following actions:

1. *Don't attempt any therapeutic intervention without sufficient knowledge, skills, training, and supervision.* You should never attempt helping actions that are outside the bounds of your qualifications and competence. Workshops, certification programs, postgraduate training, internships, and intensive supervision are the means by which you can legitimately augment your therapeutic skills and continue to grow as a professional. Make referrals to specialists and other helping professionals when appropriate.

2. *You should be free of all biases and prejudices that might interfere with the capacity for objectivity, neutrality, and positive regard in the therapeutic relationship.* This includes sexual and racial biases, as well as those directed toward any ethnic or religious group, special population, or belief system.

3. *Sexual involvement with clients is strictly prohibited.* Under no circumstances should you as a counselor ever engage in erotic contact, act seductively, or respond to overtures made by those who have offered their trust in your professional integrity.

4. *The rights of all participants in research projects should be carefully protected.* All experimental procedures that could conceivably produce side effects must be thoroughly described and informed consent obtained from all subjects.

5. *You are responsible for protecting the privacy and confidentiality of all sessions.* Except in those circumstances wherein human life is endangered, you must preserve the sanctity of the therapeutic encounter. Information regarding a case may be released only with proper client authorization or under legal compulsion.

6. *The focus of counseling is on helping the client to reach self-determined goals.* Except in those instances in which goals appear to be destructive, self-defeating, or in violation of principles of reality, you are committed to working toward the client's greater autonomy and independence. You should therefore avoid manipulating clients, as well as creating dependencies or meeting your own needs in the session.

7. *You are committed to continuing professional training and growth after completing your formal education.* The knowledge and research in the field change so rapidly that practitioners must continually update their expertise. For this reason, many professional organizations and certification/licensing boards require annual continuing-education credits of members.

8. *You have an obligation to confront colleagues engaged in unethical, illegal, or incompetent practices.* As a professional, you have a responsibility to your profession, your community, and the safety of those who seek counseling services. Your duty is to challenge directly the behavior of those who are transcending the bounds of generally accepted principles. If the problem is not sufficiently resolved, you are then required to report such behavior to appropriate authorities.

9. *You are committed to maintaining high standards of integrity, honesty, and moral fiber.* Counselors accept their responsibility as professional helpers, recognize their powerful influence, and work toward functioning as effective models for their clients.

10. *As a counselor, you act for the general welfare of clients and society.* You attempt to prevent discrimination, to help the needy and disadvantaged, to promote social justice, and to help all persons become more fully functioning.

As a counselor you must be sensitive to the cultural, ethnic, religious, gender, and philosophical differences among people of diverse backgrounds, all of whom operate by rules, values, and customs that may not be familiar to you. Recognize that, whenever you are dealing with moral issues (and counseling is most certainly a value-laden discipline), there are many different paths to "truth" and many different standards of what is "right."

LEGAL ISSUES IN COUNSELING

As if it is not complicated enough that you must be familiar with and accountable to the ethical standards of the profession and the standards of professional competence in your work setting, you must also be familiar with how your work intersects with the legal system. In situations like the following, you will be expected to apply legal principles and make difficult decisions that may conflict with your own values, the ethical principles of your profession, or the policies of your institution:

- When a client's civil rights are violated, such as in cases involving sex, age, or racial discrimination
- When clients are involved in custody battles or divorce action
- When clients are seeking eligibility for disability or unemployment compensation
- When you believe a client is a danger to himself or herself or to others
- When you receive a court referral
- When you suspect that child abuse has taken place
- When a client you are seeing is engaged in planning or carrying out criminal acts
- When you serve as an expert witness in a case
- When you are subjected to malpractice litigation because of claims that you caused harm or injury to a client or acted negligently

As frightening as these examples might appear, there are several other situations in which counselors may find themselves embroiled in legal disputes: (1) There is a charge of sexual misconduct, (2) there is a breach of confidentiality, (3) a client has committed suicide, (4) there is a violation of civil rights, (5) there are accusations of libel or slander, (6) there has been a failure to diagnose properly, (7) there is a breach of contract, (8) client abandonment is alleged, (9) the counselor has exerted undue influence, and (10) there has been an accident on the premises.

Practicing counselors are expected to familiarize themselves with three kinds of law that affect their work: *civil law* related to malpractice suits and disputes between parties; *criminal law*, in which you may be expected to serve as an expert witness; and *mental health law*, which governs the ways that various client groups must be treated (Swenson, 1997). In each of these cases, you will need to have a working mastery of the legal system and how it affects the particular work that you do. Sometime in your career, you are likely to: (1) be served a subpoena to show up in court, (2) have your records called, (3) function as a witness on behalf of or against an injured party, or (4) be threatened with legal action yourself for some perceived injustice.

The intention here is not to alarm you to the point where you select a safer occupation, but rather to convince you of the importance that legal and ethical training will have in your work. By familiarizing yourself thoroughly with the legal statutes of your state and the ethical codes of your profession and by learning to apply them in real-life situations, you will protect your clients from harm and also

VOICE FROM THE FIELD

I'm so tired of being threatened by litigation that I now limit my practice to only those clients I can trust. I know this sounds strange—that we are the ones that are supposed to earn their trust—but I think it goes both ways. Twice already this year I have been threatened with legal action because two very disturbed ex-clients of mine do not want to pay their outstanding bills. They think if they sue me for some imaginary breach they will be able to weasel their way out of their debts.

I will own the part of the problem that I'm not so good at collecting fees for service, but I have to tell you: With both of these cases I worked my butt off for them. I devoted my heart and soul to doing whatever I could to help them. Frankly, I feel betrayed. It's like I need to keep my own attorney on retainer just to deal with all these nuisance suits.

protect yourself from needless vulnerability. In addition, you will guarantee your clients' rights in a number of circumstances:

1. *The right to informed consent.* The client is entitled to receive accurate and clear information regarding the therapeutic process, expected roles, risks and benefits of treatment, costs and contractual arrangements, right to access his or her files, implications of diagnostic labeling, alternative treatment options available, and qualifications and training of the counselor.

2. *The right to privacy.* This involves helping the client to understand the meaning of confidentiality and privileged communication, as well as the circumstances under which they may be breached. It also means keeping records secure and protecting the content of counseling sessions.

3. *The right to protection against harm.* This means following the major dictum of all helping professions: Do no harm! But it involves more than not hurting a client through negligence; it also means protecting the client against himself or herself. There are certain circumstances—notably when clients are suicidal or otherwise self-destructive—that require intervention to avoid a disaster.

4. *The right to refuse treatment.* At one time, mentally ill inpatients were forced to undergo shock and chemical treatments against their will. A number of new laws were enacted to protect people from being subjected to "chemical straitjackets," especially with regard to being medicated and "medically managed" to the point where they lost their free will. Except in emergency situations, or when someone is in imminent danger of inflicting harm, laws now offer some protection against forcible mental health treatments.

5. *The right to competent treatment.* The client is entitled to a counselor who is well trained in the profession and in any specialties that are practiced (for example, substance-abuse counseling, family therapy, hypnosis, and so on). In legal language this means that you will abide by the usual and customary standards of care that are agreed on by members of the profession. You can familiarize yourself with these "standards of care" by carefully reading the ethical codes and consulting a knowledgeable supervisor when you have questions. It also means that you do not practice outside of your scope of competence, using interventions that you haven't had a course on, obtained specialized training in, or have been supervised in using correctly.

VOICE FROM THE FIELD

I've been doing this for 20 years. I've never been sued, and my records have been subpoenaed only once. I've heard horror stories from other counselors, so I wonder if I've just been lucky, or whether it's something I'm doing in my work. My hunch is that it has to do with my attitude toward my clients. I'm a believer in the idea that you create your own reality, and the reality I want to create is one where the clients I work with are good people who appreciate that counseling is hard work, and not a miracle drug that makes all your problems go away. I respect the clients I work with, and they seem to respect me. I don't do anything that would hurt a client, and I guess they don't want to hurt me in return. Could it be that simple? I don't know, but I'd like to think so.

It is the perceived violation of this right of clients to competent treatment that most often embroils counselors in the legal system, usually in the form of a malpractice suit. When a client's rights are compromised or, more specifically, when the counselor's actions may be deemed as negligent, malpractice may be claimed. Such a charge must meet several criteria: (1) A professional relationship existed between the client and counselor, (2) a demonstrable standard of care was breached, (3) the client suffered harm, and (4) the counselor's behavior was the probable cause of the client's injury (Grosso, 2009; Welfel, 2006).

Let's apply these factors to a particular case. A client comes to you complaining of anxiety and poor self-esteem. He has trouble sleeping at night and feels agitated. You attempt to treat him with weekly counseling, but his condition worsens to the point where he requires hospitalization. During routine tests at admission, it is discovered that his symptoms are not psychologically based but were, in fact, caused by an underlying neurological disease. Does this situation constitute negligence on your part and justify a malpractice suit against you?

1. No. You were not the cause of his injury—the neurological disease was.
2. No. Because you are not a physician, you are not qualified or expected to diagnose neurological problems.
3. Yes. You violated the standard of customary care. Through your negligence in not referring the client for a medical consultation, he suffered undue pain and hardship.

This last choice is the correct answer. It illustrates the kinds of professional challenges you will face and the fact that you must safeguard your client's welfare by getting adequate consultation and supervision when you even suspect the possibility of problems outside your specialty.

As frightening as these situations may be for you to consider (and as tragic as they may be for some clients), the risks can be significantly decreased by following several guidelines:

1. Study the ethical codes, state laws, and standards of care for your profession very carefully. Review some of the "casebooks" that are available (Herlihy & Corey, 2006; Wilcoxon, Remley, Gladding, & Huber, 2007) to help you to reason through professional decision making.

VOICE FROM THE FIELD

If I could only get one message across to the interns and trainees I supervise, it would be this: Come to me for help whenever you aren't sure about something. Don't pretend to know things you don't! And if you are not sure about what to do, don't just reread a chapter in your school textbook. Come talk to me. Really—that's why I love to supervise, so I can help you. The students who get in trouble, and come close to committing malpractice, are the ones who are embarrassed to admit what they don't know, and try to figure everything out for themselves. But honestly, it takes years to attain competence in all the kinds of situations you encounter. This is a difficult profession. Be patient. Be humble. Be honest with yourself. Monitor your thinking processes for every time you say to yourself, "I'm not sure, but I think I know what to do in this situation, so I'll be OK." Those are the times when you have to say, "No. I really don't know what I'm doing here. I need help."

2. Make sure that you carry liability insurance to protect yourself from malpractice claims (as a student you are eligible for coverage at very reasonable rates).

3. As a beginner in the field, do not attempt any treatments without adequate supervision by qualified experts.

4. Document carefully your case records. Be especially prudent in checking out suicidal/homicidal ideation, history, and intent.

5. Consult frequently with medical personnel and make appropriate referrals when there is a possibility of some underlying organic problem.

6. Take steps to improve your level of competence by pursuing continuing education and advanced training.

7. Alert yourself to signs of fatigue and burnout that may lead you to miss important information or make needless mistakes.

8. Avoid those high-risk situations that are most likely to result in litigation: failure to treat a needy client, sexual involvement with a client, breach of confidentiality, failure to warn someone of potential harm, negligence leading to suicide, inadequate record keeping, collecting unpaid fees, and failure to diagnose or treat properly.

9. If you believe you might be engaging in some ethical or legal violation, get some help for yourself. Often remedial therapy alone is not enough and other forms of rehabilitation may be required to counteract the chronic boundary violation, especially in the case of sexual contact.

10. Make yourself more knowledgeable about the differences and commonalities between ethical codes, the legal system, and the realities of everyday practice.

Keep in mind that this is an introductory course so it is only appropriate to cover general principles of ethical and legal conduct. As you gain more experience and work in more specialized areas, you will be expected to apply sound ethical decision making to particular kinds of situations and cases. There are, for instance, more detailed guidelines for practitioners working with: (1) minors in the mental health system (Isaacs & Stone, 2001), (2) older adults (Schwiebert, Myers, & Dice, 2000), (3) gay and lesbian clients (Greene, 2006), (4) family counseling modalities (Wilcoxon et al., 2007), (5) Internet-based treatments (Shaw & Shaw,

2006), (6) addictions (Cottone & Tarvydas, 2007), and (7) managed care settings (Sommers-Flanagan & Sommers-Flanagan, 2007). In each case, and in every setting, you will be required to assess the potential ethical and legal risks that could occur as a result of your actions—or inaction (Falvey, 2002). If you are ever called on to appear in court, seek legal counsel as well as sources that prepare you for depositions and appearances as a witness (see Barsky & Gould, 2002).

Remember, as a beginner to this field you are not expected to know everything and be able to do everything perfectly. Making mistakes is part of your growth and crucial to your learning. You are, however, responsible for making certain that you find the best possible training and supervision so that you can become the most proficient and responsible professional possible.

SUMMARY

The first step in making ethically sound decisions is to anticipate some possible dilemmas and to think through alternatives and preferred responses in an objective and analytical manner. These personal resolutions must be congruent with professional standards, state and federal laws, and institutional policies in order to be useful.

A systematic approach will yield ethical decisions that are personally meaningful, have a specific rationale for behavior, and are objectively defensible. It will also enable the counselor to respond to challenges, legal or personal, with a sense of integrity and a clear rationale for any behavior. The counselor should maintain an open, questioning attitude toward ethical decision making, recognizing the need to challenge and question decisions, values, and attitudes.

Ethical decision making is not a state counselors achieve but an ongoing process of learning, growth, and maturation. Ethical decision making means that counselors take responsibility for functioning at the highest possible level of moral behavior, both to serve clients better and to avoid legal entanglements. Periodic reflection and a full examination of ethically challenging situations are essential factors in this process. It is often helpful to consult with colleagues and supervisors. Yet in this profession, confusion has its healthy side; it helps counselors avoid rigidity and forces them to personalize the meaning of their behavior.

SELF-GUIDED EXPLORATIONS

1. List some of your strongest beliefs and values regarding how you and other people should live their lives. Include those related to religion, premarital and extramarital sex, abortion, children's discipline, drug use, war, divorce, and any others that come to mind. Then describe the values of a person who feels the opposite that you do. Now, imagine that your opposite walks in the door to see you as a client. How will you work with him or her?

2. List three of the most important moral rules that guide your life. Meet with several others to share your individual principles. Come to a consensus as to which three moral rules you can all agree with. Describe your personal reactions to this dialogue and negotiation.

3. Think of a time in your life when you faced a major ethical dilemma. Trace the internal process you went through to reach a decision. What helped you along the way to reach a satisfactory resolution?

4. Which is the ethical conflict that you fear the most? Describe a real-life example in which you are confronted by this very issue. Talk through how you would come to some decision as to what you should do.

5. View one of the following movies: *Analyze This*, *Good Will Hunting*, or *Antwone*

Fisher. All of these films depict ethical breaches. See if you can identify what they are. Ask yourself whether the ethical breaches were committed to satisfy the needs of the counselor, or instead were justified because they may have helped the client. If you feel a breach was justified, you need to ask yourself as well, was there an alternate, ethical path the counselor could have taken that would have been equally effective?

FOR HOMEWORK

Carefully read through the *Ethical Codes* of the profession. Jot down a few notes of areas that you think are particularly confusing or about which you have questions. Check with a few experienced counselors to sort out your areas of concern.

SUGGESTED READINGS

Barsky, A. E., & Gould, J. W. (2002). *Clinicians in court: A guide to subpoenas, depositions, testifying, and everything else you need to know.* New York: Guilford.

Corey, G., Corey, M. S., & Callanan, P. (2007). *Issues and ethics in the helping professions* (7th ed.). Belmont, CA: Brooks/Cole.

Cottone, R., & Tarvydas, V. M. (2007). *Ethical and professional issues in counseling* (3rd ed.). Upper Saddle River, NJ: Merrill/Prentice Hall.

Dillon, C. (2003). *Learning from mistakes in clinical practice.* Belmont, CA: Brooks/Cole.

Falvey, J. E. (2002). *Managing clinical supervision: Ethical practice and legal risk management.* Belmont, CA: Brooks/Cole.

Kottler, J. A., & Carlson, J. (2003). *Bad therapy: Master therapists share their worst failures.* New York: Brunner/Routledge.

Remley, T. P., & Herlihy, B. (2010). *Ethical, legal, and professional issues in counseling* (3rd ed.). Upper Saddle River, NJ: Prentice Hall.

Sperry, L. (2007). *The ethical and professional practice of counseling and psychotherapy.* Boston: Allyn & Bacon.

Welfel, E. R. (2006). *Ethics in counseling and psychotherapy: Standards, research, and emerging issues* (3rd ed.). Belmont, CA: Thomson Brooks/Cole.

Wilcoxon, S. A., Gladding, S. T., Remley, T. P., & Huber, C. H. (2007). *Ethical, legal, and professional issues in the practice of marriage and family therapy* (4th ed.). Upper Saddle River, NJ: Prentice Hall.

Toward Closure: Advice for the Passionately Committed Counseling Student

This chapter is for those dedicated individuals who, after completing their introductory course in counseling, have decided to devote their lives to helping other people. Your commitment to the counseling profession is not to be taken lightly, nor can you realistically expect to treat your career as a mere job in which you just put in your time. Counselors are passionately committed to helping their clients to become more productive, fully functioning beings. The counseling student, too, must be intensely motivated to pursue a path of lifelong learning. It is only through your own hunger to understand, your thirst to know, your craving to find truth, and your skill in communicating your ideas that you become able to influence people in constructive ways.

In the spirit of enthusiasm for the mission of counselors, we offer the following advice to students.

BE SELF-DIRECTED

The best way to become passionate about learning is to follow your own natural curiosity to make sense of the world. So much of counseling deals with abstractions and complex queries that defy understanding. Your teachers, supervisors, and authors you read will only begin to tantalize you with answers to the questions that plague you the most. How does counseling work? Why does counseling work? Your assigned readings, lectures, and class discussions are but stimuli for you to begin resolving many of these difficult issues. It is through personal reflection, self-directed study, and leisurely wandering through the library and Internet that you can really begin to educate yourself.

READ

We would encourage you, in your self-directed study, to research systematically the works that have had the most impact in the counseling profession. Make a list of

VOICE FROM THE FIELD

If there's one thing I miss the most from my graduate school days, it's time spent reading books related to counseling. Not just the reading, but also the moments devoted to reflecting on what I was reading. Somehow, I don't find the time to do that anymore. I work with eating disorders, so I browse through the journals in my area, but that's about it. After making my client progress notes, dealing with insurance forms, and going home to spend time with my family, sitting down with a book is simply not possible. It's really a shame. When I was in school, I felt overwhelmed by all the reading. I used to tell myself I never had time to read because of all the papers and assignments I had to do. I promised myself that once I graduated, then I'd get to all the books I meant to read. Didn't happen.

classic books in the field—and read them. Solicit nominations from teachers and peers. Notice in the literature those titles that are most frequently cited. Most of all, find a few reliable persons whose opinions you respect (such as a mentor) and read everything they recommend. Don't restrict yourself to just the books in counseling, but become familiar with the literature in related fields such as psychology, social work, psychiatry, education, nursing, sociology, and philosophy. There are also some who believe (and we are among them) that reading fiction can offer as much insight into the inner workings of the human condition as any professional book. By all means, ask for recommendations for instructive novels, as well as for professional books (see the list at the end of the chapter).

FIND A MENTOR

In all chosen professions—the arts, sciences, law, medicine, business—and especially in a people-oriented career such as counseling, it is important to have a model to emulate. A mentor, usually a teacher, senior colleague, or other benevolent friend/coach, helps the neophyte to learn the ropes during the period of apprenticeship. A mentor does more, much more, than give homespun advice or recommend books; she or he becomes an advocate. It is through this relationship that the beginning counselor receives support, encouragement, constructive feedback, and a guiding hand.

Select a mentor whom you admire, who has skills and knowledge you respect and wish to acquire for yourself, and who has a genuine, nonpossessive interest in you. Find someone you can trust and confide in, yet one who does not feel that such a commitment is a burden. A mentor can be a source not only of nurturance and wisdom during the formative years of professional development but also of invaluable assistance in securing a job.

NETWORK

This is the time to start the process of professional networking, developing friendships with students who may very well be colleagues throughout your career. We all have a need to choose friends who are most like us, with whom we intuitively feel there will be strong kinship. Those connections are important, but equally valuable are connections with peers whom you perceive as potentially talented counselors who are focused on success, and likely to be leaders in the field. These are the people who will stimulate and challenge you and who will help make your study groups effective learning opportunities. Years down the line, these may be the people who refer clients to you, tell you about job opportunities, and are even in a position to hire you.

The real action in graduate school takes place during breaks between class, over coffee or lunch, or in your program's student associations. Here is where you can seek out the classmates with whom you want to develop relationships. Here is where you can engage in some of the most interesting and enjoyable conversations of your career: talking with classmates about the theories you are learning, discussing what you relate to and don't; listening to ideas that challenge you and letting yourself taste them like a food you ordinarily would never try. If you disagree with what someone is saying, engage in debate; elevate the discourse to increasingly higher levels. These processes are what forge connections between people, creating professional and personal friendships that can last a lifetime.

Volunteer to Do Research

Getting actively involved in a research project is helpful in a number of obvious ways. It allows you to apply learning to the solution of real-life problems and personalizes the usefulness of the scientific method. Upon publication, a writing credit can be a marketable commodity for gaining entrance to a doctoral program or a competitive job. Doing research also permits interaction with professors and colleagues on a level that would not be possible in the classroom. Finally, research gives you practical experience in exploring the issues, problems, and methodology of the profession. It is an opportunity to advance the growth of counseling and your own knowledge.

Ask Questions

When you don't know the answer to a question, *ask!*

Many of the questions students ask in class are posed less to learn new ideas than to win brownie points, demonstrate what they already know, or express opinions in diplomatic ways. And that raises the following question: Are we saying that students are afraid to take risks by displaying their ignorance?

Unfortunately, yes—that's what we are saying. In our experience, it is rare that a student really feels comfortable enough to ask the questions that she or he would most like to have answered. Most of us feel too timid to admit our uncertainty—as if by questioning the professors, we might reveal to others that we were not so bright and didn't really belong in class. We appreciate that this kind of passivity is safer than putting yourself on the line in front of your classmates, but we promise you—years from now, when sitting with a client and feeling stuck, you will flash back to a time in class when you had wished you had asked the question that never got past the tip of your tongue. So we encourage you to take risks in class and ask about those things you don't understand. How, after all, can you expect your future clients to open up if you feel such reluctance? Right at this moment, make a list of the questions you never got around to asking. Good news! There are still many opportunities left in future classes.

CHALLENGE YOUR TEACHERS

Challenging those ideas presented in class that you disagree with is even riskier than questioning—but potentially more fun, too. This style of learning is critical to the development of your own ideas, especially with those teachers who don't react defensively.

There are many concepts central to the core of counseling that some beginning students accept with great difficulty. For example, the notion of avoiding absolutes, shoulds, and other moralistic "rights" and "wrongs" cannot be internalized except through active dialogue with others who have reflected on the implications and tested the principles. It is through having interesting debates and challenging new ideas that these principles can be understood and personalized.

CHALLENGE YOURSELF

The most difficult task of a student is to maintain an openness to new ideas while simultaneously retaining a critical perspective. When ideas, concepts, and theories are presented that at first seem threatening, rather than immediately leaping to defend yourself against other classmates or professors, first challenge yourself to explore the merits of the point of view. Ask yourself why you are responding so emotionally to the subject. What would it mean for you if you had to change your ideas to conform to this added information?

A related danger is that of too enthusiastically embracing a particular point of view, sowing the seeds of terminal rigidity and closing out the possibility of other ideas. Initially it is helpful to be suspicious and tentative. After exploring a theory that seems attractive and useful, do not fall into the destructive trap of confusing it with ultimate truth.

EXPERIENCE COUNSELING AS A CLIENT

In the process of challenging yourself, there is no vehicle more appropriate than experiencing counseling as a client. Many programs encourage participation in a form of counseling prior to graduation. For anyone who hopes to do counseling, it is important to know intimately the fears, joys, and apprehensions that clients experience.

Participating in counseling as a client allows you to work through inhibitions, distracting conflicts, and unresolved problems that may interfere with the ability to remain objective, focused, and therapeutic. It also helps you to believe fervently in the power of the process when you have experienced firsthand its beneficial effects.

We urge you to seek out both individual and group counseling experiences for another reason. Clearly, while a counseling student is engaged in a therapeutic relationship, there is always a part of him or her that is closely observing the process, noting the interventions that work best, and knowing—really knowing—how the

VOICE FROM THE FIELD

I pick my supervisor's brain constantly. I talk to other professionals all the time—on the phone, at lunch, in e-mail, at conferences. I subscribe to every publication I can afford. I continuously consult Web sites to check for information. I read. I survey and watch other people all the time. I question people: "So tell me, you seem to be a happy person. How do you manage that?"

Based on all this study, I try new things in my work. Right now I'm working on a new drawing technique and a different approach to use with this one adolescent who is giving me a hard time. I'm always searching for new metaphors and stories to use.

process works. If we truly believe that counseling is for everyone, then it is most certainly for us—all of us.

PERSONALIZE EVERYTHING

Counseling is a joy to study because all the abstract ideas, theoretical constructs, research hypotheses, clinical interpretations, class lectures, and textbook discourses can be personalized and applied to your own life. All of a sudden the behavior of those around you no longer appears the same. As counselors, we seem more critical yet more forgiving.

The novels we read, movies we see, and conversations we participate in become wonderful opportunities to think, act, and feel differently. Learning has more meaning to us if we can make it more relevant. And that, primarily, is the student's job—to take the nucleus of an idea from one's teacher, mentor, counselor, or colleague and apply it in such a way that it becomes personally useful.

EXPAND YOUR WORLD

The people who most likely need help the most are not like you. They come from different backgrounds, subscribe to different values, and may even have a different color of skin. They come from a variety of different religions and spiritual belief systems. Many of them have led impoverished or disadvantaged lives or suffered abuse and neglect that is unimaginable. All of them bring a unique cultural context to their worlds and their problems, shaped by their ethnicity, gender, identity, and life experiences.

A course or two in multicultural counseling or diverse populations can't put a dent in all the things you need to know in order to be helpful to clients who need you the most. All the reading in the world can't be a substitute, either, for what you can learn in the real world. While clients will help to educate you about their cultures and values, you can't depend on them to do your work for you; there is so much to learn and so little time.

One of the best ways to expand your world is through travel, not just to foreign lands but also to any novel environment that exposes you to diverse peoples, new customs and language, different values and beliefs. Push yourself, whenever

VOICE FROM THE FIELD

It's a funny thing, travel. The best things you find are those you're not really looking for. I used to think in going to conferences that the important stuff was in the programs. I was so compulsive about following a schedule, collecting handouts, hitting as many different presentations as I could. I had this misguided belief that if only I could soak up all this knowledge that I could serve my clients best when I got home.

Then I discovered one day when I skipped going to the conference that a whole new world opened up to me by trying to learn about the place that I was at from the people. I rode a subway in a big city for the first time. I talked to everyone I could. And I learned so much that I could never have found out any other way.

possible, to explore as much of the planet as you can. More importantly, don't travel like a tourist who is only interested in souvenirs, taking photographs, and seeing sanctioned sites. Interact with people and find out about their worlds. Take risks to venture into unknown territory. Monitor the internal judgments you have about the ways people act differently. Notice how critical you are of different customs you don't fully understand. Then take this learning home with you. Apply it to your work in such a way that you become more sensitive and responsive to those who are most unlike you.

BECOME ACTIVE IN PROFESSIONAL ORGANIZATIONS

The American Counseling Association, the American Association for Marriage and Family Therapy, and the American Psychological Association are a few of the groups that advance the profession of counseling. Through their lobbying activities, public relations and consumer education programs, and professional development courses, these organizations help support practitioners. They also develop written ethical codes, work toward certification and training standards, provide referral services, sponsor national and regional conventions, fund research projects, publish professional journals, run job search programs, and provide social activities for their members.

There are many opportunities for students to get actively involved in the organizations by attending conventions, contributing articles to journals, serving on committees, presenting papers and workshops, and working on special projects of interest. Participating in state, regional, and national conventions is especially interesting because of the opportunities to make lifelong friendships with colleagues around the world. Conventions are also ideal places to receive specialized training and find jobs, because many employers are present to interview candidates for positions.

Organizational activities help you to identify with the counseling profession as a whole, as well as with a number of specialty areas. The American Counseling Association or the American Psychological Association offer members a number of divisions they can join, each with its own journal and networking opportunities. Within ACA, for example, students can join, for reduced rates, specialty groups that focus on dozens of different areas, including adult development and aging, college counseling, multicultural counseling, mental health counseling, rehabilitation counseling, school counseling, and many others. You can join as many of these divisions as you have the time and inclination for, each one offering a unique perspective of the field.

DEVELOP A FLEXIBLE SPECIALTY

As we have already said, a degree in counseling does not guarantee employment in a specific career. Graduates may have to market themselves in such a way that they will fit a particular position or even tailor a job to fit their own unique skills, training, and interests.

Practically everyone knows what the psychologist, psychiatrist, or social worker can and cannot do. Counseling practitioners, however, now function in many diverse settings. Five students in the same program, with the same course work, may eventually find employment in five different settings: school counseling, industrial relations, consumer education, rehabilitation counseling, and mental health counseling. The counseling degree, then, reflects education for the generalist who, through specialized training and interests, develops a unique professional identity.

We therefore suggest to the beginning student the following course of action for finding eventual employment in a desired area:

1. Talk to counselors in the field about what they do and how they feel about their jobs.
2. Find excuses to talk to prospective employers to determine what they are looking for in candidates.
3. Discover a few particular types of client populations (disabled, gifted), age groups (preschoolers, older adults), settings (hospitals, schools), and counseling skills (consultation, group interventions) in which you can gain specialized experience.
4. Use elective courses, workshop experiences, and your internship sites to become expert in a few flexible specialties.
5. Volunteer your time at local community agencies to accumulate additional professional experiences.

RESIST BURNOUT

In recent years there has developed a considerable body of literature describing the burnout phenomenon, especially as it relates to counselors, psychologists, social workers, teachers, and other human services personnel (see Kottler, 2010; Skovholt, 2001; Young & Lambie, 2007). Symptoms of this insidious condition include fatigue, irritation, reduced work performance, apathy, boredom, and negative attitudes. In its earliest forms you will notice more subtle signs of feeling dispirited and disillusioned.

The condition is caused, in part, by such factors as an excessive workload, monotony, a lack of control, and isolation in your work. Belson (1992) facetiously

■ | VOICE FROM THE FIELD

When I go home, I go home. I have come to value the ambiguity of the work that I do. But I have to have an anchored place to retreat from it. For me, that anchor is my home, my husband, and my son. After a tough day, I answer no calls at home. I cancel any evening appointments.

Although I have learned to tolerate—even appreciate—the ambiguous, stressful nature of my work, I can't let it permeate all my life. I must be able to say, "This far, no farther!" I've just got to have my haven, my safe boundary line.

---

recommends several tried-and-true methods for achieving burnout, if that is your goal:

1. Work long hours, especially weekends and evenings. Tell yourself this doesn't really interfere with the quality of your relationships with family.
2. Think about your hardest cases even when you are not working. Worry about what you aren't doing that you should be doing.
3. Blame your clients, their families, your colleagues, your boss, or the system for the reasons why things are not going as smoothly as you would prefer.
4. Believe that you can help everyone you see, and that you can cure them within a very short time.

The only antidotes for burnout are renewed enthusiasm or a job change. Those counselors who are most committed to their jobs and to the profession may be less likely to experience the effects of burnout and disillusionment. They also tend to be practitioners who, despite having high standards of excellence for their work, are accepting of their limitations. They are able to let go of those aspects of their jobs that they can't control and focus instead on what is within their power to change.

The time to prevent burnout is now, not when you are already experiencing negative symptoms. Begin structuring your professional life so that you are surrounded by a good support system. Most importantly: Practice what you preach and take care of yourself!

CONFRONT YOUR FEARS OF FAILURE

We recall that moment sitting in our first counseling class, looking around the room, and feeling utterly despondent because everyone else seemed so much brighter and more talented than we were. Doubts assailed us: "Am I smart enough to get through this program?" "Do I have what it takes to be a counselor?" "What will my professors think when they find out how weird I really am?" These doubts, and many others like them, are not only a normal part of most students' inner thoughts, but also continue to plague practitioners in the field. Counselors often worry about failure. What if they inadvertently harm a client? What if they are confronted with a situation in which they don't know what to do? What if they are caught making a mistake? Yet these doubts become unmanageable only when they are avoided and denied; it is by confronting your fears that you are able to work through them.

Some of you may deal with issues of failure by pushing yourself to get A's in every course. Each high grade becomes more proof that you are a worthwhile, competent person, while keeping at bay the underside of perfectionism: the despair of not being good enough, the worry about not pleasing your parents, or the fear of being discovered as a fraud whose success comes from obsessive studying rather than real talent and ability. It's a perilous place in which to live, because one low grade can feel like a house of cards is collapsing.

We therefore urge you to find a support group of peers in which you can confide your doubts and fears, disclose your fantasies of being an imposter, and talk about your imperfections and misunderstandings. We can confidently reassure you that, although it is difficult to recruit confidants who are compatible in any walk of life, you are definitely not alone in your apprehensions. Even after several decades of practicing and teaching counseling, both of us still continue to confront our own fears of failure.

The implications for the beginning counselor are clear. You must work diligently to develop a sense of professional commitment to clients, colleagues, the profession, and ultimately yourselves as professional counselors. This sense of commitment will result in renewal and provide the energy base necessary to perform creatively and enthusiastically. The time to begin developing that sense of commitment is now.

Get the Most from Supervision

Just as it takes some practice and skill to be a "good" client in counseling—that is, to get the most from the experience—so too does it take a certain resolve, trust, perseverance, and commitment to get the most from your supervision experience. Much will depend, of course, on whether you trust and respect your supervisor, whether you think and feel that he or she is competent and has your best interests at heart. But even when you are forced to work with supervisors you would never have chosen, you can still gain much from their experience. Under the best circumstances, you may be fortunate to work with someone who is not only highly skilled, sensitive, and caring, but who is also well trained in the special nuances of conducting supervisory relationships.

In order to get the most from supervision, you will need to work hard on the relationship. This means doing solid preparation. It means reflecting on your cases and professional struggles, defining where you are having the most difficulty, and articulating your concerns and needs. More than anything, supervisors appreciate working with students who talk about what is working and what is not working. We don't just mean with your own cases but also in your supervision relationship. Your supervisor cannot better meet your needs or address your major concerns if you don't take responsibility for communicating what is most and least helpful.

Seize the Day

Try to be a model of the person you would like your clients to be. If you think that people are happiest, most satisfied, and most productive when they are loving and caring—when they live in the present as much as possible—then strive to do the same in your own life. Be who you want your clients to be by the way you live your life—with honesty and integrity, with compassion, with hunger to experience as much as you can in the brief time you will be residing on this planet.

Jeffrey's coauthor on previous editions of this textbook, Bob Brown, died several years ago. Jeffrey interviewed him just a few weeks before he died of cancer, and this is the advice he offered to new counselors in the field:

> What do I have to say to counselors in the field who are trying to find their way, to create meaning in their own lives? Don't take yourself seriously, but take yourself measurably. Don't take yourself in a manner that is cavalier, but take yourself in a manner that has sincerity and thoughtfulness about it.

What Bob was struggling to grasp in his last days was what meaning his career had. He had spent decades as a science teacher, a school counselor, a psychologist, and a counselor educator. He had devoted his life to helping others, yet felt regretful about the time he wasted not allowing himself to give and receive love to those who mattered the most to him.

"Dying is not that big a deal," Bob said. "I know how to die. Now I want to die with a sense of enjoyment and laughter and happiness and contentment. I want to be filled with the excitement of every precious moment I have left."

We are all dying—right this moment. The question remains, what do you want to do with the time you have left? That is the question you will help your clients struggle with. You will be a lot better prepared to do so if you have the answers for yourself.

WHAT MOST STUDENTS DON'T LEARN UNTIL IT IS WAY TOO LATE

See Companion DVD
Secrets of the
Profession

There are some secrets to this profession that are not ordinarily discussed in your training. Perhaps the reasoning is that there is no sense depressing, discouraging, or otherwise overwhelming you with realities of practice before you've had a chance to really get your feet wet—and get hooked to the point that you can't let go if you wanted to.

Our feeling on the matter is that you are better off knowing what you are likely to face so that you can take steps to prepare yourself for certain challenges. If you prefer surprise endings, then read no further.

Stop reading now if you are faint of heart.

No? We didn't think so. Courage, after all, is an important attribute for counselors.

In all honesty (and we intend to be very honest with you), we believe the following material will actually make you more intrigued with this work, more committed to doing what you can to flourish in spite of some difficult issues that lay ahead.

As a very dramatic example, one concept you have already been exposed to is the idea of "informed consent." This means that you provide people with the accurate information they need, including risks and contraindications, so that they can make good decisions about whether to undergo a particular procedure or therapeutic experience. For instance, if you were going to take a medication prescribed by your doctor she would first tell you about possible side effects that might occur. Then you decide whether you want to go ahead with the treatment. In counseling, we follow this standard procedure as well, letting our clients know what they might face so that they can decide if they wish to follow our lead in that area. It occurred to us that if we were truly to practice informed consent with respect to your training as a counselor, there are a lot of things we would tell you that might very well scare you away. For instance, are you aware that there is a decent possibility that as a result of training to be a counselor you may leave your spouse or partner behind? Just consider the consequences to a relationship when one person—you—makes a major commitment to work on himself or herself in a significant way. You read, study, attend classes, complete assignments, all of which are designed to change not only your professional demeanor but your whole being. If your loved one continues with the usual things and does not make a parallel commitment to personal growth, what effect do you think that might have on the relationship? If you guess a fairly negative one, you'd be correct. Not only is there a risk that your loved one might get left behind, but he or she may become quite threatened by your new friends, new growth, and "strange" transformations. And if you think you can get through your training without changing who you are, then you haven't been paying very close attention.

Must relationships always be left in the dust? Of course not. In fact, your education actually prepares you to make your most important relationships even more satisfying. But we'd be negligent if we didn't warn you about the risks involved.

Likewise, another probable consequence of your educational experience is that all your relationships will change—with your friends, your family members, your neighbors, and coworkers. You may find yourself bored with superficial conversations. You may feel a greater need for deeper intimacy in relationships. In some ways, you will become spoiled. After practicing your new skills, learning to get inside people's heads and hearts, working hard on developing closeness with others, you will also want to apply all this to the relationships that matter most.

Just watch a bunch of counselors hanging out together and you can immediately see that we are a strange breed. It is not that we don't enjoy talking about sports and weather and politics, it is just that because we spend our lives dealing with very deep issues, talking about the most private and intimate topics imaginable, it raises the bar considerably as far as what we like to talk about when we are off duty. Others who have not been exposed to this stuff may very well flee in terror. As you've already discovered, people are a little afraid and in awe of counselors. They think we can read minds, and in a sense we can, and do. Based on our training and experience, we can predict what people will do before they are even aware that they are headed in that direction. We are highly skilled at influencing people; we can get them to do things they don't particularly want to do. What all this adds up to is that we are treated like gods, we act like gods, and sometimes even believe we have superpowers not granted to mortal beings.

Listed below are several other secrets that are not often revealed to beginners:

- *There are very personal reasons why you entered this profession.* As we mentioned in the beginning of this book, newcomers to this field not only want to heal others but also heal themselves. Some of us have been victims of abuse, neglect, traumas, or just plain old self-doubt. We are voyeurs. We yearn for power or control. We enjoy the one-way intimacy that is part of therapeutic relationships. There is a dark side to our own narcissism.

- *Life isn't a multiple-choice exam.* The problem you will face is not a scarcity of options but far too many from which to choose. This class, or others, may offer multiple-choice exams in which you are presented with four choices, one of which is obviously the wrong one, but counseling practice overwhelms you with so many options that it often feels whichever action you take there were a hundred others you could have chosen that might have been better.

- *The answers you need most are not found in books.* You don't really learn counseling by reading about it, or listening to people talking about it. You've got to experience it yourself, from both ends. You have to immerse yourself more fully in life, explore other cultures, take constructive risks, engage more completely in relationships.

- *What we do is often absurd.* A lot about counseling doesn't make sense. We don't fully understand how and why it works. We don't agree on the best way to approach this craft. And even when we do help people, we can't always explain why it happened, or why the effects did or didn't last.

- *Your family still won't listen to you.* Perhaps it's a coincidence (or maybe not, given the personal reasons people enter this field), but one of the reasons both of us studied to be a counselor, and then attained more advanced degrees, is because we wanted the respect and approval of our families. Even with a master's degree, then a PhD, then being professors, then authors, our families still don't take us any more seriously than they did before.

- *People don't want what you are selling.* Even the clients who seem cooperative and motivated may have hidden agendas. The honest ones tell you directly they don't trust you. The really difficult clients will pretend they want counseling, and even report that they are improving, but secretly they just want to keep you from getting close.

- *You will have to empathize with people you don't like.* One of the most important skills you will learn is how to maintain a nonjudgmental stance with your clients. This is easy with nice people; the true challenge is sustaining this attitude toward clients who offend you with their attitudes, values, and behaviors. Some of your clients may even disclose to you that they have done hurtful things to others; once you start the counseling process, you can't tell them, "Sorry, now that I know the kind of person you are, I refuse to work with you anymore."

  Every client, no matter how unpleasant, has something you can connect with; it may be a desire to change, or shame for past behaviors, or the lost, hurt child you can detect somewhere behind the surface of his or her personality. Your job is to search for at least one part in every client that you can hold onto and that gives you the incentive to help him or her.

- *You will forget everything you know and learn it again.* Your program is going to cram your brain with more information than you can possibly digest. When you start your practicum and internships, you'll discover how much you've forgotten and will have to revisit your texts. If you pursue a license, you will relearn everything your professors taught you all over again to prepare for the exam. Expect this cycle to continue throughout your career.

- *You will never know enough.* You will never get it right. No matter how hard you study, how compulsively you strive for perfection, how many books you read, how many degrees you attain or workshops you attend, you will still not know as much as you need to do the job. That is one of the burdens of this profession but also one of the most exciting aspects—you could study counseling your whole life, or a dozen lifetimes, and you will still never master the discipline.

- *Failure is more important than success.* It is interesting how, when things go well, we put the incident out of our minds; it is when we fail that we are forever haunted by our mistakes. There is no shame in failing with your clients; this is inevitable. The most important thing, however, is to learn from these experiences so you can process them constructively and not make the same mistakes again.

- *Who you are is as important as what you do.* As much as you want to learn all the content and skills and fancy techniques of counseling—to fill up your bag of tricks—your essential kindness and caring and commitment are as important as what you can do. We don't mean to say that being knowledgeable and highly skilled are not important, because they are—but rather that they are not enough. You must also work hard to make yourself into the best kind of person you can be—someone who is compassionate and dedicated to making the world a better place.

- *Many changes don't last.* As hard as it seems to help people to change, that is only the first step. Look at how many times in your own life that you have started to make changes you said were important—losing weight, starting an exercise program, calling your mother regularly, saving your money, studying two hours per day. You really meant it when you promised yourself to do those things. You may have even made solid efforts to get things going. But how long did the changes last? Never forget that your job not only involves helping people get started on their personal transformations, but involves making those changes permanent.

- *You will be haunted by those you helped, and those you didn't.* The relationships you develop with clients will become so intimate, so moving, so challenging at times, that their memories will stay in your head as long as you live. For better or worse, you will be irrevocably changed as a result of these encounters. You will smile and feel all warm inside thinking about some of the people you really helped, and who were so grateful for your efforts. Then there will be others who will leave your services dissatisfied, angry, and determined to make your life miserable. What distinguishes those who do well in our field are those who accept their mistakes, learn from them, and then move on, readily able to forgive themselves for being less than perfect.

- *You will learn how not to cry, and you will still cry.* Clients fear that their pain will overwhelm us, rendering us unable to help them. Our task is to remain calm and focused even while listening to tragic stories of loss and suffering. We can do this not because we become hardened and detached, but because we appreciate that when clients disclose painful material, they are releasing a heavy burden. As our faces show a composed compassion, inside we feel a kind of happiness for them that they've been able to put their pain into words and let their tears start to flow. We feel privileged that they would share their suffering with us. But there will still be those moments when our therapeutic composure is punctured by the intensity of their pain or the terrible sadness of their lives, and we will tear up with them. Those moments are not counseling mistakes; they are experiences of deep connection and a healing message to clients that their suffering is witnessed. Those moments remind us of our humanness, and they are profound and precious.

- *You won't have enough time to do what you want, or what needs to be done.* You have to pace yourself. You have to set limits. You can't possibly do everything that needs to be done, especially in the time constraints that you must live with. In many jobs, you will be understaffed and overworked. If you hope to stay in this profession long and enjoy the work you do, you must find ways to set limits, to accept your limitations, and do what you can.

- *Supervision isn't always available when you need it most.* A lot of the time you're on your own. Even with the best possible supervision available, you will still find yourself having to figure out many things on your own. Almost every session will present you with questions that you can't answer. Every day you will feel flooded by challenges and internal conflicts. Even if you had the opportunity to talk to a supervisor about all of them, you will still have unanswered questions. Somehow, some way, you are going to have to learn to live with the complexity and ambiguity of what you do.

- *Counselors are not just trained or educated; they are grown.* You must remain committed to your own growth and development. This does not mean simply taking more classes or going to continuing education workshops. It means seeking help for yourself when you need it. Most of all, it means practicing in your own life what you ask of your clients.

VARIATIONS ON A THEME

Naturally, we wish to leave you with the appropriate balance of healthy confusion and eager enthusiasm to grow, to learn more, to find your own truth, and to continue in a profession that helps others to clarify their directions. One consequence of doing counseling that is often observed by experienced practitioners is an increase in their own self-awareness, self-assurance, and psychological sensitivity. This phenomenon is, perhaps, the best reason of all for feeling passionate about and committed to the role.

In the 16th century, a Samurai warrior and master of kendo ("he who wields the sword") wrote a manual of instruction for those who wished to learn his strategy. Musashi's *Book of Five Rings* (1982) has since become a bible for Japanese businesspeople. We believe that his wisdom also speaks to prospective counselors—to those who wish to learn "the Way of Water" of becoming calm, unbiased, with a settled spirit—and to those who follow "the Way of Fire" by researching and training diligently. Musashi prescribes the following advice for those who want to follow his way:

- Do not think dishonestly.
- The Way is in training.
- Become acquainted with every art.
- Know the Ways of all professions.
- Distinguish between gain and loss in worldly matters.
- Develop intuitive judgment and understanding for everything.
- Perceive those things which cannot be seen.
- Pay attention to trifles.
- Do nothing which is of no use.

The greatest obstacle to any significant discovery is the illusion of knowledge. Boorstein (1983) explains that it was not ignorance that precipitated our descent into the Dark Ages of history, but rather those imaginative bold strokes that temporarily pacified fears and served hopes for simple solutions. True knowledge always advances slowly, with contradictions, conflicts, and controversy. And it is precisely these furiously passionate debates among discrepant views that produce an approximation of truth. With each course you take, with each book you read, with each workshop you attend, with each supervision session you complete, and with each client you see, greater wisdom and competence will evolve if (1) you learn from mistakes, (2) you passionately search for greater mastery in personal and professional skills, and (3) you retain sufficient humility to continue asking questions that have no simple answers.

A CLOSING VOICE FROM THE FIELD

In a supervision conference, one counselor lamented her frustrations and confusions about a particular case in which she felt lost, inept, and discouraged. "How, after all," she pleaded, "can I work with this client when I have no idea what is going on?" The supervisor softly responded in a voice that rose above the chatter of advice directed at the counselor.

"Don't worry when you don't know what you're doing," he said. "Worry when you think you do."

SELF-GUIDED EXPLORATIONS

1. What are some of your most perplexing questions about counseling that you would like to be able to answer before you graduate?
2. By challenging material presented in your textbook and by your instructor, you are able to develop your own ideas and internalize novel concepts. Write down at least three ideas presented in the textbook and three ideas presented by your instructor in class that you disagree with. Explain your reasoning.
3. Make a list of the goals that you have for yourself that you wish to accomplish in the next year. Sign and date this commitment.
4. As you look back on all the things that you have reflected on and written about in these

Self-Guided Explorations, what stands out for you as being most significant?

5. Describe how you intend to educate yourself to be the best possible counselor that you can be.

6. Reflect on what you do during a typical week. How much time do you spend sitting in class, studying, working, being with family, being engaged in physical exercise, playing, relaxing, and just being still? We appreciate that, as a graduate student, it's impossible to spend sufficient, if any, time in all of these activities. But you will need to achieve some balance in your life, or you will burn out. List the things that you can do to ensure good self-care while pursuing your degree.

Personal Reflections

These exercises represent the beginning, not the end, of your self-explorations and reflections on what it means for you to be a counselor. In a journal, continue writing follow-up entries about the lingering effects of this class. Make yourself accountable to all the previous things you declared and committed yourself to during the course of the semester. Make sure you write to yourself at least once per week for the next dozen or so weeks. After that you may wish to continue this intensive search in your own unstructured journal.

Suggested Readings

Corey, M. S., & Corey, G. (2007). *Becoming a helper* (5th ed.). Belmont, CA: Brooks/Cole.

Dass, R., & Gorman, P. (1985). *How can I help? Stories and reflections on service.* New York: Knopf.

Kottler, J. A. (2001). *Making changes last.* New York: Brunner/Routledge.

Rosenthal, H. (2004). *Before you see your first client: Fifty-five things counselors and human service providers need to know.* New York: Brunner/Routledge.

Skovholt, T. M. (2010). *The resilient practitioner: Burnout prevention and self-care strategies for counselors, therapists, teachers, and health professionals* (2nd ed.). Boston: Allyn & Bacon.

Yalom, I. (2001). *Gift of therapy: An open letter to a new generation of therapists and their patients.* New York: HarperCollins.

Suggested Readings: Some Great Novels with Themes Related to Counseling

Conroy, Pat	*Prince of Tides*	Medoff, Jillian	*Good Girls Gone Bad*
Guest, Judith	*Ordinary People*	Plath, Sylvia	*The Bell Jar*
Haddon, Mark	*The Curious Incident of the Dog in the Night-Time*	Rossner, Judith	*August*
Kaysen, Susanna	*Girl, Interrupted*	Shriver, Lionel	*We Need to Talk About Kevin*
Kellerman, Jonathan	*When the Bough Breaks*	Yalom, Irvin	*Schopenhauer's Cure*

AMERICAN COUNSELING ASSOCIATION (ACA) CODE OF ETHICS

APPENDIX A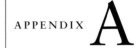

(As approved by the ACA Governing Council, 2005)

Contents

ACA members agree to abide by the rules, regulations, and enforcement of the terms of the *ACA Code of Ethics*.

AMERICAN COUNSELING ASSOCIATION
5999 Stevenson Avenue
Alexandria, VA 22304
© 2005 by the American Counseling Association. All rights reserved.
Note: This document may be reproduced without permission for educational purposes.
The American Counseling Association will not knowingly engage in any activities that discriminate on the basis of ethnic group, race, religion, gender, sexual orientation, age, and/or disability.

AMERICAN COUNSELING ASSOCIATION
ABOUT ACA

The American Counseling Association (ACA) is a nonprofit professional and educational organization dedicated to the growth and enhancement of the counseling profession. Founded in 1952, ACA is the world's largest association representing professional counselors in various practice settings. By providing professional development, leadership training, publications, continuing education opportunities, and advocacy services to nearly 45,000 members, ACA helps counseling professionals develop their skills and expand their knowledge base.

ACA is instrumental in setting professional and ethical standards for the counseling profession. The Association has also made considerable strides in accreditation, licensure, and national certification. In addition, ACA represents the interests of the profession before Congress and federal agencies and strives to promote recognition of professional counselors to the public and the media. For more information on ACA, visit our Web site at http://www.counseling.org.

ACA CODE OF ETHICS PREAMBLE

The American Counseling Association is an educational, scientific, and professional organization whose members work in a variety of settings and serve in multiple capacities. ACA members are dedicated to the enhancement of human development throughout the life span. Association members recognize diversity and embrace a cross-cultural approach in support of the worth, dignity, potential, and uniqueness of people within their social and cultural contexts.

Professional values are an important way of living out an ethical commitment. Values inform principles. Inherently held values that guide our behaviors or exceed prescribed behaviors are deeply ingrained in the counselor and developed out of personal dedication, rather than the mandatory requirement of an external organization.

ACA CODE OF ETHICS PURPOSE

The *ACA Code of Ethics* serves five main purposes:

1. The *Code* enables the association to clarify to current and future members, and to those served by members, the nature of the ethical responsibilities held in common by its members.
2. The *Code* helps support the mission of the association.
3. The *Code* establishes principles that define ethical behavior and best practices of association members.
4. The *Code* serves as an ethical guide designed to assist members in constructing a professional course of action that best serves those utilizing counseling services and best promotes the values of the counseling profession.

5. The *Code* serves as the basis for processing of ethical complaints and inquiries initiated against members of the association.

The *ACA Code of Ethics* contains eight main sections that address the following areas:

Section A: The Counseling Relationship

Section B: Confidentiality, Privileged Communication, and Privacy

Section C: Professional Responsibility

Section D: Relationships with Other Professionals

Section E: Evaluation, Assessment, and Interpretation

Section F: Supervision, Training, and Teaching

Section G: Research and Publication

Section H: Resolving Ethical Issues

Each section of the *ACA Code of Ethics* begins with an Introduction. The introductions to each section discuss what counselors should aspire to with regard to ethical behavior and responsibility. The Introduction helps set the tone for that particular section and provides a starting point that invites reflection on the ethical mandates contained in each part of the *ACA Code of Ethics*.

When counselors are faced with ethical dilemmas that are difficult to resolve, they are expected to engage in a carefully considered ethical decision-making process. Reasonable differences of opinion can and do exist among counselors with respect to the ways in which values, ethical principles, and ethical standards would be applied when they conflict. While there is no specific ethical decision-making model that is most effective, counselors are expected to be familiar with a credible model of decision making that can bear public scrutiny and its application.

Through a chosen ethical decision-making process and evaluation of the context of the situation, counselors are empowered to make decisions that help expand the capacity of people to grow and develop.

A brief glossary is given to provide readers with a concise description of some of the terms used in the *ACA Code of Ethics*.

SECTION A: THE COUNSELING RELATIONSHIP

INTRODUCTION

Counselors encourage client growth and development in ways that foster the interest and welfare of clients and promote formation of healthy relationships. Counselors actively attempt to understand the diverse cultural backgrounds of the clients they serve. Counselors also explore their own cultural identities and how these affect their values and beliefs about the counseling process.

Counselors are encouraged to contribute to society by devoting a portion of their professional activity to services for which there is little or no financial return (pro bono publico).

A.1. Welfare of Those Served by Counselors

A.1.a. Primary Responsibility

The primary responsibility of counselors is to respect the dignity and to promote the welfare of clients.

A.1.b. Records

Counselors maintain records necessary for rendering professional services to their clients and as required by laws, regulations, or agency or institution procedures. Counselors include sufficient and timely documentation in their client records to facilitate the delivery and continuity of needed services. Counselors take reasonable steps to ensure that documentation in records accurately reflects client progress and services provided. If errors are made in client records, counselors take steps to properly note the correction of such errors according to agency or institutional policies. *(See A.12.g.7., B.6., B.6.g., G.2.j.)*

A.1.c. Counseling Plans

Counselors and their clients work jointly in devising integrated counseling plans that offer reasonable promise of success and are consistent with abilities and circumstances of clients. Counselors and clients regularly review counseling plans to assess their continued viability and effectiveness, respecting the freedom of choice of clients. *(See A.2.a., A.2.d., A.12.g.)*

A.1.d. Support Network Involvement

Counselors recognize that support networks hold various meanings in the lives of clients and consider enlisting the support, understanding, and involvement of others (e.g., religious/spiritual/community leaders, family members, friends) as positive resources, when appropriate, with client consent.

A.1.e. Employment Needs

Counselors work with their clients considering employment in jobs that are consistent with the overall abilities, vocational limitations, physical restrictions, general temperament, interest and aptitude patterns, social skills, education, general qualifications, and other relevant characteristics and needs of clients. When appropriate, counselors appropriately trained in career development will assist in the placement of clients in positions that are consistent with the interest, culture, and the welfare of clients, employers, and/or the public.

A.2. Informed Consent in the Counseling Relationship

(See A.12.g., B.5., B.6.b., E.3., E.13.b., F.1.c., G.2.a.)

A.2.a. Informed Consent

Clients have the freedom to choose whether to enter into or remain in a counseling relationship and need adequate information about the counseling process and the counselor. Counselors have an obligation to review in writing and verbally with clients the rights and responsibilities of both the counselor and the client. Informed consent is an ongoing part of the counseling process, and counselors appropriately document discussions of informed consent throughout the counseling relationship.

A.2.b. Types of Information Needed

Counselors explicitly explain to clients the nature of all services provided. They inform clients about issues such as, but not limited to, the following: the purposes, goals, techniques, procedures, limitations, potential risks, and benefits of services; the counselor's qualifications, credentials, and relevant experience; continuation of services upon the incapacitation or death of a counselor; and other pertinent information. Counselors take steps to ensure that clients understand the implications of diagnosis, the intended use of tests and reports, fees, and billing arrangements. Clients have the right to confidentiality and to be provided with an explanation of its limitations (including how supervisors and/or treatment team professionals are involved); to obtain clear information about their records; to participate in the ongoing counseling plans; and to refuse any services or modality change and to be advised of the consequences of such refusal.

A.2.c. Developmental and Cultural Sensitivity

Counselors communicate information in ways that are both developmentally and culturally appropriate. Counselors use clear and understandable language when discussing issues related to informed consent. When clients have difficulty understanding the language used by counselors, they provide necessary services (e.g., arranging for a qualified interpreter or translator) to ensure comprehension by clients. In collaboration with clients, counselors consider cultural implications of informed consent procedures and, where possible, counselors adjust their practices accordingly.

A.2.d. Inability to Give Consent

When counseling minors or persons unable to give voluntary consent, counselors seek the assent of clients to services, and include them in decision making as appropriate. Counselors recognize the need to balance the ethical rights of clients to make choices, their capacity to give consent or assent to receive services, and parental or familial legal rights and responsibilities to protect these clients and make decisions on their behalf.

A.3. Clients Served by Others

When counselors learn that their clients are in a professional relationship with another mental health professional, they request release from clients to inform the other professionals and strive to establish positive and collaborative professional relationships.

A.4. Avoiding Harm and Imposing Values

A.4.a. Avoiding Harm

Counselors act to avoid harming their clients, trainees, and research participants and to minimize or to remedy unavoidable or unanticipated harm.

A.4.b. Personal Values

Counselors are aware of their own values, attitudes, beliefs, and behaviors and avoid imposing values that are inconsistent with counseling goals. Counselors respect the diversity of clients, trainees, and research participants.

A.5. ROLES AND RELATIONSHIPS WITH CLIENTS

(See F.3., F.10., G.3.)

A.5.a. Current Clients

Sexual or romantic counselor-client interactions or relationships with current clients, their romantic partners, or their family members are prohibited.

A.5.b. Former Clients

Sexual or romantic counselor-client interactions or relationships with former clients, their romantic partners, or their family members are prohibited for a period of 5 years following the last professional contact. Counselors, before engaging in sexual or romantic interactions or relationships with clients, their romantic partners, or client family members after 5 years following the last professional contact, demonstrate forethought and document (in written form) whether the interactions or relationship can be viewed as exploitive in some way and/or whether there is still potential to harm the former client; in cases of potential exploitation and/or harm, the counselor avoids entering such an interaction or relationship.

A.5.c. Nonprofessional Interactions or Relationships
(Other Than Sexual or Romantic Interactions or Relationships)

Counselor-client nonprofessional relationships with clients, former clients, their romantic partners, or their family members should be avoided, except when the interaction is potentially beneficial to the client. *(See A.5.d.)*

A.5.d. Potentially Beneficial Interactions

When a counselor-client nonprofessional interaction with a client or former client may be potentially beneficial to the client or former client, the counselor must document in case records, prior to the interaction (when feasible), the rationale for such an interaction, the potential benefit, and anticipated consequences for the client or former client and other individuals significantly involved with the client or former client. Such interactions should be initiated with appropriate client consent. Where unintentional harm occurs to the client or former client, or to an individual significantly involved with the client or former client, due to the nonprofessional interaction, the counselor must show evidence of an attempt to remedy such harm. Examples of potentially beneficial interactions include, but are not limited to, attending a formal ceremony (e.g., a wedding/commitment ceremony or graduation); purchasing a service or product provided by a client or former client (excepting unrestricted bartering); hospital visits to an ill family member; mutual membership in a professional association, organization, or community. *(See A.5.c.)*

A.5.e. Role Changes in the Professional Relationship

When a counselor changes a role from the original or most recent contracted relationship, he or she obtains informed consent from the client and explains the right of the client to refuse services related to the change. Examples of role changes include

1. changing from individual to relationship or family counseling, or vice versa;
2. changing from a nonforensic evaluative role to a therapeutic role, or vice versa;

3. changing from a counselor to a researcher role (i.e., enlisting clients as research participants), or vice versa; and
4. changing from a counselor to a mediator role, or vice versa.

Clients must be fully informed of any anticipated consequences (e.g., financial, legal, personal, or therapeutic) of counselor role changes.

A.6. ROLES AND RELATIONSHIPS AT INDIVIDUAL, GROUP, INSTITUTIONAL, AND SOCIETAL LEVELS

A.6.a. Advocacy

When appropriate, counselors advocate at individual, group, institutional, and societal levels to examine potential barriers and obstacles that inhibit access and/or the growth and development of clients.

A.6.b. Confidentiality and Advocacy

Counselors obtain client consent prior to engaging in advocacy efforts on behalf of an identifiable client to improve the provision of services and to work toward removal of systemic barriers or obstacles that inhibit client access, growth, and development.

A.7. MULTIPLE CLIENTS

When a counselor agrees to provide counseling services to two or more persons who have a relationship, the counselor clarifies at the outset which person or persons are clients and the nature of the relationships the counselor will have with each involved person. If it becomes apparent that the counselor may be called upon to perform potentially conflicting roles, the counselor will clarify, adjust, or withdraw from roles appropriately. *(See A.8.a., B.4.)*

A.8. GROUP WORK

(See B.4.a.)

A.8.a. Screening

Counselors screen prospective group counseling/therapy participants. To the extent possible, counselors select members whose needs and goals are compatible with goals of the group, who will not impede the group process, and whose well-being will not be jeopardized by the group experience.

A.8.b. Protecting Clients

In a group setting, counselors take reasonable precautions to protect clients from physical, emotional, or psychological trauma.

A.9. END-OF-LIFE CARE FOR TERMINALLY ILL CLIENTS

A.9.a. Quality of Care

Counselors strive to take measures that enable clients

1. to obtain high-quality end-of-life care for their physical, emotional, social, and spiritual needs;
2. to exercise the highest degree of self-determination possible;

3. to be given every opportunity possible to engage in informed decision making regarding their end-of-life care; and

4. to receive complete and adequate assessment regarding their ability to make competent, rational decisions on their own behalf from a mental health professional who is experienced in end-of-life care practice.

A.9.b. Counselor Competence, Choice, and Referral

Recognizing the personal, moral, and competence issues related to end-of-life decisions, counselors may choose to work or not work with terminally ill clients who wish to explore their end-of-life options. Counselors provide appropriate referral information to ensure that clients receive the necessary help.

A.9.c. Confidentiality

Counselors who provide services to terminally ill individuals who are considering hastening their own deaths have the option of breaking or not breaking confidentiality, depending on applicable laws and the specific circumstances of the situation and after seeking consultation or supervision from appropriate professional and legal parties. *(See B.5.c., B.7.c.)*

A.10. FEES AND BARTERING

A.10.a. Accepting Fees from Agency Clients

Counselors refuse a private fee or other remuneration for rendering services to persons who are entitled to such services through the counselor's employing agency or institution. The policies of a particular agency may make explicit provisions for agency clients to receive counseling services from members of its staff in private practice. In such instances, the clients must be informed of other options open to them should they seek private counseling services.

A.10.b. Establishing Fees

In establishing fees for professional counseling services, counselors consider the financial status of clients and locality. In the event that the established fee structure is inappropriate for a client, counselors assist clients in attempting to find comparable services of acceptable cost.

A.10.c. Nonpayment of Fees

If counselors intend to use collection agencies or take legal measures to collect fees from clients who do not pay for services as agreed upon, they first inform clients of intended actions and offer clients the opportunity to make payment.

A.10.d. Bartering

Counselors may barter only if the relationship is not exploitive or harmful and does not place the counselor in an unfair advantage, if the client requests it, and if such arrangements are an accepted practice among professionals in the community. Counselors consider the cultural implications of bartering and discuss relevant concerns with clients and document such agreements in a clear written contract.

A.10.e. Receiving Gifts

Counselors understand the challenges of accepting gifts from clients and recognize that in some cultures, small gifts are a token of respect and showing gratitude. When determining whether or not to accept a gift from clients, counselors take into account the therapeutic relationship, the monetary value of the gift, a client's motivation for giving the gift, and the counselor's motivation for wanting or declining the gift.

A.11. TERMINATION AND REFERRAL

A.11.a. Abandonment Prohibited

Counselors do not abandon or neglect clients in counseling. Counselors assist in making appropriate arrangements for the continuation of treatment, when necessary, during interruptions such as vacations, illness, and following termination.

A.11.b. Inability to Assist Clients

If counselors determine an inability to be of professional assistance to clients, they avoid entering or continuing counseling relationships. Counselors are knowledgeable about culturally and clinically appropriate referral resources and suggest these alternatives. If clients decline the suggested referrals, counselors should discontinue the relationship.

A.11.c. Appropriate Termination

Counselors terminate a counseling relationship when it becomes reasonably apparent that the client no longer needs assistance, is not likely to benefit, or is being harmed by continued counseling. Counselors may terminate counseling when in jeopardy of harm by the client, or another person with whom the client has a relationship, or when clients do not pay fees as agreed upon. Counselors provide pretermination counseling and recommend other service providers when necessary.

A.11.d. Appropriate Transfer of Services

When counselors transfer or refer clients to other practitioners, they ensure that appropriate clinical and administrative processes are completed and open communication is maintained with both clients and practitioners.

A.12. TECHNOLOGY APPLICATIONS

A.12.a. Benefits and Limitations

Counselors inform clients of the benefits and limitations of using information technology applications in the counseling process and in business/billing procedures. Such technologies include but are not limited to computer hardware and software, telephones, the World Wide Web, the Internet, online assessment instruments, and other communication devices.

A.12.b. Technology-Assisted Services

When providing technology-assisted distance counseling services, counselors determine that clients are intellectually, emotionally, and physically capable of using the application and that the application is appropriate for the needs of clients.

A.12.c. Inappropriate Services

When technology-assisted distance counseling services are deemed inappropriate by the counselor or client, counselors consider delivering services face to face.

A.12.d. Access

Counselors provide reasonable access to computer applications when providing technology-assisted distance counseling services.

A.12.e Laws and Statutes

Counselors ensure that the use of technology does not violate the laws of any local, state, national, or international entity and observe all relevant statutes.

A.12.f. Assistance

Counselors seek business, legal, and technical assistance when using technology applications, particularly when the use of such applications crosses state or national boundaries.

A.12.g. Technology and Informed Consent

As part of the process of establishing informed consent, counselors do the following:

1. Address issues related to the difficulty of maintaining the confidentiality of electronically transmitted communications.
2. Inform clients of all colleagues, supervisors, and employees, such as Informational Technology (IT) administrators, who might have authorized or unauthorized access to electronic transmissions.
3. Urge clients to be aware of all authorized or unauthorized users including family members and fellow employees who have access to any technology clients may use in the counseling process.
4. Inform clients of pertinent legal rights and limitations governing the practice of a profession over state lines or international boundaries.
5. Use encrypted Web sites and e-mail communications to help ensure confidentiality when possible.
6. When the use of encryption is not possible, counselors notify clients of this fact and limit electronic transmissions to general communications that are not client specific.
7. Inform clients if and for how long archival storage of transaction records are maintained.
8. Discuss the possibility of technology failure and alternate methods of service delivery.
9. Inform clients of emergency procedures, such as calling 911 or a local crisis hotline, when the counselor is not available.
10. Discuss time zone differences, local customs, and cultural or language differences that might impact service delivery.
11. Inform clients when technology-assisted distance counseling services are not covered by insurance. *(See A.2.)*

A.12.h. Sites on the World Wide Web

Counselors maintaining sites on the World Wide Web (the Internet) do the following:

1. Regularly check that electronic links are working and professionally appropriate.
2. Establish ways clients can contact the counselor in case of technology failure.
3. Provide electronic links to relevant state licensure and professional certification boards to protect consumer rights and facilitate addressing ethical concerns.
4. Establish a method for verifying client identity.
5. Obtain the written consent of the legal guardian or other authorized legal representative prior to rendering services in the event the client is a minor child, an adult who is legally incompetent, or an adult incapable of giving informed consent.
6. Strive to provide a site that is accessible to persons with disabilities.
7. Strive to provide translation capabilities for clients who have a different primary language while also addressing the imperfect nature of such translations.
8. Assist clients in determining the validity and reliability of information found on the World Wide Web and other technology applications.

SECTION B: CONFIDENTIALITY, PRIVILEGED COMMUNICATION, AND PRIVACY

INTRODUCTION

Counselors recognize that trust is a cornerstone of the counseling relationship. Counselors aspire to earn the trust of clients by creating an ongoing partnership, establishing and upholding appropriate boundaries, and maintaining confidentiality. Counselors communicate the parameters of confidentiality in a culturally competent manner.

B.1. RESPECTING CLIENT RIGHTS

B.1.a. Multicultural/Diversity Considerations

Counselors maintain awareness and sensitivity regarding cultural meanings of confidentiality and privacy. Counselors respect differing views toward disclosure of information. Counselors hold ongoing discussions with clients as to how, when, and with whom information is to be shared.

B.1.b. Respect for Privacy

Counselors respect client rights to privacy. Counselors solicit private information from clients only when it is beneficial to the counseling process.

B.1.c. Respect for Confidentiality

Counselors do not share confidential information without client consent or without sound legal or ethical justification.

B.1.d. Explanation of Limitations

At initiation and throughout the counseling process, counselors inform clients of the limitations of confidentiality and seek to identify foreseeable situations in which confidentiality must be breached. *(See A.2.b.)*

B.2. EXCEPTIONS

B.2.a. Danger and Legal Requirements

The general requirement that counselors keep information confidential does not apply when disclosure is required to protect clients or identified others from serious and foreseeable harm or when legal requirements demand that confidential information must be revealed. Counselors consult with other professionals when in doubt as to the validity of an exception. Additional considerations apply when addressing end-of-life issues. *(See A.9.c.)*

B.2.b. Contagious, Life-Threatening Diseases

When clients disclose that they have a disease commonly known to be both communicable and life threatening, counselors may be justified in disclosing information to identifiable third parties, if they are known to be at demonstrable and high risk of contracting the disease. Prior to making a disclosure, counselors confirm that there is such a diagnosis and assess the intent of clients to inform the third parties about their disease or to engage in any behaviors that may be harmful to an identifiable third party.

B.2.c. Court-Ordered Disclosure

When subpoenaed to release confidential or privileged information without a client's permission, counselors obtain written, informed consent from the client or take steps to prohibit the disclosure or have it limited as narrowly as possible due to potential harm to the client or counseling relationship.

B.2.d. Minimal Disclosure

To the extent possible, clients are informed before confidential information is disclosed and are involved in the disclosure decision-making process. When circumstances require the disclosure of confidential information, only essential information is revealed.

B.3. INFORMATION SHARED WITH OTHERS

B.3.a. Subordinates

Counselors make every effort to ensure that privacy and confidentiality of clients are maintained by subordinates, including employees, supervisees, students, clerical assistants, and volunteers. *(See F.1.c.)*

B.3.b. Treatment Teams

When client treatment involves a continued review or participation by a treatment team, the client will be informed of the team's existence and composition, information being shared, and the purposes of sharing such information.

B.3.c. Confidential Settings

Counselors discuss confidential information only in settings in which they can reasonably ensure client privacy.

B.3.d. Third-Party Payers

Counselors disclose information to third-party payers only when clients have authorized such disclosure.

B.3.e Transmitting Confidential Information

Counselors take precautions to ensure the confidentiality of information transmitted through the use of computers, electronic mail, facsimile machines, telephones, voicemail, answering machines, and other electronic or computer technology. *(See A.12.g.)*

B.3.f. Deceased Clients

Counselors protect the confidentiality of deceased clients, consistent with legal requirements and agency or setting policies.

B.4. GROUPS AND FAMILIES

B.4.a. Group Work

In group work, counselors clearly explain the importance and parameters of confidentiality for the specific group being entered.

B.4.b. Couples and Family Counseling

In couples and family counseling, counselors clearly define who is considered "the client" and discuss expectations and limitations of confidentiality. Counselors seek agreement and document in writing such agreement among all involved parties having capacity to give consent concerning each individual's right to confidentiality and any obligation to preserve the confidentiality of information known.

B.5. CLIENTS LACKING CAPACITY TO GIVE INFORMED CONSENT

B.5.a. Responsibility to Clients

When counseling minor clients or adult clients who lack the capacity to give voluntary, informed consent, counselors protect the confidentiality of information received in the counseling relationship as specified by federal and state laws, written policies, and applicable ethical standards.

B.5.b. Responsibility to Parents and Legal Guardians

Counselors inform parents and legal guardians about the role of counselors and the confidential nature of the counseling relationship. Counselors are sensitive to the cultural diversity of families and respect the inherent rights and responsibilities of parents/guardians over the welfare of their children/charges according to law. Counselors work to establish, as appropriate, collaborative relationships with parents/guardians to best serve clients.

B.5.c. Release of Confidential Information

When counseling minor clients or adult clients who lack the capacity to give voluntary consent to release confidential information, counselors seek permission from an appropriate third party to disclose information. In such instances, counselors inform clients consistent with their level of understanding and take culturally appropriate measures to safeguard client confidentiality.

B.6. RECORDS

B.6.a. Confidentiality of Records

Counselors ensure that records are kept in a secure location and that only authorized persons have access to records.

B.6.b. Permission to Record

Counselors obtain permission from clients prior to recording sessions through electronic or other means.

B.6.c. Permission to Observe

Counselors obtain permission from clients prior to observing counseling sessions, reviewing session transcripts, or viewing recordings of sessions with supervisors, faculty, peers, or others within the training environment.

B.6.d. Client Access

Counselors provide reasonable access to records and copies of records when requested by competent clients. Counselors limit the access of clients to their records, or portions of their records, only when there is compelling evidence that such access would cause harm to the client. Counselors document the request of clients and the rationale for withholding some or all of the record in the files of clients. In situations involving multiple clients, counselors provide individual clients with only those parts of records that related directly to them and do not include confidential information related to any other client.

B.6.e. Assistance with Records

When clients request access to their records, counselors provide assistance and consultation in interpreting counseling records.

B.6.f. Disclosure or Transfer

Unless exceptions to confidentiality exist, counselors obtain written permission from clients to disclose or transfer records to legitimate third parties. Steps are taken to ensure that receivers of counseling records are sensitive to their confidential nature. (See A.3., E.4.)

B.6.g. Storage and Disposal after Termination

Counselors store records following termination of services to ensure reasonable future access, maintain records in accordance with state and federal statutes governing records, and dispose of client records and other sensitive materials in a manner that protects client confidentiality. When records are of an artistic nature, counselors obtain client (or guardian) consent with regard to handling of such records or documents. *(See A.1.b.)*

B.6.h. Reasonable Precautions

Counselors take reasonable precautions to protect client confidentiality in the event of the counselor's termination of practice, incapacity, or death. *(See C.2.h.)*

B.7. RESEARCH AND TRAINING

B.7.a. Institutional Approval

When institutional approval is required, counselors provide accurate information about their research proposals and obtain approval prior to conducting their research. They conduct research in accordance with the approved research protocol.

B.7.b. Adherence to Guidelines

Counselors are responsible for understanding and adhering to state, federal, agency, or institutional policies or applicable guidelines regarding confidentiality in their research practices.

B.7.c. Confidentiality of Information Obtained in Research

Violations of participant privacy and confidentiality are risks of participation in research involving human participants. Investigators maintain all research records in a secure manner. They explain to participants the risks of violations of privacy and confidentiality and disclose to participants any limits of confidentiality that reasonably can be expected. Regardless of the degree to which confidentiality will be maintained, investigators must disclose to participants any limits of confidentiality that reasonably can be expected. *(See G.2.e.)*

B.7.d. Disclosure of Research Information

Counselors do not disclose confidential information that reasonably could lead to the identification of a research participant unless they have obtained the prior consent of the person. Use of data derived from counseling relationships for purposes of training, research, or publication is confined to content that is disguised to ensure the anonymity of the individuals involved. *(See G.2.a., G.2.d.)*

B.7.e Agreement for Identification

Identification of clients, students, or supervisees in a presentation or publication is permissible only when they have reviewed the material and agreed to its presentation or publication. *(See G.4.d.)*

B.8. CONSULTATION

B.8.a. Agreements

When acting as consultants, counselors seek agreements among all parties involved concerning each individual's rights to confidentiality, the obligation of each individual to preserve confidential information, and the limits of confidentiality of information shared by others.

B.8.b. Respect for Privacy

Information obtained in a consulting relationship is discussed for professional purposes only with persons directly involved with the case. Written and oral reports present only data germane to the purposes of the consultation, and every effort is made to protect client identity and to avoid undue invasion of privacy.

B.8.c. Disclosure of Confidential Information

When consulting with colleagues, counselors do not disclose confidential information that reasonably could lead to the identification of a client or other person or organization with whom they have a confidential relationship unless they have obtained the prior consent of the person or organization or the disclosure cannot be avoided. They disclose information only to the extent necessary to achieve the purposes of the consultation. *(See D.2.d.)*

SECTION C: PROFESSIONAL RESPONSIBILITY

INTRODUCTION

Counselors aspire to open, honest, and accurate communication in dealing with the public and other professionals. They practice in a nondiscriminatory manner within the boundaries of professional and personal competence and have a responsibility to abide by the *ACA Code of Ethics*. Counselors actively participate in local, state, and national associations that foster the development and improvement of counseling. Counselors advocate to promote change at the individual, group, institutional, and societal levels that improves the quality of life for individuals and groups and remove potential barriers to the provision or access of appropriate services being offered. Counselors have a responsibility to the public to engage in counseling practices that are based on rigorous research methodologies. In addition, counselors engage in self-care activities to maintain and promote their emotional, physical, mental, and spiritual well-being to best meet their professional responsibilities.

C.1. KNOWLEDGE OF STANDARDS

Counselors have a responsibility to read, understand, and follow the *ACA Code of Ethics* and adhere to applicable laws and regulations.

C.2. PROFESSIONAL COMPETENCE

C.2.a. Boundaries of Competence

Counselors practice only within the boundaries of their competence, based on their education, training, supervised experience, state and national professional credentials, and appropriate professional experience. Counselors gain knowledge, personal awareness, sensitivity, and skills pertinent to working with a diverse client population. *(See A.9.b., C.4.e., E.2., F.2., F.11.b.)*

C.2.b. New Specialty Areas of Practice

Counselors practice in specialty areas new to them only after appropriate education, training, and supervised experience. While developing skills in new specialty areas, counselors take steps to ensure the competence of their work and to protect others from possible harm. *(See F.6.f.)*

C.2.c. Qualified for Employment

Counselors accept employment only for positions for which they are qualified by education, training, supervised experience, state and national professional credentials, and appropriate professional experience. Counselors hire for professional counseling positions only individuals who are qualified and competent for those positions.

C.2.d. Monitor Effectiveness

Counselors continually monitor their effectiveness as professionals and take steps to improve when necessary. Counselors in private practice take reasonable steps to seek peer supervision as needed to evaluate their efficacy as counselors.

C.2.e. Consultation on Ethical Obligations

Counselors take reasonable steps to consult with other counselors or related professionals when they have questions regarding their ethical obligations or professional practice.

C.2.f. Continuing Education

Counselors recognize the need for continuing education to acquire and maintain a reasonable level of awareness of current scientific and professional information in their fields of activity. They take steps to maintain competence in the skills they use, are open to new procedures, and keep current with the diverse populations and specific populations with whom they work.

C.2.g. Impairment

Counselors are alert to the signs of impairment from their own physical, mental, or emotional problems and refrain from offering or providing professional services when such impairment is likely to harm a client or others. They seek assistance for problems that reach the level of professional impairment, and, if necessary, they limit, suspend, or terminate their professional responsibilities until such time it is determined that they may safely resume their work. Counselors assist colleagues or supervisors in recognizing their own professional impairment and provide consultation and assistance when warranted with colleagues or supervisors showing signs of impairment and intervene as appropriate to prevent imminent harm to clients. *(See A.11.b., F.8.b.)*

C.2.h. Counselor Incapacitation or Termination of Practice

When counselors leave a practice, they follow a prepared plan for transfer of clients and files. Counselors prepare and disseminate to an identified colleague or "records custodian" a plan for the transfer of clients and files in the case of their incapacitation, death, or termination of practice.

C.3. ADVERTISING AND SOLICITING CLIENTS

C.3.a. Accurate Advertising

When advertising or otherwise representing their services to the public, counselors identify their credentials in an accurate manner that is not false, misleading, deceptive, or fraudulent.

C.3.b. Testimonials

Counselors who use testimonials do not solicit them from current clients nor former clients nor any other persons who may be vulnerable to undue influence.

C.3.c. Statements by Others

Counselors make reasonable efforts to ensure that statements made by others about them or the profession of counseling are accurate.

C.3.d. Recruiting through Employment

Counselors do not use their places of employment or institutional affiliation to recruit or gain clients, supervisees, or consultees for their private practices.

C.3.e. Products and Training Advertisements

Counselors who develop products related to their profession or conduct workshops or training events ensure that the advertisements concerning these products or events are accurate and disclose adequate information for consumers to make informed choices. (See C.6.d.)

C.3.f. Promoting to Those Served

Counselors do not use counseling, teaching, training, or supervisory relationships to promote their products or training events in a manner that is deceptive or would exert undue influence on individuals who may be vulnerable. However, counselor educators may adopt textbooks they have authored for instructional purposes.

C.4. PROFESSIONAL QUALIFICATIONS

C.4.a. Accurate Representation

Counselors claim or imply only professional qualifications actually completed and correct any known misrepresentations of their qualifications by others. Counselors truthfully represent the qualifications of their professional colleagues. Counselors clearly distinguish between paid and volunteer work experience and accurately describe their continuing education and specialized training. (See C.2.a.)

C.4.b. Credentials

Counselors claim only licenses or certifications that are current and in good standing.

C.4.c. Educational Degrees

Counselors clearly differentiate between earned and honorary degrees.

C.4.d. Implying Doctoral-Level Competence

Counselors clearly state their highest earned degree in counseling or closely related field. Counselors do not imply doctoral-level competence when only possessing a master's degree in counseling or a related field by referring to themselves as "Dr." in a counseling context when their doctorate is not in counseling or a related field.

C.4.e Program Accreditation Status

Counselors clearly state the accreditation status of their degree programs at the time the degree was earned.

C.4.f. Professional Membership

Counselors clearly differentiate between current, active memberships and former memberships in associations. Members of the American Counseling Association must clearly differentiate between professional membership, which implies the possession of at least a master's degree in counseling, and regular membership, which is open to individuals whose interests and activities are consistent with those of ACA but are not qualified for professional membership.

C.5. NONDISCRIMINATION

Counselors do not condone or engage in discrimination based on age, culture, disability, ethnicity, race, religion/spirituality, gender, gender identity, sexual orientation, marital status/partnership, language preference, socioeconomic status, or any basis proscribed by law. Counselors do not discriminate against clients, students, employees, supervisees, or research participants in a manner that has a negative impact on these persons.

C.6. PUBLIC RESPONSIBILITY

C.6.a. Sexual Harassment

Counselors do not engage in or condone sexual harassment. Sexual harassment is defined as sexual solicitation, physical advances, or verbal or nonverbal conduct that is sexual in nature, that occurs in connection with professional activities or roles, and that either

1. is unwelcome, is offensive, or creates a hostile workplace or learning environment, and counselors know or are told this; or
2. is sufficiently severe or intense to be perceived as harassment to a reasonable person in the context in which the behavior occurred.

Sexual harassment can consist of a single intense or severe act or multiple persistent or pervasive acts.

C.6.b. Reports to Third Parties

Counselors are accurate, honest, and objective in reporting their professional activities and judgments to appropriate third parties, including courts, health insurance companies, those who are the recipients of evaluation reports, and others. *(See B.3., E.4.)*

C.6.c. Media Presentations

When counselors provide advice or comment by means of public lectures, demonstrations, radio or television programs, prerecorded tapes, technology-based applications, printed articles, mailed material, or other media, they take reasonable precautions to ensure that

1. the statements are based on appropriate professional counseling literature and practice,
2. the statements are otherwise consistent with the *ACA Code of Ethics*, and
3. the recipients of the information are not encouraged to infer that a professional counseling relationship has been established.

C.6.d. Exploitation of Others
Counselors do not exploit others in their professional relationships. *(See C.3.e.)*

C.6.e. Scientific Bases for Treatment Modalities
Counselors use techniques/procedures/modalities that are grounded in theory and/or have an empirical or scientific foundation. Counselors who do not must define the techniques/procedures as "unproven" or "developing" and explain the potential risks and ethical considerations of using such techniques/procedures and take steps to protect clients from possible harm. *(See A.4.a., E.5.c., E.5.d.)*

C.7. Responsibility to Other Professionals

C.7.a. Personal Public Statements
When making personal statements in a public context, counselors clarify that they are speaking from their personal perspectives and that they are not speaking on behalf of all counselors or the profession.

SECTION D: RELATIONSHIPS WITH OTHER PROFESSIONALS

Introduction

Professional counselors recognize that the quality of their interactions with colleagues can influence the quality of services provided to clients. They work to become knowledgeable about colleagues within and outside the field of counseling. Counselors develop positive working relationships and systems of communication with colleagues to enhance services to clients.

D.1. Relationships with Colleagues, Employers, and Employees

D.1.a. Different Approaches
Counselors are respectful of approaches to counseling services that differ from their own. Counselors are respectful of traditions and practices of other professional groups with which they work.

D.1.b. Forming Relationships
Counselors work to develop and strengthen interdisciplinary relations with colleagues from other disciplines to best serve clients.

D.1.c. Interdisciplinary Teamwork

Counselors who are members of interdisciplinary teams delivering multifaceted services to clients keep the focus on how to best serve the clients.

They participate in and contribute to decisions that affect the well-being of clients by drawing on the perspectives, values, and experiences of the counseling profession and those of colleagues from other disciplines. *(See A.1.a.)*

D.1.d. Confidentiality

When counselors are required by law, institutional policy, or extraordinary circumstances to serve in more than one role in judicial or administrative proceedings, they clarify role expectations and the parameters of confidentiality with their colleagues. *(See B.1.c., B.1.d., B.2.c., B.2.d., B.3.b.)*

D.1.e. Establishing Professional and Ethical Obligations

Counselors who are members of interdisciplinary teams clarify professional and ethical obligations of the team as a whole and of its individual members. When a team decision raises ethical concerns, counselors first attempt to resolve the concern within the team. If they cannot reach resolution among team members, counselors pursue other avenues to address their concerns consistent with client well-being.

D.1.f. Personnel Selection and Assignment

Counselors select competent staff and assign responsibilities compatible with their skills and experiences.

D.1.g. Employer Policies

The acceptance of employment in an agency or institution implies that counselors are in agreement with its general policies and principles. Counselors strive to reach agreement with employers as to acceptable standards of conduct that allow for changes in institutional policy conducive to the growth and development of clients.

D.1.h. Negative Conditions

Counselors alert their employers of inappropriate policies and practices. They attempt to effect changes in such policies or procedures through constructive action within the organization. When such policies are potentially disruptive or damaging to clients or may limit the effectiveness of services provided and change cannot be effected, counselors take appropriate further action. Such action may include referral to appropriate certification, accreditation, or state licensure organizations, or voluntary termination of employment.

D.1.i. Protection from Punitive Action

Counselors take care not to harass or dismiss an employee who has acted in a responsible and ethical manner to expose inappropriate employer policies or practices.

D.2. Consultation

D.2.a. Consultant Competency

Counselors take reasonable steps to ensure that they have the appropriate resources and competencies when providing consultation services. Counselors provide appropriate referral resources when requested or needed. *(See C.2.b.)*

D.2.b. Understanding Consultees

When providing consultation, counselors attempt to develop with their consultees a clear understanding of problem definition, goals for change, and predicted consequences of interventions selected.

D.2.c. Consultant Goals

The consulting relationship is one in which consultee adaptability and growth toward self-direction are consistently encouraged and cultivated.

D.2.d. Informed Consent in Consultation

When providing consultation, counselors have an obligation to review, in writing and verbally, the rights and responsibilities of both counselors and consultees. Counselors use clear and understandable language to inform all parties involved about the purpose of the services to be provided, relevant costs, potential risks and benefits, and the limits of confidentiality. Working in conjunction with the consultee, counselors attempt to develop a clear definition of the problem, goals for change, and predicted consequences of interventions that are culturally responsive and appropriate to the needs of consultees. *(See A.2.a., A.2.b.)*

SECTION E: EVALUATION, ASSESSMENT, AND INTERPRETATION

Introduction

Counselors use assessment instruments as one component of the counseling process, taking into account the client personal and cultural context. Counselors promote the well-being of individual clients or groups of clients by developing and using appropriate educational, psychological, and career assessment instruments.

E.1. General

E.1.a. Assessment

The primary purpose of educational, psychological, and career assessment is to provide measurements that are valid and reliable in either comparative or absolute terms. These include, but are not limited to, measurements of ability, personality, interest, intelligence, achievement, and performance. Counselors recognize the need to interpret the statements in this section as applying to both quantitative and qualitative assessments.

E.1.b. Client Welfare

Counselors do not misuse assessment results and interpretations, and they take reasonable steps to prevent others from misusing the information these techniques provide. They respect the client's right to know the results, the interpretations made, and the bases for counselors' conclusions and recommendations.

E.2. COMPETENCE TO USE AND INTERPRET ASSESSMENT INSTRUMENTS

E.2.a. Limits of Competence

Counselors utilize only those testing and assessment services for which they have been trained and are competent. Counselors using technology-assisted test interpretations are trained in the construct being measured and the specific instrument being used prior to using its technology-based application. Counselors take reasonable measures to ensure the proper use of psychological and career assessment techniques by persons under their supervision. *(See A.12.)*

E.2.b. Appropriate Use

Counselors are responsible for the appropriate application, scoring, interpretation, and use of assessment instruments relevant to the needs of the client, whether they score and interpret such assessments themselves or use technology or other services.

E.2.c. Decisions Based on Results

Counselors responsible for decisions involving individuals or policies that are based on assessment results have a thorough understanding of educational, psychological, and career measurement, including validation criteria, assessment research, and guidelines for assessment development and use.

E.3. INFORMED CONSENT IN ASSESSMENT

E.3.a. Explanation to Clients

Prior to assessment, counselors explain the nature and purposes of assessment and the specific use of results by potential recipients. The explanation will be given in the language of the client (or other legally authorized person on behalf of the client), unless an explicit exception has been agreed upon in advance. Counselors consider the client's personal or cultural context, the level of the client's understanding of the results, and the impact of the results on the client. *(See A.2., A.12.g., F.1.c.)*

E.3.b. Recipients of Results

Counselors consider the examinee's welfare, explicit understandings, and prior agreements in determining who receives the assessment results. Counselors include accurate and appropriate interpretations with any release of individual or group assessment results. *(See B.2.c., B.5.)*

E.4. RELEASE OF DATA TO QUALIFIED PROFESSIONALS

Counselors release assessment data in which the client is identified only with the consent of the client or the client's legal representative. Such data are released only to persons recognized by counselors as qualified to interpret the data. *(See B.1., B.3., B.6.b.)*

E.5. Diagnosis of Mental Disorders

E.5.a. Proper Diagnosis

Counselors take special care to provide proper diagnosis of mental disorders. Assessment techniques (including personal interview) used to determine client care (e.g., locus of treatment, type of treatment, or recommended follow-up) are carefully selected and appropriately used.

E.5.b. Cultural Sensitivity

Counselors recognize that culture affects the manner in which clients' problems are defined. Clients' socioeconomic and cultural experiences are considered when diagnosing mental disorders. *(See A.2.c.)*

E.5.c. Historical and Social Prejudices in the Diagnosis of Pathology

Counselors recognize historical and social prejudices in the misdiagnosis and pathologizing of certain individuals and groups and the role of mental health professionals in perpetuating these prejudices through diagnosis and treatment.

E.5.d. Refraining from Diagnosis

Counselors may refrain from making and/or reporting a diagnosis if they believe it would cause harm to the client or others.

E.6. Instrument Selection

E.6.a. Appropriateness of Instruments

Counselors carefully consider the validity, reliability, psychometric limitations, and appropriateness of instruments when selecting assessments.

E.6.b. Referral Information

If a client is referred to a third party for assessment, the counselor provides specific referral questions and sufficient objective data about the client to ensure that appropriate assessment instruments are utilized. *(See A.9.b., B.3.)*

E.6.c. Culturally Diverse Populations

Counselors are cautious when selecting assessments for culturally diverse populations to avoid the use of instruments that lack appropriate psychometric properties for the client population. *(See A.2.c., E.5.b.)*

E.7. Conditions of Assessment Administration

(See A.12.b., A.12.d.)

E.7.a. Administration Conditions

Counselors administer assessments under the same conditions that were established in their standardization. When assessments are not administered under standard conditions, as may be necessary to accommodate clients with disabilities, or when unusual behavior or irregularities occur during the administration, those conditions are noted in interpretation, and the results may be designated as invalid or of questionable validity.

E.7.b. Technological Administration

Counselors ensure that administration programs function properly and provide clients with accurate results when technological or other electronic methods are used for assessment administration.

E.7.c. Unsupervised Assessments

Unless the assessment instrument is designed, intended, and validated for self-administration and/or scoring, counselors do not permit inadequately supervised use.

E.7.d. Disclosure of Favorable Conditions

Prior to administration of assessments, conditions that produce most favorable assessment results are made known to the examinee.

E.8. MULTICULTURAL ISSUES/DIVERSITY IN ASSESSMENT

Counselors use with caution assessment techniques that were normed on populations other than that of the client. Counselors recognize the effects of age, color, culture, disability, ethnic group, gender, race, language preference, religion, spirituality, sexual orientation, and socioeconomic status on test administration and interpretation, and place test results in proper perspective with other relevant factors. *(See A.2.c., E.5.b.)*

E.9. SCORING AND INTERPRETATION OF ASSESSMENTS

E.9.a. Reporting

In reporting assessment results, counselors indicate reservations that exist regarding validity or reliability due to circumstances of the assessment or the inappropriateness of the norms for the person tested.

E.9.b. Research Instruments

Counselors exercise caution when interpreting the results of research instruments not having sufficient technical data to support respondent results. The specific purposes for the use of such instruments are stated explicitly to the examinee.

E.9.c. Assessment Services

Counselors who provide assessment scoring and interpretation services to support the assessment process confirm the validity of such interpretations. They accurately describe the purpose, norms, validity, reliability, and applications of the procedures and any special qualifications applicable to their use. The public offering of an automated test interpretations service is considered a professional-to-professional consultation. The formal responsibility of the consultant is to the consultee, but the ultimate and overriding responsibility is to the client. *(See D.2.)*

E.10. ASSESSMENT SECURITY

Counselors maintain the integrity and security of tests and other assessment techniques consistent with legal and contractual obligations. Counselors do not appropriate, reproduce, or modify published assessments or parts thereof without acknowledgment and permission from the publisher.

E.11. OBSOLETE ASSESSMENTS AND OUTDATED RESULTS

Counselors do not use data or results from assessments that are obsolete or outdated for the current purpose. Counselors make every effort to prevent the misuse of obsolete measures and assessment data by others.

E.12. ASSESSMENT CONSTRUCTION

Counselors use established scientific procedures, relevant standards, and current professional knowledge for assessment design in the development, publication, and utilization of educational and psychological assessment techniques.

E.13. FORENSIC EVALUATION: EVALUATION FOR LEGAL PROCEEDINGS

E.13.a. Primary Obligations

When providing forensic evaluations, the primary obligation of counselors is to produce objective findings that can be substantiated based on information and techniques appropriate to the evaluation, which may include examination of the individual and/or review of records. Counselors are entitled to form professional opinions based on their professional knowledge and expertise that can be supported by the data gathered in evaluations. Counselors will define the limits of their reports or testimony, especially when an examination of the individual has not been conducted.

E.13.b. Consent for Evaluation

Individuals being evaluated are informed in writing that the relationship is for the purposes of an evaluation and is not counseling in nature, and entities or individuals who will receive the evaluation report are identified. Written consent to be evaluated is obtained from those being evaluated unless a court orders evaluations to be conducted without the written consent of individuals being evaluated. When children or vulnerable adults are being evaluated, informed written consent is obtained from a parent or guardian.

E.13.c. Client Evaluation Prohibited

Counselors do not evaluate individuals for forensic purposes they currently counsel or individuals they have counseled in the past. Counselors do not accept as counseling clients individuals they are evaluating or individuals they have evaluated in the past for forensic purposes.

E.13.d. Avoid Potentially Harmful Relationships

Counselors who provide forensic evaluations avoid potentially harmful professional or personal relationships with family members, romantic partners, and close friends of individuals they are evaluating or have evaluated in the past.

SECTION F: SUPERVISION, TRAINING, AND TEACHING

INTRODUCTION

Counselors aspire to foster meaningful and respectful professional relationships and to maintain appropriate boundaries with supervisees and students. Counselors have theoretical and pedagogical foundations for their work and aim to be fair, accurate, and honest in their assessments of counselors-in-training.

F.1. COUNSELOR SUPERVISION AND CLIENT WELFARE

F.1.a. Client Welfare
A primary obligation of counseling supervisors is to monitor the services provided by other counselors or counselors-in-training. Counseling supervisors monitor client welfare and supervisee clinical performance and professional development. To fulfill these obligations, supervisors meet regularly with supervisees to review case notes, samples of clinical work, or live observations. Supervisees have a responsibility to understand and follow the *ACA Code of Ethics*.

F.1.b. Counselor Credentials
Counseling supervisors work to ensure that clients are aware of the qualifications of the supervisees who render services to the clients. *(See A.2.b.)*

F.1.c. Informed Consent and Client Rights
Supervisors make supervisees aware of client rights including the protection of client privacy and confidentiality in the counseling relationship. Supervisees provide clients with professional disclosure information and inform them of how the supervision process influences the limits of confidentiality. Supervisees make clients aware of who will have access to records of the counseling relationship and how these records will be used. *(See A.2.b., B.1.d.)*

F.2. COUNSELOR SUPERVISION COMPETENCE

F.2.a. Supervisor Preparation
Prior to offering clinical supervision services, counselors are trained in supervision methods and techniques. Counselors who offer clinical supervision services regularly pursue continuing education activities including both counseling and supervision topics and skills. *(See C.2.a., C.2.f.)*

F.2.b. Multicultural Issues/Diversity in Supervision
Counseling supervisors are aware of and address the role of multiculturalism/diversity in the supervisory relationship.

F.3. SUPERVISORY RELATIONSHIPS

F.3.a. Relationship Boundaries with Supervisees
Counseling supervisors clearly define and maintain ethical professional, personal, and social relationships with their supervisees. Counseling supervisors avoid nonprofessional relationships with current supervisees. If supervisors must assume other professional roles (e.g., clinical and administrative supervisor, instructor) with supervisees, they work to minimize potential conflicts and explain to supervisees the expectations and responsibilities associated with each role. They do not engage in any form of nonprofessional interaction that may compromise the supervisory relationship.

F.3.b. Sexual Relationships

Sexual or romantic interactions or relationships with current supervisees are prohibited.

F.3.c. Sexual Harassment

Counseling supervisors do not condone or subject supervisees to sexual harassment. *(See C.6.a.)*

F.3.d. Close Relatives and Friends

Counseling supervisors avoid accepting close relatives, romantic partners, or friends as supervisees.

F.3.e. Potentially Beneficial Relationships

Counseling supervisors are aware of the power differential in their relationships with supervisees. If they believe nonprofessional relationships with a supervisee may be potentially beneficial to the supervisee, they take precautions similar to those taken by counselors when working with clients. Examples of potentially beneficial interactions or relationships include attending a formal ceremony; hospital visits; providing support during a stressful event; or mutual membership in a professional association, organization, or community. Counseling supervisors engage in open discussions with supervisees when they consider entering into relationships with them outside of their roles as clinical and/or administrative supervisors. Before engaging in nonprofessional relationships, supervisors discuss with supervisees and document the rationale for such interactions, potential benefits or drawbacks, and anticipated consequences for the supervisee. Supervisors clarify the specific nature and limitations of the additional role(s) they will have with the supervisee.

F.4. SUPERVISOR RESPONSIBILITIES

F.4.a. Informed Consent for Supervision

Supervisors are responsible for incorporating into their supervision the principles of informed consent and participation. Supervisors inform supervisees of the policies and procedures to which they are to adhere and the mechanisms for due process appeal of individual supervisory actions.

F.4.b. Emergencies and Absences

Supervisors establish and communicate to supervisees procedures for contacting them or, in their absence, alternative on-call supervisors to assist in handling crises.

F.4.c. Standards for Supervisees

Supervisors make their supervisees aware of professional and ethical standards and legal responsibilities. Supervisors of postdegree counselors encourage these counselors to adhere to professional standards of practice. *(See C.1.)*

F.4.d. Termination of the Supervisory Relationship

Supervisors or supervisees have the right to terminate the supervisory relationship with adequate notice. Reasons for withdrawal are provided to the other party. When cultural, clinical, or professional issues are crucial to the viability of the supervisory relationship, both parties make efforts to resolve differences. When termination is warranted, supervisors make appropriate referrals to possible alternative supervisors.

F.5. COUNSELING SUPERVISION EVALUATION, REMEDIATION, AND ENDORSEMENT

F.5.a. Evaluation

Supervisors document and provide supervisees with ongoing performance appraisal and evaluation feedback and schedule periodic formal evaluative sessions throughout the supervisory relationship.

F.5.b. Limitations

Through ongoing evaluation and appraisal, supervisors are aware of the limitations of supervisees that might impede performance. Supervisors assist supervisees in securing remedial assistance when needed. They recommend dismissal from training programs, applied counseling settings, or state or voluntary professional credentialing processes when those supervisees are unable to provide competent professional services. Supervisors seek consultation and document their decisions to dismiss or refer supervisees for assistance. They ensure that supervisees are aware of options available to them to address such decisions. *(See C.2.g.)*

F.5.c. Counseling for Supervisees

If supervisees request counseling, supervisors provide them with acceptable referrals. Counselors do not provide counseling services to supervisees. Supervisors address interpersonal competencies in terms of the impact of these issues on clients, the supervisory relationship, and professional functioning. *(See F.3.a.)*

F.5.d. Endorsement

Supervisors endorse supervisees for certification, licensure, employment, or completion of an academic or training program only when they believe supervisees are qualified for the endorsement. Regardless of qualifications, supervisors do not endorse supervisees whom they believe to be impaired in any way that would interfere with the performance of the duties associated with the endorsement.

F.6. RESPONSIBILITIES OF COUNSELOR EDUCATORS

F.6.a. Counselor Educators

Counselor educators who are responsible for developing, implementing, and supervising educational programs are skilled as teachers and practitioners. They are knowledgeable regarding the ethical, legal, and regulatory aspects of the profession, are skilled in applying that knowledge, and make students and supervisees aware of their responsibilities. Counselor educators conduct counselor education and training programs in an ethical manner and serve as role models for professional behavior. *(See C.1., C.2.a., C.2.c.)*

F.6.b. Infusing Multicultural Issues/Diversity

Counselor educators infuse material related to multiculturalism/diversity into all courses and workshops for the development of professional counselors.

F.6.c. Integration of Study and Practice

Counselor educators establish education and training programs that integrate academic study and supervised practice.

F.6.d. Teaching Ethics

Counselor educators make students and supervisees aware of the ethical responsibilities and standards of the profession and the ethical responsibilities of students to the profession. Counselor educators infuse ethical considerations throughout the curriculum. *(See C.1.)*

F.6.e. Peer Relationships

Counselor educators make every effort to ensure that the rights of peers are not compromised when students or supervisees lead counseling groups or provide clinical supervision. Counselor educators take steps to ensure that students and supervisees understand they have the same ethical obligations as counselor educators, trainers, and supervisors.

F.6.f. Innovative Theories and Techniques

When counselor educators teach counseling techniques/procedures that are innovative, without an empirical foundation, or without a well-grounded theoretical foundation, they define the counseling techniques/procedures as "unproven" or "developing" and explain to students the potential risks and ethical considerations of using such techniques/procedures.

F.6.g. Field Placements

Counselor educators develop clear policies within their training programs regarding field placement and other clinical experiences. Counselor educators provide clearly stated roles and responsibilities for the student or supervisee, the site supervisor, and the program supervisor. They confirm that site supervisors are qualified to provide supervision and inform site supervisors of their professional and ethical responsibilities in this role.

F.6.h. Professional Disclosure

Before initiating counseling services, counselors-in-training disclose their status as students and explain how this status affects the limits of confidentiality. Counselor educators ensure that the clients at field placements are aware of the services rendered and the qualifications of the students and supervisees rendering those services. Students and supervisees obtain client permission before they use any information concerning the counseling relationship in the training process. *(See A.2.b.)*

F.7. STUDENT WELFARE

F.7.a. Orientation

Counselor educators recognize that orientation is a developmental process that continues throughout the educational and clinical training of students. Counseling faculty provide prospective students with information about the counselor education program's expectations:

1. the type and level of skill and knowledge acquisition required for successful completion of the training;

2. program training goals, objectives, and mission, and subject matter to be covered;
3. bases for evaluation;
4. training components that encourage self-growth or self-disclosure as part of the training process;
5. the type of supervision settings and requirements of the sites for required clinical field experiences;
6. student and supervisee evaluation and dismissal policies and procedures; and
7. up-to-date employment prospects for graduates.

F.7.b. Self-Growth Experiences

Counselor education programs delineate requirements for self-disclosure or self-growth experiences in their admission and program materials. Counselor educators use professional judgment when designing training experiences they conduct that require student and supervisee self-growth or self-disclosure. Students and supervisees are made aware of the ramifications their self-disclosure may have when counselors whose primary role as teacher, trainer, or supervisor requires acting on ethical obligations to the profession. Evaluative components of experiential training experiences explicitly delineate predetermined academic standards that are separate and do not depend on the student's level of self-disclosure. Counselor educators may require trainees to seek professional help to address any personal concerns that may be affecting their competency.

F.8. STUDENT RESPONSIBILITIES

F.8.a. Standards for Students

Counselors-in-training have a responsibility to understand and follow the *ACA Code of Ethics* and adhere to applicable laws, regulatory policies, and rules and policies governing professional staff behavior at the agency or placement setting. Students have the same obligation to clients as those required of professional counselors. *(See C.1., H.1.)*

F.8.b. Impairment

Counselors-in-training refrain from offering or providing counseling services when their physical, mental, or emotional problems are likely to harm a client or others. They are alert to the signs of impairment, seek assistance for problems, and notify their program supervisors when they are aware that they are unable to effectively provide services. In addition, they seek appropriate professional services for themselves to remediate the problems that are interfering with their ability to provide services to others. *(See A.1., C.2.d, C.2.g.)*

F.9. EVALUATION AND REMEDIATION OF STUDENTS

F.9.a. Evaluation

Counselors clearly state to students, prior to and throughout the training program, the levels of competency expected, appraisal methods, and timing of evaluations for both didactic and clinical competencies. Counselor educators provide students with ongoing performance appraisal and evaluation feedback throughout the training program.

F.9.b. Limitations

Counselor educators, throughout ongoing evaluation and appraisal, are aware of and address the inability of some students to achieve counseling competencies that might impede performance. Counselor educators

1. assist students in securing remedial assistance when needed,
2. seek professional consultation and document their decision to dismiss or refer students for assistance, and
3. ensure that students have recourse in a timely manner to address decisions to require them to seek assistance or to dismiss them and provide students with due process according to institutional policies and procedures. *(See C.2.g.)*

F.9.c. Counseling for Students

If students request counseling or if counseling services are required as part of a remediation process, counselor educators provide acceptable referrals.

F.10. Roles and Relationships between Counselor Educators and Students

F.10.a. Sexual or Romantic Relationships

Sexual or romantic interactions or relationships with current students are prohibited.

F.10.b. Sexual Harassment

Counselor educators do not condone or subject students to sexual harassment. *(See C.6.a.)*

F.10.c. Relationships with Former Students

Counselor educators are aware of the power differential in the relationship between faculty and students. Faculty members foster open discussions with former students when considering engaging in a social, sexual, or other intimate relationship. Faculty members discuss with the former student how their former relationship may affect the change in relationship.

F.10.d. Nonprofessional Relationships

Counselor educators avoid nonprofessional or ongoing professional relationships with students in which there is a risk of potential harm to the student or that may compromise the training experience or grades assigned. In addition, counselor educators do not accept any form of professional services, fees, commissions, reimbursement, or remuneration from a site for student or supervisee placement.

F.10.e. Counseling Services

Counselor educators do not serve as counselors to current students unless this is a brief role associated with a training experience.

F.10.f. Potentially Beneficial Relationships

Counselor educators are aware of the power differential in the relationship between faculty and students. If they believe a nonprofessional relationship with a student may be potentially beneficial to the student, they take precautions similar to those taken by counselors when working with clients. Examples of potentially beneficial interactions or relationships include, but are not limited to, attending a formal ceremony; hospital visits; providing support during a stressful event; or mutual membership in a professional association, organization, or community. Counselor educators engage in open discussions with students when they consider entering into relationships with students outside of their roles as teachers and supervisors. They discuss with students the rationale for such interactions, the potential benefits and drawbacks, and the anticipated consequences for the student. Educators clarify the specific nature and limitations of the additional role(s) they will have with the student prior to engaging in a nonprofessional relationship. Nonprofessional relationships with students should be time-limited and initiated with student consent.

F.11. MULTICULTURAL/DIVERSITY COMPETENCE IN COUNSELOR EDUCATION AND TRAINING PROGRAMS

F.11.a. Faculty Diversity

Counselor educators are committed to recruiting and retaining a diverse faculty.

F.11.b. Student Diversity

Counselor educators actively attempt to recruit and retain a diverse student body. Counselor educators demonstrate commitment to multicultural/diversity competence by recognizing and valuing diverse cultures and types of abilities students bring to the training experience. Counselor educators provide appropriate accommodations that enhance and support diverse student well-being and academic performance.

F.11.c. Multicultural/Diversity Competence

Counselor educators actively infuse multicultural/diversity competency in their training and supervision practices. They actively train students to gain awareness, knowledge, and skills in the competencies of multicultural practice. Counselor educators include case examples, role-plays, discussion questions, and other classroom activities that promote and represent various cultural perspectives.

SECTION G: RESEARCH AND PUBLICATION

INTRODUCTION

Counselors who conduct research are encouraged to contribute to the knowledge base of the profession and promote a clearer understanding of the conditions that lead to a healthy and more just society. Counselors support efforts of researchers by participating fully and willingly whenever possible. Counselors minimize bias and respect diversity in designing and implementing research programs.

G.1. RESEARCH RESPONSIBILITIES

G.1.a. Use of Human Research Participants

Counselors plan, design, conduct, and report research in a manner that is consistent with pertinent ethical principles, federal and state laws, host institutional regulations, and scientific standards governing research with human research participants.

G.1.b. Deviation from Standard Practice

Counselors seek consultation and observe stringent safeguards to protect the rights of research participants when a research problem suggests a deviation from standard or acceptable practices.

G.1.c. Independent Researchers

When independent researchers do not have access to an Institutional Review Board (IRB), they should consult with researchers who are familiar with IRB procedures to provide appropriate safeguards.

G.1.d. Precautions to Avoid Injury

Counselors who conduct research with human participants are responsible for the welfare of participants throughout the research process and should take reasonable precautions to avoid causing injurious psychological, emotional, physical, or social effects to participants.

G.1.e. Principal Researcher Responsibility

The ultimate responsibility for ethical research practice lies with the principal researcher. All others involved in the research activities share ethical obligations and responsibility for their own actions.

G.1.f. Minimal Interference

Counselors take reasonable precautions to avoid causing disruptions in the lives of research participants that could be caused by their involvement in research.

G.1.g. Multicultural/Diversity Considerations in Research

When appropriate to research goals, counselors are sensitive to incorporating research procedures that take into account cultural considerations. They seek consultation when appropriate.

G.2. RIGHTS OF RESEARCH PARTICIPANTS

(See A.2., A.7.)

G.2.a. Informed Consent in Research

Individuals have the right to consent to become research participants. In seeking consent, counselors use language that

1. accurately explains the purpose and procedures to be followed,
2. identifies any procedures that are experimental or relatively untried,
3. describes any attendant discomforts and risks,

4. describes any benefits or changes in individuals or organizations that might be reasonably expected,
5. discloses appropriate alternative procedures that would be advantageous for participants,
6. offers to answer any inquiries concerning the procedures,
7. describes any limitations on confidentiality,
8. describes the format and potential target audiences for the dissemination of research findings, and
9. instructs participants that they are free to withdraw their consent and to discontinue participation in the project at any time without penalty.

G.2.b. Deception

Counselors do not conduct research involving deception unless alternative procedures are not feasible and the prospective value of the research justifies the deception. If such deception has the potential to cause physical or emotional harm to research participants, the research is not conducted, regardless of prospective value. When the methodological requirements of a study necessitate concealment or deception, the investigator explains the reasons for this action as soon as possible during the debriefing.

G.2.c. Student/Supervisee Participation

Researchers who involve students or supervisees in research make clear to them that the decision regarding whether or not to participate in research activities does not affect one's academic standing or supervisory relationship. Students or supervisees who choose not to participate in educational research are provided with an appropriate alternative to fulfill their academic or clinical requirements.

G.2.d. Client Participation

Counselors conducting research involving clients make clear in the informed consent process that clients are free to choose whether or not to participate in research activities. Counselors take necessary precautions to protect clients from adverse consequences of declining or withdrawing from participation.

G.2.e. Confidentiality of Information

Information obtained about research participants during the course of an investigation is confidential. When the possibility exists that others may obtain access to such information, ethical research practice requires that the possibility, together with the plans for protecting confidentiality, be explained to participants as a part of the procedure for obtaining informed consent.

G.2.f. Persons Not Capable of Giving Informed Consent

When a person is not capable of giving informed consent, counselors provide an appropriate explanation to, obtain agreement for participation from, and obtain the appropriate consent of a legally authorized person.

G.2.g. Commitments to Participants

Counselors take reasonable measures to honor all commitments to research participants. (See A.2.c.)

G.2.h. Explanations after Data Collection

After data are collected, counselors provide participants with full clarification of the nature of the study to remove any misconceptions participants might have regarding the research. Where scientific or human values justify delaying or withholding information, counselors take reasonable measures to avoid causing harm.

G.2.i. Informing Sponsors

Counselors inform sponsors, institutions, and publication channels regarding research procedures and outcomes. Counselors ensure that appropriate bodies and authorities are given pertinent information and acknowledgment.

G.2.j. Disposal of Research Documents and Records

Within a reasonable period of time following the completion of a research project or study, counselors take steps to destroy records or documents (audio, video, digital, and written) containing confidential data or information that identifies research participants. When records are of an artistic nature, researchers obtain participant consent with regard to handling of such records or documents. *(See B.4.a., B.4.g.)*

G.3. Relationships with Research Participants (When Research Involves Intensive or Extended Interactions)

G.3.a. Nonprofessional Relationships

Nonprofessional relationships with research participants should be avoided.

G.3.b. Relationships with Research Participants

Sexual or romantic counselor–research participant interactions or relationships with current research participants are prohibited.

G.3.c. Sexual Harassment and Research Participants

Researchers do not condone or subject research participants to sexual harassment.

G.3.d. Potentially Beneficial Interactions

When a nonprofessional interaction between the researcher and the research participant may be potentially beneficial, the researcher must document, prior to the interaction (when feasible), the rationale for such an interaction, the potential benefit, and anticipated consequences for the research participant. Such interactions should be initiated with appropriate consent of the research participant. Where unintentional harm occurs to the research participant due to the nonprofessional interaction, the researcher must show evidence of an attempt to remedy such harm.

G.4. Reporting Results

G.4.a. Accurate Results

Counselors plan, conduct, and report research accurately. They provide thorough discussions of the limitations of their data and alternative hypotheses. Counselors do not engage in misleading or fraudulent research, distort data, misrepresent data, or deliberately bias their results. They explicitly mention all variables and conditions known to the investigator that may have affected the outcome of a study or the interpretation of data. They describe the extent to which results are applicable for diverse populations.

G.4.b. Obligation to Report Unfavorable Results

Counselors report the results of any research of professional value. Results that reflect unfavorably on institutions, programs, services, prevailing opinions, or vested interests are not withheld.

G.4.c. Reporting Errors

If counselors discover significant errors in their published research, they take reasonable steps to correct such errors in a correction erratum, or through other appropriate publication means.

G.4.d. Identity of Participants

Counselors who supply data, aid in the research of another person, report research results, or make original data available take due care to disguise the identity of respective participants in the absence of specific authorization from the participants to do otherwise. In situations where participants self-identify their involvement in research studies, researchers take active steps to ensure that data are adapted/changed to protect the identity and welfare of all parties and that discussion of results does not cause harm to participants.

G.4.e. Replication Studies

Counselors are obligated to make available sufficient original research data to qualified professionals who may wish to replicate the study.

G.5. PUBLICATION

G.5.a. Recognizing Contributions

When conducting and reporting research, counselors are familiar with and give recognition to previous work on the topic, observe copyright laws, and give full credit to those to whom credit is due.

G.5.b. Plagiarism

Counselors do not plagiarize; that is, they do not present another person's work as their own work.

G.5.c. Review/Republication of Data or Ideas

Counselors fully acknowledge and make editorial reviewers aware of prior publication of ideas or data where such ideas or data are submitted for review or publication.

G.5.d. Contributors

Counselors give credit through joint authorship, acknowledgment, footnote statements, or other appropriate means to those who have contributed significantly to research or concept development in accordance with such contributions. The principal contributor is listed first, and minor technical or professional contributions are acknowledged in notes or introductory statements.

G.5.e. Agreement of Contributors

Counselors who conduct joint research with colleagues or students/supervisees establish agreements in advance regarding allocation of tasks, publication credit, and types of acknowledgment that will be received.

G.5.f. Student Research

For articles that are substantially based on students' course papers, projects, dissertations or theses, and on which students have been the primary contributors, they are listed as principal authors.

G.5.g. Duplicate Submission

Counselors submit manuscripts for consideration to only one journal at a time. Manuscripts that are published in whole or in substantial part in another journal or published work are not submitted for publication without acknowledgment and permission from the previous publication.

G.5.h. Professional Review

Counselors who review material submitted for publication, research, or other scholarly purposes respect the confidentiality and proprietary rights of those who submitted it. Counselors use care to make publication decisions based on valid and defensible standards. Counselors review article submissions in a timely manner and based on their scope and competency in research methodologies. Counselors who serve as reviewers at the request of editors or publishers make every effort to only review materials that are within their scope of competency and use care to avoid personal biases.

SECTION H: RESOLVING ETHICAL ISSUES

INTRODUCTION

Counselors behave in a legal, ethical, and moral manner in the conduct of their professional work. They are aware that client protection and trust in the profession depend on a high level of professional conduct. They hold other counselors to the same standards and are willing to take appropriate action to ensure that these standards are upheld.

Counselors strive to resolve ethical dilemmas with direct and open communication among all parties involved and seek consultation with colleagues and supervisors when necessary. Counselors incorporate ethical practice into their daily professional work. They engage in ongoing professional development regarding current topics in ethical and legal issues in counseling.

H.1. STANDARDS AND THE LAW

(See F.9.a.)

H.1.a. Knowledge

Counselors understand the *ACA Code of Ethics* and other applicable ethics codes from other professional organizations or from certification and licensure bodies of which they are members. Lack of knowledge or misunderstanding of an ethical responsibility is not a defense against a charge of unethical conduct.

H.1.b. Conflicts between Ethics and Laws

If ethical responsibilities conflict with law, regulations, or other governing legal authority, counselors make known their commitment to the *ACA Code of Ethics* and take steps to resolve the conflict. If the conflict cannot be resolved by such means, counselors may adhere to the requirements of law, regulations, or other governing legal authority.

H.2. SUSPECTED VIOLATIONS

H.2.a. Ethical Behavior Expected

Counselors expect colleagues to adhere to the *ACA Code of Ethics*. When counselors possess knowledge that raises doubts as to whether another counselor is acting in an ethical manner, they take appropriate action. *(See H.2.b., H.2.c.)*

H.2.b. Informal Resolution

When counselors have reason to believe that another counselor is violating or has violated an ethical standard, they attempt first to resolve the issue informally with the other counselor if feasible, provided such action does not violate confidentiality rights that may be involved.

H.2.c. Reporting Ethical Violations

If an apparent violation has substantially harmed, or is likely to substantially harm, a person or organization and is not appropriate for informal resolution or is not resolved properly, counselors take further action appropriate to the situation. Such action might include referral to state or national committees on professional ethics, voluntary national certification bodies, state licensing boards, or to the appropriate institutional authorities. This standard does not apply when an intervention would violate confidentiality rights or when counselors have been retained to review the work of another counselor whose professional conduct is in question.

H.2.d. Consultation

When uncertain as to whether a particular situation or course of action may be in violation of the *ACA Code of Ethics*, counselors consult with other counselors who are knowledgeable about ethics and the *ACA Code of Ethics*, with colleagues, or with appropriate authorities.

H.2.e. Organizational Conflicts

If the demands of an organization with which counselors are affiliated pose a conflict with the *ACA Code of Ethics*, counselors specify the nature of such conflicts and express to their supervisors or other responsible officials their commitment to the *ACA Code of Ethics*. When possible, counselors work toward change within the organization to allow full adherence to the *ACA Code of Ethics*. In doing so, they address any confidentiality issues.

H.2.f. Unwarranted Complaints

Counselors do not initiate, participate in, or encourage the filing of ethics complaints that are made with reckless disregard or willful ignorance of facts that would disprove the allegation.

H.2.g. Unfair Discrimination against Complainants and Respondents

Counselors do not deny persons employment, advancement, admission to academic or other programs, tenure, or promotion based solely upon their having made or their being the subject of an ethics complaint. This does not preclude taking action based upon the outcome of such proceedings or considering other appropriate information.

H.3. COOPERATION WITH ETHICS COMMITTEES

Counselors assist in the process of enforcing the *ACA Code of Ethics*. Counselors cooperate with investigations, proceedings, and requirements of the ACA Ethics Committee or ethics committees of other duly constituted associations or boards having jurisdiction over those charged with a violation. Counselors are familiar with the *ACA Policy and Procedures for Processing Complaints of Ethical Violations* and use it as a reference for assisting in the enforcement of the *ACA Code of Ethics*.

GLOSSARY OF TERMS

Advocacy—promotion of the well-being of individuals and groups and of the counseling profession within systems and organizations. Advocacy seeks to remove barriers and obstacles that inhibit access, growth, and development.

Assent—to demonstrate agreement, when a person is otherwise not capable or competent to give formal consent (e.g., informed consent) to a counseling service or plan.

Client—an individual seeking or referred to the professional services of a counselor for help with problem resolution or decision making.

Counselor—a professional (or a student who is a counselor-in-training) engaged in a counseling practice or other counseling-related services. Counselors fulfill many roles and responsibilities such as counselor educators, researchers, supervisors, practitioners, and consultants.

Counselor Educator—a professional counselor engaged primarily in developing, implementing, and supervising the educational preparation of counselors-in-training.

Counselor Supervisor—a professional counselor who engages in a formal relationship with a practicing counselor or counselor-in-training for the purpose of overseeing that individual's counseling work or clinical skill development.

Culture—membership in a socially constructed way of living, which incorporates collective values, beliefs, norms, boundaries, and lifestyles that are cocreated with others who share similar worldviews comprising biological, psychosocial, historical, psychological, and other factors.

Diversity—the similarities and differences that occur within and across cultures, and the intersection of cultural and social identities.

Documents—any written, digital, audio, visual, or artistic recording of the work within the counseling relationship between counselor and client.

Examinee—a recipient of any professional counseling service that includes educational, psychological, and career appraisal utilizing qualitative or quantitative techniques.

Forensic Evaluation—any formal assessment conducted for court or other legal proceedings.

Multicultural/Diversity Competence—a capacity whereby counselors possess cultural and diversity awareness and knowledge about self and others, and how this awareness and knowledge is applied effectively in practice with clients and client groups.

Multicultural/Diversity Counseling—counseling that recognizes diversity and embraces approaches that support the worth, dignity, potential, and uniqueness of individuals within their historical, cultural, economic, political, and psychosocial contexts.

Student—an individual engaged in formal educational preparation as a counselor-in-training.

Supervisee—a professional counselor or counselor-in-training whose counseling work or clinical skill development is being overseen in a formal supervisory relationship by a qualified trained professional.

Supervisor—counselors who are trained to oversee the professional clinical work of counselors and counselors-in-training.

Teaching—all activities engaged in as part of a formal educational program designed to lead to a graduate degree in counseling.

Training—the instruction and practice of skills related to the counseling profession. Training contributes to the ongoing proficiency of students and professional counselors.

INDEX

ACA MEMBER BENEFITS AND ADDITIONAL ETHICS RESOURCES

Free Consultation on Ethics for ACA Members

ACA members receive free access to consultation services on ethical practice and professional issues such as licensure; third-party reimbursement; testing; managed care; practice issues such as opening, enhancing, or closing a practice; and many other counseling-related issues. Consultation is offered by experienced, credentialed professional counselors and is designed to assist members in making ethical decisions. Members may call 800-347-6647 x314 during regular business hours for consultation.

Online Access to the 2005 ACA Code of Ethics

A free copy of the 2005 *ACA Code of Ethics* may be downloaded from the ACA Web site at http://www.counseling.org/ethics. Multiple copies for classroom use can be purchased from ACA at http://www.counseling.org or 800-422-2648 x222.

Policies and Procedures for Processing Complaints of Ethical Violations

For a copy of the *ACA Policies and Procedures for Processing Complaints of Ethical Violations*, visit http://www.counseling.org/ethics or contact the ACA Ethics and Professional Standards Department at 800-347-6647 x314.

RELATED PUBLICATIONS AND ONLINE ETHICS COURSE

Visit http://www.counseling.org or call Member Services at 800-422-2648 x222 to order the publications and online course below.

ACA ETHICAL STANDARDS CASEBOOK, SIXTH EDITION

Barbara Herlihy and Gerald Corey

A resource no counselor or counselor-in-training can afford to be without—the *ACA Ethical Standards Casebook* assists you in making sound ethical decisions. Through enlightening case studies and vignettes, the *Casebook* provides the foundation for analytic evaluation of the 2005 *ACA Code of Ethics* and guidance in applying these standards in work with diverse clients. The sixth edition of this book reflects the latest changes in the 2005 *Code*, including modifications to thinking on dual relationships, online counseling, and the nuances of culturally sensitive counseling.

BUILDING A FOUNDATION FOR ETHICAL PRACTICE IN COUNSELING, ONLINE COURSE

Rocco Cottone, Harriet Glosoff, and Michael Kocet

Learn the ethical principles that form the basis for codes of ethics—including the 2005 *ACA Code of Ethics*—in the helping professions. This course covers key concepts in ethical practice and provides decision-making models, case studies, examples, principle ethics, virtue ethics, conflicts between law and ethics, and learning exercises. Designed as a primer, this course offers a foundation of knowledge that can be applied immediately to your work regardless of your work setting. *The course is approved for continuing education credit by NBCC and APA.*

BOUNDARY ISSUES IN COUNSELING: MULTIPLE ROLES AND RESPONSIBILITIES, SECOND EDITION

Barbara Herlihy and Gerald Corey

Fully updated and expanded, the second edition of this best seller reflects the profession's most current thinking on dual or multiple relationships. Revised in accordance with the 2005 *ACA Code of Ethics* and the most recent ethical codes of related professional associations including APA, ACES, ASCA, AAMFT, ASGW, and NASW, this book is a necessity for all counselors seeking to make sense of and develop a clear personal stance on this controversial topic. It is also an outstanding supplementary text for courses on ethical and professional issues.

AMERICAN COUNSELING ASSOCIATION
5999 Stevenson Avenue
Alexandria, VA 22304
http://www.counseling.org • 800-422-2648 x222

Note: This document may be reproduced without permission for educational purposes.

REFERENCES

Abreu, J. M., Chung, R. H. G., & Atkinson, D. R. (2000). Multicultural counseling training: Past, present, and future directions. *Counseling Psychologist, 28*(5), 641–656.

Adler, A. (1958). *What life should mean to you.* New York: Putnam.

Aklin, W. M., & Turner, S. M. (2006). Toward understanding ethnic and cultural factors in the interviewing process. *Psychotherapy: Theory, Research, Practice, Training, 43,* 50–64.

Alexander, F., & French, T. M. (1980). *Psychoanalytic therapy: Principles and applications.* Lincoln: University of Nebraska Press.

Allen, W. (1976). *Without feathers.* New York: Warner.

Altekruse, M. K., Harris, H. L., & Brandt, M. A. (2001). The role of the professional counselor in the 21st century. *Counseling and Human Development, 34*(4), 1–10.

American Counseling Association. (2005). *Code of ethics.* Washington, D.C.: Author.

American Psychological Association. (2002). Ethical principles of psychologists and code of conduct. *American Psychologist, 57,* 1060–1075.

Anderson, P., & Vandehey, M. (2006). *Career counseling and development in a global economy.* Boston: Lahaska Press.

Andrews, B. (2007). Doing what counts. *Human Givens Journal, 14,* 32–37.

Annesi, J. J. (2005). Changes in depressed mood associated with 10 weeks of moderate cardiovascular exercise in formerly sedentary adults. *Psychological Reports, 96,* 855–862.

Anton, R. F., O'Malley, S. S., Ciraulo, D. A., Cisler, R. A., Couper, D., Donovan, D. M., et al. (2006). Combined pharmacotherapies and behavioral interventions for alcohol dependence. *The Journal of the American Medical Association, 295,* 2003–2017.

Archer Jr., J., & McCarthy, C. J. (Eds.) (2007). *Theories of counseling and psychotherapy: Contemporary applications.* Upper Saddle River, NJ: Pearson Merrill Prentice Hall.

Argyris, C. (1974). *Theory in practice: Increasing professional effectiveness.* San Francisco: Jossey-Bass.

Argyris, C., & Schon, D. A. (1992). *Theory in action: Increasing professional effectiveness.* San Francisco: Jossey-Bass.

Arkowitz, H., & Miller, W. R. (2008). Learning, applying, and extending motivational interviewing. In H. Arkowitz, H. A. Westra, W. R. Miller, & S. R. Rollnick (Eds.), *Motivational interviewing in the treatment of psychological problems.* New York: Guilford.

Arredondo, P. (1999). Multicultural counseling competencies as tools to address oppression and racism. *Journal of Counseling & Development, 77,* 101–123.

Arredondo, P., & Perez, P. (2003). Expanding multicultural competence through social justice. *The Counseling Psychologist, 31,* 282–289.

Arredondo, P., & Perez, P. (2006). Historical perspectives on the multicultural guidelines and contemporary applications. *Professional Psychology: Research and Practice, 37,* 1–5.

Association for Specialists in Group Work (2007). *Best practices guidelines.* Washington, D.C.: American Counseling Association.

Association for Specialists in Group Work. (2000). Professional standards for the training of group leaders. *Journal for Specialists in Group Work, 25,* 327–342.

Atkinson, B. (2005). *Emotional intelligence in couples therapy: Advances from neurobiology and the science of intimate relationships.* New York: W. W. Norton.

Austin, W., Bergum, V., Nuttgens, S., & Peternelj-Taylor, C. (2006). A re-visioning of boundaries in professional helping relationships: Exploring other metaphors. *Ethics & Behavior, 16,* 77–94.

Bacaigalupe, G. (2002). Reflecting teams: Creative, integrative, and collaborative practices. *Journal of Systemic Therapies*, 21(1), 78.

Baer, R. A. & Huss, D. B. (2008). Mindfulness- and acceptance-based therapy. In J. L. Lebow (Ed.), *Twenty-first century psychotherapies: Contemporary approaches to theory and practice* (pp. 123–166). Hoboken, NJ: Wiley.

Bagby, M. R., Costa, P. T., Widiger, T. A., Ryder, A. G., & Marshall, M. (2005). DSM-IV personality disorders and the five-factor model of personality: A multi-method examination of domain and facet-level predictions. *European Journal of Personality*, 19, 307–324.

Baker, S. B., & Gerler, E. R. (2007). *School counseling for the 21st century* (5th ed.) Upper Saddle River, NJ: Merrill.

Ballou, M., West, C., & Hill, M. (2007). *Feminist therapy theory and practice: A contemporary perspective.* New York: Springer.

Bandura, A. (1977). *Social learning theory*. Englewood Cliffs, NJ: Prentice Hall.

Barret, B., & Logan, C. (2002). *Counseling gay men and lesbians: A practice primer.* Pacific Grove, CA: Brooks/Cole.

Barsky, A. E., & Gould, J. W. (2002). *Clinicians in court: A guide to subpoenas, depositions, testifying, and everything else you need to know.* New York: Guilford.

Baruth, L., & Manning, M. L. (2006). *Multicultural counseling and psychotherapy: A lifespan perspective* (4th ed.). Upper Saddle River, NJ: Merrill Prentice Hall.

Bass, E. (1994). *The courage to heal* (3rd ed.). New York: HarperPerennial.

Bateson, G. (1979). *Mind and nature.* New York: Bantam Books.

Beck, A. T. (1967). *Depression: Causes and treatments.* Philadelphia: University of Pennsylvania Press.

Beck, A. T. (1976). *Cognitive therapy and the emotional disorders.* New York: International Universities Press.

Beck, A. T., & Weishaar, M. (2005). Cognitive therapy. In R. J. Corsini & D. Wedding (Eds.), *Current psychotherapies* (7th ed.) (pp. 238–268). Belmont, CA: Thomson Brooks/Cole.

Beck, A. T., Rush, A. J., Shaw, B. F., & Emery, G. (1979). *Cognitive therapy of depression.* New York: Guilford.

Beck, A. T., Steer, R. A., & Brown, G. K. (2004). *Beck Depression Inventory, II.* San Antonio, TX: Harcourt Assessment.

Becvar, D. S. (2008). The legacy of Michael White. *Contemporary Family Therapy*, 30, 139–140.

Beers, C. (1945). *A mind that found itself.* New York: Doubleday.

Behar, R. (2006). Gender-related aspects of eating disorders: A psychological view. In P. I. Swain (Ed.), *New developments in eating disorders research* (pp. 37–63). Hauppauge, NY: Nova Science Publishers.

Belson, R. (1992, September/October). Ten tried-and-true methods to achieve therapist burnout. *Family Therapy Networker*, 22.

Bemak, F., & Epp, L. R. (1996). The 12th curative factor: Love as an agent of healing in group psychotherapy. *Journal for Specialists in Group Work*, 21, 118–127.

Bemak, F., & Epp, L. R. (2001). Countertransference in the development of graduate student group counselors. *Journal for Specialists in Group Work*, 26(4), 305–318.

Berg, I. K., & White, M. (2007). Constructivist therapies. In J. O. Prochaska & J. C. Norcross (Eds.), *Systems of psychotherapy* (6th ed.) (pp. 451–473). Belmont, CA: Brooks/Cole.

Berg, I. S., & DeJong, P. (2005). Engagement through complimenting. *Journal of Family Psychotherapy*, 16, 51–56.

Berrios, R., & Lucca, N. (2006). Qualitative methodology in counseling research: Recent contributions and challenges for a new century. *Journal of Counseling and Development*, 84, 174–186.

Betts, G. R., & Remer, R. (1993). The impact of paradoxical interventions on perceptions of the therapist and ratings of treatment acceptability. *Professional Psychology: Research and Practice*, 24, 164–170.

Beutler, L. E., Machado, P. P., & Neufeldt, S. A. (1994). Therapist variables. In A. E. Bergin & S. L. Garfield (Eds.), *Handbook of psychotherapy and behavior change* (4th ed.) (pp. 229–269). New York: John Wiley & Sons.

Biancoviso, A. N., Fuertes, J. N., & Bishop-Towle, W. (2001). Planned group counseling: A single-session intervention for reluctant, chemically dependent individuals. *Journal for Specialists in Group Work*, 26(4), 319–338.

Blazina, C., & Watkins, C. E., Jr. (1996). Masculine gender role conflict: Effects on college men's psychological well-being, chemical substance usage, and attitudes toward help seeking. *Journal of Counseling Psychology*, 43, 461–465.

Blennerhassett, R. C., & O'Raghallaigh, J. W. (2005). Dialectical behavior therapy in the treatment of borderline personality disorder. *British Journal of Psychiatry*, 186, 278–280.

Blocher, D. H. (2000). *Counseling: A developmental approach* (4th ed.). New York: John Wiley & Sons.

Bloom, B. L. (1997). *Planned short-term psychotherapy: A clinical handbook.* Boston: Allyn & Bacon.

Blume, A. W. (2005). *Treating drug problems.* New York: John Wiley & Sons.

Boggs, C. D., Morey, L. C., Skodol, A. E., Shea, T. M., Sanislow, C. A., Grilo, C. M., et al. (2005). Differential impairment as an indicator of sex bias in DSM-IV criteria for four personality disorders. *Psychological Assessment*, 17, 492–496.

Bohart, A. C. (2005). Evidence-based psychotherapy means evidence-informed, not evidence-driven. *Journal of Contemporary Psychotherapy*, 35, 39–53.

Bohart, A. C. (2006). The client as active self-healer. In G. Stricker & J. Gold (Eds.), *A casebook of psychotherapy integration* (pp. 214–251). Washington, D.C.: American Psychological Association.

Book, H. E. (1998). *How to practice brief, psychodynamic psychotherapy.* Washington, D.C.: American Psychological Association.

Boorstein, D. (1983). *The discoverers.* New York: Random House.

Boy, A. V. (1989). Psychodiagnosis: A person-centered perspective. *Person-Centered Review*, 4(2), 132–151.

Boy, A. V., & Pine, G. J. (1999). *A person-centered foundation for counseling and psychotherapy*

(2nd ed.). Springfield, IL: Charles C. Thomas.

Boy, A. V., & Pine, G. J. (1982). The effectiveness of a counseling theory. *Michigan Personnel and Guidance Journal, 4,* 39–42.

Breuer, J., & Freud, S. (1893). On the psychological mechanism of hysterical phenomena: Preliminary communication. In J. Strachey (Ed. and Trans.), *The standard edition of the complete psychological works of Sigmund Freud, Vol. 2.* London Hogarth Press.

Briggs, M. K., & Rayle, A. D. (2005). Incorporating spirituality into core counseling courses: Ideas for classroom application. *Counseling and Values, 50,* 63–75.

Britt, E., Blampied, N. M., & Hudson, S. M. (2003). Motivational interviewing: A review. *Australian Psychologist, 38,* 193–201.

Broderick, P. C., & Blewitt, P. (2006). *The lifespan: Human development for helpers and professionals* (2nd ed.). Upper Saddle River, NJ: Merrill Prentice Hall.

Brooks, D. K., & Gerstein, L. H. (1990). Counselor credentialing and interpersonal collaboration. *Journal of Counseling and Development, 68,* 477–484.

Brott, P. E. (2001). The storied approach: A postmodern perspective for career counseling. *The Career Development Quarterly, 49,* 304–313.

Brown, C., & Augusta-Scott, T. (Eds.). (2006). *Narrative therapy: Making meaning, making lives.* Thousand Oaks, CA: Sage.

Brown, D. (2007). *Career information, career counseling, and career development* (9th ed.). Boston: Allyn & Bacon.

Brown, L. (2004). *Subversive dialogues: Theory in feminist therapy.* New York: Basic Books.

Brown, L. (2009). *Feminist therapy.* Washington, D.C.: American Psychological Association.

Brown, L.S. (2005). Still subversive after all these years: The relevance of feminist therapy in the age of evidence-based practice. *Psychology of Women Quarterly, 30,* 15–24.

Brown, M. T., Lum, J. L., & Voyle, K. (1997). Roe revisited: A call for the reappraisal of the theory of personality development and career

choice. *Journal of Vocational Behavior, 51,* 283–294.

Brown, R. T., & Sammons, M. T. (2002). Pediatric psychopharmacology: A review of new developments and recent research. *Professional Psychology: Research and Practice, 33,* 135–147.

Bugental, J. F. T. (1991). Outcomes of an existential-humanistic psychotherapy. *Humanistic Psychologist, 19,* 2–9.

Bugental, J. F. T., Peirson, J. F., & Schneider, K. J. (2001). Closing statements. In K. J. Schneider, J. F. T. Bugental, & J. F. Peirson (Eds.), *The handbook of humanistic psychology.* Thousand Oaks, CA: Sage.

Buhrke, R. A., & Douce, L. A. (1991). Training issues for counseling psychologists in working with lesbian women and gay men. *Counseling Psychology, 19,* 216–234.

Burkard, A. W., Knox, S., & Groen, M. (2006). European-American therapist self-disclosure in cross-cultural counseling. *Journal of Counseling Psychology, 53,* 15–25.

Burkhard, A. W., Pruitt, N. T., Medler, B. R., & Stark-Booth, A. M. (2009). Validity and reliability of the lesbian, gay, bisexual working alliance self-efficacy scales. *Training and Education in Professional Psychology, 3*(1), 37–46.

Burks, H. M., Jr., & Steffire, B. (1979). *Theories of counseling* (3rd ed.). New York: McGraw-Hill.

Burns, D. D. (1999). *Feeling good: The new mood therapy.* New York: HarperCollins.

Burrow-Sanchez, J. J. (2006). Understanding adolescent substance abuse: Prevalence risk factors and clinical implications. *Journal of Counseling and Development, 84,* 283–290.

Bush, R. A. & Folger, J. (2004). *The promise of mediation: The transformative approach to conflict.* San Francisco: Jossey-Bass.

Butcher, J. N., Perry, J., & Hahn, J. (2004). Computers in clinical assessment: Historical developments, present status, and future challenges. *Journal of Clinical Psychology, 60,* 331–345.

Butler, A. C., Chapman, J. E., Forman, E. M., & Beck, A. T. (2006). The empirical status of cognitive-behavioral therapy: A review of

meta-analyses, *Clinical Psychology Review 26,* 17–31.

Campbell, C., & Ungar, M. (2004). Constructing a life that works: Part 2, an approach to practice. *The Career Development Quarterly, 53,* 28–40.

Campos, P. E., & Goldfried, M. R. (2001). Perspectives on therapy with gay, lesbian, and bisexual clients. *Journal of Clinical Psychology, 57*(5), 609–613.

Caplow, T. (1954). *The sociology of work.* Minneapolis: University of Minnesota Press.

Capuzzi, D., & Gross, D. R. (Eds.). (2007). *Counseling and psychotherapy: Theories and interventions* (4th ed.). Upper Saddle River, NJ: Prentice Hall.

Capuzzi, D., Gross, D. R., & Staffer, M. D. (2009). *Introduction to group work* (5th ed.). Denver, CO: Love.

Carkhuff, R. R., & Berenson, B. G. (1977). *Beyond counseling and therapy* (2nd ed.). New York: Holt, Rinehart & Winston.

Carlson, J. D., & Englar-Carlson, M. (2007). Adlerian therapy. In J. Frew & M. Spengler (Eds.), *Contemporary psychotherapy for a diverse world.* Boston: Lahaska Press.

Carlson, J., Sperry, L., & Lewis, J. (2003). *Family therapy techniques.* New York: Brunner-Routledge.

Carlson, J., Watts, R. E., & Maniacci, M. (2005). *Adlerian therapy: Theory and practice.* Washington, D.C.: American Psychological Association.

Carnes, P. J., Delmonico, D. L., & Griffin, E. J. (2001). *In the shadows of the Net: Breaking free of compulsive online sexual behavior.* Center City, MN: Hazelden.

Carroll, K. M., Ball, S. A., Nich, C., Martino, S., Frankfort, T. L., Farentinos, C., & Woody, G. E. (2006). Motivational interviewing to improve treatment engagement and outcome in individuals seeking treatment for substance abuse: A multisite effectiveness study. *Drug and Alcohol Dependence, 81,* 301–312.

Case, C., & Dalley, T. (2006). *The handbook of art therapy* (2nd ed.). New York: Routledge.

Castongury, L. G., Constantino, M. J., & Holtforth, M. G. (2006). The working alliance: Where are we and where should we go? *Psychotherapy: Theory, Research, Practice, Training, 43*, 271–279.

Caviola, A. A., & Colford, J. E. (2006). *A practical guide to crisis intervention*. Boston: Lahaska Press.

Celenza, A. (2005). Sexual boundary violations: How do they happen? *Directions in Psychiatry, 25*, 141–149.

Cepeda, L. M., & Davenport, D. S. (2006). Person-centered therapy and solution-focused brief therapy: An integration of present and future awareness. *Psychotherapy: Theory, Research, Practice, Training, 43*, 1–12.

Chen, C. P. (2006). Strengthening career human agency. *Journal of Counseling and Development, 84*, 131–138.

Chomsky, N. (1968/2006). *Language and mind*. Cambridge, UK: Cambridge University Press.

Chrisler, J. C., & Ulsh, H. M. (2001). Feminist bibliotherapy: Report on a survey of feminist therapies. *Women and Therapy, 23*(4), 71–84.

Christensen, T. M., & Kline, W. B. (2001). Anxiety as a condition for learning in group supervision. *Journal for Specialists in Group Work, 26*(4), 385–396.

Christenson, J. (2009, February). Finding hope after losing a job. *Counseling Today*, 38–41.

Chung, R., & Bemak, F. (2002). The relationship of culture and empathy in cross-cultural counseling. *Journal of Counseling and Development, 80*, 154–159.

Claiborn, C. D. (1987). Science and practice: Reconsidering the Pepinskys. *Journal of Counseling and Development, 65*, 286–288.

Clark, M. A., Severy, L., & Sawyer, S. A. (2004). Creating connections: Using a narrative approach in career group counseling with college students from diverse populations. *Journal of College Counseling, 7*, 24–31.

Cochran, S. V., & Rabinowitz, F. E. (2003). Gender-sensitive recommendations for assessment and treatment of depression in men. *Professional Psychology: Research and Practice, 34*, 132–140.

Combs, A. W., & Gonzalez, D. W. (1994). *Helping relationships* (4th ed.). Boston: Allyn & Bacon.

Comstock, D. L. (2005). Women's development. In D. L. Comstock (Ed.), *Diversity in development: Critical contexts that shape our lives and relationships*. Belmont, CA: Thomson Wadsworth.

Confresi, N. J., & Gorman, A. A. (2004). Testing and assessment issues with Spanish-English bilingual Latinos. *Journal of Counseling and Development, 82*, 99–106.

Conger, R., Conger, K., Elder, G., & Lorenz, F. (1992). A family process model of economic hardship and adjustment of early adolescent boys. *Child Development, 63*, 526–541.

Conger, R. D., & Donellan, M. B. (2007). An interactionist perspective on the socioeconomic context of human development. *Annual Review of Psychology, 58*, 175–199.

Constantine, M. G., Hage, S. M., Kindachi, M. M., & Bryant, R. M. (2007). Social justice and multicultural issues: Implications for the practice and training of counselors and counseling psychologists. *Journal of Counseling & Development, 85*, 24–29.

Conyne, R., Rapin, L., & Rand, J. (1997). A model for leading task groups. In H. Forester-Miller & J. Kottler (Eds.), *Issues and challenges for group practitioners*. Denver, CO: Love.

Cooper, C. C., & Gottlieb, M. C. (2000). Ethical issues in managed care: Challenges facing counseling psychology. *Counseling Psychologist, 28*(2), 179–236.

Cooper, M. (2003). *Existential therapies*. Thousand Oaks, CA: Sage.

Corey, G. (2004). *Theory and practice of counseling and psychotherapy* (7th ed.). Pacific Grove, CA: Brooks/Cole.

Corey, G., Corey, M. S., & Callanan, P. (2007). *Issues and ethics in the helping professions* (7th ed.). Belmont, CA: Thomson Brooks/Cole.

Corey, M. S., & Corey, G. (2006). *Groups: Process and practice* (7th ed.). Belmont, CA: Thomson Brooks/Cole.

Cormier, S., & Hackney, H. (2008). *Counseling strategies and interventions* (7th ed.). Boston: Allyn & Bacon.

Cormier, W. H., Nurius, P. S. , & Osborne, J. O. (2009). *Interviewing and change strategies for helpers: Fundamental skills and cognitive behavioral interventions*. (6th ed.). Pacific Grove, CA: Brooks/Cole.

Corrigan, M. J., Jones, C. A., & McWhirter, J. J. (2001). College students with disabilities: An access employment group. *Journal for Specialists in Group Work, 26*(4), 339–349.

Cottone, R. R. (1992). *Theories and paradigms of counseling and psychotherapy*. Boston: Allyn & Bacon.

Cottone, R., & Travydas, V. M. (2007). *Counseling ethics and decision making* (3rd ed.). Upper Saddle River, NJ: Prentice Hall.

Coughlin, P., Della Selva, D., & Malan, D. (2007). *Lives transformed: A revolutionary method of dynamic psychotherapy*. London: Karnac.

Craig, R. J. (2004). *Counseling the alcohol- and drug-dependent client: A practical approach*. Boston: Allyn & Bacon.

Creswell, J. (2007). *Qualitative inquiry and research design: Choosing among five approaches*. Thousand Oaks, CA: Sage.

Crethar, H. C., Rivera, E. T., & Nash, S. In search of common threads; Linking multicultural, feminist, and social justice counseling paradigms. *Journal of Counseling & Development, 86*, 269–278.

Crocket, K. (2008). Narrative therapy. In J. Frew & M. D. Spiegler (Eds.) Contemporary psychotherapies for a diverse world (pp. 489–533). Boston: Lahaska Press.

Crowell, S., Beauchaine, T. , & Linehan, M. (2009). A biosocial developmental model of borderline personality: Elaborating and extending Linehan's theory. *Psychological Bulletin, 135*, 495–510.

D'Andrea, M. (2000). Postmodernism, constructivism, and multiculturalism: Three forces reshaping and expanding our thoughts about counseling. *Journal of Mental Health Counseling, 22*(1), 1–16.

Daniels, J. A. (2001). Managed care, ethics, and counseling. *Journal of Counseling and Development, 79*, 119–122.

Daniels, J. A. (2002). Assessing threats of school violence: Implications for counselors. *Journal of Counseling and Development, 80*, 215–218.

Davanloo, H. (1992). *Short-term dynamic psychotherapy*. New York: Jason Aronson.

David, D. S., & Brannon, R. (1976). *The forty-nine percent majority: The male sex role*. Reading, MA: Addison Wesley.

Davis, K. M. (2001). Structural-strategic family counseling: A case study in elementary school counseling. *Professional School Counseling*, 4(3), 180–186.

Davis, K. M., & Lambie, G. W. (2005). Family engagement: A collaborative, systemic approach for middle school counselors. *Professional School Counseling*, 9(2), 144–148.

Day, S. X. (2007). *Groups in practice*. Boston: Houghton Mifflin.

Day, S. X. (2009). *Theory and design in counseling and psychotherapy* (2nd ed.). Boston: Lahaska Press.

De Jong, P., & Berg, I. K. (2008). *Interviewing for solutions* (3rd ed.). Pacific Grove, CA: Brooks/Cole.

de Shazer, S. (1988). *Clues: Investigating solutions in brief therapy*. New York: W. W. Norton.

DeAngelis, T. (2009). Tools for tough times. *Monitor on Psychology*, 40(1), 32–35.

DeLucia-Waack, J., Bridbord, K. H., Kleiner, J. S., & Nitza, A. G. (2006). *Group work experts share their favorite activities*. Alexandria, VA: Association for Specialists in Group Work.

Demos, J. N. (2005). *Getting started with neurofeedback*. New York: W. W. Norton.

DeYoung, P. A. (2003). *Relational psychotherapy: A primer*. New York: Brunner-Routledge.

Dillon, C. (2003). *Learning from mistakes in clinical practice*. Pacific Grove, CA: Brooks/Cole.

Dimidjian, S., Martell, C. R., & Christensen, A. (2008). Integrative behavioral couple therapy. In A. S. Gurman (Ed.), *Clinical handbook of couple therapy* (pp. 73–106). New York: Guilford.

Doherty, W. J. (2009). How therapists harm marriages and what we can do about it. *The National Registry of Marriage Friendly Therapists*. Retrieved from http://www.marriagefriendlytherapists.com/therapistsharmmarriages.php.

Dole, S., & McMahan, J. (2005). Using videotherapy to help adolescents cope with social and emotional problems. *Intervention in School and Clinic*, 40, 151–155.

Dollard, J., & Miller, N. (1950). *Personality and psychotherapy*. New York: McGraw-Hill.

Donigian, J., & Malnati, R. (1999). *Critical incidents in group therapy* (2nd ed.). Pacific Grove, CA: Brooks/Cole.

Donigian, J., & Malnati, R. (2005). *Systematic group therapy: A triadic model*. Belmont, CA: Wadsworth.

Doweiko, H. E. (2009). *Concepts of chemical dependency* (7th ed.). Belmont, CA: Brooks/Cole.

Drake, R. E., Goldman, H. H., Leff, S. H., Lehman, A. F., Dixon, L., & Torrey, W. C. (2001). Implementing evidence-based practices in routine mental health service settings. *Psychiatric Services*, 52, 179–182.

Drewes, A. A. (2009). *Blending play therapy with cognitive behavioral therapy*. Hoboken, NJ: Wiley.

Drug Policy Alliance (2003, September). *State of the states: Drug policy reforms 1996–2002: A report by the Drug Policy Alliance*. New York: Author.

Dublin, H. S., & Ulman, K. H. (2005). Axis II me spinning. In L. Motherwell (Ed.), *Complex dilemmas in group therapy: Pathways to resolution* (87–95). New York: Brunner-Routledge.

Duffy, M., Gillig, S. E., Tureen, R. M., & Ybarra, M. A. (2002). A critical look at the DSM-IV. *The Journal of Individual Psychology*, 58, 363–373.

Duncan, B. L., Miller, S. D., & Sparks, J. A. (2004). *The heroic client*. San Francisco: Jossey-Bass.

Duncan, B., & Miller, S. (2006). Treatment manuals do not improve outcomes. In J. Norcross, Levant, R., & Beutler, L. (Eds.) Evidence-based practices in mental health. Washington D.C.: American Psychological Association Press.

Duncan, B., Miller, S., & Hubble, M. (2007). How being bad can make you better. *Psychotherapy Networker*, 31, 36–45.

Dworkin, S. H., & Gutierrez, F. (1989). Introduction to the special issue. Counselors be aware: Clients come in every size, shape, color, and sexual orientation. *Journal of Counseling and Development*, 68, 6–8.

Eaves, S. H., & Erford, B. T. (2010). Outcome research in counseling. In B. T. Erford (Ed.) *Orientation to the counseling profession: Advocacy, ethics, and essential professional foundations* (pp. 390–418). Boston: Pearson.

Ecker, B., & Hulley, L. (1996). *Depth-oriented brief therapy*. San Francisco: Jossey-Bass.

Edwards, R. B. (1982). Mental health as rational autonomy. In R. B. Edwards (Ed.), *Psychiatry and ethics* (pp. 68–78). Buffalo, NY: Prometheus.

Egan, G. (2007). *The skilled helper: A problem management and opportunity development approach to helping* (8th ed.). Belmont, CA: Thomson Brooks/Cole.

Eldridge, W. D. (1982). A perspective on similarities among selected concepts of traditional scientific research and clinical counseling. *Journal of Clinical Psychology*, 38, 452–460.

Elliot, R., Watson, J. C., Goldman, R. N., & Greenberg, L. S. (2004). Introduction. In R. Elliot, J. C. Watson, R. N. Goldman, & L. S. Greenberg (Eds.), *Learning emotion-focused therapy: The process-experiential approach to change* (pp. 3–16). Washington, D.C.: American Psychological Association.

Ellis, A. (1962). *Reason and emotion in psychotherapy*. New York: Lyle Stuart.

Ellis, A. (1988, September). Albert Ellis on the essence of RET. *Psychology Today*, 5–8.

Ellis, A. (1994). *Reason and emotion in psychotherapy* (Rev. ed.). New York: Carol Publishing Corporation.

Ellis, A. (1995). *Better, deeper, and more enduring brief therapy: The rational emotive behavior therapy approach*. New York: Brunner/Mazel.

Ellis, A. (2001). *Overcoming destructive beliefs, feelings, and behaviors: New directions for rational emotive behavior therapy*. New York: Prometheus.

Ellis, A., & Grieger, R. (Eds.) (1986). *Handbook of rational-emotive therapy*. New York: Springer.

Ellis, A., & Joffe, D. (2002). A study of volunteer clients who experienced live sessions of rational emotive behavior therapy in front of a public audience. *Journal of Rational-Emotive & Cognitive Behavior Therapy*, 20, 151–158.

Ellis, A., & Whiteley, J. M. (Eds.) (1979). *Theoretical and empirical foundations of rational emotive therapy*. Pacific Grove, CA: Brooks/Cole.

Ellis, A., & Wilde, J. (2002). *Case studies in rational emotive behavior therapy with children and adolescents*. Upper Saddle River, NJ: Prentice Hall.

Englar-Carlson, M., & Shepard, D. S. (2003, March). *Counseling men: What we can learn (and shouldn't learn) from Hollywood*. Paper presented at the annual meeting of the American Counseling Association, Anaheim, CA.

Englar-Carlson, M., & Shepard, D. S. (2005). Engaging men in couples counseling: Strategies for overcoming ambivalence and inexpressiveness. *The Family Journal, 13*, 383–391.

Epston, D., White, M., & Murray, K. (1992). A proposal for a re-authoring therapy: Rose's revisioning of her life and commentary. In S. McNamee & K. J. Gergen (Eds.), *Therapy as social construction* (pp. 96–115). Newbury Park, CA: Sage.

Erford, B. T. (2008). *Research and evaluation in counseling*. Boston: Lahaska Press.

Eriksen, K., & Kress, V. E. (2008). Gender and diagnosis: Struggles and suggestions for counselors. *Journal of Counseling & Development, 86*, 152–162.

Erikson, E. (1950). *Childhood and society*. New York: W. W. Norton.

Erlanger, M. A. (1990). Using the genogram with the older client. *Journal of Mental Health Counseling, 12*(3), 321–331.

Etchinson, M., & Kleist, D. M. (2000). Review of narrative therapy: Research and utility. *The Family Journal, 8*, 61–66.

Evans, J. (2009). *Online counseling and guidance skills: A practical resource for trainees and practitioners*. Thousand Oaks, CA: Sage.

Evans, K. M., Kincade, E. A., Marbley, A. F., & Seem, S. R. (2005). Feminism and feminist therapy: Lessons from the past and hopes for the future. *Journal of Counseling and Development, 83*, 269–277.

Evans, K., & Gilbert, M. (2005). *An introduction to integrative psychotherapy*. New York: Palgrave Macmillan.

Fall, K. A., Holden, J. M., & Marquis, A. (2010). *Theoretical models of counseling and psychotherapy* (2nd ed.). New York: Brunner-Routledge.

Falvey, J. E. (2002). *Managing clinical supervision: Ethical practice and legal risk management*. Pacific Grove, CA: Brooks/Cole.

Fassinger, R. E. (1991). The hidden minority: Issues and challenges in working with lesbian women and gay men. *Counseling Psychologist, 19*, 157–176.

Fearing, J. (1996, March). New addiction finds people hooked on the Net. *Counseling Today*, 26.

Feldman, D. C., & Lankau, M. J. (2005). Executive coaching: A review and agenda for future research. *Journal of Management, 31*, 829–848.

Fiedler, F. E. (1950). A comparison of therapeutic relationships in psychoanalytic, nondirective, and Adlerian therapy. *Journal of Consulting Psychology, 14*, 436–445.

Filer, R. D., & Filer, P. A. (2000). Practical considerations for counselors working with hearing children of deaf parents. *Journal of Counseling and Development, 78*, 38–43.

Fiorentine, R. U., & Hillhouse, M. P. (2003). Why extensive participation in treatment and *twelve-step programs* is associated with the cessation of addictive behaviors: An application of the Addicted-Self Model of recovery. *Journal of Addictive Diseases, 22*, 35–55.

Fish, J. (1973). *Placebo therapy*. San Francisco: Jossey-Bass.

Fiske, S. (2005). Social cognition and the normality of prejudgment. In J. F. Dovidio, P. Glick, & L. A. Rudman (Eds.), *On the nature of prejudice: Fifty years after Allport* (pp. 36–53). Malden, MA: Blackwell Publishing.

Flores, L. Y., & Heppner, M. J. (2002). Multicultural career counseling: Ten essentials for training. *Journal of Career Development, 28*(3), 181–202.

Forester-Miller, H., & Gressard, C. F. (1997). The tao of group work. In H. Forester-Miller & J. Kottler (Eds.), *Issues and challenges for group practitioners*. Denver, CO: Love.

Fosha, D., Siegel, D., & Solomon, M. (Eds.) (2009). *The healing power of emotion: Affective neuroscience, development & clinical practice*. New York: W. W. Norton.

Fowler, J. W. (1981). *Stages of faith: The psychology of human development and the quest for meaning*. New York: Harper & Row.

Frank, J. D. (1973). *Persuasion and healing*. Baltimore: Johns Hopkins University Press.

Frankl, V. (1962). *Man's search for meaning*. Boston: Beacon.

Freedman, J., & Combs, G. (2008). Narrative couple therapy. In A. S. Gurman (Ed.), *Clinical handbook of couple therapy* (4th ed.) (pp. 229–258). New York: Guilford.

Freire, E. S., Koller, S. H., Piason, A., & da Silva, R. B. (2005). Person-centered therapy with impoverished, maltreated, and neglected children and adolescents in Brazil. *Journal of Mental Health Counseling, 27*, 225–238.

French, T. M. (1933). Interrelations between psychoanalysis and the experimental work of Pavlov. *American Journal of Psychiatry, 89*, 1165–1203.

Freud, S. (1912). The dynamics of transference. In J. Strachey (Ed.), *The standard edition of the complete psychological works of Sigmund Freud* (Vol. 12, pp. 97–108). London: Hogarth.

Freud, S. (1924). *A general introduction to psychoanalysis*. New York: Washington Square.

Freud, S. (1954). *The origins of psychoanalysis*. New York: Basic Books.

Frew, J., & Spiegler, M. D. (Eds.) (2008). *Contemporary psychotherapies for a diverse world*. Boston: Lahaska.

Fromme, K., & Corbin, W. (2004). Prevention of heavy drinking and associated negative consequences among mandatory and voluntary students. *Journal of Consulting and Clinical Psychology, 72*, 1038–1049.

Fuchs, T. (2004). Neurobiology and psychotherapy: An emerging dialogue. *Current Opinion in Psychiatry, 17*, 479–485.

Fugate, M., Landis, L., Riordan, K., Naureckas, S., & Engel, B. (2005). Barriers to domestic violence help seeking. *Violence Against Women, 11*, 290–310.

Galluzzo, G. R., Hilldrup, J., Hays, D. G., & Erford, B. T. (2008). The nature of research and inquiry.

In B. T. Erford (Ed.), *Research and evaluation in counseling* (pp. 2–24). Boston: Lahaska Press.

Garb, H. N. (2000). Computers will become increasingly important for psychological assessment: Not that there's anything wrong with that! *Psychological Assessment, 12*(1), 31–39.

Gardner, B. C., Burr, B. K., & Wiedower, S. E. (2006). Reconceptualizing strategic family therapy: Insights from a dynamic systems perspective. *Contemporary Family Therapy, 28,* 339–352.

Gehart, D. R., & Tuttle, A. R. (2003). *Theory-based treatment planning for marriage and family therapists.* Pacific Grove, CA: Brooks/Cole.

Geis, H. J. (1973). Effectively leading a group in the present moment. *Educational Technology, 13*(1), 76–88.

Geisenger, K. F., Spies, R. P., & Plake, B. S. (2007). *The seventeenth mental measurements yearbook.* Lincoln, NE: Buros Institute.

Gergen, K. J. (1991). *The saturated self.* New York: Basic Books.

Gergen, K. J. (1994). *Toward transformation in social knowledge* (3rd ed.). Thousand Oaks, CA: Sage.

Gergen, K. J., & Kaye, J. (1992). *Beyond narrative in the negotiation of therapeutic meaning.* Thousand Oaks, CA: Sage.

Gerrity, D. A., & Matthews, L. (2006). Leader training and practices in groups for survivors of childhood sexual abuse. *Group Dynamics: Theory, Research, and Practice, 10,* 100–115.

Gershoff, E. T. (2002). Corporal punishment by parents and associated child behaviors and experiences: A theoretical review. *Psychological Bulletin, 128,* 539–579.

Gibbons, R. D., Brown, H., Hur, K., Marcus, S. M., Bhaumik, D. K., Erkens, J. A., & Mann. J. J. (2007). Early evidence on the effects of regulators' suicidality warnings on SSRI prescriptions and suicide in children and adolescents. *American Journal of Psychiatry, 164,* 1356–1363.

Gibbs, L. (2003). *Evidence-based practice for the helping professions: A practical guide with integrated multimedia.* Pacific Grove, CA: Brooks/Cole.

Gilbert, P., & Leahy, R. (Eds.) (2007). *The therapeutic relationship in the cognitive behavioral psychotherapies.* New York: Routledge.

Gill, M. (1982). *The analysis of transference.* New York: International Universities Press.

Gilligan, C. (1982). *In a different voice.* Cambridge, MA: Harvard University Press.

Ginger, S., Spargo, S., Colean, S. R., & Evans, K. (2007). *Gestalt therapy: The art of contact.* London: Karnac.

Giordano, M., Landreth, G., & Jones, L. (2005). *A practical handbook for building the play therapy relationship.* Lanham, MD: Aronson.

Gladding, S. T. (2004). *Community and agency counseling* (2nd ed.). Upper Saddle River, NJ: Merrill Prentice Hall.

Gladding, S. T. (2005). *Counseling as an art: The creative arts in counseling* (3rd ed.). Upper Saddle River, NJ: Merrill.

Gladding, S. T. (2006). *Family therapy: History, theory, and practice.* (4th ed.). Upper Saddle River, NJ: Prentice Hall.

Gladding, S. T. (2007). *Group work: A counseling specialty* (5th ed.). Englewood Cliffs, NJ: Merrill.

Gladding, S. T. (2008). *Counseling: A comprehensive profession* (6th ed.). Upper Saddle River, NJ: Merrill Prentice Hall.

Glantz, K., & Pearce, J. K. (1989). *Exiles from Eden: Psychotherapy from an evolutionary perspective.* New York: W. W. Norton.

Glasser, W. (1965). *Reality therapy.* New York: Harper and Row.

Glasser, W. (1976). *Positive addiction.* New York: HarperCollins.

Glasser, W. (1990). *The quality school.* New York: HarperCollins.

Glasser, W. (1998). *Choice theory: A new psychology of personal freedom.* New York: HarperCollins.

Glasser, W. (2000). *Reality therapy in action.* New York: HarperCollins.

Glasser, W., & Breggin, P. R. (2001). *Counseling with choice theory.* New York: Quill.

Glosoff, H. L. (2005). Early historical perspectives. In D. Capuzzi & D. R. Gross (Eds.), *Introduction to the counseling profession.* Boston: Allyn & Bacon.

Glosoff, H. L. (2009). The counseling profession: A historical perspective. In D. Capuzzi & D. Gross (Eds.) *Introduction to the counseling profession* (5th ed.). Upper Saddle River, N.J: Merrill.

Goldenberg, I., & Goldenberg, H. (2008). *Family therapy: An overview* (6th ed.). Belmont, CA: Brooks/Cole.

Goldfried, M. R. (Ed.) (1982). *Converging themes in psychotherapy.* New York: Springer.

Goodheart, C. D., Kazdin, A. E., & Sternberg, R. J. (2006). *Evidence-based psychotherapy: Where practice and research meet.* Washington, D.C.: American Psychological Association.

Goodman, J., Schlossberg, N. K., & Anderson, M. (2006). *Counseling adults in transition* (3rd ed.). New York: Springer.

Gordon, T. G. (1970). *Parent effectiveness training.* New York: Peter Wyden.

Gordon, T. G. (1974). *Teacher effectiveness training.* New York: Peter Wyden.

Gottfredson, L. S. (2002). Gottfredson's theory of circumscription and compromise. In D. Brown, L. Brooks, & Associates (Eds.), *Career choice and development* (3rd ed.) (pp. 85–148). San Francisco: Jossey-Bass.

Gottman, J. M. (1999). *The marriage clinic: A scientifically-based marital therapy.* New York: W. W. Norton.

Gottman, J. M., & Leiblum, S. R. (1974). *How to do psychotherapy and how to evaluate it.* New York: Holt, Rinehart & Winston.

Gottman, J. M., & Levenson, R. W. (2000). The timing of divorce: Predicting when a couple will divorce over a 14-year period. *Journal of Marriage and the Family, 62,* 737–745.

Gottman, J. M., & Gottman, J. S. (2008). Gottman Method couple therapy. In A. S. Gurman (Ed.), *Clinical handbook of couple therapy* (pp. 138–166). New York: Guilford.

Green, S. L., & Hansen, J. C. (1989). Ethical dilemmas faced by family therapists. *Journal of Marital and Family Therapy, 15*(2), 149–158.

Greenberg, L. (2002). Emotion-focused therapy: *Clinical Psychology and Psychotherapy, 11,* 3–16.

Greenberg, L. S. (2002). *Emotion-focused therapy: Coaching clients to work through feelings.* Washington,

D.C.: American Psychological Association.

Greenberg, L. S., & Watson, J. (1998). Experiential therapy of depression: Differential effects of client-centered relationship conditions and process experiential interventions. *Psychotherapy Research, 8,* 210–224.

Greenberg, L. S., & Watson, J. C. (2006). Introduction: The nature and experience of depression and its treatment. In L. S. Greenberg & J. C. Watson (Eds.), *Emotion-focused therapy for depression* (pp. 3–16). Washington, D.C.: American Psychological Association.

Greenberg, L. S., Rice, L. N., & Elliott, R. (1993). *Facilitating emotional change: The moment-to-moment process.* New York: Guilford.

Greenberg, L., & Pascual-Leone, A. (2006). Emotion in psychotherapy: A practice-friendly research review. *Journal of Clinical Psychology, 62,* 611–630.

Greenberg, R. P., Constantino, M. J., & Bruce, N. (2006). Are patient expectations still relevant for psychotherapy process and outcome? *Clinical Psychology Review, 26,* 657–678.

Greene, B. (2006). Delivering ethical psychological services to lesbian, gay, and bisexual clients. In K. J. Bieschke, R. M. Perez, & K. A. DeBord (Eds.), *Handbook of counseling and psychotherapy with lesbian, gay, bisexual, and transgender clients* (2nd ed.). Washington, D.C.: American Psychological Association.

Greenfield, S. (2000). *Brain story.* London: BBC Worldwide Limited.

Gregory, R. J., Canning, S. S., Lee, T. W., & Wise, J. C. (2004). Cognitive bibliotherapy for depression: A meta-analysis. *Professional Psychology: Research and Practice, 35,* 275–280.

Griffiths, M. (2001). Sex on the Internet: Observations and implications for Internet sex addiction. *Journal of Sex Research. 38,* 333–343.

Gross, D. R., & Robinson, S. E. (1987). Ethics, violence, and counseling: Hear no evil, see no evil, speak no evil? *Journal of Counseling and Development, 65,* 340–344.

Grosso, F. C. (2009). *Complete applications of law and ethics: A workbook for California Marriage and Family Therapists* (8th ed.). Santa Barbara, CA: Author.

Guterman, J. T., & Rudes, J. (2005). A narrative approach to strategic eclecticism. *Journal of Mental Health Counseling, 27,* 1–11.

Hackney, H., & Cormier, S. (2009). *The professional counselor* (5th ed.). Upper Saddle River, NJ: Merrill.

Hage, S. M. (2006). A closer look at the role of spirituality in psychology training programs. *Professional Psychology: Research and Practice, 37,* 303–310.

Hage, S. M., Hopson, A., Siegel, M., Payton, G., & DeFanti, E. (2006). Multicultural training in spirituality: An interdisciplinary review. *Counseling and Values, 50,* 217–234.

Halbur, D. A., & Halbur, K. V. (2006). *Developing your theoretical orientation in counseling and psychotherapy.* Boston: Allyn & Bacon.

Haley, J. (1973). *Uncommon therapy.* New York: W. W. Norton.

Haley, J. (1976). *Problem-solving therapy.* New York: Harper & Row.

Haley, J. (1980). How to be a marriage therapist without knowing practically anything. *Journal of Marital and Family Counseling, 6*(4), 385–392.

Haley, J. (1984). *Ordeal therapy: Unusual ways to change behavior.* San Francisco: Jossey-Bass.

Haley, J. (1989). *The first therapy session.* San Francisco: Jossey-Bass.

Haley, J., & Richeport-Haley, M. (2003). *The art of strategic therapy.* New York: Taylor & Francis.

Hall, E. (1983, June). A conversation with Erik Erikson. *Psychology Today,* 22–30.

Halstead, R. W. (2007). *Assessment of client core issues.* Alexandria, VA: American Counseling Association.

Hartling, L. , & Sparks, E. (2008). Relational-cultural practice: Working in a nonrelational world. *Women & Therapy, 31*(2–4), 165–188.

Hayes, J. A., & Mahalik, J. R. (2000). Gender role conflict and psychological distress in male counseling center clients. *Psychology of Men & Masculinity, 1,* 116–125.

Hazler, R. J., Stanard, R., Conkey, V., & Granello, P. (1997). Mentoring group leaders. In H. Forester-Miller & J. Kottler (Eds.), *Issues and challenges for group practitioners.* Denver, CO: Love.

Hazler, R., & Kottler, J. A. (2005). *The emerging professional counselor:* *Student dreams to professional realities.* Alexandria, VA: American Counseling Association.

Heard, H. L., & Linehan, M. M. (2005). Integrative therapy for borderline personality disorder. In J. C. Norcross & M. R. Goldfried (Eds.). *Handbook of psychotherapy integration* (pp. 299–320). Oxford: Oxford University Press.

Heath, M. A., Sheen, D., Leavy, D., Young, E., & Money, K. (2005). Bibliotherapy: A resource to facilitate emotional healing and growth. *School Psychology International, 26,* 563–580.

Heather, N. (2005). Motivational interviewing: Is it all our clients need? *Addiction Research and Theory, 13,* 1–18.

Heitzman, D., Schmidt, A. K., & Hurley, F. W. (1986). Career encounters: Career decision making through on-site visits. *Journal of Counseling and Development, 66,* 209–210.

Held, B. S. (1984). Toward a strategic eclecticism. *Psychotherapy: Theory, Research, and Practice, 21*(2), 232–241.

Hendrix, H. (1988). *Getting the love you want: A guide for couples.* New York: Harper Perennial.

Hendrix, H. (2007) *Getting the love you want.* New York: Henry Holt.

Heppner, P. P., Kivlighan, D. M., & Wampold, B. E. (2008). *Research design in counseling* (4th ed.). Belmont, CA: Brooks/Cole.

Herbeck, D. M., Yihing, H., & Teruyam, C. (2008). Empirically supported substance abuse treatment approaches: A survey of treatment providers' perspectives and practices. *Addictive Behaviors, 33,* 699–712

Herlihy, B., & Corey, G. (2006). *Ethical standards casebook* (6th ed.). Alexandria, VA: American Counseling Association.

Herper, M. & Karno, P. (2009, July 1). The world's ten best-selling drugs. *Forbes.* Retrieved from http://www. forbes.com/2006/03/21html.

Herron, W. G., & Rouslin, S. (1984). *Issues in psychotherapy.* Washington, D.C.: Oryn.

Hesley, J., & Hesley, J. (2001). *Rent two films and let's talk in the morning* (2nd ed.). Washington, D.C.: American Psychiatric Press.

Hettama, J., Steele, J., & Miller, W. R. (2005). Motivational interviewing.

Annual Review of Clinical Psychology, 1, 91–111.

Hill, C. E. (1990). Is individual therapy process really different from group therapy process? The jury is still out. *Counseling Psychologist, 18,* 126–130.

Hill, C. L., & Ridley, C. R. (2001). Diagnostic decision making: Do counselors delay final judgments? *Journal of Counseling and Development, 79,* 98–104.

Hill, M., & Ballou, M. (Eds.) (2005). *The foundation and future of feminist therapy.* Binghamton, NY: Haworth.

Ho, B. S. (2001). Family-centered, integrated services: Opportunities for school counselors. *Professional School Counseling 4(5),* 357–361.

Hohenshil, T. H. (2000). High-tech counseling. *Journal of Counseling and Development, 78,* 365–368.

Holland, J. (1973). *Making vocational choices: A theory of careers.* Englewood Cliffs, NJ: Prentice Hall.

Holland, J. L. (1996). Exploring careers with a typology: What we have learned and some new directions. *American Psychologist, 51,* 397–406.

Hood, A. B., & Johnson, R. W. (2007). *Assessment in counseling: A guide to the use of psychological assessment procedures* (4th ed.). Alexandria, VA: American Counseling Association.

Hoppock, R. (1976). *Occupational information* (4th ed.). New York: McGraw-Hill.

Horner, A. (1995). *Psychoanalytic object relations therapy.* New York: Jason Aronson.

Horowitz, J. L. & Newcomb, M. D. (2001). A multidimensional approach to homosexual identity. *Journal of Homosexuality, 42(2)* 1–19.

Horsfall, J. (2001). Gender and mental illness: An Australian overview. *Issues in Mental Health Nursing, 22,* 421–438.

Hosford, R. E. (1969). Behavioral counseling: A contemporary overview. *Counseling Psychologist, 1,* 1–33.

Hoshmand, L. T., & Polkinghorne, D. E. (1992). Redefining the science-practice relationship and professional training. *American Psychologist, 47,* 55–66.

Huber, C. H. (1994). *Ethical, legal, and professional issues in the practice of marriage and family therapy.* New York: Merrill.

Hunsley, J. (2007). Training psychologists for evidence-based practice. *Canadian Psychology, 48(1),* 32–42.

International Association of Coaching (2009). *IAC ethical principles.* Retrieved from http://www.certified coach.org/ethics/principles.html.

Isaacs, M. L. (1997). The duty to warn and protect: Tarasoff and the elementary school counselor. *Elementary School Guidance and Counseling, 31,* 326–342.

Isaacs, M. L., & Stone, C. (2001). Confidentiality with minors: Mental health counselors' attitudes toward breaching or preserving confidentiality. *Journal of Mental Health Counseling, 23(4),* 342–356.

Ivey, A., & Ivey, M. B. (1998). Reframing DSM-IV: Positive strategies from developmental counseling and therapy. *Journal of Counseling & Development, 76,* 334–350.

Ivey, A., & Ivey, M. B. (2007). *Intentional interviewing and counseling: Facilitating development in a multicultural society* (6th ed.). Pacific Grove, CA: Brooks/Cole.

Ivey, A., D'Andrea, M., Ivey, M., & Simek-Morgan, L. (2007). *Theories of counseling and psychotherapy: A multicultural perspective* (6th ed.). Boston: Allyn & Bacon.

Ivey, A., Ivey, M., Myers, J., & Sweeney, T. (2004). *Developmental counseling and therapy: Promoting wellness over the life-span* (2nd ed.). Mahwah, NJ: Lawrence Erlbaum Associates.

Jackson, A. P., & Scharman, J. S. (2002). Constructing family-friendly careers: Mothers' experiences. *Journal of Counseling and Development, 80,* 180–187.

Jacobs, E. E. (2006). *Group counseling: Strategies and skills* (5th ed.). Belmont, CA: Thomson Brooks/Cole.

Jacobs, E., Masson, R. L., & Harvill, R. L. (2009). *Group counseling: Strategies and skills* (6th ed.). Belmont, CA: Brooks/Cole.

Jacobson, N. S., & Christensen, A. (1999). *Acceptance and change in couples therapy: A therapist's guide to transforming relationships.* New York: W. W. Norton.

James, R. K., & Gilliland, B. E. (2008). *Crisis intervention strategies* (6th ed.). Belmont, CA: Thomson Brooks/Cole.

James, W. (1907). *Pragmatism.* New York: New American Library.

Jellinek, E. M. (1952). Phases of alcohol addiction. *Quarterly Journal of Studies on Alcohol, 13,* 673–674.

Jellinek, E. M. (1960). *The disease concept of alcoholism.* New Haven, CT: College and University Press.

Joanning, H., & Keoughan, P. (2005). Enhancing marital sexuality. *The Family Journal, 13,* 351–355.

Johnson, D. W., & Johnson, F. P. (2006). *Joining together: Group theory and group skills* (9th ed.). Boston: Allyn & Bacon.

Johnson, J. E., Finney, J. W., & Moos, R. H. (2006). End-of-treatment outcomes in cognitive-behavioral treatment and twelve-step substance use treatment programs: Do they differ and do they predict one-year outcomes? *Journal of Substance Abuse Treatment, 31,* 41–50.

Johnson, S. M. (2004). *The practice of emotionally focused couple therapy: Creating connection* (2nd ed.). New York: Brunner-Routledge.

Johnson, S., & Lebow, J. (2000). The coming of age of couple therapy: A decade review. *Journal of Marital and Family Therapy, 26(1),* 23–38.

Johnson, S. M. (2008). Emotionally focused couple therapy. In A. S. Gurman (Ed.), *Clinical handbook of couple therapy* (pp. 107–137). New York: Guilford.

Jones, W. P., & Kottler, J. A. (2005). *Understanding research: Becoming a competent and critical consumer.* Upper Saddle River, NJ: Prentice Hall.

Jordan, J. V. (1997). Relational development through mutual empathy. In A. C. Bohart & L. S. Greenberg (Eds.), *Empathy reconsidered: New directions in psychotherapy.* Washington, D.C.: American Psychological Association.

Jordan, J. V. (2001). A relational-cultural model: Healing through mutual empathy. *Bulletin of the Menninger Clinic, 65,* 92–104.

Jordan, J. V. (2003). Relational-cultural therapy. In M. Kopala & M. A. Keitel (Eds.), *Handbook of counseling women* (pp. 22–30). Thousand Oaks, CA: Sage.

Joshua, J., & DeMenna, D. (2000). *Read two books and let's talk next week: Using bibliotherapy in clinical practice*. New York: John Wiley & Sons.

Josselson, R. (1992). *The space between us: Exploring the dimensions of human relationships*. San Francisco: Jossey-Bass.

Julien, R. M. (2008). *A primer of drug action* (11th ed.). New York: Worth.

Kabat-Zinn, J. (2005). *Wherever you go, there you are: Mindfulness meditation in everyday life*. New York: Hyperion.

Kagan, N. (1973). Can technology help us toward reliability in influencing human interaction? In J. Vriend & W. Dyer (Eds.), *Counseling effectively in groups*. Englewood Cliffs, NJ: Educational Technology.

Kahn, M. (2002). *Basic Freud: Psychoanalytic thought for the 21st century*. New York: Basic Books.

Kalivas, P. W. (2003). Predisposition to addiction: Pharmacokinetics, pharmacodynamics, and brain circuitry. *American Journal of Psychiatry, 160*, 1–3.

Kalodner, C. R., & DeLucia-Waack, J. L. (2003). Theory and research in eating disorders and disturbances in women: Suggestions for practice. In M. Kopala & M. A. Keitel (Eds.), *Handbook of counseling for women* (pp. 506–534). Thousand Oaks, CA: Sage.

Kanel, K. (2007). *A guide to crisis intervention* (3rd ed.). Belmont, CA: Thomson Brooks/Cole.

Kanfer, F. H., & Goldstein, A. P. (1991). *Helping people change* (4th ed.). New York: Pergamon.

Kanfer, F. H., & Phillips, J. S. (1970). *Learning foundations of behavior therapy*. New York: John Wiley & Sons.

Kaplan, M. (1983). A woman's view of DSM-III. *American Psychologist, 38*(7), 786–792.

Karver, M. S., Handelsman, J. B., Fields, S., & Bickman, L. (2005). A theoretical model of common process factors in youth and family therapy. *Mental Health Services Research, 7*, 35–51.

Kaslow, F., & Lebow, J. (2004). *Comprehensive handbook of psychotherapy: Integrative/eclectic* (Vol. 4). New York: John Wiley & Sons.

Kazden, A. E. (2006). Arbitrary metrics: Implications for identifying evidence-based treatments. *American Psychologist, 61*, 42–49.

Keene, M., & Erford, B. T. (2007). *Group activities: Firing up for performance*. Upper Saddle River, NJ: Prentice Hall.

Kelly, E. W., Jr. (1997). Relationship-centered counseling: A humanistic model of integration. *Journal of Counseling and Development, 75*, 337–345.

Kernberg, O. (1984). *Severe personality disorders*. New Haven, CT: Yale University Press.

King, J. H., & Anderson, S. M. (2004). Therapeutic implications of pharmacotherapy: Current trends and ethical issues. *Journal of Counseling and Development, 82*, 329–335.

Kirschenbaum, H. (2007). *The Life and Work of Carl Rogers*. Ross-on-Wye, England: PCCS Books.

Kiselica, M. S. (2003). Transforming psychotherapy in order to succeed with adolescent boys: Male-friendly practices. *Journal of Clinical Psychology, 59*, 1225–1236.

Kiselica, M. S., Englar-Carlson, M., & Horne, A. M. (Eds.) (2008). *Counseling troubled boys: A guidebook for professionals*. New York: Routledge.

Kleinke, C. L. (1994). *Common principals of psychotherapy*. Pacific Grove, CA: Brooks/Cole.

Kline, W. B. (2003). *Interactive group counseling and therapy*. Upper Saddle River, NJ: Prentice Hall.

Koffka, K. (1935). *Principles of Gestalt psychology*. New York: Harcourt Brace & World.

Kohlberg, L. (1969). *Stages in the development of moral thought and action*. New York: Holt, Rinehart & Winston.

Kohler, W. (1929). *Gestalt psychology*. New York: Liveright.

Kohut, H. (1984). *How does analysis cure?* Chicago: The University of Chicago Press.

Koocher, G. P. (2007). Twenty-first century ethical challenges for psychology. *American Psychologist, 62*, 375–384.

Kottler, J. A. (1992). *Compassionate therapy: Working with difficult clients*. San Francisco: Jossey-Bass.

Kottler, J. A. (1995). *Growing a therapist*. San Francisco: Jossey-Bass.

Kottler, J. A. (2000). *Doing good: Passion and commitment for helping others*. New York: Brunner-Routledge.

Kottler, J. A. (2001). *Making changes last*. New York: Brunner-Routledge.

Kottler, J. A. (2006). *Divine madness: Ten stories of creative struggle*. San Francisco: Jossey-Bass.

Kottler, J. A. (2010). *On being a therapist* (3rd ed.). San Francisco: Jossey-Bass.

Kottler, J. A., & Carlson, J. (2003). *Bad therapy: Master therapists share their worst failures*. New York: Brunner-Routledge.

Kottler, J. A., & Carlson, J. (2005a). *The client who changed me: Stories of therapist personal transformation*. New York: Brunner-Routledge.

Kottler, J. A., & Carlson, J. (2005b). *Their finest hour: Master therapists share their greatest success stories*. Boston: Pearson.

Kottler, J. A., & Englar-Carlson, M. (2009). *Learning group leadership*. Thousand Oaks, CA: Sage.

Kottler, J. A., & Hazler, R. (1997). *What you never learned in graduate school*. New York: W. W. Norton.

Kottler, J. A., & Markos, P. (1997). The group leader's uses of self. In H. Forester-Miller & J. Kottler (Eds.), *Issues and challenges for group practitioners*. Denver, CO: Love.

Kottler, J. A., & Marriner, M. (2009). *Changing people's lives while transforming your own: Paths to social justice and global human rights*. Hoboken, NJ: Wiley.

Kottler, J. A., & Smart, R. (2006). Reciprocal influences: How clients change their therapists. *Psychotherapy in Australia, 12*(3), 22–28.

Kottler, J. A., Montgomery, M., & Shepard, D. S. (2004). Acquisitive desire: Assessment and treatment. In T. Kasser & A. D. Kramer (Eds.), *Psychology and consumer culture: The struggle for a good life in a materialistic world*. Washington, D.C.: American Psychological Association.

Kottler, J. A., Sexton, T., & Whiston, S. (1994). *The heart of healing: Relationships in therapy*. San Francisco: Jossey-Bass.

Kovacs, A. L. (1982). Survival in the 1980s on the theory and practice of brief psychotherapy. *Psychotherapy: Theory, Research, and Practice, 19*(2), 142–159.

Kraemer, S. (2006). Something happens: Elements of therapeutic change. *Clinical Child Psychology and Psychiatry, 11,* 239–248.

Kress, V. E. W., Eriksen, K. P., Rayle, A. D., & Ford, S. J. W. (2005). The DSM-IV-TR and culture: Considerations for counselors. *Journal of Counseling and Development, 83,* 97–104.

Kroll, J. (1988). *The challenge of the borderline patient.* New York: W. W. Norton. Krumboltz, J. D. (1965). Behavioral counseling: Rationale and research. *Personnel and Guidance Journal, 44,* 373–387.

Kubie, L. S. (1934). Relation of the conditioned reflex to psychoanalytic technique. *Archives of Neurology and Psychiatry, 32,* 1137–1142.

Lambert, M. J. (1992). Implications of outcome research for psychotherapy integration. In J. N. Norcross & M. R. Goldstein (Eds.), *Handbook of psychotherapy integration* (pp. 94–129). New York: Basic Books.

Lambert, M. J. (2003). *Bergin and Garfield's handbook of psychotherapy and behavior change* (5th ed.). New York: John Wiley & Sons.

Lampropoulos, G. K., & Spengler, P. M. (2005). Helping and change without traditional therapy: Commonalities and opportunities. *Counselling Psychology Quarterly, 18,* 47–59.

Lampropoulos, G. K., Kazantzis, N., & Deane, F. P. (2004). Psychologists' use of motion pictures in clinical practice. *Professional Psychology: Research and Practice, 35,* 535–541.

Langs, R. (2009). *Managing managed care: Psychotherapy and medication management in the modern era.* Lanham, MD: Jason Aronson.

Layman, M. J., & McNamara, J. R. (1997). Remediation for ethics violations: Focus on psychotherapists' sexual contact with clients. *Professional Psychology: Research and Practice, 28,* 281–292.

Lazarus, A. A. (1981). *The practice of multimodal therapy.* New York: McGraw-Hill.

Lazarus, A. A. (1993). Tailoring the therapeutic relationship, or being an authentic chameleon. *Psychotherapy, 30,* 404–414.

Lazarus, A. A. (1995). Multimodal therapy. In R. J. Corsini &

D. Wedding (Eds.), *Current psychotherapies* (5th ed.). Itasca, IL: F. E. Peacock.

Lazarus, A. A. (2006). *Brief but comprehensive psychotherapy: The multimodal way.* New York: Springer.

Lazarus, A. A. (2008). Multimodal therapy. In R. J. Corsini & D. Wedding (Eds.) *Current psychotherapies* (8th ed.). Belmont, CA: Brooks/Cole.

Lebow, J. L. (Ed.) (2008). *Twenty-first psychotherapies: Contemporary approaches to theory and practice.* Hoboken, NJ: Wiley.

Lester, D. (2008). The use of the Internet for counseling the suicidal individual: Possibilities and drawbacks. *Omega, 58,* 233–250.

Levant, R. F., & Hasan, N. (2008). *Professional Psychology: Research and Practice, 39,* 658–662.

Lewis, J. H., Arnold, M. S., House, R., & Toporek, R. I. (2002). *ACA advocacy competencies.* Retrieved from http://counseling.org/Publications/.

Lewis, T. F., & Osborn, C. J. (2004). Solution-focused counseling and motivational interviewing: A consideration of confluence. *Journal of Counseling and Development, 82,* 38–48.

Lichtenberger, E. O. (2006). Computer utilization and clinical judgment in psychological assessment reports. *Journal of Clinical Psychology, 62,* 19–32.

Lieber, T., Archer, J., Munson, J., & York, G. (2006). An exploratory study of client perceptions of Internet counseling and the therapeutic alliance. *Journal of Mental Health Counseling, 28,* 69–83.

Lieberman, M., Yalom, L., & Miles, M. (1973). *Encounter groups: First facts.* New York: Basic Books.

Liu, W. M., & Iwamoto, D. K. (2006). Asian-American men's gender role conflict: The role of Asian values, self-esteem, and psychological distress. *Psychology of Men & Masculinity, 7,* 153–164.

Lobb, M., & Amendt-Lyon, N. (2004). *Creative license: The art of Gestalt therapy.* New York: Springer.

Loevinger, J. (1976). *Ego development.* San Francisco: Jossey-Bass.

Long, V. (1996). *Communication skills in helping relationships.* Pacific Grove, CA: Brooks/Cole.

Loyd, B. D. (2005). The effects of reality therapy/choice theory principles on high school students' perception of needs satisfaction and behavioral change. *International Journal of Reality Therapy, 25,* 5–9.

Lum, D. (2007). *Culturally competent practice.* Belmont, CA: Thomson Brooks/Cole.

Lum, W. (2002). The use of the self of the therapist. *Contemporary Family Therapy, 24*(1), 181–197.

Lundin, R. W. (1989). *Alfred Adler's basic concepts and implications.* Muncie, IN: Accelerated Development.

Lyness, A. (2006). *Politics of the personal in feminist family therapy.* New York: Haworth.

MacDougall, C. (2002). Rogers's person-centered approach: Consideration for use in multicultural counseling. *Journal of Humanistic Psychology, 42*(2), 48–65.

Madanes, C. (1983). *Strategic family therapy.* San Francisco: Jossey-Bass.

Madanes, C. (1984). *Beyond the one-way mirror.* San Francisco: Jossey-Bass.

Maddux, R. E. & Riso, L. P (2007). Promoting the scientist-practitioner mindset in clinical training. *Journal of Contemporary Psychotherapy, 37,* 213–220.

Madson, M. B., Loignon, A. C., & Lane, C. (2009). Training in motivational interviewing: A systematic review. *Journal of Substance Abuse Treatment, 36,* 101–109.

Mahoney, M. J. (2005). *Constructive psychotherapy: Theory and practice.* New York: Guilford.

Mahrer, A. R. (1996). Discovering how to do psychotherapy. *Journal of Humanistic Psychotherapy, 36*(3), 31–48.

Mahrer, A. R. (2008). *Psychotherapeutic change: An alternative approach to meaning and measurement.* New York: W. W. Norton.

Maione, P. V., & Chenail, R. J. (1999). Qualitative inquiry in psychotherapy: Research on common factors. In M. A. Hubble, B. L. Duncan, & S. D. Miller (Eds.), *The heart and soul of change: What works in therapy.* Washington, D.C.: American Psychological Association.

Malhi, G. S., Adams, D., Lampe, L., Paton, M., O'Connor, N., Newton, L. A., & Berk, M. (2009). Clinical practice recommendations for bipolar disorder. *Acta Psychiatra Scandinavica, 119*, 27–46.

Mann, J. (1973). *Time-limited psychotherapy*. Cambridge, MA: Harvard University Press.

Maples, M. F., & Abney, P. C. (2006). Baby boomers mature and gerontological counseling comes of age. *Journal of Counseling and Development, 84*, 3–9.

Marlatt, G. A. (1985). Relapse prevention: Theoretical rationale and overview of the model. In G. A. Marlatt & J. R. Gordon (Eds.), *Relapse prevention* (pp. 250–280). New York: Guilford.

Marlatt, G. A., & Gordon, K. R. (1985). *Relapse prevention: Maintenance strategies in the treatment of addictive behaviors*. New York: Guilford.

Marmarosh, C., Holtz, A., & Schottenbauer, M. (2005). Group cohesiveness, group-derived collective self-esteem, group-derived hope, and the well-being of group therapy members. *Group Dynamics: Theory, Research, and Practice, 9*, 32–44.

Marmarosh, C. L., Gelso, C. J., Marken, R. D., Mallery, C., & Choi, J. (2009). The real relationship in psychotherapy: Relationship to adult attachments, working alliance, transference, and therapy outcome. *Journal of Counseling Psychology, 56*, 337–350.

Maroda, K. J. (2004). *The power of countertransference* (2nd ed.). New York: Analytic Press.

May, R. (1958). *Existence*. New York: Simon & Schuster.

May, R. (1981). *Freedom and destiny*. New York: W. W. Norton.

May, R. (1983). *The discovery of being*. New York: W. W. Norton.

May, R., & Yalom, I. (1995). Existential psychotherapy. In R. J. Corsini & D. Wedding, *Current psychotherapies* (5th ed.). Itasca, IL: F. E. Peacock.

McGlothlin, J. (2008). *Developing clinical skills in suicide assessment, prevention and treatment*. Alexandria, VA: American Counseling Association.

McGoldrick, M., & Gerson, R. (1985). *Genograms in family assessment*. New York: W. W. Norton.

McNeece, C. A., & DiNitto, D. M. (2005). *Chemical dependency: A systems approach* (3rd ed.). Boston: Allyn & Bacon.

McRae, B. (1998). *Negotiating and influencing skills*. Thousand Oaks, CA: Sage.

McWilliams, N. (2007). *Psychoanalytic therapy*. Washington, D.C.: American Psychological Association.

Melton, J. L., Nofzinger-Collins, D., Wynne, M. E., & Susman, M. (2005). Exploring the affective inner experiences of therapists in training: The qualitative interaction between session experience and session content. *Counselor Education and Supervision, 45*, 82–96.

Messer, S. B. (2001). Evidence-based practice: Beyond empirically supported treatments. *Professional Psychology: Research and Practice, 6*, 580–588.

Miller, G. M. (1982). Deriving meaning from standardized tests: Interpreting results to clients. *Measurement and Evaluation in Guidance, 15*, 87–94.

Miller, J. (2008). How change happens: Controlling images, mutuality, and power. *Women & Therapy, 31*(2–4), 109–127.

Miller, S., Duncan, B. L., et al. (2006). Using formal client feedback to improve retention and outcome. *Journal of Brief Therapy, 5*, 5–22.

Miller, S., Hubble, M. & Duncan, B. L. (2007). Supershrinks: What's the secret of their success? *Psychotherapy Networker, 31*, 26–35.

Miller, T. W., Veltkamp, L. J., Lane, T., Bilyeu, J., & Elzie, N. (2002). Care pathway guidelines for assessment and counseling for domestic violence. *The Family Journal, 10*(1), 41–48.

Miller, W. R., & Hester, R. (1986). Inpatient alcoholism treatment: Who benefits? *American Psychologist, 41*, 794–805.

Miller, W. R., & Rollnick, S. (2002). *Motivational interviewing* (2nd ed.). New York: Guilford.

Miller, W. R., & Thoresen, C. E. (2003). Spirituality, religion, and health: An emerging research field. *American Psychologist, 58*, 24–35.

Miller, W. R., Meyers, R. J., & Tonigan, J. S. (1999). Engaging the unmotivated in treatment for alcohol problems. *Journal of Consulting and Clinical Psychology, 67*(5), 688–697.

Miller, W. R., Zweben, J., & Johnson, W. R. (2005). Evidence-based treatment: Why, what, where, when, and how? *Journal of Substance Abuse Treatment, 29*, 267–276.

Milne, A. L., Folberg, J., & Salem, P. (2004). In J. Folberg & A. Milne (Eds.), *Divorce and family mediation: Models, techniques, and applications* (pp. 3–25). New York: Guilford.

Minichiello, V., & Kottler, J. A. (2009). *Qualitative Journeys: Student and Mentor Experiences with Research*. Thousand Oaks, CA: Sage.

Minuchin, S. (1974). *Families and family therapy*. Cambridge, MA: Harvard University Press.

Minuchin, S., & Fishman, H. C. (1981). *Family therapy techniques*. Cambridge, MA: Harvard University Press.

Minuchin, S., Lee, W., & Simon, G. M. (2006). *Mastering family therapy: Journeys of growth and transformation*. San Francisco: Wiley.

Mitchell, K. J., Becker-Blease, K. A., & Finkelhor, D. (2005). Inventory of problematic Internet experiences encountered in clinical practice. *Professional Psychology: Research and Practice, 36*, 498–509.

Mitchell, L. K., & Krumboltz, J. D. (1987). The effects of cognitive restructuring and decision-making training on career indecision. *Journal of Counseling and Development, 66*, 171–174.

Moleski, S. M., & Kiselica, M. S. (2005). Dual relationships: A continuum ranging from the destructive to the therapeutic. *Journal of Counseling and Development, 83*, 3–11.

Monk, G., Winslade, J., Crocket, K., & Epston, D. (1997). *Narrative therapy in practice*. San Francisco: Jossey-Bass.

Morgan, Alice (2000). *What is narrative therapy? An easy-to-read introduction*. Dulwich, Australia: Dulwich Centre Publications.

Morison, J., Bromfield, L., & Cameron, H. (2003). A therapeutic model for supporting families of children with chronic illness or disability. *Child & Adolescent Mental Health, 8*, 125–130.

Mortenson, G., & Relin, D. O. (2006). *Three cups of tea: One man's mission to promote peace . . . one school at a time*. New York: Viking.

Mosak, H. H. (2005). Adlerian psychotherapy. In R. J. Corsini & D. Wedding (Eds.), *Current psychotherapies* (7th ed.) (pp. 52–95). Belmont, CA: Thomson Brooks/Cole.

Mosher, J., Goldsmith, J., Stiles, W., & Greenberg, L. (2008). Assimilation of two critic voices in a person-centered therapy for depression. *Person-Centered and Experiential Psychotherapies*, 7(1), 1–19.

Moss, D. (2002). Biofeedback. In S. Shannon (Ed.), *Handbook of complementary and alternative therapies in mental health* (pp. 135–158). San Diego, CA: Academic Press.

Murdock, N. L. (2008). *Theories of counseling and psychotherapy: A case approach* (2nd ed.). Upper Saddle River, NJ: Merrill Prentice Hall.

Murphy, B. C., & Dillon, C. (2003). *Interviewing in action: Process and practice* (2nd ed.). Belmont, CA: Thomson Brooks/Cole.

Murphy, J. A., Rawlings, E. I., & Howe, S. R. (2002). A survey of clinical psychologists on treating lesbian, gay, and bisexual clients. *Professional Psychology: Research and Practice*, 33(2), 183–189.

Murphy, J., & Duncan, B. L. (2007). *Brief intervention for school problems: Outcome-informed strategies*. New York: Guilford.

Myers, J. E., & Harper, M. C. (2004). Evidence-based effective practices with older adults. *Journal of Counseling and Development*, 82, 207–218.

National Association of Counties (2005). *The meth epidemic in America: Two surveys of U.S. counties: The criminal effect of meth on communities: The impact of meth on children*. Washington, D.C.: Author.

National Career Development Association Professional Standards Committee (1997). *Career counseling competencies*. Alexandria, VA: National Career Development Association.

National Institute for Health Care Management (2002, March 29). *Prescription drug expenditures 2001: Another year of escalating costs*. Retrieved October 1, 2006, from http://www.nihcm.org.

National Institute on Alcohol Abuse and Alcoholism (2001). *Alcohol alert: New advances in alcohol treatment*. No. 49–2000. Rockville, MD: Author.

National Institute on Drug Abuse (2009). *NIDA InfoFacts: High school and youth trends*. Retrieved from http://www.drugabuse.gov/infofacts/HSYouthtrends.html.

Naus, M., Philipp, L., & Samsi, M. (2009). From paper to pixels: A comparison of paper and computer formats in psychological assessment. *Computers in Human Behavior*, 25, 1–7.

Neimeyer, R. A. (2002). *Lessons of loss: A guide to coping* (2nd ed.). New York: Brunner-Routledge.

Neimeyer, R. A., & Mahoney, M. J. (Eds.) (1999). *Constructivism in psychotherapy*. Washington, D.C.: American Psychological Association.

Nelson, J. (2006). For parents only: A strategic family therapy approach to school counseling. *The Family Journal*, 14, 180–183.

Nestoriuc, Y., Rief, W., & Martin, A. (2008). Meta-analysis of biofeedback for tension-type headache: Efficacy, specificity, and treatment moderators. *Journal of Consulting & Clinical Psychology*, 76, 379–396.

Neukrug, E. S., & Fawcett, R. C. (2010). *Essentials of testing and assessment: A practical guide for counselors, social workers, and psychologists* (2nd ed.). Belmont, CA: Thomson Brooks/Cole.

Newman, B. M., & Newman. P. R. (2009). *Development through life: A psychosocial approach* (10th ed.). Belmont, CA: Brooks/Cole.

Newport, F. (2006). *Who believes in God and who doesn't*. Princeton, NJ: The Gallup Organization.

Nichols, P. M., & Schwartz, R. C. (2007). *The essentials of family therapy* (3rd ed.). Boston: Allyn & Bacon.

Niles, S. G., & Harris-Bowlsbey, J. H. (2009). *Career development interventions in the 21st century* (3rd ed.). Upper Saddle River, NJ: Merrill Prentice Hall.

Norcross, J. (2005). The psychotherapist's own psychotherapy: Educating and developing psychologists. *American Psychologist*, 60, 840–850.

Norcross, J. C., Karpiak, C. P., & Lister, M. (2005). What's an integrationist? A study of self-identified integrative and (occasionally) eclectic psychologists. *Journal of Clinical Psychology*, 61, 1587–1594.

Norcross, J. C., Beutler, L. E., & Levant, R. F. (Eds.) (2006). *Evidence-based practices in mental health: Debate and dialogue on the fundamental questions*. Washington, D.C.: American Psychological Association.

Nugent, F. A., & Jones, K. D. (2005). *An introduction to the profession of counseling* (4th ed.). Upper Saddle River, NJ: Merrill Prentice Hall.

Nugent, F. A., & Jones, K. D. (2009). *An introduction to the counseling profession* (5th ed.). Upper Saddle River, NJ: Merrill.

O'Hanlon, W. H. (1986). Fragments for a therapeutic autobiography. In D. E. Efron (Ed.), *Journeys: Expansion of the strategic-systemic therapies* (pp. 30–39). New York: Brunner/Mazel.

O'Hanlon, W. H. (1994, November/December). The third wave. *Family Therapy Networker*, 18–26.

O'Hanlon, W. H., & Weiner-Davis, M. (2003). *In search of solutions* (Rev. ed.). New York: W. W. Norton.

Oaklander, V. (2006). *Hidden treasure: A map to the child's inner self*. London: Karnac Books.

Ogles, B. M., Lunnen, K. M., & Bonesteel, K. (2001). Clinical significance: History, application, and current practice. *Clinical Psychology Review*, 21(3), 421–446.

Okun, B. F., & Kantrowitz, R.E. (2002). *Effective helping: Interviewing and counseling techniques* (7th ed.). Pacific Grove, CA: Brooks/Cole.

Orlinsky, D. E. (2005). Becoming and being a psychotherapist: A psychodynamic memoir and meditation. *Journal of Clinical Psychology*, 61, 999–1007.

Osatuke, K., Glick, M. J., Stiles, W. B., Greenberg, L. S., Shapiro, D. A., & Barkham, M. (2005). Temporal patterns of improvement in client-centered therapy and cognitive-behavioral therapy. *Counseling Psychology Quarterly*, 18, 95–108.

Palmer, S. (2006). *Brief multimodal therapy*. Thousand Oaks, CA: Sage.

Pardeck, J. T., & Pardeck, J. A. (1993). *Bibliotherapy: A clinical approach for helping children*. New York: Gordon & Breach.

Parsons, F. (1909). *Choosing a vocation*. Boston: Houghton Mifflin.

Parsons, R. D. (2007). *Counseling strategies that work: Evidence-based interventions for school counselors*. Boston: Pearson.

Pascarelli, E. F. (1981). Drug abuse and the elderly. In J. H. Lowinson & P. Ruiz (Eds.), *Substance abuse: Clinical problems and perspectives.* Baltimore: Williams & Wilkins.

Patterson, L. E., & Welfel, E. R. (2005). *The counseling process* (6th ed.). Belmont, CA: Thomson Brooks/Cole.

Payne, M. (2006). *Narrative therapy: An introduction for counselors.* Thousand Oaks, CA: Sage.

Pedersen, P. B. (2001). Multiculturalism and the paradigm shift in counseling: Controversies and alternative futures. *Canadian Journal of Counseling, 35,* 15–25.

Pedersen, P. B., & Carey, J. C. (2003). *Multicultural counseling in the schools.* Boston: Allyn & Bacon.

Perls, F. (1969a). *Gestalt therapy verbatim.* Lafayette, CA: Real People Press.

Perls, F. (1969b). *In and out of the garbage pail.* Lafayette, CA: Real People Press.

Perosa, S. L., & Perosa, L. M. (1987). Strategies for counseling mid-career changers: A conceptual framework. *Journal of Counseling and Development, 65,* 558–561.

Peterson, K. (2005). Biomarkers for alcohol use and abuse: A summary. *Alcohol Research & Health, 28,* 30–37.

Pfaffenberger, A. (2007). Different conceptualizations of optimum development. *Journal of Humanistic Psychology, 47,* 501–523.

Philaretou, A. G., Mahfouz, A. Y., & Allen, K. R. (2005). Use of Internet pornography and men's well-being. *International Journal of Men's Health, 4,* 149–169.

Phillips, S. D., Christopher-Sisk, E. K., & Gravino, K. L. (2001). Making career decisions in a relational context. *Counseling Psychologist, 29*(2), 193–213.

Piaget, J. (1926). *The language and thought of the child.* New York: Harcourt Brace Jovanovich.

Pieterse, A. L., Evans, S. A., Risner-Butner, A., Collins, N. M., & Mason, L. M. (2009). Multicultural competence and social justice training in counseling psychology and counselor education: A review and analysis of a sample of multicultural course syllabi. *The Counseling Psychologist, 17,* 93–115.

Piran, N., & Cormier, H. C. (2005). The social construction of women and disordered eating patterns. *Journal of Counseling Psychology, 52,* 549–558.

Plummer, D. (1999). *One of the boys: Masculinity, homophobia, and modern manhood.* New York: Haworth.

Polivy, J., & Herman, C. P. (2002). If at first you don't succeed: False hopes of self-change. *American Psychologist, 57,* 677–689.

Polkinghorne, D. E. (2005). Language and meaning: Data collection in qualitative research. *Journal of Counseling Psychology, 52,* 137–145.

Pollack, W. (1998). *Real boys: Rescuing our sons from the myths of boyhood.* New York: Henry Holt and Company.

Polster, E. (2006). *Uncommon ground: Creating a system of lifetime guidance.* Phoenix, AZ: Zeig, Tucker.

Pomerantz, A. M., & Handelsman, M. M. (2004). Informed consent revisited: An updated written-question format. *Professional Psychology: Research and Practice. 35,* 201–205.

Ponterotto, J. G. (2005). Qualitative research in counseling psychology: A primer on research paradigms and philosophy of science. *Journal of Counseling Psychology, 52,* 126–136.

Ponterotto, J. G., Alexander, C. M., & Grieger, I. (1995). A multicultural competency checklist for counseling training programs. *Journal of Multicultural Counseling and Development, 23,* 11–20.

Pope, K. S., & Vasquez, M. J. (2007). *Ethics in psychotherapy and counseling* (3rd ed.). San Francisco: Jossey-Bass.

Posthuma, B. W. (2001). *Small groups in counseling and therapy* (4th ed.). Boston: Allyn & Bacon.

Powell, L. H., Shahabi, L., & Thoresen, C. E. (2003). Religion and spirituality: Linkages to physical health. *American Psychologist, 58,* 36–52.

Prah, P. M. (2005, July 15). Methamphetamine. *CQ Researcher, 15.* Retrieved February 12, 2006, from file: http://E:\meth%20use%20 review%20%20CQ%20 Researcher%2005.htm.

Prediger, D. J. (1993). *Multicultural assessment standards: A compilation*

for counselors. Alexandria, VA: American Counseling Association.

Prochaska, J. O., & Norcross, J. C. (2010). *Systems of psychotherapy: A transtheoretical analysis* (7th ed.). Belmont, CA: Brooks/Cole.

Prochaska, J. O., DiClemente, C. C., & Norcross, J. C. (1992). In search of how people change. *American Psychologist, 47,* 1102–1114.

Quick, E. K. (1996). *Doing what works in brief therapy.* San Diego: Academic Press.

Rabinowitz, F. E., & Shepard, D. S. (2002, July). *Deepening psychotherapy with men.* Paper presented at Alliant University, Alhambra, CA.

Ratts, M. J. & Hutchins, A. M. (2009). ACA advocacy competencies: Social justice advocacy at the client/student level. *Journal of Counseling & Development, 87,* 269–275.

Raz, A. (2006). Perspective on the efficacy of antidepressants for child and adolescent depression. *PLoS Medicine, 3*(1), e9.

Redding, R., Herbert, J., Forman, E., & Gaudiano, B. (2008). Popular self-help books for anxiety, depression, and trauma: How scientifically grounded and useful are they? *Professional Psychology: Research and Practice, 39,* 537–545.

Reese, R. J., Conoley, C. W., & Brossart, D. F. (2006). The attractiveness of telephone counseling: An empirical investigation of client perceptions. *Journal of Counseling and Development, 84,* 54–60.

Remley, T. P., & Herlihy, B. (2010). *Ethical, legal, and professional issues in counseling* (3rd ed.). Upper Saddle River, NJ: Merrill Prentice Hall.

Ridley, C. R., Tracy, M. L., Pruitt-Stephens, L., Wimsatt, M. K., & Beard, J. (2008). Multicultural assessment validity: The preeminent ethical issue in psychological assessment. In L. A. Suzuki & J. G. Ponterotto (Eds.), *Handbook of multicultural assessment: Clinical, psychological, and educational applications* (3rd ed.). San Francisco: Jossey-Bass.

Riordan, R. J., & Walsh, L. (1994). Guidelines for professional referral to Alcoholics Anonymous and other twelve-step groups. *Journal of Counseling and Development, 72,* 351–355.

Robb, C. (2006). *This changes everything: The relational revolution in psychology.* New York: Farrar, Straus, & Giroux.

Robertiello, R. C. (1978). The occupational disease of psychotherapists. *Journal of Contemporary Psychotherapy, 9,* 123–129.

Robertson, J., & Shepard, D. S. (2008). The psychological development of boys. In M. S. Kiselica, M. Englar-Carlson, & A. M. Horne (Eds.), *Counseling troubled boys: A guidebook for professionals* (pp. 3–30). New York: Routledge.

Robiner, W. N. (2006). The mental health professions: Workforce supply and demand, issues, and challenges. *Clinical Psychology Review, 26,* 600–625.

Robinson, T. E. (2007). *The consequences of race, ethnicity, and gender: Multiple identities in counseling* (2nd ed.). Upper Saddle River, NJ: Prentice Hall.

Rochlen, A. B., Zack, J. S., & Speyer, C. (2004). Online therapy: Review of relevant definitions, debates, and current empirical support. *Journal of Clinical Psychology, 60,* 269–283.

Roe, A. (1957). Early determinants of vocational choice. *Journal of Counseling Psychology, 4,* 212–217.

Rogers, C. R. (1942). *Counseling and psychotherapy.* Boston: Houghton Mifflin.

Rogers, C. R. (1951). *Client-centered therapy.* Boston: Houghton Mifflin.

Rogers, C. R. (1957). The necessary and sufficient conditions of therapeutic personality change. *Journal of Consulting Psychology, 21,* 93–103.

Rogers, C. R. (1961). *On becoming a person.* Boston: Houghton Mifflin.

Rogers, C. R. (1969). *Freedom to learn.* Columbus, OH: Charles E. Merrill.

Rollins, J. (2009, February). A reality too horrible to consider. *Counseling Today,* 32–37.

Romano, D. M. (2005). Virtual reality therapy. *Developmental Medicine & Child Neurology, 47,* 580.

Rosenthal, D. A., & Berven, N. L. (1999). Effects of client race on clinical judgment. *Rehabilitation Counseling Bulletin, 42,* 243–264.

Rosenzweig, S. (1936). Some implicit common factors in diverse methods in psychotherapy. *American Journal of Orthopsychiatry, 6,* 412–415.

Roth, A., & Fonagy, P. (2006). *What works for whom? A critical review of psychotherapy research* (2nd ed.). New York: Guilford.

Roysircar, G. (2009). The big picture of advocacy: Counselor, heal society and thyself. *Journal of Counseling & Development, 87,* 288–294.

Rubenfeld, S. (2001). Group therapy and complexity theory. *International Journal of Group Psychotherapy, 51*(4), 449–471.

Rule, W., & Bishop, M. (2005). *Adlerian lifestyle counseling.* New York: Routledge.

Russell, J. M. (2007). Existential psychotherapy. In A. B. Rochlen (Ed.), *Applying counseling theories.* Upper Saddle River, NJ: Pearson.

Russell, S. R., & Yarhouse, M. A. (2006). Training in religion/spirituality within APA-accredited psychology predoctoral internships. *Professional Psychology: Research and Practice, 37,* 430–436.

Rutter, P. (1989). *Sex in the forbidden zone.* Los Angeles: Jeremy Tarcher.

Rychlak, J. F. (1981). *Introduction to personality and psychotherapy: A theory-construction approach* (2nd ed.). Boston: Houghton Mifflin.

Sampson, J. P., Jr. (2000). Using the Internet to enhance testing in counseling. *Journal of Counseling and Development, 78,* 348–356.

Sanderson, W. C. (1998). The case for evidence-based psychotherapy treatment guidelines. *American Journal of Psychotherapy, 52,* 382–387.

Sapienza, B. G., & Bugental, J. F. T. (2000). Keeping our instruments finely tuned: An existential perspective. *Professional Psychology: Research and Practice, 31,* 458–460.

Sartre, J. P. (1957). *Existentialism and human emotions.* New York: The Wisdom Library.

Satir, V., & Baldwin, M. (1984). *Satir step by step: A guide to creating change in families.* Palo Alto, CA: Science and Behavior Books.

Scaramella, L., Neppl, T., Ontai, L., & Conger, R. (2008). Consequences of socioeconomic disadvantage across three generations: Parenting behavior and child externalizing problems. *Journal of Family Psychology, 22,* 725–733.

Scharff, J., & Scharff, D. (2005). *The primer of object relations* (2nd ed.). New York: Jason Aronson.

Scharff, J., & Scharff, D. (2006). *New paradigms for treating relationships.* New York: Jason Aronson.

Schmidt, J. J. (2006). *Social and cultural foundations of counseling and human services: Multiple influences on self-concept development.* Boston: Allyn & Bacon.

Schneider, K. J. (1998). Toward a science of the heart: Romanticism and the revival of psychology. *American Psychologist, 53,* 277–289.

Schofield, W. (1964). *Psychotherapy: The purchase of friendship.* Englewood Cliffs. NJ: Prentice Hall.

Schuckit, M. A. (2000). Genetics of the risk for alcoholism. *The American Journal on Addictions, 9,* 103–112.

Schultheiss, D. E. P. (2003). A relational approach to career counseling: Theoretical integration and practical application. *Journal of Counseling and Development, 81,* 310–310.

Schwartz, R. C., & Feisthamel, K. P. (2009). Disproportionate diagnosis of mental disorders among African American versus European American clients: Implications for counseling theory, research, and practice. *Journal of Counseling & Development, 87,* 295–301.

Schwiebert, V. L., Myers, J. E., & Dice, C. (2000). Ethical guidelines for counselors working with older adults. *Journal of Counseling and Development, 78*(2), 123–129.

Seligman, L. (1998). *Selecting effective treatments* (2nd ed.). San Francisco: Jossey-Bass.

Seligman, L. (2004). *Diagnosis and treatment planning in counseling* (3rd ed.). New York: Springer.

Seligman, M. (1983). Sources of psychological disturbance among siblings of handicapped children. *Personnel and Guidance Journal, 61,* 529–531.

Selman, R. L. (1980). *The growth of interpersonal understanding: Developmental and clinical analyses.* Orlando, FL: Academic Press.

Senior, J. (2007). Life coaching: Origins, directions and potential risk: Why the contribution of psychologists is needed more than ever. *Special Group in Coaching Psychology, 3,* 19–22.

Shaffer, H. J., Hall, M. N., & Bilt, J. V. (2000). "Computer addiction": A critical consideration. *American Journal of Orthopsychiatry, 70,* 162–168.

Shallcross, L. (2009). Regaining life balance. *Counseling Today, 51*(12), 28–33.

Shapiro, F. (1995). *Eye movement desensitization and reprocessing: Basic principles, protocols, and procedures.* New York: Guilford.

Shapiro, F. (2001). *Eye movement desensitization and reprocessing: Basic principles, protocols, and procedures* (2nd ed.). New York: Guilford.

Shapiro, F., & Forrest, M. F. (2004). *EMDR: The breakthrough "eye movement" therapy for overcoming anxiety, stress, and trauma: Updated edition.* New York: Basic Books.

Shapiro, F., Kaslo, F. W., & Maxfield, L. (2007). *Handbook of EMDR and family therapy processes.* Hoboken, NJ: Wiley.

Sharf, R. S. (2006). *Applying career development theory to counseling* (4th ed.). Belmont, CA: Thomson Brooks/Cole.

Sharf, R. S. (2008). *Theories of psychotherapy and counseling: Concepts and cases* (4th ed.). Thomson Brooks/Cole.

Shaver, K. G. (1985). *The attribution of blame.* New York: Springer-Verlag.

Shaw, H. E., & Shaw, S. F. (2006). Critical ethical issues in online counseling: Assessing current practices with an ethical intent checklist. *Journal of Counseling and Development, 84,* 41–53.

Shechtman, Z. (2006). *Group counseling and psychotherapy with children and adolescents: Theory, research, and practice.* Mahwah, NJ: Lawrence Erlbaum Associates.

Shechtman, Z., & Pastor, R. (2005). Humanistic group treatment for children with learning disabilities: A comparison of outcome and process. *Journal of Counseling Psychology, 51,* 322–336.

Sheehy, G. (1995). *New passages: Mapping your life across time.* New York: Random House.

Shepard, D. S. (2004). A negative state of mind: Patterns of depressive symptoms among men with high gender role conflict. *Psychology of Men & Masculinity, 3,* 3–8.

Shepard, D. S. (2005). Male development and the journey toward disconnection. In D. L. Comstock (Ed.), *Diversity in development: Critical contexts that shape our lives and relationships* (pp. 133–160). Belmont, CA: Thomson Brooks/Cole.

Shirk, S. R., & Karver, M. (2003). Prediction of treatment outcome from relationship variables in child and adolescent therapy: A meta-analytic review. *Journal of Consulting and Clinical Psychology, 7,* 452–464.

Siegel, D. J. (1999). *The developing mind: Toward a neurobiology of interpersonal experience.* New York: Guilford.

Siegel, D. J., & Hartzell, M. (2003). *Parenting from the inside out.* New York: Tarcher Penguin.

Siegel, D. (2007). *The mindful brain: Reflection and attunement in the cultivation of well-being.* New York: W. W. Norton.

Simon, G. M. (2004). An examination of the integrative nature of emotionally focused therapy. *The Family Journal, 12,* 254–262.

Simon, R. I., & Hales, R. E. (2006). *The American psychiatric publisher textbook of suicide assessment and management.* Washington, D.C.: American Psychiatric Association.

Sinacola, R. S., & Peters-Strickland, R. (2006). *Basic psychopharmacology for counselors and psychotherapists.* Boston: Allyn & Bacon.

Sinacore-Guinn, A. L. (1995). The diagnostic window: Culture- and gender-sensitive diagnosis and training. *Counselor Education and Supervision, 35,* 18–31.

Skinner, B. F. (1938). *The behavior of organisms: An experimental analysis.* New York: Appleton-Century-Crofts.

Skinner, B. F. (1953). *Science and human behavior.* New York: Macmillan.

Skinner, B. F. (1983). Intellectual self-management in old age. *American Psychologist, 38,* 239–244.

Sklare, G. (2004). *Brief counseling that works: A solution-focused approach for school counselors* (2nd ed.). Thousand Oaks, CA: Corwin Press.

Skovholt, T. M. (2001). *The resilient practitioner: Burnout prevention and self-care strategies for counselors, therapists, teachers, and health professionals.* Boston: Allyn & Bacon.

Skovholt, T. M., & Jennings, L. (2004). *Master therapists: Exploring expertise in therapy and counseling.* Boston: Allyn & Bacon.

Slattery, J. M. (2004). *Counseling diverse clients: Bringing context into therapy.* Belmont, CA: Thomson Brooks/Cole.

Sloan, D. M. (2004). Emotion-focused therapy: An interview with Leslie Greenberg. *Journal of Contemporary Psychotherapy, 34,* 105–116.

Smart, J. F., & Smart, D. W. (2006). Models of disability: Implications for the counseling profession. *Journal of Counseling and Development, 84,* 29–40.

Society of Clinical Psychology (2009). *Website on research-supported psychological treatments.* Retrieved from http://www.psychology.sunysb.edu/eklonsky-/division12/.

Somer, E., & Nachman, I. (2005). Constructions of therapist-client sex: A comparative analysis of retrospective victim reports. *Sexual Abuse: Journal of Research and Treatment, 17,* 47–62.

Sommers-Flanagan, J., & Sommers-Flanagan, R. (2004). *Counseling and psychotherapy theories in context and practice.* Hoboken, NJ: John Wiley & Sons.

Sommers-Flanagan, J., & Sommers-Flanagan, R. (2007). *Becoming an ethical helping professional: Cultural and philosophical foundations.* Hoboken, NJ: John Wiley & Sons.

Sommers-Flanagan, J., & Sommers-Flanagan, R. (2009). *Clinical interviewing* (4th ed.). New York: John Wiley & Sons.

Southern, S., Smith, R. L., & Oliver, M. (2005). Marriage and family counseling: Ethics in context. *The Family Journal, 13,* 459–466.

Sparks, J. A., Duncan, B. L., & Miller, S. D. (2008). Common factors in psychotherapy. In J. L. Lebow, *Twenty-first century psychotherapies: Contemporary approaches to theory and practice* (pp. 453–497). Hoboken, NJ: Wiley.

Sperry, L. (2008). Executive coaching: An intervention, role function, or profession? *Consulting Psychology Journal: Practice and Research, 60*(1), 33–37.

Sperry, L., Carlson, J., & Peluso, P. R. (2006). *Couples therapy: Integrating theory and technique* (2nd ed.). Denver, CO: Love.

Spiegler, M. D., & Guevremont, D. C. (2003). *Contemporary behavior therapy* (4th ed.). Pacific Grove, CA: Brooks/Cole.

Spitzer, R. L., Skodol, A. E., Gibbon, M., & Williams, J. (1994). *DSM-III case book*. Washington, D.C.: American Psychiatric Association.

Stadter, M. (2009). *Object relations brief therapy: The therapeutic relationship in short-term work*. Lanham, MD: Jason Aronson.

Standard, R., & Hazler, R. (1995). Legal and ethical implications of HIV and duty to warn for counselors. *Journal of Counseling and Development, 73*, 397–400.

Stanford Internet Study (2009). *The internet study*. Retrieved from http://www.stanford.edu/group/siqss/Press_Release/press_detail.html.

Stathopoulou, G., Powers, M. B., Berry, A. C., Smits, J. A. J., & Otto, M. W. (2006). Exercise interventions for mental health: A quantitative and qualitative review. *Clinical Psychology, 13*, 179–193.

Steinman, S. O., Richardson, N. F., & McEnroe, T. (1998). *The ethical decision-making manual for helping professionals*. Pacific Grove, CA: Brooks/Cole.

Stevens, M. J., & Morris, S. J. (1995). A format for case conceptualization. *Counselor Education and Supervision, 35*, 35–93.

Stevens, P., & Smith, R. L. (2008). *Substance abuse counseling: Theory and practice* (4th ed.). Upper Saddle River, NJ: Merrill Prentice Hall.

Stoltenberg, C. D. & Pace, R. M. (2008). The scientist-practitioner model: Now more than ever. *Journal of Contemporary Psychotherapy, 37*, 195–203.

Stone, D. (2004). The historiography of genocide: Beyond "uniqueness" and ethnic competition. *Rethinking History, 8*, 127–143.

Stossel, J. (Correspondent) (2004, April 16). *ABC News 20/20* [Television broadcast]. New York: American Broadcasting Company.

Strohl, J. E. (1998). Transpersonalism: Ego meets soul. *Journal of Counseling and Development, 76*, 397–403.

Strohle, A. (2009). Physical activity, exercise and anxiety disorders. *Journal of Neural Transmission, 116*, 777–784.

Strupp, H. (1973). On the basic ingredients of psychotherapy. *Journal of Consulting and Clinical Psychology, 41*(1), 1–8.

Strupp, H. (1989). Can the practitioner learn from the researcher? *American Psychologist, 44*(4), 717–724.

Strupp, H. H., & Binder, J. L. (1984). *Psychotherapy in a new key*. New York: Basic Books.

Sue, D. W. & Sue, D. (2008). *Counseling the culturally different: Theory and practice* (5th ed.). New York: Wiley.

Suler, J. (2004). The online disinhibition effect. *The Psychology of Cyberspace 2.2*. Retrieved September 27, 2006, from http://www.rider.edu/~suler/psycyber/disinhibit.html.

Sullivan, S. E. (1999). The changing nature of careers: A review and research agenda. *Journal of Management, 25*, 457–484.

Super, D. E. (1953). A theory of vocational development. *American Psychologist, 8*, 185–190.

Super, D. E. (1957). *The psychology of careers*. New York: Harper & Row.

Super, D. E. (1990). A life span, life space approach to career development. In D. Brown & L. Brooks (Eds.), *Career choice and development* (2nd ed.). San Francisco: Jossey-Bass.

Suzuki, L. A., & Ponterotto, J. G. (2007). *Handbook of multicultural assessment: Clinical, psychological, and educational implications* (3rd ed.). San Francisco: Jossey-Bass.

Sweeney, T. J. (2009). *Adlerian counseling and psychotherapy: A practitioner's approach* (5th ed.). New York: Routledge.

Swenson, L. C. (1997). *Psychology and the law* (2nd ed.). Pacific Grove, CA: Brooks/Cole.

Swift, R. M. (1999). Drug therapy for alcohol dependence. *New England Journal of Medicine, 340*(19), 1482–1490.

Tarragona, M. (2008). Postmodern/poststructuralist therapies. In J. Lebow (Ed.), *Twenty-first century psychotherapies: Contemporary approaches to theory and practice* (pp. 167–205). Hoboken, NJ: Wiley.

Tate, D. F., & Zabinski, M. F. (2004). Computer and Internet applications for psychological treatment: Update for clinicians. *Journal of Clinical Psychology, 60*, 209–220.

Terkel, S. (1972). *Working*. New York: Avon.

Teyber, E. (2006). *Interpersonal process in therapy: An integrative model* (5th ed.). Belmont, CA: Thomson Brooks/Cole.

Thoresen, C. E. (1969). The counselor as an applied behavioral scientist. *Personnel and Guidance Journal, 47*, 841–848.

Thorne, F. C. (1950). *The principles of personal counseling*. Brandon, VT: Clinical Psychology Publishing.

Tinsley, H. E., & Bradley, R. W. (1986). Test interpretation. *Journal of Counseling and Development, 64*, 462–466.

Truax, C. B., & Carkhuff, R. R. (1967). *Toward effective counseling and psychotherapy*. Chicago: Aldine.

Trull, T. (2007). Expanding the aperture of psychological assessment: Introduction to the special section on innovative clinical assessment technologies and methods. *Psychological Assessment, 19*, 1–3.

Tryon, G. S. (2002). Engagement in counseling. In G. S. Tryon (Ed.), *Counseling based on process research*. Boston: Allyn & Bacon.

Tudor, K., & Worrall, M. (2006). *Person-centered therapy: A critical philosophy*. New York: Routledge.

Turner, K. (2009). Mindfulness: The present moment in clinical social work. *The Journal of Clinical Social Work, 37*, 95–103.

Tyler, L. (1970). Thoughts about theory. In W. H. Van Hoose & J. J. Pietrofesa (Eds.), *Counseling and guidance in the twentieth century* (pp. 298–305). Boston: Houghton Mifflin.

U.S. Equal Employment Opportunity Commission (n.d.). *Sexual harassment*. Retrieved October 1, 2006, from http://www.eeoc.gov/types/sexual_harassment.html.

United States Department of Health and Human Services (2008). Health, United States, 2008.

Vacc, N. A., & Juhnke, G. A. (1997). The use of structured clinical interviews for assessment in counseling. *Journal of Counseling and Development, 75*, 470–480.

Vaillant, G. E. (2005). Alcoholics Anonymous: Cult or cure? *Australian and New Zealand Journal of Psychiatry, 35,* 431–436.

Van der Walde, H., Urgenson, F. T., Weltz, S. H., & Hanna, F. J. (2002). Women and alcoholism: A biopsychosocial perspective and treatment approaches. *Journal of Counseling and Development, 80,* 145–153.

Van Deurzen-Smith, E. (2002). *Existential counseling in practice* (2nd ed.). London: Sage.

Van Kalmthout, M. (2008). Meaning in a godless universe: A challenge for person-centered therapy. *Person-Centered and Experiential Psychotherapies, 7*(1), 56–69.

Vanderbleek, L. M. (2004). Engaging families in school-based mental health treatment. *Journal of Mental Health Counseling, 26*(3), 211–214.

Vujanovic, A. A., Youngwirth, N. E., Johnson, K. A., & Zvolensky, M. J. (2009). Mindfulness-based acceptance and posttraumatic stress symptoms among trauma-exposed adults without axis I psychopathology. *Journal of Anxiety Disorders, 23,* 297–303.

Vygotsky, L. S. (1934/1986). *Thought and language* (Rev. ed.). Cambridge, MA: MIT Press.

Vygotsky, L. S. (1978/2006). *Mind in society: The development of higher psychological processes.* Cambridge, MA: Harvard University Press.

Wachtel, P. (1977). *Psychoanalysis and behavior therapy: Toward an integration.* New York: Basic Books.

Wakefield, J. C. (1997). Diagnosing DSM-IV-Part I: DSM-IV and the concept of disorder. *Behavior Research and Therapy, 35,* 633–649.

Walker, D. F., Gorsuch, R. L., and Tan, S. (2004). Therapists' integration of religion and spirituality in counseling: A meta-analysis. *Counseling and Values, 49,* 69–80.

Waller, D. (2006). Art therapy for children: How it leads to change. *Clinical Child Psychology and Psychiatry, 11,* 271–282.

Wallin, D. J. (2007). *Attachment in psychotherapy.* New York: Guilford.

Wampold, B. E. (2001). *The great psychotherapy debate: Models, methods, and findings.* Hillsdale, NJ: Erlbaum.

Wampold, B. E., & Bhati, K. S. (2004). Attending to the omissions: A historical examination of evidence-based practice movements. *Professional Psychology: Research and Practice, 35,* 563–570.

Watson, J. C., & Bohart, A. (2001). Humanistic-existential therapies in the era of managed care. In K. J. Schneider, J. F. T. Bugental, & J. F. Pierson (Eds.), *The handbook of humanistic psychology.* Thousand Oaks, CA: Sage.

Watson, J. C., Goldman, R. N., & Greenberg, L. S. (2007). *Case studies in emotion-focused treatment of depression: A comparison of good and poor outcome.* Washington, D.C.: American Psychological Association.

Wedding, D., & Corsini, R. J. (2008). *Case studies in psychotherapy* (5th ed.). Itasca, IL: F. E. Peacock.

Wedding, D., & Niemec, R. M. (2003). The clinical use of films in psychotherapy. *Journal of Clinical Psychology, 59,* 207–215.

Weil, A. (1972). *The natural mind.* Boston: Houghton Mifflin.

Weil, A. (1998). *Self-healing.* Watertown, MA: Thorne Communications.

Welfel, E. R. (2006). *Ethics in counseling and psychotherapy: Standards, research, and emerging issues* (3rd ed.). Belmont, CA: Thomson Brooks/Cole.

Weltner, J. (1988, May/June). Different strokes: A pragmatist's guide to intervention. *Family Therapy Networker,* 53–57.

Wertz, F. J. (1998). The role of the humanistic movement in the history of psychology. *Journal of Humanistic Psychology, 38,* 42–70.

Whaley, A. L., & Geller, P. A. (2007). Toward a cognitive process model of ethnic/racial biases in clinical judgment. *Review of General Psychology, 11,* 75–96.

White, M. (2008). *Maps of narrative practice.* New York: W. W. Norton.

White, M., & Epston, D. (1990). *Narrative means to therapeutic ends.* New York: W. W. Norton.

Widiger, T. A., & Samuel, D. B. (2005). Diagnostic categories or dimensions: A question for the Diagnostic and Statistical Manual of Mental Disorders—5th Edition. *Journal of Abnormal Psychology, 114,* 494–504.

Wilbur, K. (2000). *Integral psychology: Consciousness, spirit, psychology, therapy.* Boston: Shambala.

Wilcoxon, S. A., Remley, T. P., Gladding, S. T., & Huber, C. H. (2007). *Ethical, legal, and professional issues in the practice of marriage and family therapy* (4th ed.). Upper Saddle River, NJ: Merrill Prentice Hall.

Wile, D. B. (1993). *After the fight: Using your disagreements to build a stronger relationship.* New York: Guilford.

Wile, D. B. (1999). Collaborative couple therapy. In J. M. Donovan (Ed.), *Short-term couple therapy* (pp. 201–225). New York: Guilford.

Williams, C., & Abeles, N. (2004). Issues and implications of deaf culture in therapy, *Professional Psychology: Research and Practice, 35,* 643–648.

Williams, P., & Davis, D. C. (2002). *Therapist as a life coach.* New York: W. W. Norton.

Windle, M. (2001). Substance abuse among children and adolescents. In E. R. Welfel & R. E. Ingersoll (Eds.), *The mental health desk reference.* New York: John Wiley & Sons.

Winkeleman, M. (2001). Alternative and traditional medicine approaches for substance abuse programs: A shamanic perspective. *International Journal of Drug Policy, 12,* 337–351.

Winnicott, D. W. (1958). *Collected papers: Through pediatrics to psychoanalysis.* London: Tavistock.

Winslade, J., & Monk, G. (2008). *Practicing narrative mediation: Loosening the grip of conflict.* San Francisco: Jossey-Bass.

Wishne, H. A. (2005). *Working in the countertransference: Necessary entanglements.* New York: Jason Aronson.

Witkiewitz, K., & Marlatt, G. A. (2004). Relapse prevention for alcohol and drug problems: That was Zen, this is Tao. *American Psychologist, 59,* 224–235.

Wolf, E. S. (1988). *Treating the self: Elements of clinical self psychology.* New York: Guilford.

Wolpe, J. (1958). *Psychotherapy by reciprocal inhibition.* Palo Alto, CA: Stanford University Press.

Wolpe, J. (1982). *The practice of behavior therapy* (2nd ed.). Elmsford, NY: Pergamon.

Wood, J. (2007). *Leaving Microsoft to change the world.* New York: HarperCollins.

Worrell, J., & Remer, P. (2003). *Feminist perspectives in therapy.* New York: John Wiley & Sons.

Wright, R. (1994). *The moral animal.* New York: Pantheon.

Wright, S. (2008, September). Positive psychology courses, authentic happiness coaching, Martin Seligman, and Ben Dean. *Meaning and happiness.com.* Retrieved from http://www.meaningandhappiness.com/positive-psychology-courses-authentic-happiness-coaching/142/.

Wubbolding, R. (1990). *Expanding reality therapy.* Cincinnati, OH: Real World.

Wubbolding, R. (2000). *Reality therapy for the 21st century.* New York: Brunner-Routledge.

Wubbolding, R. E. (2008). Reality therapy. In J. Frew & M. D. Spiegler (Eds.), *Contemporary psychotherapies for a diverse world* (pp. 360–398). Boston: Lahaska Press.

Wylie, M. S. (1995, May/June). Diagnosing for dollars. *Family Therapy Networker,* 22–33, 65–69.

Yalom, I. (1980). *Existential psychotherapy.* New York: Basic Books.

Yalom, I. (1989). *Love's executioner and other tales of psychotherapy.* New York: Basic Books.

Yalom, I. (1995). *The theory and practice of group psychotherapy* (4th ed.). New York: Basic Books.

Yalom, I. (2001). *Momma and the meaning of life: Tales of psychotherapy.* New York: HarperCollins.

Yalom, I. (2008). *Staring at the sun: Overcoming the terror of death.* San Francisco: Wiley.

Yalom, I., & Leszcz, M. (2005). *The theory and practice of group psychotherapy* (5th ed.). New York: Basic Books.

Yang, J., Milleren, A., & Blagen, M. (2009). *The psychology of courage: An Adlerian handbook for healthy social living.* New York: Routledge.

Young, K. S. (2004). Internet addiction: A new clinical phenomenon and its consequences. *The American Behavioral Scientist, 48,* 402–416.

Young, K. S. (2008). Internet sex addiction: Risk factors, stages of development, and treatment. *American Behavioral Scientist, 52*(1), 21–37.

Young, M. A. & Basham, A. (2010). Consultation and supervision. In B. T. Erford (Ed.), *Orientation to the Counseling Profession* (pp. 193–212). Boston: Pearson.

Young, M. E. (2009). *Learning the art of helping: Building blocks and techniques* (4th ed.). Upper Saddle River, NJ: Merrill Prentice Hall.

Young, M. E., & Lambie, G. W. (2007). Wellness in school and mental health settings. *Journal of Humanistic Counseling, Education and Development, 46,* 9–16.

Zakalik, R. A., & Wei, M. (2006). Adult attachment, perceived discrimination based on sexual orientation, and depression in gay males: Examining the mediation and moderation effects. *Journal of Counseling Psychology, 53,* 302–313.

Zunker, V. G. (2006). *Career counseling: Applied concepts of life planning* (7th ed.). Belmont, CA: Thomson Brooks/Cole.

INDEX

$$\underline{10} + \textcircled{1} = \underline{1}\textcircled{1}$$

$$\underline{10} + \textcircled{3} = 1\textcircled{3}$$

$$5 + 6 =$$

$$\begin{array}{r} +5 \\ \underline{+5} \\ 10 \\ \underline{-1} \\ 11 \end{array}$$

scared

Carl Rogers